Critical Care Challenges

DISORDERS, TREATMENTS, AND PROCEDURES

Critical Care Challenges

DISORDERS, TREATMENTS, AND PROCEDURES

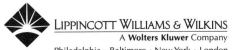
LIPPINCOTT WILLIAMS & WILKINS
A **Wolters Kluwer** Company
Philadelphia • Baltimore • New York • London
Buenos Aires • Hong Kong • Sydney • Tokyo

STAFF

Publisher
Judith A. Schilling McCann, RN, MSN

Editorial Director
H. Nancy Holmes

Clinical Director
Joan M. Robinson, RN, MSN

Senior Art Director
Arlene Putterman

Clinical Project Manager
Beverly Ann Tscheschlog, RN, BS

Clinical Editors
Joanne Bartelmo, RN, MSN;
Maryann Foley, RN, BSN

Designers
Debra Moloshok (interior design),
Lynn Foulk (project manager)

Editors
Jennifer P. Kowalak (senior associate
editor), William Welsh (associate editor),
Elizabeth Jacqueline Mills

Copy Editors
Kimberly Bilotta (supervisor), Scotti Cohn,
Tom DeZego, Shana Harrington,
Dona Hightower, Irene Pontarelli,
Marcia Ryan, Dorothy P. Terry,
Pamela Wingrod

Cover Photo
Courtesy of Division of Trauma Anesthesia
and Critical Care, University of Miami/
Jackson Memorial Medical Center

Digital Composition Services
Diane Paluba (manager), Joyce Rossi Biletz
(senior desktop assistant), Donna S. Morris

Manufacturing
Patricia K. Dorshaw (senior manager),
Beth Janae Orr (book production
coordinator)

Editorial Assistants
Danielle J. Barsky, Carol Caputo,
Arlene Claffee, Beverly Lane, Linda Ruhf

Indexer
Barbara E. Hodgson

CCC – D N O S A J J M A
05 04 03   10 9 8 7 6 5 4 3 2 1

**Library of Congress
Catalog-in-Publication Data**
Critical care challenges : disorders, treatments, and procedures.
    p. ; cm.
    Includes index.
    1. Intensive care nursing.
    [DNLM: 1. Critical Illness—nursing. 2. Critical Care—methods. WY 154 C9322 2003] I. Lippincott Williams & Wilkins.
    RT120.I5C734 2003
    610.73'61—dc21
ISBN 1-58255-241-X (pbk. : alk. paper)   2003002026

Contents

Contributors and consultants

Elizabeth (Libby) Archer, RN, EdD(c)
Assistant Professor
Baptist College of Health Sciences
Memphis

W. Chad Barefoot, MSN, ACNP, CRNP
Critical Care Nurse Practitioner
Abington (Pa.) Memorial Hospital

Mary Bouchaud, RN, MSN, CNS, CRRN
Faculty
Thomas Jefferson University
College of Health Professionals
Philadelphia

Laurie Donaghy, RN
Emergency Department Charge Nurse
Nazareth Hospital
Philadelphia

Shelba Durston, RN, MSN, CCRN
Adjunct Faculty
San Joaquin Delta College
Stockton, Calif.

Ellie Z. Franges, RN, MSN, CNRN
Director of Neuroscience Services
Sacred Heart Hospital
Allentown, Pa.

Mary Gerard, RN, BSN, CCRN
Medical Information Specialist
Johnson & Johnson
Skillman, N.J.

Karen Ann Hamel, RN, BSN
Assistant Nurse Manager
Transplant Unit
New York University Medical Center
New York

Sandy Hamilton, RN, BSN, MEd, CRNI
*Regional Coordinator of Pharmacy
    Nursing Services*
Kindred Pharmacy Services
Las Vegas

Gary R. Jones, MSN, ARNP
ARNP Coordinator
Mercy Disease Management Program
    and Heart Failure Program
Mercy Health Center
Fort Scott, Kans.

JoAnne Konick-McMahan, RN,
    MSN, CCRN
Advance Practice Nurse
Inglis Foundation
School of Nursing
University of Pennsylvania
Philadelphia

Lynda A. Mackin, RN, MS, ANP,
    CN, CNS
Assistant Clinical Professor
University of California
San Francisco

Jeanne U. Magrath, RN, MSN
*Cardiothoracic Clinical Nurse Specialist,
    Legal Nurse Consultant*
St. Louis

Deanna H. McCarthy, RN, BSN, CCRN
Critical Care Clinical Nurse Educator
Albert Einstein Medical Center
Philadelphia

Jennifer McWha, RN, MSN
Vocational Nursing Instructor
Delmar College
Corpus Christi, Tex.

Concha Carrollo Sitter, MS, APN,
    CGRN, FNP
GI Nurse Practitioner
Sterling (Ill.) Rock Falls Clinic

Linda Wood, RN, MSN
Director of Practical Nursing
Massanutten Technical Center
Harrisburg, Va.

Karen Zulkowski, RN, DNSc, CWS
Assistant Professor
Montana State University
College of Nursing
Bozeman

Foreword

Today, more than ever before, critical care nursing is undergoing unparalleled and rapid change. The intensity of the work that critical care nurses face on a daily basis requires unrelenting vigilance and high levels of physical and emotional energy. We can easily become overwhelmed by the severity of our patients' conditions and the frequency of death, the rising patient loads, increasing demands by patients' families, coworkers who are pushed to their limits, reduced presence and support from management, short-staffed ancillary services, inadequate preparation of new staff, and limited resources for ongoing professional development. Furthermore, the persistent shortage of nurses is a challenge to every critical care nurse.

And yet, while critical care nurses do indeed find their abilities and resources tested by their work, they also find their work stimulating and rewarding. Most critical care nurses would agree that challenges are the essence of our practice.

One way to assist in meeting our patients' needs is to gain access to the necessary tools and skills that enable us to provide this optimal care. *Critical Care Challenges* is one such tool, providing resources for new and experienced critical care nurses alike.

In Part I of *Critical Care Challenges,* you'll find the latest information on many critical care disorders, diagnostic tests, drug therapies, procedures, and medical treatments. Evidence-based interventions and technological advances are also covered.

Organized A-to-Z in Part II, "Quick reference to vital facts" includes respiratory panel results, calculations for cardiac output, life-threatening diagnostic test results, conversion tables, I.V. drip rates — and much, much more. This quick reference section provides time-saving essentials for fast review and retrieval.

The format of *Critical Care Challenges* provides for rapid retrieval and quick and easy interventions in a rapid-paced CCU. Flowcharts, graphs, bullet points, and diagrams help you quickly gain access to vital information.

Illustrations are used to enhance your understanding of pathophysiology, assessment techniques, and essential procedural steps. The nurse new to critical care will find this book a "must-have" resource for learning new conditions, treatments, and nursing interventions. Experienced critical care nurses will find the book an excellent resource for less commonly occurring conditions or technologies that aren't encountered every day.

Critical Care Challenges includes "alerts" that clue you in to special precautions and warnings. In addition, the book includes special "age issue" icons that highlight disease variations and procedural changes necessitated by patient age. Also, "multisystem disorder" identifies entries that commonly involve problems in multiple body systems, such as burns, trauma, and multiple organ dysfunction syndrome.

This essential book includes both basic critical care information, such as arterial pressure monitoring, and detailed guidelines for complex skills, such as cerebral blood flow monitoring. Flowcharts and guidelines from the American Heart Association and the Agency for Healthcare Research & Quality as well as from other standard-setting organizations, are just a few of the invaluable resources you'll find at your fingertips in this book.

Critical Care Challenges provides a forum to enhance your knowledge, bolster your critical thinking, and offset the emotional stress inherent in managing the challenges in your practice. You'll find *Critical Care Challenges* a great addition to your personal library and a valuable resource for your practice for years to come!

Michael L. Williams, RN, MSN, CCRN
Assistant Professor of Nursing
Eastern Michigan University
Past-President
American Association of Critical-Care
    Nurses

PART ONE

Disorders, treatments, and procedures

1 | *Cardiovascular system challenges*

Imagine a patient who presents with chest pain. Does the pain signal an acute myocardial infarction (MI) or some other disorder such as pericarditis? What would you do first? What if a 12-lead electrocardiogram (ECG) was done and you needed to interpret it — could you decipher the information for each lead? Could you interpret the ECG recording to determine if the patient was experiencing a Q-wave infarction or non–Q-wave infarction? Are ST-segment changes present and if so, what do they mean and how would they affect your care? Could you determine if axis deviation was present? Would you know how to intervene if a hemostatic device was used to close the insertion site after a cardiac catheterization? How would you care for the patient who needs a pacemaker? Do you know how to level the transducer for a patient receiving continuous cardiac output (CO) monitoring? Could you determine the CO accurately? Suppose you see what you think is an abnormal hemodynamic waveform. Is there a problem with the patient, is the catheter blocked or clotted, or is the equipment malfunctioning? How would you prepare the patient who requires intra-aortic balloon-pump counterpulsation? Could you interpret the waveforms accurately? Do you know how early inflation

might affect the patient? In this chapter, you'll find answers to these and other questions that will allow you to address the major cardiovascular system challenges commonly encountered by critical care nurses.

Acute coronary syndromes

Acute coronary syndromes (ACSs) are clinical conditions that involve the rupture or erosion of plaque — an unstable and lipid-rich substance — as the initiating event. The rupture results in platelet adhesions, fibrin clot formation, and activation of thrombin. Acute MI (Q-wave and non–Q-wave) and unstable angina are now recognized as part of this group.

In cardiovascular disease, the leading cause of death in the United States and Western Europe, death usually results from cardiac damage or complications of MI. Each year, approximately 900,000 people in the United States experience MI. Mortality is high when treatment is delayed, and almost one-half of sudden deaths due to MI occur before hospitalization, within 1 hour of the onset of symptoms. The prognosis improves if vigorous treatment begins immediately.

Viewing the coronary vessels

If an occlusion in a coronary artery causes a myocardial infarction (MI), the amount of damage to the myocardium depends on several factors. The area of the heart supplied by the affected vessel is a concern as well as the demand for oxygen in the affected area of the heart. In addition, the collateral circulation in the affected area of the heart affects the outcome. Collateral circulation is an alternate circulation that develops when blood flow to a tissue is blocked. The illustration below shows the major coronary vessels that may be involved in an MI.

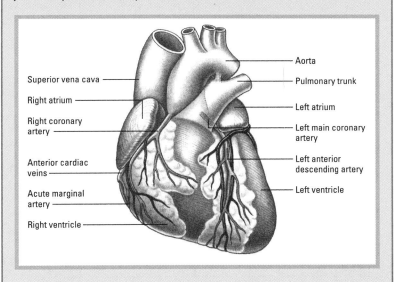

Superior vena cava

Right atrium

Right coronary artery

Anterior cardiac veins

Acute marginal artery

Right ventricle

Aorta

Pulmonary trunk

Left atrium

Left main coronary artery

Left anterior descending artery

Left ventricle

Pathophysiology

An ACS most commonly results when a thrombus progresses and occludes blood flow (recall that an early thrombus doesn't necessarily block blood flow.) The degree of blockage and the time that the affected vessel remains occluded are major determinants for the type of infarct that occurs. (See *Viewing the coronary vessels.*) The underlying effect is an imbalance in myocardial oxygen supply and demand.

For patients with unstable angina, a thrombus partially occludes a coronary vessel. This thrombus is full of

platelets. The partially occluded vessel may have distal microthrombi that cause necrosis in some myocytes. The smaller vessels infarct, and patients are at higher risk for MI. These patients may progress to a non–Q-wave MI.

If a thrombus fully occludes the vessel for a prolonged time, this is known as a Q-wave MI. In this type of MI, a greater concentration of thrombin and fibrin is noted.

Occlusion of a vessel progresses through three stages:
- *Ischemia* occurs first. It indicates that blood flow and oxygen demand

Release of cardiac enzymes and proteins

Because they're released by damaged tissue, serum proteins and isoenzymes (catalytic proteins that vary in concentration in specific organs) can help identify the compromised organ and assess the extent of damage. After acute myocardial infarction (MI), cardiac enzymes and proteins rise and fall in a characteristic pattern, as shown in the graph below.

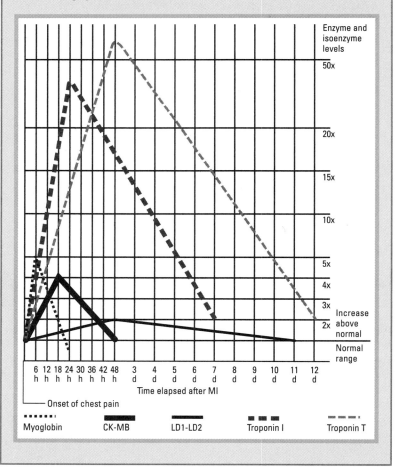

are out of balance. Ischemia can be resolved by improving flow or reducing oxygen needs.

■ *Injury* is the next stage, when the ischemia is prolonged enough to damage the area of the heart.

■ In *infarct,* the third stage, myocardial cells have died.

All MIs have a central area of necrosis or infarction surrounded by an area of potentially viable hypoxic injury. This zone may be salvaged if circulation is restored, or it may progress to necrosis. An area of viable ischemic tissue, in turn, surrounds the zone of injury. Although ischemia begins immediately, the size of the infarct can be limited if circulation is restored within 6 hours.

When the heart muscle is damaged, the integrity of the cell membrane is impaired and intracellular contents — including cardiac enzymes and proteins — are released and can be measured in the bloodstream. The release follows a characteristic rising and falling of values. The released enzymes include creatine kinase, lactate dehydrogenase, and aspartate aminotransferase; the proteins released include troponin T, troponin I, and myoglobin. (See *Release of cardiac enzymes and proteins.*)

Within 24 hours, the infarcted muscle becomes edematous and cyanotic. During the next several days, leukocytes infiltrate the necrotic area and begin to remove necrotic cells, thinning the ventricular wall. Scar formation begins by the 3rd week after MI, and by the 6th week, scar tissue is well established.

The scar tissue that forms on the necrotic area inhibits contractility. When this occurs, the compensatory mechanisms (vascular constriction, increased heart rate, and renal retention of sodium and water) try to maintain cardiac output (CO). Ventricular dilation may also occur in a process called remodeling. Functionally, an MI may cause reduced contractility with abnormal wall motion, altered left ventricular compliance, reduced stroke volume, reduced ejection fraction, and elevated left ventricular end-diastolic pressure.

Comprehensive assessment

A thorough assessment is essential for a patient with ACS. It must be done quickly — especially if the patient's condition appears unstable. After the patient is stabilized, further information can be developed regarding the patient's lifestyle and presence of the following risk factors:

■ positive family history
■ gender (Men and postmenopausal women are more susceptible to MI than premenopausal women, although the incidence is rising among women, especially those who smoke and take oral contraceptives.)
■ hypertension
■ smoking
■ elevated serum triglyceride, total cholesterol, and low-density lipoprotein levels
■ obesity
■ excessive intake of saturated fats
■ sedentary lifestyle
■ aging
■ stress or type A personality
■ drug use, especially cocaine and amphetamines.

Although chest pain may be a symptom of some other disorder, retrosternal chest discomfort, pain, or pressure is a prime symptom of infarction. Patients typically describe the following symptoms of acute ischemia and MI:

■ uncomfortable pressure, squeezing, pain, or fullness in the center of the

ACS algorithm

The acute coronary syndrome (ACS) algorithm shows the assessment steps and actions for the patient complaining of chest pain. It outlines the three syndromes of which you should be aware and their respective treatments.

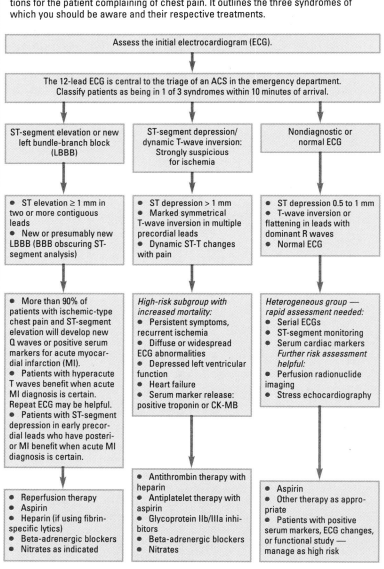

Assess the initial electrocardiogram (ECG).

The 12-lead ECG is central to the triage of an ACS in the emergency department. Classify patients as being in 1 of 3 syndromes within 10 minutes of arrival.

ST-segment elevation or new left bundle-branch block (LBBB)

- ST elevation ≥ 1 mm in two or more contiguous leads
- New or presumably new LBBB (BBB obscuring ST-segment analysis)

- More than 90% of patients with ischemic-type chest pain and ST-segment elevation will develop new Q waves or positive serum markers for acute myocardial infarction (MI).
- Patients with hyperacute T waves benefit when acute MI diagnosis is certain. Repeat ECG may be helpful.
- Patients with ST-segment depression in early precordial leads who have posterior MI benefit when acute MI diagnosis is certain.

- Reperfusion therapy
- Aspirin
- Heparin (if using fibrin-specific lytics)
- Beta-adrenergic blockers
- Nitrates as indicated

ST-segment depression/ dynamic T-wave inversion: Strongly suspicious for ischemia

- ST depression > 1 mm
- Marked symmetrical T-wave inversion in multiple precordial leads
- Dynamic ST-T changes with pain

High-risk subgroup with increased mortality:
- Persistent symptoms, recurrent ischemia
- Diffuse or widespread ECG abnormalities
- Depressed left ventricular function
- Heart failure
- Serum marker release: positive troponin or CK-MB

- Antithrombin therapy with heparin
- Antiplatelet therapy with aspirin
- Glycoprotein IIb/IIIa inhibitors
- Beta-adrenergic blockers
- Nitrates

Nondiagnostic or normal ECG

- ST depression 0.5 to 1 mm
- T-wave inversion or flattening in leads with dominant R waves
- Normal ECG

Heterogeneous group — rapid assessment needed:
- Serial ECGs
- ST-segment monitoring
- Serum cardiac markers
  Further risk assessment helpful:
- Perfusion radionuclide imaging
- Stress echocardiography

- Aspirin
- Other therapy as appropriate
- Patients with positive serum markers, ECG changes, or functional study — manage as high risk

chest lasting several minutes (usually longer than 15 minutes)

■ pain radiating to the shoulders, neck, arms, or jaw, or pain in the back between the shoulder blades

■ accompanying symptoms of light-headedness, fainting, sweating, nausea, or shortness of breath; feeling of impending doom.

Other manifestations may include palpitations, fatigue, nausea or vomiting, jugular vein distention, reduced urine output (secondary to reduced renal perfusion and increased aldosterone and antidiuretic hormone), systolic murmur (indicating papillary muscle dysfunction), and a decrease in or abnormal heart sounds, such as an S_3, S_4, or paradoxical splitting of S_2.

The ACS algorithm can be used to quickly classify patients so that treatment can be directed appropriately. (See *ACS algorithm.*)

AGE ISSUE *Many older adults don't have chest pain with MI but experience atypical signs and symptoms, such as fatigue, low body temperature, dyspnea, falls, tingling of the extremities, nausea, vomiting, weakness, syncope, and confusion. This is what's known as a "silent MI."*

The initial step in assessing a patient complaining of chest pain is to obtain a 12-lead electrocardiogram (ECG), which should be done within 10 minutes of the patient's arrival at your unit. Interpreting the ECG is the next step in identifying an ACS; your findings will direct the treatment plan. The patient should be classified as having ST-segment elevation or new left bundle-branch block (LBBB), ST-segment depression or dynamic T-wave inversion, or nondiagnostic or normal ECG. These changes indicate an event is occurring to the heart that may be due to occlusion of a vessel. If the ECG is nondiagnostic or normal, the patient will be monitored over several hours, with repeated testing, to either confirm or rule out MI — enzyme levels will be the key.

Diagnosis

The following tests help diagnose ACS:

■ Serial 12-lead ECG may reveal characteristic changes, such as serial ST-segment depression in non–Q-wave MI (subendocardial MI that affects the innermost myocardial layer) and ST-segment elevation in Q-wave MI (transmural MI with damage extending through all myocardial layers). The Q waves are considered abnormal when they appear greater than or equal to 0.04 second wide and their height is greater than 25% of the R wave height in that lead. An ECG can also identify the location of MI, arrhythmias, hypertrophy, and pericarditis. (See *Pinpointing myocardial infarction*, page 8.) Remember that the more combinations of leads affected with ECG changes, the more myocardium damage and the worse the prognosis. In addition, if a bundle-branch block (BBB) is present, it may make the diagnosis of MI very difficult because the BBB distorts the ST segment (an LBBB distorts the ST segment more than a right BBB). Moreover, a new onset of BBB accompanied by "typical" symptoms suggests an acute MI.

■ Serial cardiac enzymes and proteins may show a characteristic rise and fall of cardiac enzymes, specifically CK-MB, and the proteins troponin T and I, and myoglobin to confirm the diagnosis of MI.

Pinpointing myocardial infarction

Depending on location, ischemia or infarction causes changes in the following electrocardiographic leads.

Type of myocardial infarction	Leads
Inferior	II, III, aV$_F$
Anterior	V$_3$, V$_4$
Septal	V$_1$, V$_2$
Lateral	I, aV$_L$, V$_5$, V$_6$
Anterolateral	I, aV$_L$, V$_3$ to V$_6$
Posterior	V$_1$ or V$_2$
Right ventricular	II, III, aV$_F$, V$_{1R}$ to V$_{4R}$

■ When assessing CK-MB levels, be sure to compare with other cardiac markers.

■ Pay special attention to troponin levels because they're a good indicator about recurrent cardiac events and mortality. Because troponin levels generally rise sooner and remain elevated longer than CK-MB levels, troponin can be a precise indicator of myocardial damage and can reveal smaller amounts of myocardial necrosis.

■ In addition to CK-MB and troponin, be sure to consider the patient's myoglobin level because doubling within 2 hours of onset of symptoms strongly suggests infarction; on the other hand, a decrease in myoglobin within 4 to 8 hours eliminates MI.

■ Laboratory testing may reveal elevated white blood cell count and erythrocyte sedimentation rate due to inflammation, increased glucose levels following the release of catecholamines, and changes in electrolytes — all of which provide information about the patient's potential for developing arrhythmias and can identify the cause of an arrhythmia that accompanies chest discomfort.

■ Echocardiography may show ventricular wall motion abnormalities and may detect septal or papillary muscle rupture.

■ Transesophageal echocardiography can be used to provide more definitive views of the heart.

■ Chest X-rays may show left-sided heart failure or cardiomegaly.

■ Nuclear imaging scanning using thallium 201 and technetium 99m can be used to identify areas of infarction and areas of viable muscle cells.

■ Multiple-gated acquisition scanning is used to determine left ventricular function and identify aneurysms, problems with wall motion, and intracardiac shunting.

■ Cardiac catheterization may be used to identify the involved coronary artery as well as to provide information on ventricular function and pressures and volumes within the heart.

Collaborations

For the patient with ACS, a multidisciplinary approach to care is essential. Typically, outside of the hospital, emergency medical service personnel are involved. When the patient reaches the emergency department (ED), one physician assumes the "team leader" role and directs the team. The secondary ABCD survey is reapplied, including vital signs, oxygen saturation, brief and targeted history, 12-lead ECG, I.V. access, and a decision regarding thrombolytic therapy. The focus is on rapid but accurate diagnosis.

Treatment and care

The goals for patients experiencing an ACS include the following:

■ Reduce the amount of myocardial necrosis in those with ongoing infarction.

■ Prevent major adverse cardiac events.

■ Provide for rapid defibrillation when ventricular fibrillation is present.

Most patients with ST-segment elevation will develop Q-wave MI. Fifty-two percent of patients with MI die before reaching the hospital, and another 19% die within the first 24 hours of hospitalization. Therefore, initiating the algorithm for ischemic chest pain is essential whenever patients experience chest discomfort. (See *Ischemic chest pain algorithm,* pages 10 and 11.) This algorithm contains three scenarios, one of them being care for patients experiencing acute MI. The goal for treating patients with acute MI is to make sound — but rapid — decisions and reestablish blood flow to halt the ischemic process.

Generally, treatment of unstable angina consists of glycoprotein IIb and glycoprotein IIIa inhibitors and aspirin, which affect platelet formation and decrease platelet adhesion. It has been found that fibrinolytics aren't effective in these patients.

Administration of fibrinolytics or percutaneous coronary intervention (PCI), which may decrease or limit the amount of necrosis, are the preferred treatments for patients experiencing a Q-wave infarction. Typically, PCI is superior to fibrinolytic administration; restoration of vessel patency occurs in more than 90% of patients. In addition, reocclusion rates are lower when PCI is an initial form of therapy.

If the patient is a candidate for thrombolytic therapy, the time interval from arrival to the ED to the start of thrombolytic therapy should be 30 minutes or less. In some situations, where transfer time to an ED is greater than 60 minutes or where a physician is present, fibrinolysis will be started before the patient's arrival at the hospital. (See *Using thrombolytics,* page 12.)

The major determinants in saving myocardial tissue and improving long-term survival outcomes include:

■ a short time to reperfusion

■ early and sustained vessel patency

■ normal microvascular perfusion.

Research shows that the greatest benefits in survival and preservation of left ventricular function occur when therapy is initiated within the first 3 hours of onset of symptoms. However, because patients don't always seek help immediately or may have had intermittent chest pain, time determination may be difficult. Survival rates are still significant with treatment even 12 hours after onset of signs and symptoms.

MONA

Use the memory device, MONA — which stands for morphine, oxygen, nitroglycerin, and aspirin — to institute treatment of any patient experiencing ischemic chest pain or suspected ACS.

Morphine   Morphine is indicated for central anxiety and is the drug of choice to relieve pain associated with acute MI. The dosage is 2 to 4 mg I.V. push with repeat doses every 5 to 10 minutes until pain is relieved. Pain affects heart rate, contractility, and sys-

(Text continues on page 12.)

Ischemic chest pain algorithm

The ischemic chest pain algorithm reviews initial assessment and actions for a patient with possible ischemic chest pain. It also shows electrocardiogram (ECG) changes you may encounter in the patient. Base your treatments on ECG findings and patient status.

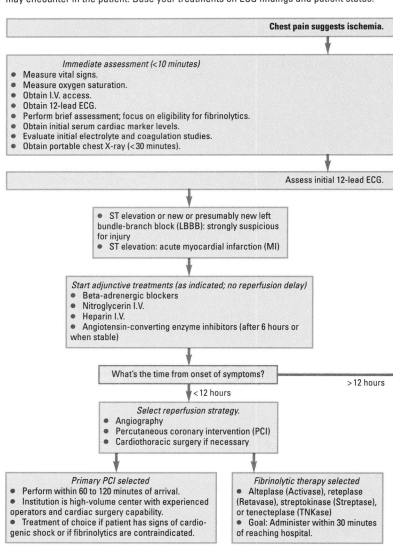

Chest pain suggests ischemia.

Immediate assessment (<10 minutes)
- Measure vital signs.
- Measure oxygen saturation.
- Obtain I.V. access.
- Obtain 12-lead ECG.
- Perform brief assessment; focus on eligibility for fibrinolytics.
- Obtain initial serum cardiac marker levels.
- Evaluate initial electrolyte and coagulation studies.
- Obtain portable chest X-ray (<30 minutes).

Assess initial 12-lead ECG.

- ST elevation or new or presumably new left bundle-branch block (LBBB): strongly suspicious for injury
- ST elevation: acute myocardial infarction (MI)

Start adjunctive treatments (as indicated; no reperfusion delay)
- Beta-adrenergic blockers
- Nitroglycerin I.V.
- Heparin I.V.
- Angiotensin-converting enzyme inhibitors (after 6 hours or when stable)

What's the time from onset of symptoms?

>12 hours

<12 hours

Select reperfusion strategy.
- Angiography
- Percutaneous coronary intervention (PCI)
- Cardiothoracic surgery if necessary

Primary PCI selected
- Perform within 60 to 120 minutes of arrival.
- Institution is high-volume center with experienced operators and cardiac surgery capability.
- Treatment of choice if patient has signs of cardiogenic shock or if fibrinolytics are contraindicated.

Fibrinolytic therapy selected
- Alteplase (Activase), reteplase (Retavase), streptokinase (Streptase), or tenecteplase (TNKase)
- Goal: Administer within 30 minutes of reaching hospital.

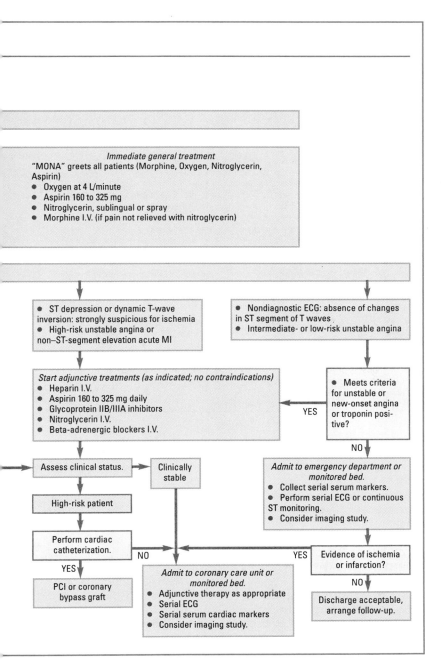

Immediate general treatment
"MONA" greets all patients (Morphine, Oxygen, Nitroglycerin, Aspirin)
● Oxygen at 4 L/minute
● Aspirin 160 to 325 mg
● Nitroglycerin, sublingual or spray
● Morphine I.V. (if pain not relieved with nitroglycerin)

● ST depression or dynamic T-wave inversion: strongly suspicious for ischemia
● High-risk unstable angina or non–ST-segment elevation acute MI

● Nondiagnostic ECG: absence of changes in ST segment of T waves
● Intermediate- or low-risk unstable angina

Start adjunctive treatments (as indicated; no contraindications)
● Heparin I.V.
● Aspirin 160 to 325 mg daily
● Glycoprotein IIB/IIIA inhibitors
● Nitroglycerin I.V.
● Beta-adrenergic blockers I.V.

● Meets criteria for unstable or new-onset angina or troponin positive?

YES

NO

Assess clinical status.

Clinically stable

High-risk patient

Perform cardiac catheterization.

NO

YES

PCI or coronary bypass graft

Admit to emergency department or monitored bed.
● Collect serial serum markers.
● Perform serial ECG or continuous ST monitoring.
● Consider imaging study.

YES

Evidence of ischemia or infarction?

NO

Admit to coronary care unit or monitored bed.
● Adjunctive therapy as appropriate
● Serial ECG
● Serial serum cardiac markers
● Consider imaging study.

Discharge acceptable, arrange follow-up.

Using thrombolytics

Thrombolytics are considered a Class I intervention (a universal standard of care) for acute myocardial infarction. Inclusion criteria are:

- ST elevation greater than or equal to 1 mm in at least two contiguous leads
- age less than 75 years
- no contraindications present
- signs and symptoms consistent with ischemic-type chest pain.

If the patient is over age 75, or symptoms have existed for more than 12 hours, thrombolytics are a Class IIa intervention (indicated when data support usefulness and efficacy). Percutaneous coronary intervention for patients under age 75 with signs of shock is a Class I intervention.

Contraindications for thrombolytic agents are separated into absolute and relative categories. These contraindications are heeded because of the inherent action of thrombolytic agents and the potential to cause excessive bleeding.

Absolute contraindications include:

- previous hemorrhagic stroke
- uncontrolled hypertension (180/110 mm Hg or higher)

- other strokes at any time or cerebrovascular events within 1 year
- known intracranial neoplasm
- active internal bleeding
- suspected aortic dissection.

Relative contraindications include:

- severe uncontrolled hypertension at presentation (greater than 180/110 mm Hg)
- other intracerebral pathology
- current use of anticoagulants (International Normalized Ratio greater than 2), known bleeding diathesis
- recent trauma (2 to 4 weeks), including head trauma
- prolonged (more than 10 minutes) and potentially traumatic cardiopulmonary resuscitation
- major surgery (less than 3 weeks)
- noncompressible vascular punctures
- recent (2 to 4 weeks) internal bleeding
- prior exposure (less than 2 years) for streptokinase or anistreplase
- pregnancy
- active peptic ulcer
- history of chronic severe hypertension.

tolic blood pressure, thereby adversely increasing myocardial oxygen demand. Evaluate the patient's pain response and his vital signs. Frequent blood pressure monitoring is especially important because morphine can cause hypotension.

Oxygen   Oxygen has been proven to reduce ST elevation and limit ischemic myocardial injury and should be administered to anyone experiencing chest discomfort. Oxygen may be administered by nasal cannula or mask. The type and amount of oxygen to be administered is determined by oxygen

saturation. Lower concentrations of oxygen (less than 40%) can be delivered by nasal cannula, whereas higher concentrations (over 40%) can be delivered by mask. If equipment to measure pulse oximetry is available, oxygen saturation should be maintained at more than 90%.

Nitroglycerin   Sublingual nitroglycerin is the initial treatment for a patient with chest pain that suggests ischemia because nitrates result in coronary dilation and allow greater perfusion. Venodilation improves preload because it increases venous capacitance. Systemic arteriolar dilation improves afterload as it reduces the workload of the left ventricle. Both of these actions reduce the heart's oxygen requirements.

A dose of 0.3 to 0.4 mg nitroglycerin sublingually may be given three times at 5-minute intervals as long as blood pressure is stable (usually greater than 90 mm Hg systolic). When nitroglycerin use will be prolonged, the I.V. route allows active titration. Nitrates are contraindicated with right ventricular infarct or when the heart rate is less than 50 beats/minute.

Aspirin Aspirin is considered a Class I action in the treatment of the patient with MI. Aspirin 160 to 325 mg is given by mouth as soon as possible. Chewed aspirin is absorbed the fastest and is preferred.

Additional therapies
When a patient is being evaluated for ischemic chest pain, simultaneous treatment is performed while the secondary survey is underway. This includes oxygen administration, nitroglycerin sublingually (may be followed by I.V.), morphine I.V., aspirin by mouth, thrombolytic agents, heparin I.V., beta-adrenergic blockers, lidocaine (if ectopy is present), magnesium sulfate I.V., and coronary angiography.

Adjunctive therapy can be started while reperfusion strategies are being considered, and may include:
■ beta-adrenergic blockers (decrease the workload of the heart)
■ I.V. nitroglycerin (dilates coronary arteries, improves preload and afterload)

■ heparin (indicated for patients receiving tissue plasminogen activator or reteplase [Retavase] and for patients who are candidates for percutaneous transluminal coronary angioplasty [PTCA] or surgical revascularization)
■ angiotensin-converting enzyme inhibitors (block conversion of angiotensin; should be given within 12 to 24 hours of symptoms).
Reperfusion strategies include:
■ angiography
■ PCI, which includes angioplasty with or without stents
■ cardiothoracic surgery
■ fibrinolytic therapy.

Complications
Complications may include:
■ arrhythmias
■ cardiogenic shock
■ heart failure causing pulmonary edema
■ pericarditis
■ rupture of the atrial or ventricular septum, ventricular wall, or valves
■ mural thrombi causing cerebral or pulmonary emboli
■ ventricular aneurysms
■ myocardial rupture
■ extensions of the original infarction
■ death.
Any patient with ACS is at risk for complications for up to 12 weeks following the acute episode. In addition, for approximately the next 6 months, the patient is at risk for additional episodes until the area of the initiating plaque heals.

Nursing considerations
■ On admission to the critical care unit (CCU), monitor and record the patient's ECG, blood pressure, temperature, and heart and breath sounds.

Also, assess and record the pain's severity, location, type, and duration. Obtain a 12-lead ECG and assess heart rate and blood pressure when the patient experiences acute chest pain.

■ Monitor the patient's hemodynamic status closely and be alert for indicators suggesting decreased CO, such as decreased blood pressure, increased heart rate, increased pulmonary artery pressure, increased pulmonary artery wedge pressure, decreased CO measurements, and decreased right atrial pressure.

■ Assess urine output hourly for at least the first 4 hours, and then according to your facility's policy.

■ Monitor the patient's oxygen saturation levels and continue oxygen administration as ordered. Notify the physician if oxygen saturation falls below 90%.

■ Check the patient's blood pressure after giving nitroglycerin, especially after the first dose.

■ Frequently monitor ECG rhythm strips to detect heart rate changes and arrhythmias.

■ During episodes of chest pain, monitor the ECG and blood pressure and pulmonary artery catheter measurements (if applicable) to determine changes.

■ Obtain serial measurements of cardiac enzyme levels as ordered.

■ Watch for crackles, cough, tachypnea, and edema, which may indicate impending left-sided heart failure. Carefully monitor daily weight, intake and output, respiratory rate, serum enzyme levels, ECG waveforms, and blood pressure. Auscultate for adventitious breath sounds periodically. Also auscultate for S_3 or S_4 gallops.

■ Prepare the patient for reperfusion therapy as indicated.

■ Administer and titrate medications as ordered. Avoid giving I.M. injections because absorption from muscles is unpredictable and I.V. administration provides more rapid symptomatic relief.

■ Organize patient care and activities to allow periods of uninterrupted rest. Assist with range-of-motion exercises. If the patient is immobilized, turn him often and use antiembolism stockings or intermittent compression devices. Gradually increase the patient's activity level as tolerated and as indicated by acceptable monitoring parameters.

■ Provide a clear-liquid diet until nausea subsides. Anticipate the possibility for a low-cholesterol, low-sodium diet without caffeine.

■ Provide a stool softener to prevent straining during defecation. Allow the patient to use a bedside commode if appropriate, and provide as much privacy as possible.

■ Provide emotional support, and help reduce stress and anxiety; administer antianxiety agents as needed.

Patient teaching

■ Explain procedures and answer questions for the patient and his family. Explain the unit environment and routine. Instruct the patient and his family about specific interventions, such as PTCA, coronary artery bypass grafting, or reperfusion therapies.

■ Thoroughly explain the medication and treatment regimen. Inform the patient of the drug's adverse effects and advise him to watch for and report any signs (for example, headache, dizziness, hypotension, nausea, and vomiting associated with nitroglycerin;

bleeding or bruising associated with thrombolytics). Teach the patient self-monitoring techniques such as pulse monitoring.

■ Advise the patient about appropriate responses to new or recurring symptoms, including what actions he should take.

■ Advise the patient to report typical or atypical chest pain. Post-MI syndrome may develop, producing chest pain that must be differentiated from recurrent MI, pulmonary infarction, and heart failure.

■ Review dietary restrictions with the patient. If he must follow a low-sodium or low-fat and low-cholesterol diet, provide a list of foods to avoid. Ask the facility's dietitian to speak to the patient and his family.

■ Encourage the patient to participate in a cardiac rehabilitation exercise program that includes progressive activities.

■ Advise the patient to resume sexual activity gradually. He may need to take nitroglycerin before sexual intercourse to prevent chest pain caused by the increased activity.

■ Stress the need to stop smoking. If necessary, refer the patient to a support group.

Aortic aneurysm

An aortic aneurysm is a localized out-pouching or abnormal dilation in the weakened arterial wall that typically occurs in the aorta between the renal arteries and the iliac branches. However, the abdominal, thoracic, or ascending arch of the aorta may be affected. These slow-developing aneurysms can be fusiform (spindle-shaped) or saccular (pouchlike).

About 95% of aortic aneurysms result from arteriosclerosis or atherosclerosis (85% of thoracic aneurysms and most abdominal aneurysms); the rest result from congenital cystic medial necrosis, trauma, syphilis, and other inflammatory or infectious causes. Aortic aneurysms occur most commonly in white males with hypertension between ages 50 and 80. With involvement of the aorta, the potential exists for severe compromise in blood flow to major organs of the body, such as the brain, heart, kidneys, and GI tract, if rupture occurs. Thus, complications can be life-threatening.

Although the prognosis for patients with aortic aneurysm is grim if surgical repair isn't done, prognosis improves significantly if the surgical repair is performed as an elective nonemergency procedure. Otherwise, the aneurysm will continue to enlarge until it ruptures.

Pathophysiology

Aneurysms result from a defect in the middle layer of the arterial wall (tunica media). When the elastic fibers and collagen in the tunica media are damaged, stretching and segmental dilation occur and the medial layer loses some of its elasticity, leading to fragmentation. Smooth-muscle cells are lost and the media thins. The thinned wall may be brittle due to the presence of calcium deposits and atherosclerotic plaque. As a person ages, the elastin in the wall decreases, further weakening the vessel. If hypertension is present, blood flow slows, resulting in ischemia and additional weakening.

Lateral pressure increases as the aneurysm develops, causing the vessel lumen to widen and blood flow to slow. Over time, mechanical stressors contribute to elongation of the aneurysm, and the aorta becomes bowed and tortuous. Hemodynamic forces may also play a role, causing pulsatile stresses on the weakened wall and pressing on the small vessels that supply the arterial wall with nutrients.

Although the cause of aortic aneurysms is unclear, several factors have been identified as placing a person at risk. These include:

- advancing age
- history of hypertension
- smoking
- atherosclerosis
- connective tissue disorders
- diabetes mellitus
- trauma.

Comprehensive assessment

Most patients with aortic aneurysms are asymptomatic until the aneurysm enlarges and compresses surrounding tissue. Be aware that a large aneurysm may produce signs and symptoms that mimic those of myocardial infarction (MI), renal calculi, lumbar disk disease, and duodenal compression. Usually, patients' symptoms are caused by rupture, expansion, embolization, thrombosis, or pressure from the mass on surrounding structures.

If the patient has a thoracic aortic aneurysm, assess for complaints of substernal pain possibly radiating to the neck, back, abdomen, or shoulders.

AGE ISSUE *Because of the normal age-related changes in the older adult's vasculature, a patient over age 65 should be assessed for aneurysms. Rupture is more common if the patient also has hypertension or if the aneurysm is larger than 6 cm.*

ALERT *Be alert for complaints of sharp, sternal pain between the scapulae. Be ready to intervene quickly — this type of pain may indicate an impending rupture.*

The patient may also exhibit hoarseness or coughing due to pressure on the laryngeal nerve; in addition, he may have difficulty swallowing if the mass is compressing the esophagus. Difficulty breathing or hemoptysis suggests rupture with subsequent bleeding into the tracheobronchial tree. Hematemesis suggests rupture with bleeding into the esophagus.

Assess the patient's vital signs, specifically blood pressure and pulse in both arms, and compare the findings bilaterally. If unequal, suspect a thoracic aortic aneurysm. Also, auscultate heart sounds and note the presence of an aortic insufficiency murmur. In a patient with acute expansion of a thoracic aortic aneurysm, severe hypertension, neurologic changes, and a new murmur of aortic insufficiency may be present. Physical examination may also reveal a right sternoclavicular lift, jugular vein distention, or tracheal deviation.

The patient with an abdominal aortic aneurysm may complain of gnawing, generalized, steady abdominal pain or low back pain that's unaffected by movement. He may have a sensation of gastric or abdominal fullness caused by pressure on the GI structures.

ALERT *Be alert for complaints of sudden, severe abdominal pain or lumbar pain that radiates to the* *flank and groin from pressure on lumbar nerves. This may signify enlargement and imminent rupture. If the aneurysm ruptures into the peritoneal cavity, severe and persistent abdominal and back pain, mimicking renal or ureteral colic pain, occurs. If it ruptures into the duodenum, GI bleeding occurs with massive hematemesis and melena.*

Inspection of the patient with an intact abdominal aortic aneurysm usually reveals no significant findings. However, if the person isn't obese, you may note a pulsating mass in the periumbilical area. Auscultation of the abdomen, the most important diagnostic indicator, may reveal a systolic bruit over the aorta caused by turbulent blood flow in the widened arterial segment. A bruit may also be heard over the femoral arteries. Hypotension occurs with aneurysm rupture.

Palpation of the abdomen may disclose some tenderness over the affected area. A pulsatile mass may be felt in about 80% of patients.

ALERT *If a pulsatile mass is felt on palpation, avoid deep palpation to locate the mass because this may cause the aneurysm to rupture.*

Diagnosis

Because an aortic aneurysm seldom produces symptoms, it's typically detected inadvertently on a routine X-ray or during a physical examination. No specific laboratory tests are available to assist in the diagnosis of aortic aneurysms. However, if blood is leaking from the aneurysm, leukocytosis and a decrease in hemoglobin level and hematocrit may be noted.

Several diagnostic tests are available to help confirm a suspected aortic aneurysm:

■ Transesophageal echocardiogram allows for visualization of the thoracic aorta and is usually combined with Doppler flow studies to provide information about blood flow.
■ Abdominal ultrasonography or echocardiography can determine the aneurysm's size, shape, length, and location.
■ Anteroposterior and lateral X-rays of the chest or abdomen can detect aortic calcification and widened areas of the aorta.
■ Computed tomography scan and magnetic resonance imaging can identify the aneurysm's size and effect on nearby organs.
■ Serial ultrasonography at 6-month intervals shows any growth of small aneurysms.
■ Aortography helps in determining the aneurysm's approximate size and patency of the visceral vessels.

Collaborations

A multidisciplinary approach is needed to care for the patient with an aortic aneurysm. Medical and nursing health care providers should focus on administering medications to treat hypertension and pain, ensuring bed rest, and providing a calm, quiet environment. Surgical health care providers are commonly consulted to plan for resection of the aneurysm. Nutritional consultation may be necessary to help with dietary measures to control atherosclerosis and hypertension.

Treatment and care

Aortic aneurysms usually require resection with replacement of the aortic section using a vascular or Dacron graft. If the aneurysm is small and produces no symptoms, surgery may be delayed, with regular physical examination and ultrasonography performed to monitor its progression. Large or symptomatic aneurysms may rupture and need immediate repair.

Patients with abdominal aortic aneurysms that aren't extremely tortuous and don't begin at the left renal artery level are candidates for endovascular grafting, which is considered a minimally invasive procedure. In this procedure, which can be done using local or regional anesthesia, the walls of the aorta are reinforced to prevent rupture and expansion of the aneurysm. Endovascular grafting is performed under fluoroscopy. A delivery catheter with an attached compressed graft is inserted through a small incision in the femoral or iliac artery over a guide wire. The delivery catheter is advanced to the aorta, where it's positioned across the aneurysm. A balloon on the catheter expands the graft and affixes it to the vessel wall. In addition to surgery, patients usually receive medications to control blood pressure, relieve anxiety, and control pain. (See *Endovascular grafting for repair of AAA.*)

Rupture of an aortic aneurysm is a medical emergency requiring prompt treatment, including resuscitation with fluid and blood replacement, I.V. propranolol to reduce myocardial contractility, I.V. nitroprusside to reduce blood pressure and maintain it at 100 to 120 mm Hg systolic, and analgesics to relieve pain. An arterial line and indwelling urinary catheter will monitor the patient's condition until the patient is taken to surgery.

Complications

More than 50% of patients with untreated abdominal aneurysms die of hemorrhage and shock from aneurysmal rupture within 2 years of diagnosis. More than 85% die within 5 years. If the aortic aneurysm ruptures and goes untreated, the mortality rate is near 100%.

Complications that can occur after surgical repair of an aortic aneurysm include left-sided heart failure, arrhythmias, MI, renal failure, acute tubular necrosis, ileus, pancreatitis, ischemia of the left colon, paralysis due to spinal cord ischemia, lower extremity ischemia, and hemorrhage. Possible complications after endovascular grafting include bleeding, hematoma formation or wound infection at the catheter insertion site, distal ischemia or embolization, dissection or perforation of the aorta, graft thrombosis, graft infection, graft migration, breaks or leaks, delayed rupture, and bowel ischemia.

Nursing considerations

■ Assess the patient's vital signs, especially blood pressure, every 2 to 4 hours or more frequently, depending on the severity of his condition. Monitor blood pressure and pulse in extremities and compare findings bilaterally. If the difference in systolic blood pressure exceeds 10 mm Hg, notify the physician immediately.
■ Assess cardiovascular status frequently, including heart rate, rhythm, electrocardiogram, and cardiac enzyme levels (an MI can occur if an aneurysm ruptures along the coronary arteries).
■ Evaluate kidney function by obtaining blood samples for blood urea nitrogen, creatinine, and electrolyte levels. Measure intake and output regularly — hourly if necessary — as indicated by the patient's condition.

■ Monitor complete blood count for evidence of blood loss, reflected in decreased hemoglobin level, hematocrit, and red blood cell count.

■ If the patient's condition is acute, obtain an arterial sample for arterial blood gas analysis as ordered and monitor cardiac rhythm. Insert an arterial line to allow for continuous blood pressure monitoring. Assist with insertion of a pulmonary artery catheter to assess hemodynamic balance.

■ Observe the patient for signs of rupture, which may be immediately fatal. Watch closely for signs of acute blood loss: decreasing blood pressure, increasing pulse and respiratory rates, cool, clammy skin, restlessness, and decreased sensorium.

■ Administer ordered medications to control aneurysm progression. Provide analgesics to relieve pain if present.

■ If rupture occurs, insert a large-bore I.V. catheter, begin fluid resuscitation, and administer nitroprusside I.V. as ordered, usually to maintain a mean arterial pressure of 70 to 80 mm Hg. Also administer propranolol I.V. (to reduce left ventricular ejection velocity) at a rate of 1 mg every 5 minutes (to a maximum initial dose not exceeding 0.15 mg/kg of body weight) until the heart rate ranges from 60 to 80 beats/minute. Expect to administer additional doses of 2 to 6 mg every 4 to 6 hours until oral medications can be used.

■ If the patient is experiencing acute pain, administer morphine 2 to 10 mg I.V. as ordered.

■ Prepare the patient for elective surgery as indicated or emergency surgery, if rupture occurs. In an emergency, a pneumatic antishock garment

Endovascular grafting for repair of AAA

Endovascular grafting is a minimally invasive procedure for the patient who requires repair of an abdominal aortic aneurysm (AAA).

The patient is instructed to walk the first day after surgery and is discharged from the hospital in 1 to 3 days.

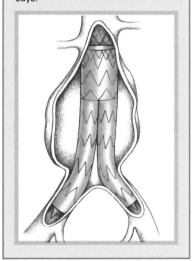

may be used while transporting him to surgery.

■ Allow the patient to express his fears and concerns about the diagnosis, and provide support to the patient and his family.

After surgery

■ Administer nitroprusside or nitroglycerin and titrate to maintain blood pressure within acceptable parameters.

■ Perform meticulous pulmonary hygiene measures, including suctioning, chest physiotherapy, and deep-breathing exercises.

■ Provide continuous cardiac monitoring.
■ Assess urine output hourly.
■ Maintain nasogastric tube patency to ensure gastric decompression.
■ Assist with serial Doppler examination of extremities to evaluate adequacy of vascular repair and presence of embolization.
■ Assess for signs of poor arterial perfusion, such as pain, paresthesia, pallor, pulselessness, paralysis, and poikilothermia (coldness).

Patient teaching

■ Provide psychological support for the patient and his family. On admission to the critical care unit, help ease their fears about this type of care, the threat of impending rupture, and any planned surgery. Take time to provide appropriate explanations and to answer questions.
■ Explain the surgical procedure and the expected postoperative care on the unit for patients undergoing surgery (such as I.V. lines, endotracheal and nasogastric intubation, and mechanical ventilation).
■ Reinforce instructions for controlling hypertension — stress the importance of medications and diet therapy and the need for smoking cessation.
■ Instruct the patient to take all medications as prescribed and to carry a list of them at all times in case of an emergency.
■ Advise the patient about activity restrictions, such as no pushing, pulling, or lifting heavy objects until the physician allows him to do so.

Arterial pressure monitoring

Arterial pressure monitoring measures arterial pressure directly using an indwelling arterial catheter connected to an external pressure transducer and fluid-filled tubing. The tubing is attached to a pressure bag of saline or heparin flush solution and the transducer is attached to a monitor. The pressure transducer converts the pressure into an electrical signal that's filtered and displayed on a monitor screen as a continuous waveform. The pressure may also be shown as a digital readout. (See *Understanding the arterial waveform*.)

Most commonly, the radial artery is the site of catheter insertion because this artery is readily accessible. However, the axillary, femoral, brachial, or pedal arteries may also be used.

ALERT *If the radial artery is to be used, always perform Allen's test before insertion to ensure collateral circulation in the hand.*

Direct arterial pressure monitoring permits continuous measurement of systolic, diastolic, and mean pressures and allows arterial blood sampling. Because direct measurement reflects systemic vascular resistance as well as blood flow, it's generally more accurate than indirect methods (such as palpation and auscultation of Korotkoff's, or audible pulse, sounds), which are based on blood flow. Moreover, direct arterial pressure monitoring permits mean arterial pressure determination, an important indicator of tissue perfusion, especially of the major organs.

In contrast to indirect monitoring, which carries few associated risks and

Understanding the arterial waveform

Normal arterial blood pressure produces a characteristic waveform, representing ventricular systole and diastole. The waveform has five distinct components: the anacrotic limb, systolic peak, dicrotic limb, dicrotic notch, and end diastole.

The anacrotic limb marks the waveform's initial upstroke, which results as blood is rapidly ejected from the ventricle through the open aortic valve into the aorta. The rapid ejection causes a sharp rise in arterial pressure, which appears as the waveform's highest point. This is called the systolic peak.

As blood continues into the peripheral vessels, arterial pressure falls and the waveform begins a downward trend, called the dicrotic limb. Arterial pressure will usually continue to fall until pressure in the ventricle is less than the pressure in the aortic root. This event appears as a small notch, called the dicrotic notch, on the waveform's downside. When the aortic valve closes, diastole begins progressing until the aortic root pressure gradually descends to its lowest point. On the waveform, this is known as end diastole.

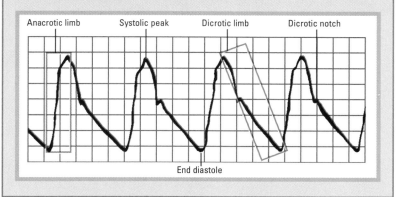

is commonly performed by applying pressure to an artery (such as by inflating a blood pressure cuff around the arm) to decrease blood flow, direct monitoring is indicated when highly accurate or frequent blood pressure measurements are required — for example, in patients with low cardiac output (CO) and high systemic vascular resistance. Also, direct monitoring may be used for patients who are receiving doses of vasoactive drugs requiring titration or who need frequent blood sampling.

Equipment

For waveform monitoring

Pressurized bag of saline or heparin flush solution ▪ indwelling arterial catheter ▪ fluid-filled tubing connected to an external pressure transducer ▪ monitor

For arterial line tubing changes

Gloves ▪ gown ▪ mask ▪ protective eyewear ▪ sheet protector ▪ preassembled arterial pressure tubing with flush device and disposable pressure transducer ▪ sterile gloves ▪ 500-ml bag of I.V. flush solution (such as dextrose 5% in water or normal saline solution) ▪ 500 or 1,000 units of heparin ■ syringe and 21G to 25G 1″ needle ■ alcohol pad ■ medication label ■ pressure bag ■ site care kit ■ tubing labels

For arterial catheter removal
Gloves ■ mask ■ gown ■ protective eyewear ■ two sterile 4″ × 4″ gauze pads ■ sheet protector ■ sterile suture removal set ■ dressing ■ hypoallergenic tape

For femoral line removal
Additional sterile 4″ × 4″ gauze pads ■ small sandbag (which you may wrap in a towel or place in a pillowcase) ■ adhesive bandage

Essential steps
■ After the catheter has been inserted and the system has been set up, observe the drip chamber of the pressurized bag to verify that the continuous flush rate is as desired. Also, check to ensure that a waveform appears on the monitor.
■ Be sure to cover the insertion site with a dressing as specified by the facility's policy.
■ Keep the site of insertion immobilized. For the radial or brachial artery, use an arm board and soft wrist restraint if necessary. For the femoral artery, assess the need for an ankle restraint and keep the patient on bed rest, with the head of the bed elevated 15 to 30 degrees to prevent catheter kinking.
■ Be sure to level the zeroing stopcock of the transducer with the phlebostatic axis (approximately the level of the right atrium located at the intersection of the fourth intercostal space and the midanterior posterior chest).

ALERT *Be sure to mark the phlebostatic axis on the patient's skin using tape or indelible ink and always use the same, marked point for taking readings. Otherwise, the readings may be inaccurate.*

■ Relevel the transducer any time the patient or the transducer is moved; for example, after raising or lowering the head of the bed or when the patient's condition changes.
■ Set the alarms for systolic and diastolic pressure on the monitor approximately 10 to 20 mm Hg above and below the patient's baseline pressure. Make sure that the alarms are on at all times to allow for prompt detection and identification of changes or possible disconnection.
■ Ensure that the pressurized bag is inflated to 300 mm Hg. This helps keep the pressure in the arterial line higher than the patient's systolic pressure, thus keeping blood from backing up into the tubing. Also, make sure that there are no air bubbles in the tubing, because air can dampen the waveform, thereby causing inaccurate results.
■ When observing the waveform on the monitor, look for normal waveform characteristics, including the sharp rise indicating systole, the systolic peak, and the dicrotic notch.

ALERT *When observing the waveform, the dicrotic notch should be approximately one-third or more of the height of the systolic peak; if it's less, suspect a decrease in CO. If the anacrotic limb appears as a steep rise, the systolic peak is very high, and the dicrotic notch is difficult to define or detect, suspect aortic insufficiency. If the anacrotic limb shows a delay in rising, suspect a problem with myocardial contractility, aortic stenosis or, possibly, a problem with catheter position or catheter clotting.*

■ Periodically check the patient's blood pressure using a sphygmomanometer and compare with the values on the monitor. Keep in mind that these values may be different; pressures obtained via arterial monitoring are generally higher than those obtained indirectly. However, if indirect measurements are higher than arterial line pressures, suspect a malfunction in the equipment or a technical error with the indirect measurement.

Check the facility's policy about tubing changes and, if permitted, check the facility's procedure manual to determine how much tubing length to change. Then follow these steps:

■ When changing tubing, first wash your hands and follow standard precautions. Assemble the new pressure monitoring system.

■ Inflate the pressure bag to 300 mm Hg and check for air leaks. Release the pressure.

■ Prepare the I.V. flush solution, and prime the pressure tubing and transducer system. At this time, add medication and tubing labels. Apply 300 mm Hg of pressure to the system. Hang the I.V. bag on a pole.

■ Place the sheet protector under the affected extremity. Remove the dressing from the catheter insertion site, taking care not to dislodge the catheter or cause vessel trauma. If your facility permits, turn off or temporarily silence the monitor alarms; otherwise, leave the alarms on.

■ Turn off the flow clamp of the tubing segment you'll be changing. Disconnect the tubing from the catheter hub, taking care not to dislodge the catheter. Immediately insert new tubing into the catheter hub. Secure the tubing, and then activate the fast-flush release to clear it.

■ Reactivate the monitor alarms. Apply an appropriate dressing.

■ Level the zeroing stopcock of the transducer with the phlebostatic axis, and zero the system to atmospheric pressure.

Consult facility policy to determine whether you're permitted to remove an arterial line. If permitted, follow these steps:

■ Explain the procedure to the patient.

■ Assemble all equipment. Wash your hands. Observe standard precautions, including wearing personal protective equipment, for this procedure.

■ Record the patient's systolic, diastolic, and mean blood pressures. If a manual, indirect blood pressure hasn't been assessed recently, obtain one now to establish a new baseline.

■ Turn off the monitor alarms. Then turn off the flow clamp to the flush solution.

■ Carefully remove the dressing over the insertion site. Remove any sutures using the suture removal kit, and then carefully check that all sutures have been removed.

■ Withdraw the catheter using a gentle, steady motion. Keep the catheter parallel to the artery during withdrawal to reduce the risk of traumatic injury.

■ Immediately after withdrawing the catheter, apply pressure to the site with a sterile 4″ × 4″ gauze pad. Maintain pressure for at least 10 minutes (longer if bleeding or oozing persists). Apply additional pressure to a femoral site or if the patient has coagulopathy or is receiving anticoagulants.

■ Cover the site with an appropriate dressing and secure the dressing with tape. If stipulated by facility policy, make a pressure dressing for a femoral site by folding in half four sterile 4″ × 4″ gauze pads, and apply the dressing. Cover the dressing with a tight adhesive bandage; then cover the bandage with a sandbag.

■ Maintain the patient on bed rest for 6 hours with the sandbag in place.

■ If the physician has ordered a culture of the catheter tip (to diagnose a suspected infection), gently place the catheter tip on a sterile 4″ × 4″ gauze pad. When the bleeding is under control, hold the catheter over the sterile container. Using sterile scissors, cut the tip so that it falls into the sterile container. Label the specimen and send it to the laboratory.

■ Observe the site for bleeding. Assess circulation in the extremity distal to the site by evaluating color, pulses, and sensation. Repeat this assessment every 15 minutes for the first 4 hours, every 30 minutes for the next 2 hours, and then hourly for the next 6 hours.

Complications

Direct arterial pressure monitoring can cause complications, such as arterial bleeding, infection, air embolism, arterial spasm, vessel damage, or thrombosis.

Nursing considerations

■ Observing the pressure waveform on the monitor can enhance assessment of arterial pressure. An abnormal waveform may reflect an arrhythmia (such as atrial fibrillation) or other cardiovascular problems, such as aortic stenosis, aortic insufficiency, pulsus al-

ternans, or pulsus paradoxus. (See *Recognizing abnormal waveforms.*)

■ Change the pressure tubing every 2 to 3 days, according to facility policy. Change the dressing at the catheter site at intervals specified by facility policy. Regularly assess the site for signs of infection, such as redness and swelling. Notify the physician immediately if you note any such signs.

■ Be aware that erroneous pressure readings may result if a catheter becomes blocked or if its flow is affected by shoulder or arm positioning, loose connections, an addition of extra stopcocks or extension tubing, inadvertent entry of air into the system, or improper calibration, leveling, or zeroing of the monitoring system. If the catheter lumen clots, the flush system may be improperly pressurized. Regularly assess the amount of flush solution in the I.V. bag and maintain 300 mm Hg of pressure in the pressure bag.

■ Document the date of system setup so that caregivers will know when to change the components. Also record systolic, diastolic, and mean pressure readings, being sure to note the patient's position when each blood pressure reading is obtained. This is important for determining trends.

■ Carefully document the amount of flush solution infused to avoid hypervolemia and volume overload, and to ensure accurate assessment of the patient's fluid status. In addition, document evidence of circulation in the extremity distal to the site by assessing color, pulses, and sensation. Most important, be sure to include a description of any abnormalities noted and measures used to resolve them.

Recognizing abnormal waveforms

Recognizing a normal arterial waveform is relatively straightforward. An abnormal waveform, however, is more difficult to decipher. Abnormal patterns and markings may provide important diagnostic clues to the patient's cardiovascular status, or they may simply signal trouble in the monitor. Use this chart to help recognize and resolve waveform abnormalities.

Abnormality	Possible causes	Nursing considerations
Alternating high and low waves in a regular pattern 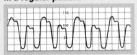	Ventricular bigeminy	● Check the patient's electrocardiogram to confirm ventricular bigeminy. The tracing should reflect premature ventricular contractions every second beat.
Flattened waveform 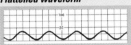	Overdamped waveform or hypotensive patient	● Check the patient's blood pressure with a sphygmomanometer. If you obtain a higher reading, suspect overdamping. Correct the problem by trying to aspirate the arterial line. If you succeed, flush the line. If the reading is very low or absent, suspect hypotension.
Slightly rounded waveform with consistent variations in systolic height 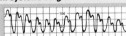	Patient on ventilator with positive end-expiratory pressure	● Check the patient's systolic blood pressure regularly. The difference between the highest and lowest pressure reading should be less than 10 mm Hg. If the difference exceeds that amount, suspect pulsus paradoxus, possibly from cardiac tamponade.
Slow upstroke 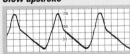	Aortic stenosis	● Check the patient's heart sounds for signs of aortic stenosis. Also, notify the physician, who will document suspected aortic stenosis in his notes.
Diminished amplitude on inspiration 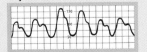	Pulsus paradoxus, possibly from cardiac tamponade, constrictive pericarditis, or lung disease	● Note systolic pressure during inspiration and expiration. If inspiratory pressure is at least 10 mm Hg less than expiratory pressure, notify the physician. ● If you are also monitoring pulmonary artery pressure, observe for a diastolic plateau, which occurs when the mean central venous pressure (right atrial pressure), mean pulmonary artery pressure, and mean pulmonary artery wedge pressure are within 5 mm Hg of one another.

Comparing normal and abnormal conduction

Normal cardiac conduction

The conduction system of the heart, shown below, begins at the heart's pacemaker, the sinoatrial (SA) node. When an impulse leaves the SA node, it travels through the atria along Bachmann's bundle and the internodal pathways to the atrioventricular (AV) node and then down the bundle of His, along the bundle branches and, finally, down the Purkinje fibers to the ventricles.

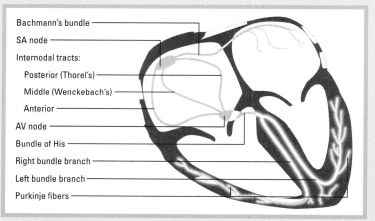

Bachmann's bundle
SA node
Internodal tracts:
Posterior (Thorel's)
Middle (Wenckebach's)
Anterior
AV node
Bundle of His
Right bundle branch
Left bundle branch
Purkinje fibers

Abnormal cardiac conduction

Altered automaticity, reentry, or conduction disturbances may cause cardiac arrhythmias.

Altered automaticity

Altered automaticity is the result of partial depolarization, which may increase the intrinsic rate of the SA node or latent pacemakers, or may induce ectopic pacemakers to reach threshold and depolarize.

Automaticity may be altered by drugs such as epinephrine, atropine, and digoxin, and by conditions such as acidosis, alkalosis, hypoxia, myocardial infarction (MI), hypokalemia, and hypocalcemia. Examples of arrhythmias caused by altered automaticity include atrial fibrillation and flutter, supraventricular tachycardia, ventricular tachycardia and fibrillation, accelerated idioventricular and junctional rhythms, and premature

Cardiac arrhythmias

Cardiac arrhythmias are variations in the normal pattern of electrical stimulation of the heart. Arrhythmias vary in severity, from those that are mild,

asymptomatic, and require no treatment (such as sinus arrhythmia, in which heart rate increases and decreases with respiration) to catastrophic ventricular fibrillation, which requires immediate resuscitation. Arrhythmias are generally classified according to their origin (ventricular or supraven-

atrial, junctional, and ventricular complexes.

Reentry
Reentry occurs when ischemia or deformation causes an abnormal circuit to develop within conductive fibers. Although current flow is blocked in one direction within the circuit, the descending impulse can travel in the other direction. By the time the impulse completes the circuit, the previously depolarized tissue within the circuit is no longer refractory to stimulation.

Conditions that increase the likelihood of reentry include hyperkalemia, myocardial ischemia, and the use of certain antiarrhythmic drugs. Reentry may be responsible for arrhythmias such as paroxysmal supraventricular tachycardia, ventricular tachycardia, and premature atrial, junctional, and ventricular complexes.

An alternative reentry mechanism depends on the presence of a congenital accessory pathway linking the atria and the ventricles outside the AV junction; for example, Wolff-Parkinson-White syndrome.

Conduction disturbances
Conduction disturbances occur when impulses are conducted too quickly or too slowly. Possible causes include trauma, drug toxicity, myocardial ischemia, MI, and electrolyte abnormalities. The AV blocks occur as a result of conduction disturbances.

tricular). Their effect on cardiac output and blood pressure, partially affected by the site of origin, determines their clinical significance. Lethal arrhythmias such as ventricular tachycardia and ventricular fibrillation are a major cause of sudden cardiac death.

Pathophysiology
Arrhythmias may result from enhanced automaticity, reentry, escape beats, or abnormal electrical conduction. (See *Comparing normal and abnormal conduction.*)

Common causes of arrhythmias include:
- congenital defects
- myocardial ischemia or infarction
- organic heart disease
- drug toxicity
- degeneration of the conductive tissue
- connective tissue disorders
- electrolyte imbalances
- cellular hypoxia
- hypertrophy of the heart muscle
- acid-base imbalances
- emotional stress.

However, each arrhythmia may have its own specific causes. (See discussion of specific arrhythmias later in this section.)

Comprehensive assessment
Identifying the specific arrhythmia the patient has is crucial to ensure proper treatment. However, remember to treat the entire patient, not just the disturbance. For any arrhythmia that could result in hemodynamic compromise, the primary action is to assess the patient. When the patient is stabilized, a complete analysis of the cardiac rhythm can be done.

When a patient presents with a history of symptoms suggestive of arrhythmias, or has been treated for an arrhythmia, be alert for the following:
- reports of precipitating factors, such as exercise, smoking, emotional stress, exposure to heat or cold, caffeine intake, position changes (from sitting to standing, for example), recent illness-

es, or sleep (Do the symptoms occur at night, awakening the patient?)

■ attempts to alleviate the symptoms, such as coughing, rest, medications, or deep breathing

■ reports of sensing the heart's rhythm, such as palpitations, irregular beating, skipped beats, or rapid or slow heart rate.

Physical examination findings will vary depending on the arrhythmia and the degree of hemodynamic compromise. Circulatory failure along with an absence of pulse and respirations is found with asystole, ventricular fibrillation and, occasionally, with ventricular tachycardia. Additional findings may include:

■ pallor

■ cold and clammy extremities

■ reduced urine output

■ dyspnea

■ hypotension

■ weakness

■ chest pains

■ dizziness

■ syncope (with severely impaired cerebral circulation).

Diagnosis

A definitive diagnosis and identification of the arrhythmia is based on careful examination of the electrocardiogram (ECG). The 12-lead ECG is considered the standard for identifying arrhythmias. In addition, a 15-lead ECG (in which additional leads are applied to the right side of the chest) or an 18-lead ECG (in which additional leads are also added to the posterior scapular area) may be done to provide more definitive information about the patient's right ventricle and the posterior wall of the left ventricle. The ECG recording demonstrates specific wave-

forms changes associated with the arrhythmia. (Specific ECG findings are described in more detail later in this section.)

Other test findings may include:

■ laboratory testing that reveals electrolyte abnormalities, hypoxemia or acid-base abnormalities (via arterial blood gas study results), or drug toxicities as the cause of arrhythmias

■ continuous ambulatory ECG (Holter) monitoring that reveals arrhythmias and effectiveness of drug therapy during a patient's daily activities

■ exercise testing that reveals exercise-induced arrhythmias

■ electrophysiologic testing that identifies the mechanism of an arrhythmia and the location of accessory pathways. (It also assesses the effectiveness of antiarrhythmic drugs.)

Collaborations

A multidisciplinary approach to treatment is necessary for the patient experiencing an arrhythmia. Prompt detection and early intervention are essential. The focus is on maintaining cardiac output (CO), promoting cardiac perfusion, and controlling the arrhythmia. Important aspects of care include medication therapy, cardioversion, defibrillation, pacemaker insertion, and ablation therapy.

Treatment and care

The goals in treating arrhythmias are to return pacer function to the sinus node, increase or decrease ventricular rate to normal, regain atrioventricular synchrony, and maintain normal sinus rhythm. Such treatment corrects abnormal rhythms through therapy with antiarrhythmic drugs, electrical conversion with defibrillation and cardioversion, physical maneuvers such as carotid massage and Valsalva's maneuver, temporary or permanent placement of a pacemaker to maintain heart rate, implantable cardioverter defibrillation (if indicated), and surgical removal or cryotherapy of an irritable ectopic focus to prevent recurring arrhythmias.

Arrhythmias may respond to treatment of the underlying disorder such as correction of hypoxia. However, arrhythmias associated with heart disease may require continuing and complex treatment. Regardless of the type of arrhythmia, treatment must be individualized to the patient's clinical presentation. (See discussion later in this section.)

Complications
Possible complications of arrhythmias include:
- sudden cardiac death
- myocardial infarction (MI)
- heart failure
- thromboembolism.

Nursing considerations
Be sure to include the following for any patient experiencing an arrhythmia:
- Evaluate the monitored patient's ECG regularly for arrhythmia and assess hemodynamic parameters as indicated. Document any arrhythmias and notify the physician immediately.
- Assess an unmonitored patient for rhythm disturbances. If the patient's pulse rate is abnormally rapid, slow, or irregular, watch for signs of hypoperfusion, such as hypotension and diminished urine output.
- Notify the physician if a change in pulse pattern or rate occurs in an un-monitored patient or if a monitored patient exhibits an arrhythmia.
- As ordered, obtain an ECG tracing in an unmonitored patient to confirm and identify the type of arrhythmia present.
- When life-threatening arrhythmias develop, rapidly assess the patient's level of consciousness, pulse and respiratory rates, and hemodynamic parameters. Be alert for trends. Monitor his ECG continuously. Be prepared to initiate cardiopulmonary resuscitation if indicated.
- Assess the patient for predisposing factors, such as fluid and electrolyte imbalance, and signs of drug toxicity, especially with digoxin.
- If an arrhythmia occurs, carefully monitor the patient's cardiac, electrolyte, and overall clinical status to determine the effect on CO.
- Administer medications as ordered, monitor for adverse effects, and perform nursing interventions related to monitoring vital signs, hemodynamic monitoring (as appropriate), and appropriate laboratory work. Prepare to assist with or perform medical procedures, if indicated (for example, cardioversion).
- If you suspect drug toxicity, report it to the physician immediately and withhold the next dose.
- To prevent arrhythmias postoperatively, provide adequate oxygen and reduce heart workload while carefully maintaining metabolic, neurologic, respiratory, and hemodynamic status.
- If the patient needs a temporary pacemaker, make sure that a fresh battery is installed to avoid temporary pacemaker malfunction, and carefully secure the external catheter wires and

the pacemaker box. (See "Pacemakers," page 122.)

■ After pacemaker insertion, monitor the patient's pulse rate regularly and watch for signs of pacemaker failure and decreased CO. Watch closely for premature contractions, a sign of myocardial irritation, and check threshold daily.

Patient teaching

■ Explain to the patient the importance of taking ordered medications at the proper time intervals.

■ Teach the patient how to take his pulse and recognize an irregular rhythm, and instruct him to report alterations from his baseline to the physician.

■ Emphasize the importance of keeping laboratory and physician's appointments.

■ Teach the adverse effects of medication and signs to report. Warn the patient not to take over-the-counter medications unless he has talked with his physician first.

■ If the patient has a permanent pacemaker, warn him about environmental and electrical hazards as indicated by the pacemaker manufacturer. Although hazards may not present a problem, in doubtful situations a 24-hour ambulatory ECG (Holter monitoring) may be helpful. Tell the patient to report light-headedness or syncope. Stress the importance of scheduling and keeping appointments for regular checkups.

Sinus tachycardia

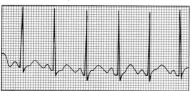

ECG characteristics

■ Regular atrial and ventricular rhythms, rates usually greater than 100 beats/minute but rarely greater than 160 beats/minute

■ Normal P wave before each QRS complex

■ QRS complex of normal duration

■ PR interval normal

Causes

With this arrhythmia, the impulse originates in the sinus node, but more quickly than normal. Causes may include:

■ normal physiologic response to fever, exercise, anxiety, pain, dehydration

■ possibly accompanying shock, left-sided heart failure, cardiac tamponade, hyperthyroidism, anemia, hypovolemia, pulmonary embolism, or anterior wall MI

■ also possible with atropine, epinephrine, isoproterenol, quinidine, caffeine, alcohol, or nicotine use.

Treatment

Treatment of sinus tachycardia focuses on correcting the underlying cause.

Sinus bradycardia

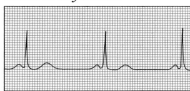

ECG characteristics
■ Regular atrial and ventricular rhythms, rates usually below 60 beats/minute
■ P wave occurring before each QRS complex
■ QRS complex of normal duration
■ PR interval normal

Causes
With this arrhythmia, the impulse originates in the sinus node, but more slowly than normal. Possible causes include:
■ normal occurrence in athletes who are well conditioned.
■ increased intracranial pressure, increased vagal tone due to bowel straining, vomiting, intubation, or mechanical ventilation, sick sinus syndrome, hypothyroidism, or inferior wall MI
■ possible secondary to use of anticholinesterase agents, beta-adrenergic blockers, digoxin, or morphine.

Treatment
No treatment is necessary unless the patient's blood pressure drops or he experiences changes in his level of consciousness (LOC). If the patient demonstrates a low CO or complains of dizziness, weakness, or altered LOC, expect any or all of the following:
■ administration of atropine, 0.5 to 1 mg

■ temporary or permanent pacemaker insertion
■ dopamine 5 to 20 µg/kg/minute
■ epinephrine 2 to 10 µg/minute.

Sinus arrhythmia

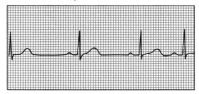

ECG characteristics
■ Irregular atrial and ventricular rhythms, with atrial and ventricular rates ranging from 60 to 100 beats/ minute
■ QRS shape and duration usually normal but possibly regularly abnormal
■ Normal P wave occurring before each QRS complex
■ Normal PR interval

Causes
With this arrhythmia, the rate increases with inspirations to accommodate for the increased venous return to the right side of the heart; the rate then decreases with expiration as the return decreases. Possible causes may include:
■ possible normal finding in children, athletes, and older adults
■ heart and valvular disease (rare).

Treatment
Usually no treatment is required unless the patient's rate drops below 40 beats/minute, and then atropine is given.

Sinus arrest or block

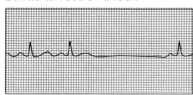

ECG characteristics
- Atrial and ventricular rhythms normal except for missing complex
- Normal P wave occurring before each QRS complex
- Pause not equal to a multiple of the previous sinus rhythm

Causes
With this arrhythmia, a temporary failure occurs in the sinus node's ability to initiate a stimulus. This can result in a dropping of one or more PQRS waves. Causes may include:
- acute infection
- coronary artery disease (CAD) or acute inferior wall MI
- vagal stimulation, Valsalva's maneuver, or carotid sinus massage
- digoxin, quinidine, or salicylate toxicity
- pesticide poisoning
- pharyngeal irritation due to endotracheal intubation
- sick sinus syndrome.

Treatment
If the patient is symptomatic, administer I.V. atropine. In addition, a temporary or permanent pacemaker may be inserted when the patient experiences repeated episodes.

Wandering atrial pacemaker

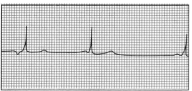

ECG characteristics
- Slight variation in atrial and ventricular rates
- PR interval irregular
- P waves irregular with changing configuration indicating that all aren't from sinoatrial node or single atrial focus; possibly appearing after the QRS complex
- Uniform shape of QRS complexes; irregular rhythm

Causes
This arrhythmia results from a slowing of the sinus node activity due to vagal stimulation, which allows other atrial sites to reach threshold and initiate a beat. Causes may include:
- drug toxicity, especially digoxin toxicity
- sick sinus syndrome
- chronic obstructive pulmonary disease (COPD)
- inflammatory disorders such as rheumatic carditis.

Treatment
If the patient is asymptomatic, no treatment is necessary. If the patient is symptomatic, treatment involves correcting the underlying cause. Digoxin levels are indicated if the patient is receiving digoxin.

Premature atrial contraction

Premature atrial contraction is also known as premature atrial complex.

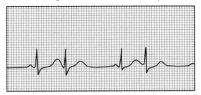

ECG characteristics
- Irregular rhythm
- Premature abnormal looking P waves differing in configuration from normal P waves (for example, early beat P wave)
- QRS complexes occurring after P waves
- P wave possibly buried or identified in preceding T wave

Causes
With this arrhythmia, an ectopic site within the atrium initiates a beat before the next sinus beat. Possible causes may include:
- coronary or valvular heart disease, atrial ischemia, heart failure, acute respiratory failure, COPD, electrolyte imbalance, or hypoxia
- digoxin toxicity
- use of aminophylline, adrenergics, or caffeine
- anxiety.

Treatment
Usually no treatment is needed unless the patient is symptomatic. In this case, treatment focuses on correcting the underlying cause, such as limiting caffeine intake. In addition, beta-adrenergic blockers, verapamil, or diltiazem may be given if the patient is symptomatic because this arrhythmia may progress to atrial fibrillation or atrial tachycardia.

Paroxysmal atrial tachycardia

Paroxysmal atrial tachycardia is also known as paroxysmal supraventricular tachycardia.

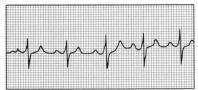

ECG characteristics
- Regular atrial and ventricular rhythms
- Heart rate greater than 160 beats/ minute, rarely exceeding 250 beats/ minute
- Regular P waves, but aberrant and difficult to differentiate from preceding T wave; occurring before QRS complexes

Causes
Causes may include:
- intrinsic abnormality of atrioventricular (AV) conduction with sudden onset and termination
- physical or psychological stress, hypoxia, hypokalemia, cardiomyopathy, congenital heart disease, MI, valvular disease, Wolff-Parkinson-White syndrome, cor pulmonale, hyperthyroidism, or systemic hypertension
- digoxin toxicity
- use of caffeine, marijuana, or central nervous system stimulants.

Treatment
Treatment includes:
- vagal maneuvers, Valsalva's maneuver, and carotid sinus massage
- if patient's cardiac function is preserved, calcium channel blocker, beta-adrenergic blocker, digoxin, and car-

Narrow-complex tachycardia algorithm

Narrow-complex tachycardia includes junctional tachycardia, paroxysmal supraventricular tachycardia (PSVT), and multifocal atrial tachycardia. Treatment of each type of rhythm depends on how well the patient is tolerating the rhythm.

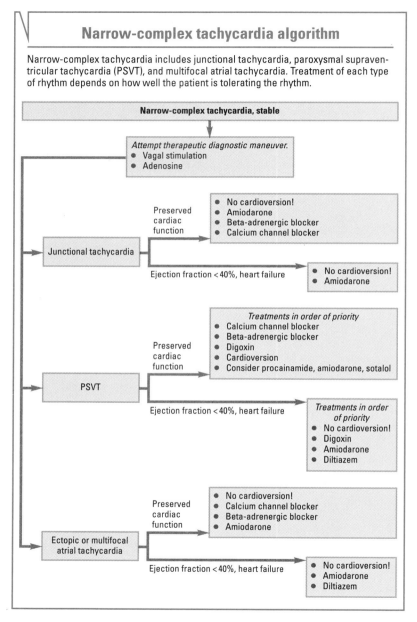

dioversion; possibly followed by procainamide, amiodarone, or sotalol if first treatment is ineffective in converting rhythm (see *Narrow-complex tachycardia algorithm*)

- digoxin, amiodarone, and then dilti-azem if patient is in heart failure or has an ejection fraction of less than 40%.

Atrial flutter

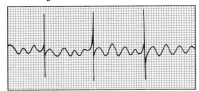

ECG characteristics
- Atrial rhythm regular but possibly irregular ranging from 240 to 400 beats/minute
- Variable ventricular rate depending on AV conduction, usually 60 to 100 beats/minute
- Saw-toothed P-wave configuration (F waves)
- QRS uniform in shape but commonly irregular in rate

Causes
This arrhythmia is due to a reentry focus within the atria. Possible causes include:
- heart failure
- pulmonary embolism
- mitral or tricuspid valve disease
- digoxin toxicity.

Treatment
If the patient has experienced atrial flutter for more than 48 hours but his heart function is normal, calcium channel blockers or beta-adrenergic blockers are given to control the rate. If the patient has experienced atrial flutter for less than 48 hours and his heart function is normal, amiodarone, ibutilide, flecainide, propafenone, or procainamide may be used to convert the rhythm. If the patient has experienced atrial flutter for longer than 48

hours and his heart function is impaired, digoxin, diltiazem, or amiodarone may be given. If the patient's heart rate is greater than 240 beats/minute, anticoagulant therapy may be initiated to prevent the formation of thrombi in the atrium.

Atrial fibrillation

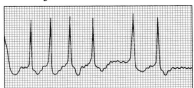

ECG characteristics
- Atrial rhythm grossly irregular with atrial rate greater than 400 beats/minute
- Ventricular rhythm grossly irregular
- P waves absent or appearing as erratic, irregular, baseline fibrillatory P waves
- PR interval indiscernible and not measurable
- Uniform configuration and duration of QRS complexes

Causes
With this arrhythmia, multiple foci in the atria simultaneously initiate impulses with only a small area of tissue responding to each impulse. Instead of contracting in a coordinated fashion, the atria quiver.

Possible causes include:
- heart failure, COPD, thyrotoxicosis, constrictive pericarditis, ischemic heart disease, sepsis, pulmonary embolism, hypertension, mitral stenosis, or atrial irritation
- possible complication of coronary bypass or valve replacement surgery
- use of nifedipine or digoxin.

Treatment

Treatment focuses on the underlying cause. For the patient whose heart is functioning normally but is experiencing a new onset of atrial fibrillation that has lasted longer than 48 hours, calcium channel blockers or beta-adrenergic blockers are used to control the rate. If the onset of atrial fibrillation is less than 48 hours and heart function is normal, amiodarone, ibutilide, flecainide, propafenone, or procainamide may be used to control the rate. For the patient with impaired heart function and atrial fibrillation over 48 hours, digoxin, diltiazem, or amiodarone may be used. Elective cardioversion may be necessary to control rapid ventricular rates. In addition, anticoagulant therapy may be needed to prevent atrial thrombi.

Atrial fibrillation is one of four types of arrhythmia addressed by the tachycardia algorithm. Use this algorithm to guide your actions. (See *Tachycardia algorithm,* pages 38 and 39.)

Junctional rhythm

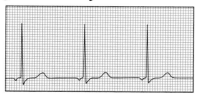

ECG characteristics
■ Regular atrial and ventricular rhythms, rates ranging from 40 to 60 beats/minute
■ P waves appearing before, hidden in, or after QRS complex; possibly inverted if visible
■ PR interval less than 0.12 second
■ Normal QRS complex

Causes

With this arrhythmia, the sinus node is suppressed which allows the AV junction to initiate beats at its intrinsic rate. Possible causes may include:
■ inferior wall MI
■ ischemia, hypoxia, or vagal stimulation
■ valvular surgery
■ digoxin toxicity.

Treatment

If the patient is symptomatic, atropine is given to increase the rate and a pacemaker may be inserted if the patient doesn't respond to atropine therapy. If digoxin toxicity is the cause, the drug is discontinued.

Premature junctional contractions and complexes

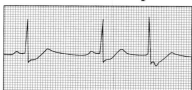

ECG characteristics
■ Irregular atrial and ventricular rhythms
■ P waves occurring before, hidden in, or after QRS complex; possibly inverted if visible
■ Shortened PR interval (less than normal) if P wave occurring before QRS complex
■ Normal QRS shape and duration

Causes

With this arrhythmia, an ectopic beat within the AV junction initiates a beat before the sinus beat. Conduction to the atria is in a retrograde fashion. Possible causes may include:

- MI
- digoxin toxicity and excessive caffeine or amphetamine use.

Treatment
Treatment focuses on correcting the underlying cause; for example, discontinuation of digoxin or limitation of caffeine intake. If necessary, antiarrhythmics may be given.

Junctional tachycardia

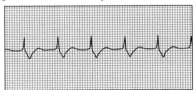

ECG characteristics
- Atrial and ventricular rate greater than 100 beats/minute
- P wave absent or hidden in QRS complex or occurring before T wave
- Inverted P wave
- Normal QRS complex
- Onset typically sudden or occurring in bursts

Causes
With this arrhythmia, an increase in the rate in spontaneous depolarization in the AV junction or reentrant tachycardia involving the AV node occurs. It may be due to catecholamines or ischemia at the AV junction.

Possible causes may include:
- myocarditis
- cardiomyopathy
- inferior wall MI or ischemia
- valve replacement surgery
- digoxin toxicity.

Treatment
Treatment depends on how well the patient is tolerating the rhythm. Because junctional tachycardia is one type of narrow-complex tachycardia, consult the algorithm for narrow-complex tachycardia for treatment options. (See *Narrow-complex tachycardia algorithm,* page 34.)

First-degree AV block

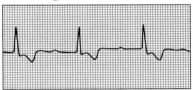

ECG characteristics
- Regular atrial and ventricular rhythms
- Prolonged PR interval greater than 0.20 second
- P wave preceding each QRS complex
- Normal QRS complex

Causes
Causes (possible in healthy adults) may include:
- inferior wall MI, ischemia, or infarction
- hypothyroidism, hypokalemia, or hyperkalemia
- digoxin toxicity or use of quinidine, procainamide, or propranolol.

Treatment
Treatment focuses on correcting the underlying cause. If the patient is experiencing symptomatic bradycardia, atropine may be·used.

(Text continues on page 40.)

Tachycardia algorithm

The algorithm for tachycardia is quite complex. Remember to base your actions on the type of tachycardia that the patient is experiencing and how the patient is tolerating the rhythm.

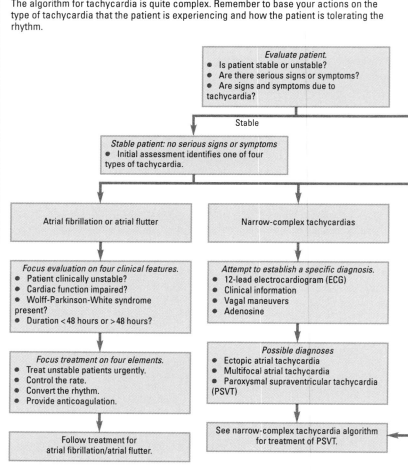

Evaluate patient.
- Is patient stable or unstable?
- Are there serious signs or symptoms?
- Are signs and symptoms due to tachycardia?

Stable

Stable patient: no serious signs or symptoms
- Initial assessment identifies one of four types of tachycardia.

Atrial fibrillation or atrial flutter

Narrow-complex tachycardias

Focus evaluation on four clinical features.
- Patient clinically unstable?
- Cardiac function impaired?
- Wolff-Parkinson-White syndrome present?
- Duration < 48 hours or > 48 hours?

Attempt to establish a specific diagnosis.
- 12-lead electrocardiogram (ECG)
- Clinical information
- Vagal maneuvers
- Adenosine

Focus treatment on four elements.
- Treat unstable patients urgently.
- Control the rate.
- Convert the rhythm.
- Provide anticoagulation.

Possible diagnoses
- Ectopic atrial tachycardia
- Multifocal atrial tachycardia
- Paroxysmal supraventricular tachycardia (PSVT)

Follow treatment for atrial fibrillation/atrial flutter.

See narrow-complex tachycardia algorithm for treatment of PSVT.

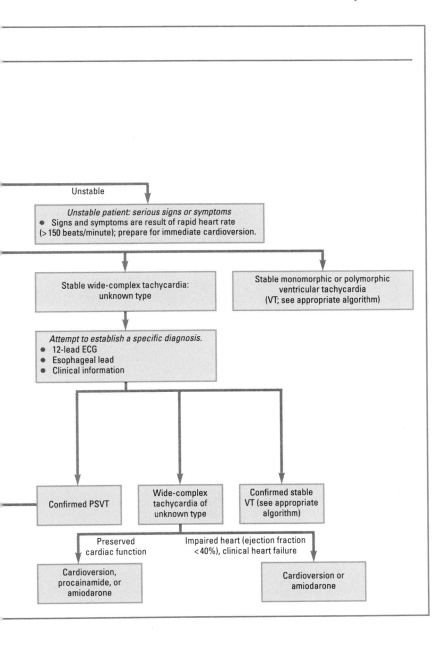

Unstable

Unstable patient: serious signs or symptoms
- Signs and symptoms are result of rapid heart rate
(> 150 beats/minute); prepare for immediate cardioversion.

Stable wide-complex tachycardia:
unknown type

Stable monomorphic or polymorphic
ventricular tachycardia
(VT; see appropriate algorithm)

Attempt to establish a specific diagnosis.
- 12-lead ECG
- Esophageal lead
- Clinical information

Confirmed PSVT

Wide-complex
tachycardia of
unknown type

Confirmed stable
VT (see appropriate
algorithm)

Preserved
cardiac function

Impaired heart (ejection fraction
<40%), clinical heart failure

Cardioversion,
procainamide, or
amiodarone

Cardioversion or
amiodarone

Second-degree AV block Type I

A second-degree AV block Type I is also known as a Mobitz I or Wenckebach block.

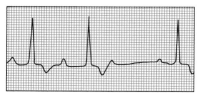

ECG characteristics

- Regular atrial rhythm
- Irregular ventricular rhythm
- Atrial rate greater than ventricular rate
- PR interval progressively and slightly longer with each cycle until QRS eventually disappears (dropped beat), with PR interval then becoming shorter

Causes

Causes may include:
- inferior wall MI, cardiac surgery, or vagal stimulation
- digoxin toxicity or use of propranolol, quinidine, or procainamide.

Treatment

Treatment focuses on the correcting the underlying cause. However, if the patient is bradycardic and experiencing symptoms, atropine may be given or a temporary pacemaker may be inserted.

Second-degree AV block Type II

A second-degree AV block Type II is also called a Mobitz II block.

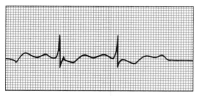

ECG characteristics

- Regular atrial rhythm
- Ventricular rhythm regular or irregular depending on extent of block
- P-P interval constant
- Periodically absent QRS complexes

Causes

Causes may include:
- severe CAD, anterior MI, or acute myocarditis
- digoxin toxicity.

Treatment

If the patient is experiencing symptomatic bradycardia, follow the bradycardia algorithm. (See *Bradycardia algorithm.*) If digoxin toxicity is the cause, discontinue the drug.

Third-degree AV block

A third-degree AV block is a complete heart block.

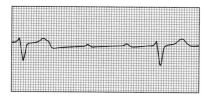

ECG characteristics

- Regular atrial rhythm
- Regular rhythm but slow ventricular rate

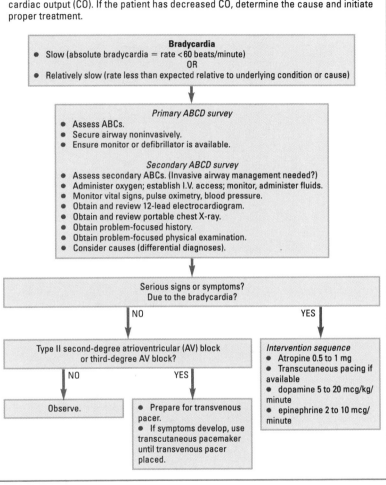

Bradycardia algorithm

A patient with bradycardia may show few symptoms or show symptoms of decreased cardiac output (CO). If the patient has decreased CO, determine the cause and initiate proper treatment.

Bradycardia
- Slow (absolute bradycardia = rate < 60 beats/minute)
  OR
- Relatively slow (rate less than expected relative to underlying condition or cause)

Primary ABCD survey
- Assess ABCs.
- Secure airway noninvasively.
- Ensure monitor or defibrillator is available.

Secondary ABCD survey
- Assess secondary ABCs. (Invasive airway management needed?)
- Administer oxygen; establish I.V. access; monitor, administer fluids.
- Monitor vital signs, pulse oximetry, blood pressure.
- Obtain and review 12-lead electrocardiogram.
- Obtain and review portable chest X-ray.
- Obtain problem-focused history.
- Obtain problem-focused physical examination.
- Consider causes (differential diagnoses).

Serious signs or symptoms?
Due to the bradycardia?

NO

Type II second-degree atrioventricular (AV) block
or third-degree AV block?

NO → Observe.

YES →
- Prepare for transvenous pacer.
- If symptoms develop, use transcutaneous pacemaker until transvenous pacer placed.

YES

Intervention sequence
- Atropine 0.5 to 1 mg
- Transcutaneous pacing if available
- dopamine 5 to 20 mcg/kg/minute
- epinephrine 2 to 10 mcg/minute

- Absence of relationship between P waves and QRS complexes
- Inconsistency of PR interval
- QRS interval normal (nodal pacemaker) or wide and bizarre (with ventricular pacemaker)

Causes

Causes may include:
- inferior or anterior wall MI, rheumatic fever, hypoxia, or postoperative complication of mitral valve surgery
- digoxin toxicity.

Treatment

If the patient is experiencing symptomatic bradycardia, atropine may be used. Pacemaker insertion may be necessary.

Premature ventricular contraction

Premature ventricular contraction (PVC) is also known as premature ventricular complex.

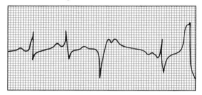

ECG characteristics

- Regular atrial rhythm
- Irregular ventricular rhythm
- Early occurring QRS complex, usually followed by a complete compensatory pause; appearing wide and distorted, usually greater than 0.14 second
- Premature QRS complexes occurring singly, in pairs, or in threes, alternating with normal beats (with a focus from one or more sites)

Causes

With this arrhythmia, an ectopic focus in the ventricles fires before the next sinus beat. Possible causes may include:

- heart failure
- old or acute myocardial ischemia, MI, or contusion
- myocardial irritation such as from a pacemaker
- hypercapnia, hypokalemia, or hypocalcemia

- drug toxicity (digoxin, tricyclic antidepressants, or beta-adrenergic blockers such as isoproterenol or dopamine)
- caffeine, tobacco, or alcohol use
- exercise, pain, psychological stress, or anxiety.

Treatment

Some controversy exists about treating a patient with PVC. If the cause is identifiable, treatment focuses on correcting it; for example, discontinuing the drug, limiting intake of caffeine or alcohol, and reducing stress. Potassium chloride may be given to correct hypokalemia. If the patient is symptomatic, administer I.V. procainamide, amiodarone, or lidocaine.

Idioventricular rhythm

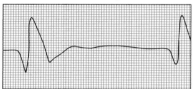

ECG characteristics

- Regular rhythm
- Absence of P waves
- Ventricular rate of 10 to 40 beats/ minute
- Wide QRS complex, greater than 0.10 second

Causes

This arrhythmia results from a failure of the higher pacemakers (the sinus node and AV junction). It's an escape rhythm originating in the Purkinje fibers.

PEA algorithm

After confirming pulseless electrical activity (PEA), determine its cause and treat it quickly. Supportive measures include epinephrine and atropine.

Pulseless electrical activity
(PEA = rhythm on monitor, without detectable pulse)

↓

Primary ABCD survey

Focus: Basic cardiopulmonary resuscitation and defibrillation
- Check responsiveness.
- Activate emergency response system.
- Call for defibrillator.
- **A** Airway: Open the airway.

- **B** Breathing: Provide positive-pressure ventilations.
- **C** Circulation: Give chest compressions.
- **D** Defibrillation: Assess for and shock ventricular fibrillation or pulseless ventricular tachycardia.

↓

Secondary ABCD survey

- **A** Airway: Place airway device as soon as possible.
- **B** Breathing: Confirm airway device placement by examination plus confirmation device.
- **B** Breathing: Secure airway device; purpose-made tube holders are preferred.
- **B** Breathing: Confirm effective oxygenation and ventilation.

- **C** Circulation: Establish I.V. access.
- **C** Circulation: Identify rhythm and monitor.
- **C** Circulation: Administer drugs appropriate for rhythm and condition.
- **C** Circulation: Assess for occult blood flow.
- **D** Differential diagnosis: Search for and treat identified reversible causes.

↓

Review for most frequent causes

- Hypovolemia
- Hypoxia
- Hydrogen ion (acidosis)
- Hyperkalemia or hypokalemia
- Hypothermia
- "Tablets" (drug overdose, accidents)

- Tamponade, cardiac
- Tension pneumothorax
- Thrombosis, coronary (acute coronary syndrome)
- Thrombosis, pulmonary (embolism)

↓

Epinephrine 1 mg I.V. push; repeat every 3 to 5 minutes

↓

Atropine 1 mg I.V. (if PEA rate is slow);
repeat every 3 to 5 minutes as needed, to a total dose of 0.04 mg/kg

---

Possible causes may include:
- MI
- severe hypoxia
- severe acidosis.

Treatment

If the patient is pulseless and displaying an idioventricular rhythm, institute the pulseless electrical activity (PEA) algorithm. (See *PEA algorithm*.)

Accelerated idioventricular rhythm

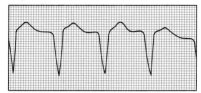

ECG characteristics
■ Regular ventricular rhythm with a ventricular rate between 40 and 100 beats/minute
■ Absence of P waves
■ Absence of PR interval
■ Wide QRS complex, greater than 0.10 second

Causes
With this arrhythmia, the higher pacemakers are suppressed or the rate of spontaneous discharge of the Purkinje fibers is increased.

Possible causes may include:
■ vagal or drug suppression of higher pacemakers
■ ischemia, MI, or myocardial reperfusion.

Treatment
Treatment is instituted only if the patient is symptomatic from the rate or loss of AV synchrony, in which case atropine may be used to restore the function of the higher pacemakers.

Ventricular tachycardia

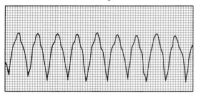

ECG characteristics
■ Irregular or regular ventricular rhythm, rate ranging from 140 to 220 beats/minute
■ Wide, bizarre QRS complexes independent of P waves
■ P waves indiscernible
■ Possible sudden onset and sudden termination

Causes
With ventricular tachycardia (VT), a reentry mechanism is occurring in the ventricles. The arrhythmia may suddenly start and stop just as suddenly. Possible causes include:
■ myocardial ischemia, MI, or aneurysm
■ CAD
■ mitral valve prolapse, heart failure, or cardiomyopathy
■ hypercalcemia or hypokalemia
■ pulmonary embolism
■ drug toxicity, such as from digoxin, procainamide, epinephrine, or quinidine.

Treatment
Treatment varies depending on whether the rhythm is monomorphic or polymorphic and if the patient is stable or not. If the arrhythmia is considered stable, follow the stable monomorphic or polymorphic VT algorithm. (See *Stable monomorphic or polymorphic VT algorithm.*) If the patient becomes pulseless, institute the PEA algorithm.

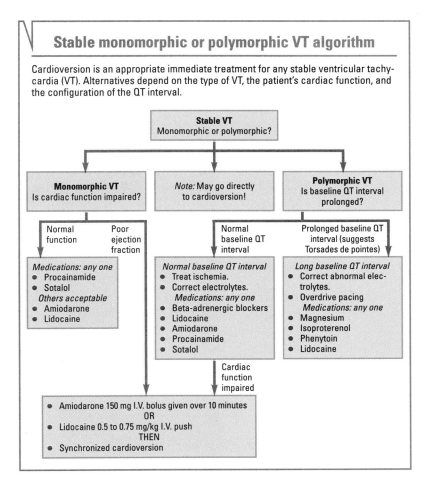

Stable monomorphic or polymorphic VT algorithm

Cardioversion is an appropriate immediate treatment for any stable ventricular tachycardia (VT). Alternatives depend on the type of VT, the patient's cardiac function, and the configuration of the QT interval.

Stable VT
Monomorphic or polymorphic?

Monomorphic VT
Is cardiac function impaired?

Note: May go directly to cardioversion!

Polymorphic VT
Is baseline QT interval prolonged?

Normal function | Poor ejection fraction

Normal baseline QT interval

Prolonged baseline QT interval (suggests Torsades de pointes)

Medications: any one
- Procainamide
- Sotalol
Others acceptable
- Amiodarone
- Lidocaine

Normal baseline QT interval
- Treat ischemia.
- Correct electrolytes.
  Medications: any one
- Beta-adrenergic blockers
- Lidocaine
- Amiodarone
- Procainamide
- Sotalol

Long baseline QT interval
- Correct abnormal electrolytes.
- Overdrive pacing
  Medications: any one
- Magnesium
- Isoproterenol
- Phenytoin
- Lidocaine

Cardiac function impaired

- Amiodarone 150 mg I.V. bolus given over 10 minutes
  OR
- Lidocaine 0.5 to 0.75 mg/kg I.V. push
  THEN
- Synchronized cardioversion

Ventricular fibrillation

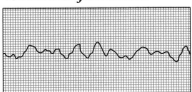

ECG characteristics
- Rapid and chaotic ventricular rhythm
- Wide, irregular QRS complexes
- Absence of visible P waves

Causes
With ventricular fibrillation (VF), multiple foci in the ventricles are initiating beats but the contraction isn't coordinated, so CO is zero. Possible causes include:
- myocardial ischemia or MI
- untreated VT, R-on-T phenomenon
- hypokalemia, alkalosis, hyperkalemia, or hypercalcemia
- electric shock or hypothermia.

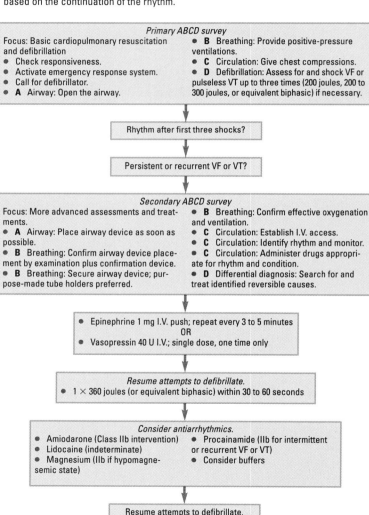

VF or VT algorithm

If a defibrillator is available and you confirm ventricular fibrillation (VF) or pulseless ventricular tachycardia (VT), perform three defibrillations. If this measure is unsuccessful and you complete the secondary survey, follow the appropriate guidelines based on the continuation of the rhythm.

Primary ABCD survey

Focus: Basic cardiopulmonary resuscitation and defibrillation
- Check responsiveness.
- Activate emergency response system.
- Call for defibrillator.
- **A** Airway: Open the airway.

- **B** Breathing: Provide positive-pressure ventilations.
- **C** Circulation: Give chest compressions.
- **D** Defibrillation: Assess for and shock VF or pulseless VT up to three times (200 joules, 200 to 300 joules, or equivalent biphasic) if necessary.

↓

Rhythm after first three shocks?

↓

Persistent or recurrent VF or VT?

↓

Secondary ABCD survey

Focus: More advanced assessments and treatments.
- **A** Airway: Place airway device as soon as possible.
- **B** Breathing: Confirm airway device placement by examination plus confirmation device.
- **B** Breathing: Secure airway device; purpose-made tube holders preferred.

- **B** Breathing: Confirm effective oxygenation and ventilation.
- **C** Circulation: Establish I.V. access.
- **C** Circulation: Identify rhythm and monitor.
- **C** Circulation: Administer drugs appropriate for rhythm and condition.
- **D** Differential diagnosis: Search for and treat identified reversible causes.

↓

- Epinephrine 1 mg I.V. push; repeat every 3 to 5 minutes
  OR
- Vasopressin 40 U I.V.; single dose, one time only

↓

Resume attempts to defibrillate.
- 1 × 360 joules (or equivalent biphasic) within 30 to 60 seconds

↓

Consider antiarrhythmics.
- Amiodarone (Class IIb intervention)
- Lidocaine (indeterminate)
- Magnesium (IIb if hypomagnesemic state)
- Procainamide (IIb for intermittent or recurrent VF or VT)
- Consider buffers

↓

Resume attempts to defibrillate.

Treatment
Initiation of the algorithm for VF is indicated. (See *VF or VT algorithm*.)

Asystole

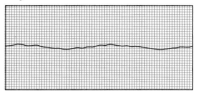

ECG characteristics
■ Absence of atrial or ventricular rate or rhythm
■ Absence of discernible P waves, QRS complexes, or T waves

Causes
This arrhythmia results from the failure of all pacemakers. Possible causes include:
■ myocardial ischemia, MI, or cardiac tamponade
■ aortic valve disease or heart failure
■ hypoxemia, hypokalemia, or severe acidosis
■ electric shock
■ ventricular arrhythmias
■ pulmonary embolism.

Treatment
Immediately begin the algorithm for asystole. (See *Asystole algorithm,* page 48.)

Cardiac catheterization

Cardiac catheterization is the passing of a catheter into the right, left, or both sides of the heart. The procedure permits measurement of blood pressure and blood flow in the heart's chambers to determine valve competence and cardiac wall contractility and to detect intracardiac shunts. The procedure also enables collection of blood samples and taking of diagnostic films of the ventricles (contrast ventriculography) and arteries (coronary arteriography or angiography).

Use of thermodilution catheters allows calculation of cardiac output. The purpose of the calculations is to evaluate valvular insufficiency or stenosis, septal defects, congenital anomalies, myocardial function and blood supply, and cardiac wall motion.

Cardiac catheterization should reveal no abnormalities of heart chamber size or configuration, wall motion or thickness, or direction of blood flow or valve motion; the coronary arteries should have a smooth and regular outline. Common abnormalities and defects that can be confirmed by cardiac catheterization include coronary artery disease, myocardial incompetence, valvular heart disease, and septal defects.

In left-sided heart catheterization, the catheter is inserted into the brachial or femoral artery through a puncture or cutdown procedure and, guided by fluoroscopy, is advanced retrograde through the aorta into the coronary artery ostium, the left ventricle, or both. Then a contrast medium is injected into the ventricle, permitting radiographic visualization of the ventricle and coronary arteries as well as filming (cineangiography) of heart activity.

Left-sided heart catheterization assesses the patency of the coronary arteries, mitral and aortic valve function, and left ventricular function. It aids diagnosis of left ventricular enlargement, aortic stenosis and insufficiency, aortic

Asystole algorithm

A diagnosis of asystole indicates a poor chance of survival for the patient. Still, after completing the primary and secondary survey, your goal is to reestablish a heart rhythm. Treatments include pacing and appropriate medications to stimulate impulse conduction.

Primary ABCD survey

Focus: Basic cardiopulmonary resuscitation and defibrillation
- Check responsiveness.
- Activate emergency response system.
- Call for defibrillator.
- **A** Airway: Open the airway.
- **B** Breathing: Provide positive-pressure ventilations.
- **C** Circulation: Give chest compressions.
- **D** Defibrillation: Assess for ventricular fibrillation (VF) or pulseless ventricular tachycardia (VT); shock if indicated.
- Rapid scene survey: Any evidence personnel shouldn't attempt resuscitation?

Secondary ABCD survey

Focus: More advanced assessments and treatments.
- **A** Airway: Place airway device as soon as possible.
- **B** Breathing: Confirm airway device placement by examination plus confirmation device.
- **B** Breathing: Secure airway device; purpose-made tube holders preferred.
- **B** Breathing: Confirm effective oxygenation and ventilation.
- **C** Circulation: Confirm true asystole.
- **C** Circulation: Establish I.V. access.
- **C** Circulation: Identify rhythm via monitor.
- **C** Circulation: Give medications appropriate for rhythm and condition.
- **D** Differential diagnosis: Search for and treat identified reversible causes.

Transcutaneous pacing.
If considered, perform immediately.

Epinephrine 1 mg I.V. push; repeat every 3 to 5 minutes

Atropine 1 mg I.V.; repeat every 3 to 5 minutes up to a total of 0.04 mg/kg

Asystole persists
Withhold or cease resuscitation efforts?
- Consider quality of resuscitation?
- Atypical clinical features present?
- Support for cease-efforts protocols in place?

root enlargement, mitral insufficiency, aneurysm, and intracardiac shunt.

In right-sided heart catheterization, the catheter is inserted into an antecubital vein or into the femoral vein and advanced through the inferior vena cava or right atrium into the right side of the heart and into the pulmonary artery. Right-sided heart catheterization assesses tricuspid and pulmonic valve function and pulmonary artery pressures.

Procedure

The patient is placed in the supine position on a padded table. Electrocardiogram (ECG) leads are applied for continuous monitoring, and an I.V. line is started (if not in place) with dextrose 5% in water or normal saline solution at a keep-vein-open rate. After the local anesthetic is injected at the catheterization site, a small incision or percutaneous puncture is made into the artery or vein, depending on whether left-side or right-side studies are to be performed, and the catheter is passed through the sheath into the vessel. The catheter is guided to the cardiac chambers or coronary arteries using fluoroscopy. When the catheter is in place, the contrast medium is injected through it to visualize the cardiac vessels and structures.

The patient may be asked to cough or breathe deeply. Coughing helps counteract nausea or light-headedness caused by the contrast medium and can correct arrhythmias produced by the medium's depressant effect on the myocardium; deep breathing can ease catheter placement into the pulmonary artery or the wedge position and moves the diaphragm downward, making the heart easier to visualize. During the procedure, the patient may be given nitroglycerin to eliminate catheter-induced spasm or to measure nitroglycerin's effect on the coronary arteries. Heart rate and rhythm, respiratory and pulse rates, and blood pressure are monitored frequently during the procedure.

Complications

Cardiac catheterization can cause many complications. Complications of left-sided catheterization include arterial embolus or thrombus in the limb and stroke. Complications of right-sided catheterization include thrombophlebitis, pulmonary embolism, and vagal response. Left-sided or right-sided catheterization complications include myocardial infarction (MI), arrhythmias, cardiac tamponade, systemic or local infection, hematoma, hypovolemia, pulmonary edema, and reaction to the contrast medium.

Nursing considerations

Instruct the patient about the procedure and events after it and institute measures to prevent postoperative complications.

Before the procedure

■ Explain to the patient that this test evaluates the function of the heart and its vessels. Instruct the patient to restrict food and fluids for at least 6 hours before the test. Discuss who will perform the test and where, and tell the patient it takes 1 to 2 hours. Inform him that he may receive a mild sedative but will remain conscious during the procedure.

■ Advise the patient that he'll lie on a padded table as the camera rotates so that his heart can be examined from different angles. Tell him that the catheterization team will wear gloves, masks, and gowns to protect him from infection. Inform him that an I.V. needle will be inserted into his arm to allow administration of medication. Assure him that the electrodes attached to his chest during the procedure will cause no discomfort.

■ Tell the patient that the catheter is inserted into an artery or vein in the arm or leg; if the skin above the vessel is hairy, it will be shaved and cleaned with an antiseptic. Tell him he'll experience a transient stinging sensation

Hemostatic devices

Hemostatic devices are beneficial primarily because their use speeds the patient's recovery and improves his comfort. The patient spends only 1 to 2 hours on bed rest and continuous compression at the insertion site — whether by hand, sandbags, or C-clamp — is unnecessary. However, use of this type of device is inappropriate for a patient with the following conditions:

- peripheral arterial disease
- hypertension
- history of blood clots.

These devices are associated with risk for the same complications as those involving traditional sheaths. Research by the American College of Cardiology has indicated that the use of a hemostatic device was associated with a greater rate of complications after the procedure than that for traditional (sheath) methods.

when a local anesthetic is injected to numb the incision site for catheter insertion. Assure him that this sensation is normal.

■ Inform the patient that injection of the contrast medium through the catheter may produce a hot, flushing sensation or nausea that quickly passes; instruct him to follow directions to cough or breathe deeply. Explain that medication will be given if he experiences chest pain during the procedure, and he may also be given nitroglycerin periodically to dilate coronary vessels and aid visualization. Reassure him that complications, such as MI and thromboemboli, are rare.

■ Make sure the patient or a responsible member of the family has signed a consent form. Check for patient hypersensitivity to shellfish, iodine, or contrast media used in other diagnostic tests; notify the physician if such hypersensitivities exist.

■ Discontinue anticoagulant therapy as ordered to reduce the risk of complications from bleeding. Just before the procedure, ask the patient to empty his bladder.

■ Review activity restrictions that may be required of the patient after the procedure, such as lying flat with the limb extended for 4 to 6 hours and use of sandbags, if a femoral sheath is used.

After the procedure

■ Determine whether hemostatic devices, such as a collagen plug or suture closure system, were used to close the vessel puncture site. (See *Hemostatic devices*.) If either method was used, inspect the site for bleeding or oozing, redness, swelling, or hematoma formation. Maintain the patient on bed rest for 1 to 2 hours.

■ If hemostatic devices weren't used, remove the catheter after the procedure and apply direct pressure to the incision site for at least 30 minutes using sandbags as necessary. Apply a dressing when hemostasis is achieved. Pressure can be applied manually or by using a C-clamp.

■ Enforce bed rest for 8 hours if no hemostatic device was used. If the femoral route was used for catheter insertion, keep the patient's leg extended for 6 to 8 hours; if the antecubital fossa route was used, keep the arm extended for at least 3 hours.

■ Monitor vital signs every 15 minutes for 2 hours, then every 30 minutes for the next 2 hours, and then every hour for 2 hours. If no hematoma or other problems arise, continue to monitor the patient every 4 hours. If vital signs are unstable, check every 5 minutes and notify the physician.

■ Continually assess the insertion site for a hematoma or blood loss and reinforce the pressure dressing as needed.

■ Check the patient's color, skin temperature, and peripheral pulse below the puncture site. The brachial approach is associated with a higher incidence of vasospasm (characterized by cool fingers and hand and weak pulses on the affected side); this usually resolves within 24 hours.

■ Confirm that a posttest ECG is scheduled to check for possible myocardial damage or, if indicated, institute continuous cardiac monitoring.

■ Consult the physician about when the patient can resume medications withheld before the test. Administer analgesics as ordered.

■ Unless the patient is scheduled for surgery, encourage intake of fluids high in potassium, such as orange juice, to counteract the diuretic effect of the contrast medium.

■ Be alert for chest pain, shortness of breath, abnormal heart rate, dizziness, diaphoresis, nausea or vomiting, or extreme fatigue. Notify the physician immediately if any of these symptoms are present.

 MULTISYSTEM DISORDER

Cardiac tamponade

Cardiac tamponade is a rapid, unchecked rise in pressure in the pericardial sac that compresses the heart, impairs diastolic filling, and reduces cardiac output (CO). The rise in pressure usually results from blood or fluid accumulation in the pericardial sac. Even a small amount of fluid (50 to 100 ml) can cause a serious tamponade if it accumulates rapidly.

Prognosis depends on the rate of fluid accumulation. If fluid accumulates rapidly, cardiac tamponade requires emergency lifesaving measures to prevent death. A slow accumulation and rise in pressure may not produce immediate symptoms because the fibrous wall of the pericardial sac can gradually stretch to accommodate as much as 1 to 2 L of fluid.

Pathophysiology

In cardiac tamponade, the progressive accumulation of fluid in the pericardial sac causes compression of the heart chambers. This compression obstructs blood flow into the ventricles and reduces the amount of blood that can be pumped out of the heart with each contraction. (See *Understanding cardiac tamponade,* pages 52 and 53.)

Cardiac tamponade may result from the following:

■ idiopathic causes (for example, Dressler's syndrome)

■ effusion (from cancer, bacterial infections, tuberculosis and, rarely, acute rheumatic fever)

■ hemorrhage from trauma (such as gunshot or stab wounds to the chest)

■ hemorrhage from nontraumatic causes (such as anticoagulant therapy in patients with pericarditis or rupture of the heart or great vessels)

■ viral or postirradiation pericarditis

■ chronic renal failure requiring dialysis

■ drug reaction from procainamide, hydralazine, minoxidil, isoniazid, penicillin, methysergide, or daunorubicin

Understanding cardiac tamponade

The pericardial sac, which surrounds and protects the heart, is composed of several layers. The fibrous pericardium is the tough outermost membrane; the inner membrane, called the serous membrane, consists of the visceral and parietal layers. The visceral layer clings to the heart and is also known as the epicardial layer. The parietal layer lies between the visceral layer and the fibrous pericardium. The pericardial space — between the visceral and parietal layers — contains 10 to 30 ml

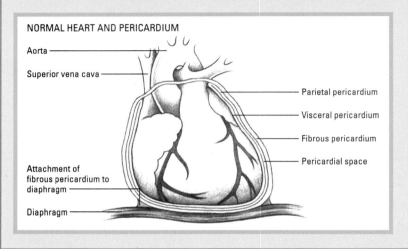

NORMAL HEART AND PERICARDIUM

Aorta

Superior vena cava

Parietal pericardium

Visceral pericardium

Fibrous pericardium

Pericardial space

Attachment of fibrous pericardium to diaphragm

Diaphragm

- connective tissue disorders (such as rheumatoid arthritis, systemic lupus erythematosus, rheumatic fever, vasculitis, and scleroderma)
- acute myocardial infarction.

Comprehensive assessment

The patient's history may reveal an underlying disorder that can lead to cardiac tamponade. He may report acute pain and dyspnea, which forces him to sit upright and lean forward to ease breathing and lessen the pain. Cough, orthopnea, and tachypnea may be present resulting from compression of the lungs by an expanding pericardial sac. Diaphoresis, cool, clammy skin, anxiety, restlessness, and syncope may be noted secondary to a decrease in CO. You may observe cyanosis due to reduced oxygenation of the tissues. Neck vein distention produced by increased venous pressure and impaired venous return may also be seen; however, this may not be present if the patient is hypovolemic. Typically, central venous pressure (CVP) is elevated to greater than 12 mm Hg because atrial compression impairs diastolic filling.

Palpation of the peripheral pulses may disclose rapid, weak pulses. Palpation of the upper quadrant may reveal hepatomegaly.

of pericardial fluid. This fluid lubricates the layers and minimizes friction when the heart contracts.

In cardiac tamponade, blood or fluid fills the pericardial space, compressing the heart chambers, increasing intracardiac pressure, and obstructing venous return. As blood flow into the ventricles falls, so does cardiac output (CO). Without prompt treatment, low CO can be fatal.

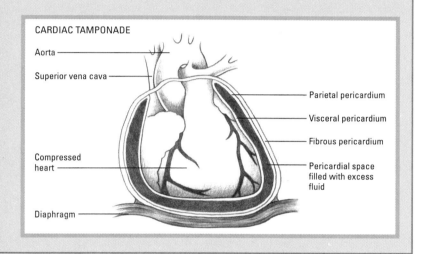

CARDIAC TAMPONADE

Aorta

Superior vena cava

Parietal pericardium

Visceral pericardium

Fibrous pericardium

Compressed heart

Pericardial space filled with excess fluid

Diaphragm

Percussion may detect a widening area of flatness across the anterior chest wall, indicating a large effusion. Hepatomegaly may also be noted.

Auscultation of the blood pressure may demonstrate a decreased arterial blood pressure (due to reduced ventricular filling), pulsus paradoxus, and narrow pulse pressure.

Heart sounds may be muffled due to accumulation of fluid in the pericardial sac that diminishes the sounds of the valves closing. Typically, the lungs are clear.

ALERT *A quiet heart with faint sounds usually accompanies only severe tamponade and occurs within minutes of the tamponade, as happens with cardiac rupture or trauma. However, be alert for the presence of Beck's triad — distended neck veins, hypotension, and muffled heart tones. These are classic signs of cardiac tamponade.*

Diagnosis

■ Electrocardiogram (ECG) may show low-amplitude QRS complex and electrical alternans, an alternating beat-to-beat change in amplitude of the P wave, QRS complex, and T wave. Generalized ST-segment elevation is noted in all leads. An ECG is used to rule out other cardiac disorders; it may reveal changes produced by acute pericarditis.

■ Pulmonary artery catheterization detects increased right atrial pressure, right ventricular diastolic pressure, and CVP.

■ Echocardiography may reveal pericardial effusion with signs of right ventricular and atrial compression.

■ Computed tomography scan or magnetic resonance imaging may identify pericardial effusions or pericardial thickening caused by constrictive pericarditis.

Collaborations

Because cardiac tamponade is considered a multisystem problem, a multidisciplinary approach to care is needed focusing on relieving the intracardial pressure and cardiac compression, thereby enhancing tissue perfusion to all organs. The patient requires intense monitoring and close scrutiny on a critical care unit (CCU).

Treatment and care

The goal of treatment is to relieve intrapericardial pressure and cardiac compression by removing accumulated blood or fluid. Pericardiocentesis (needle aspiration of the pericardial cavity) or pericardectomy (surgical creation of an opening) dramatically improve systemic arterial pressure and CO with aspiration of as little as 25 ml of fluid. A drain may be inserted into the pericardial sac to draw off the effusion. The drain may be left in until the effusion process stops or the corrective action (pericardial window) is performed. In case of infection, antibiotics can be instilled through the drain, clamped, and later drained off. If the repeated pericardiocentesis fails to prevent a recurrence, a portion or all of the pericardium may be resected to al-

low full communication with the pleura.

If the patient is hypotensive, trial volume loading with crystalloids such as I.V. normal saline solution may be used to maintain systolic blood pressure. Inotropic drugs such as isoproterenol or dopamine may be necessary to improve myocardial contractility until fluid in the pericardial sac can be removed. Throughout, continuous cardiac and hemodynamic monitoring are necessary to evaluate the patient's cardiovascular and hemodynamic status for trends.

Depending on the cause, additional treatment may include:

■ blood transfusion or a thoracotomy to drain reaccumulating fluid or to repair bleeding sites from traumatic-injury-induced tamponade

■ administration of heparin antagonist protamine to stop bleeding from heparin-induced tamponade

■ use of vitamin K to stop bleeding from warfarin-induced tamponade.

Complications

Pressure resulting from fluid accumulation in the pericardium decreases ventricular filling and CO, resulting in cardiogenic shock and death if untreated.

Nursing considerations

■ Monitor the patient's cardiovascular status at least every hour, noting extent of jugular vein distention, quality of heart sounds, and blood pressure.

■ Assess hemodynamic status, including CVP, right atrial pressure, and pulmonary artery pressure, and determine CO.

■ Monitor for pulsus paradoxus.

- Institute continuous cardiac monitoring, being alert for ST-segment and T-wave changes. Note rate and rhythm and report evidence of any arrhythmias.
- Watch closely for signs of increasing tamponade, increasing dyspnea, and arrhythmias and report immediately.
- Infuse I.V. solutions and inotropic drugs such as dopamine as ordered to maintain the patient's blood pressure.
- Administer oxygen therapy as needed and assess oxygen saturation levels. Monitor the patient's respiratory status for signs of respiratory distress, such as severe tachypnea and changes in the patient's level of consciousness (LOC). Anticipate the need for endotracheal intubation and mechanical ventilation should the patient's respiratory status deteriorate.
- Prepare the patient for pericardiocentesis, thoracotomy, or CVP line insertion as indicated.

⚡ **ALERT** *Be alert for a decrease in CVP and a concomitant rise in blood pressure following treatment, which indicate relief of cardiac compression.*

- Provide supportive care as indicated by the patient's condition and the tamponade's underlying cause.
- If the patient has trauma-induced tamponade, be sure to assess for other signs of trauma and institute appropriate care, including the use of colloids, crystalloids, and blood component therapy via pressure or rapid volume infusers if massive fluid replacement is needed. Expect to administer protamine sulfate for heparin-induced tamponade and vitamin K for warfarin-induced tamponade.
- Assess renal function status closely, monitoring urine output every hour

and notifying the physician if output is less than 0.5 mg/kg/hour. Also, check urine specific gravity at least every 4 hours to aid in determining fluid status and renal perfusion.
- Monitor capillary refill, LOC, peripheral pulses, and skin temperature for evidence of diminished tissue perfusion.
- Reassure the patient to reduce anxiety.

Patient teaching

- Provide brief explanations about the patient's condition and why it's occurring. Inform the patient and his family about how the condition will be treated, being sure to explain new procedures before beginning.
- Review signs and symptoms of a worsening condition, stressing the importance of alerting the nurse if any such signs occur.

 MULTISYSTEM DISORDER

Cardiac transplantation

Cardiac transplantation involves the replacement of a person's heart with that of a donor heart. It's the treatment of choice for a patient with end-stage cardiac disease; that is, for the patient who has a poor prognosis, estimated survival of 6 to 12 months, and poor quality of life. Typically, a cardiac transplant candidate has symptoms that aren't controlled by medical therapy and has no other surgical options available.

To be considered for a cardiac transplant, the patient must meet specific criteria, such as:
- diagnosis of end-stage heart failure

- refractory and intolerable symptoms
- failure of medical therapies (all options used to the greatest extent possible without success)
- less than a 50% chance of surviving less than 12 months
- less than age 65

AGE ISSUE *Although studies have neither proven nor disproved age as a problem factor in cardiac transplantation, operative morbidity and mortality rates and long-term survival rates following other types of cardiac surgery increase with advancing age. Thus, it's assumed that the success of cardiac transplantation would also be affected by age.*

- ejection fraction less than 35%
- history of chronic stable angina
- atrial fibrillation or ventricular arrhythmias unresponsive to treatment
- decreased cardiac output (CO)
- good health exclusive of the heart disease.

However, even if the patient meets any of the above criteria, other conditions could contraindicate the use of cardiac transplantation. Absolute contraindications include:

- insulin-dependent diabetes mellitus (complicated) with end-organ damage
- active infection (until infection resolved), including human immunodeficiency virus
- active drug addiction, including alcohol
- irreversible pulmonary hypertension
- cancer with metastasis or with a high risk of recurrence
- irreversible liver or kidney dysfunctions
- comorbid conditions, such as renal, pulmonary, neurologic, or vascular disease

- severe obesity.

After the patient is identified as a candidate, he's given a status code and placed on a waiting list. The status code indicates the severity of the patient's need; for example, status 1A identifies a patient who's acutely ill, hospitalized on the critical care unit (CCU), and receiving multiple inotropic medications, mechanical circulatory or ventilatory support, or a ventricular assist device (inserted within the past 30 days), and whose life expectancy is less than 1 week without a transplant. A patient is considered status 2 if he's stable and at home awaiting the transplant.

Following a cardiac transplant, the 1-year survival rate ranges from 80% to 90%. After 5 years, the survival rate is approximately 70%; it decreases to 50% to 60% after 10 years.

Procedure

Two major types of cardiac transplantation may be done: orthotopic and heterotopic. Orthotopic heart transplantation (OHT) is the most commonly performed procedure. OHT involves removal of most of the patient's heart (native heart), retaining a large portion of the right and left atria.

OHT involves a median sternotomy and use of cardiopulmonary bypass. The donor heart is attached (anastomosed) to the native atrial cusps, and direct end-to-end anastomoses of the aorta and pulmonary artery are performed. (See *Understanding orthotopic cardiac transplantation.*)

In OHT, the transplanted heart is denervated so it can't respond normally to stimuli from the autonomic nervous system. Initially, electrical activity in the new heart is slow, requiring the

Understanding orthotopic cardiac transplantation

The illustration below shows how the donor heart is anastomosed to the recipient's right atrium in an orthotopic heart transplant.

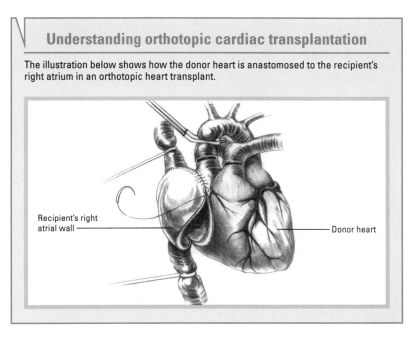

Recipient's right atrial wall

Donor heart

use of a temporary pacemaker in the immediate postoperative period. Bradycardia due to chronotropic incompetence may occur as a result of either primary sinus node dysfunction or the use of preoperative negative chronotropic agents such as amiodarone.

The denervated transplanted heart also has a blunted response to exercise because it relies on circulating catecholamines to respond to the demands of an increased heart rate. Although there have been reports of reinnervation of the recipient heart 1 year post-transplant, the response to exercise is generally considered diminished in all cases.

Heterotopic heart transplantation is less commonly performed and involves grafting a donor heart to a recipient heart without removing the recipient heart. The donor heart is used to assist the pumping ability of the native heart. This procedure is also referred to as "piggyback" heart transplantation.

Complications

The major complication following cardiac transplant is rejection, in which the recipient's body detects the transplanted heart as a foreign body (antigen), triggering the immune response. This leads to fibrosis and scar formation in the heart muscle. If untreated, the entire heart is destroyed. In addition, infection, decreased CO, and arrhythmias, such as supraventricular and ventricular arrhythmias, atrial fibrillation, and ventricular conduction defects are also major complications in the immediate postoperative period.

Nursing considerations

When caring for the patient undergoing a cardiac transplant, nursing care focuses on preparing the patient and his family physically and emotionally for the procedure. This includes instructing the patient about the procedure and events after it as well as instituting measures to prevent postoperative complications. Be ready to act rapidly when a donor heart becomes available.

Before the procedure

■ Instruct the patient and his family about the transplant and necessary diagnostic tests such as antigen typing.

■ Reinforce the surgeon's explanation of the surgery, equipment, and procedures used on the CCU or postanesthesia care unit. If one hasn't been inserted, inform the patient that he'll awaken from surgery with an endotracheal tube in place and be connected to a mechanical ventilator. Review other equipment, such as continuous cardiac monitoring, nasogastric tube, chest tube, indwelling urinary catheter, arterial lines, pacing wires and, possibly, pulmonary artery catheter. Tell him that discomfort will be minimal and the equipment will be removed as soon as possible.

■ Administer immunosuppressant agents as ordered.

■ Review techniques of incentive spirometry and range of motion with the patient.

■ Make sure that the patient or a responsible family member has signed a consent form.

■ Instruct family members in measures used to control infection and minimize rejection after transplant.

■ Provide emotional support to the patient and his family, particularly during the waiting period, because waiting for a donor heart may seem endless.

After the procedure

■ Assess cardiopulmonary and hemodynamic status closely at least every 15 minutes in the immediate postoperative period and then hourly or more frequently, as indicated by the patient's condition.

⚡ **ALERT** *Be alert for the following signs suggestive of rejection: a cardiac index less than 2.2, hypotension, atrial or other arrhythmias, fever above 99.5° F (37.5° C), evidence of an S_3 or S_4, peripheral edema, jugular vein distention, and crackles. Notify the physician or transplant coordinator immediately.*

■ Institute continuous cardiac monitoring, evaluating waveforms frequently. Keep in mind that the transplanted heart's electrocardiogram (ECG) waveform appears a bit different from the waveform of the patient's native heart. (See *ECG waveform after cardiac transplantation.*)

⚡ **ALERT** *Abnormalities of the donor sinoatrial (SA) node's conduction and automaticity usually occur as a result of injury to the donor heart during procurement, transportation, or transplantation. If the conduction system is damaged or if the SA node fails to function properly after the heart is transplanted, the ECG will reflect the abnormality.*

■ Monitor atrial and ventricular pacing as necessary, keeping heart rate greater than 110 beats/minute.

■ Administer analgesics as ordered for pain relief.

ECG waveform after cardiac transplantation

An orthotopic heart transplantation (OHT) leads to characteristic findings on an electrocardiogram (ECG); because the procedure provides the patient with a second functioning heart, the ECG shows two distinct cardiac rhythms—that of the native heart, and that of the donor heart. These can be differentiated by analyzing the recipient's preoperative ECG. In addition, the QRS complex of the donor heart usually has a higher amplitude. Remember that in OHT, the sinus node of the native heart remains intact. This accounts for the two P waves commonly seen on the post-transplant ECG. However, only the sinus node of the donor heart conducts through to the ventricles.

Initially, the atrial and ventricular rates are slow, requiring the use of a temporary pacemaker in the immediate postoperative period or therapy with drugs such as theophylline. The patient's native P waves will have a regular rhythm unrelated to the donor heart's QRS complexes. The donor atrial and ventricular rhythms are usually regular. Typically, two separate P waves are seen and the QRS complex may be widened secondary to ventricular conduction defects. Pacemaker activity should appear as long as the patient requires pacemaker support for chronotropic incompetence.

Orthotopic heart transplantation
This waveform shows two distinct types of P waves. P waves caused by the native heart's sinoatrial (SA) node are unrelated to the QRS complexes (first shaded area). P waves caused by the donor heart's SA node precede each QRS complex (second shaded area).

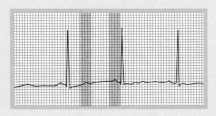

Heterotopic heart transplantation
This waveform shows the ECG of the recipient's own heart (first shaded area) and the donor heart (second shaded area).

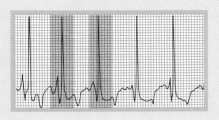

■ In the immediate postoperative period, monitor laboratory test results including complete blood count, hemoglobin level, hematocrit, platelet count, serum chemistry, serum electrolyte levels, blood urea nitrogen (BUN) and creatinine levels, arterial blood gas levels, and 12-lead ECG. Anticipate the following tests daily: serum electrolyte analysis; liver and renal function studies; coagulation studies, such as prothrombin time and partial thromboplastin time; chest X-ray; BUN and creatinine levels; urine and sputum cultures such as for cytomegalovirus (CMV) and toxoplasmosis; and immunosuppressant drug level.

■ Institute strict infection control precautions; perform meticulous handwashing.

ALERT *The postoperative cardiac transplant patient is continuously at dual risk for infection and rejection. CMV is the major cause of morbidity and mortality with the cardiac transplant patient. Expect to administer ganciclovir prophylactically and for treatment of CMV.*

■ Assist with extubating as soon as possible (usually within 4 to 6 hours) and administer supplemental oxygen as needed, based on mixed venous oxygen saturation or pulse oximetry levels. Encourage coughing, deep breathing, and the use of incentive spirometry after extubation, and splinting and premedicating for pain as necessary.

■ Monitor intake and output at least hourly and notify the physician if output is less than 30 ml/hour. Maintain fluids at 2,000 to 3,000 ml/day or as ordered to prevent fluid overload.

■ Administer postoperative drugs, such as methylprednisolone or prednisone (corticosteroids) (used to suppress T- and B-cell function, to reduce or prevent edema, promote normal capillary permeability, and prevent vasodilation), cyclosporine (immunosuppressant), azathioprine (immunosuppressant), OKT3 (an immunosuppressant used in place of cyclosporine), or tacrolimus (a highly potent immunosuppressant used in place of cyclosporine when multiple rejections occur while on cyclosporine).

■ Maintain nothing by mouth status with nasogastric decompression to low intermittent suction until bowel sounds return. Administer histamine blockers to suppress gastric acid secretion. Begin clear liquids after patient is extubated and bowel sounds are active. Advance to low-fat, sodium-restricted diet as ordered.

■ Change the patient's position at least every 2 hours, getting him out of bed to the chair within 24 hours if his condition is stable. Gradually increase the patient's activity as tolerated.

■ Monitor chest tubes attached to suction (usually for the first 24 hours or until drainage is less than 100 ml in 8 hours). While chest tubes are in place, expect to administer antibiotic as ordered to prevent infection. Assess drainage amount, color, and characteristics. Assess for bleeding. Notify the physician if chest tube drainage is greater than 400 ml in 1 hour or a sudden stop in drainage occurs.

■ Administer inotropic medications as ordered including nitroglycerin (to decrease preload), nitroprusside (to decrease afterload), dobutamine (to increase contractility and CO), epinephrine (to increase heart rate and contractility), norepinephrine (to increase blood pressure), dopamine (low doses to improve renal perfusion; high doses to increase heart rate and blood pressure), and calcium channel blockers (to control hypertension).

■ Prepare the patient for myocardial biopsy at approximately 7 days and again at 14 days postsurgery, and then as indicated by the physician. Explain the procedure to the patient and his family.

■ To ease emotional stress, plan care to allow frequent rest periods and provide as much privacy as possible. Allow family members to visit and comfort the patient as much as possible.

■ Allow the family to express their anger, anxiety, and fear.

MULTISYSTEM DISORDER

Cardiac trauma

Cardiac trauma, commonly dramatic in presentation, is usually associated with other thoracic injuries, possibly occurring secondary to blunt or penetrating trauma. Thoracic injuries — cardiac trauma included — account for approximately 25% of all trauma deaths. Although cardiac trauma can be severe, not all injuries are apparent on admission to the emergency department (ED) or critical care unit, especially when the patient exhibits no external signs of chest wall damage. It may be several hours before signs are manifested, and several days before complications are evident. As a result, keen observation and assessment are essential to identify cardiac injuries and potential complications early.

The prognosis for a patient with cardiac trauma largely depends on the extent of the patient's cardiac damage and that of his other injuries. Age and preexisting conditions also affect the prognosis.

Pathophysiology

Cardiac trauma may occur secondary to blunt or penetrating trauma. Blunt trauma typically results from vehicular accidents or falls. Cardiac concussion, a less severe form of blunt cardiac injury, occurs when rapid deceleration causes the heart to strike the anterior chest wall and sternum, thereby resulting in myocardial contusion. (See *Myocardial contusion.*) Rapid deceleration may also result in shearing forces that tear cardiac structures and cause great-vessel disruption. Falls may cause a rapid increase in intra-abdominal and

Myocardial contusion

A myocardial contusion — bruising to the myocardium — is the most common type of injury sustained from blunt trauma. It should be suspected whenever a blow to the chest occurs. The contusion usually results from a fall or from impact with a steering wheel or other object. The right ventricle is the most common site of injury because of its location directly behind the sternum.

Here's what happens:
● During deceleration injuries, the myocardium strikes the sternum as the heart and aorta move forward.
● In addition, the aorta may be lacerated by shearing forces.
● Direct force also may be applied to the sternum, causing injury.

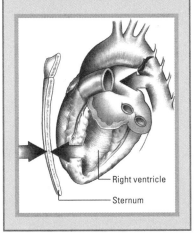

Right ventricle
Sternum

intrathoracic pressures, which can result in myocardial rupture, valvular rupture, or both. Crushing and compression forces may result in contusion or rupture as the heart is compressed between the sternum and vertebral column.

Penetrating trauma to the heart, typically due to knife or gunshot wounds or foreign bodies in the heart, carries a high mortality and usually requires immediate thoracotomy and surgical repair. This type of cardiac trauma commonly leads to cardiac tamponade. In most cases involving penetrating cardiac trauma, death occurs before the patient reaches the hospital.

Comprehensive assessment

Cardiac trauma may initially be overlooked as other life-threatening and more apparent injuries are treated. In addition, signs and symptoms of myocardial contusion or cardiac tamponade may not occur for several hours. Therefore, astute assessment skills are needed for early detection and prompt treatment.

Typically, the patient with cardiac trauma is in pain and apprehensive. Attempt to ascertain the following information:

■ mechanism of injury; for example, an automobile accident including how the accident occurred, patient location and use of seat belts, and extent of internal car damage; a fall, including how far the patient fell, onto what type of surface and how he landed; a gunshot wound, including the gun caliber and distance from which the patient was shot; a stab wound, including the size and type of the weapon
■ history of cardiac or pulmonary problems
■ pain location, onset, character, and severity
■ complaints of shortness of breath.

◄ **ALERT** *Be especially suspicious of cardiac trauma if the patient has experienced any of the following: head or spine (cervical or thoracic) injury, other thoracic injuries (such as to* the lungs, trachea, great vessels, or esophagus), upper abdominal injuries, chest wall trauma, or fractured ribs.

During physical examination, look for the following signs and symptoms associated with blunt trauma:
■ precordial chest pain
■ bradycardia or tachycardia
■ shortness of breath
■ contusion marks on the chest
■ flail chest
■ murmurs.

◄ **ALERT** *Be alert for cyanosis of the upper body. If present in conjunction with signs and symptoms of cardiac tamponade, cardiac rupture may have occurred.*

If the patient experienced penetrating trauma, look for the following:
■ tachycardia
■ shortness of breath
■ weakness
■ diaphoresis
■ acute anxiety
■ cool, clammy skin
■ evidence of an external puncture wound or protrusion of the penetrating instrument
■ cardiac tamponade.

For the patient who has a cardiac contusion, the following may be present:
■ hemodynamic instability
■ arrhythmias due to ventricular irritability
■ heart failure or cardiogenic shock
■ pericardial friction rub
■ cardiac tamponade. (See "Cardiac tamponade," page 51.)

If the patient is experiencing a cardiac concussion, many of the signs and symptoms listed above will be present. However, evidence of cellular injury is absent.

Diagnosis

Several diagnostic tests are helpful in identifying cardiac trauma:

■ Electrocardiogram (ECG): rhythm disturbances such as premature ventricular contractions, premature atrial contractions, ventricular tachycardia, atrial tachycardia, and ventricular fibrillation along with nonspecific ST-segment or T-wave changes (with cardiac contusion) occurring within 24 to 48 hours after the injury

■ Chest X-ray: widened mediastinum (with cardiac tamponade); pulmonary engorgement (with septal defect)

■ Echocardiogram: evidence of cardiac tamponade and valvular abnormalities; abnormal ventricular wall movement and decreased ejection fraction (with myocardial contusion)

■ Transesophageal echocardiogram: evidence of aortic disruptions, cardiac tamponade, atrial and septal defects

■ Multiple-gated acquisition scan: detection of decreased ability of effective heart pumping (with cardiac contusion)

■ Cardiac enzyme levels: elevations of CP-MB to greater than 8% of total CP within 3 to 4 hours after the injury (in conjunction with ECG changes suggestive of cardiac contusion)

■ Cardiac troponin I: elevations 24 hours after the injury (suggestive of cardiac injury).

Collaborations

Because cardiac trauma is a multisystem disorder, a multidisciplinary approach to care is essential to maximize the patient's cardiac function and maintain hemodynamic stability. Emergency medical services personnel at the scene of the trauma or in the ED are the first persons to intervene. Medical management and, if necessary, surgical intervention, are key components of care. In addition, other services, such as respiratory therapy, may be necessary to assist with pulmonary function. Social service may be required to facilitate care for specific trauma-related cases.

Treatment and care

Maintaining hemodynamic stability is crucial to the patient's care. Penetrating trauma may be associated with massive hemorrhage leading to acute hypotension and shock. In addition, cardiac output (CO) is affected if the patient develops cardiac tamponade or arrhythmias occurring with myocardial contusion. Hemodynamic monitoring is key to evaluating the patient's status and maintaining its adequacy. I.V. fluid therapy, including blood component therapy, may be necessary. Continuous ECG monitoring is important to detect possible arrhythmias. Lidocaine may be used to treat ventricular arrhythmias. Digoxin may be given for pump failure. Inotropic agents may be used to assist with improving CO and ejection fraction.

The patient with cardiac trauma must be monitored closely for signs and symptoms of cardiopulmonary compromise because cardiac trauma is commonly associated with pulmonary trauma. Supplemental oxygen administration and assessment of oxygen saturation are important. If the degree of associated pulmonary trauma is great, endotracheal intubation and mechanical ventilation may be warranted to maintain adequate oxygenation.

If the patient is experiencing severe pain, I.V. morphine is administered in small amounts unless the patient is hypotensive (in which case, other less potent analgesics are used). In addition, corrective surgery may be indicated to correct septal or valvular defects, penetrating injuries or rupture. Pericardiocentesis is used to treat cardiac tamponade.

Complications

Potential fatal complications may follow cardiac trauma. These may include:

■ heart failure (due to septal or valvular damage or myocardial necrosis)
■ ventricular aneurysm (due to ligation of coronary artery or suture of ventricular laceration)
■ cardiac herniation (reopening of a pericardial incision after surgery)
■ pneumopericardium (air within the pericardium creating a tamponade)
■ posttraumatic pericarditis (due to irritation of epicardium and pericardium by blood leading to inflammation and edema or due to effusion development).

Nursing considerations

■ Assess the patient's cardiopulmonary status at least every 4 hours—or more frequently if indicated—to detect signs and symptoms of possible injury. Auscultate breath sounds at least every 4 hours, reporting any signs of congestion or fluid accumulation. Evaluate peripheral pulses and capillary refill to detect decreased peripheral tissue perfusion.
■ Monitor heart rate and rhythm, heart sounds, and blood pressure every hour for changes; institute hemodynamic monitoring, including central venous pressure, pulmonary artery wedge pressure, and CO as indicated at least every 1 to 2 hours.

■ Administer fluid replacement therapy including blood component therapy as prescribed, typically to maintain systolic blood pressure above 90 mm Hg.
■ Monitor urine output every hour, notifying physician if output is less than 30 ml/hour.
■ Institute continuous cardiac monitoring for the first 48 to 72 hours to detect arrhythmias or conduction defects. If arrhythmias occur, administer antiarrhythmic agents as ordered.
■ Assess the patient's degree of pain and administer analgesic therapy as ordered, monitoring him for effectiveness. Position the patient comfortably, usually with the head of the bed elevated 30 to 45 degrees.
■ Encourage coughing and deep breathing, splinting the chest as necessary.
■ If the patient has undergone surgery, monitor and assess chest tubes for patency, volume and color of drainage, and presence of air leak.
■ Assess vital signs postoperatively, especially temperature.
■ Inspect the surgical site for evidence of infection at least every 4 hours, noting redness, drainage, warmth, edema, or localized pain at the site.
■ Arrange for possible social service consultation depending on the cause of the injury; for example, alcohol-related automobile accident, gang-related gunshot injury.

Patient teaching

■ Provide brief explanations about the patient's condition and why it's occurring. Inform the patient and his family about how the condition will be treated, being sure to explain new procedures before beginning.

■ Review signs and symptoms of a worsening condition, stressing the importance of alerting the nurse if any occur.

■ Teach the patient about signs and symptoms of complications and the need for follow-up.

Cardiogenic shock

Sometimes called pump failure, cardiogenic shock is a condition of diminished cardiac output (CO) that severely impairs tissue perfusion. Cardiogenic shock occurs as a serious complication in nearly 15% of patients who are hospitalized with acute myocardial infarction (MI). It typically affects patients whose area of infarction involves 40% or more of left ventricular muscle mass; in such patients, mortality rates may exceed 85%. Most patients with cardiogenic shock die within 24 hours of onset. The prognosis for those who survive is poor.

Pathophysiology

Cardiogenic shock is one of three major categories of shock. It can result from any condition that causes significant left ventricular dysfunction with reduced CO, such as MI (the most common cause), myocardial ischemia, papillary muscle dysfunction, and end-stage cardiomyopathy.

Other causes include myocarditis and depression of myocardial contractility after cardiac arrest and prolonged cardiac surgery. Mechanical abnormalities of the ventricle, such as acute mitral or aortic insufficiency or an acutely acquired ventricular septal defect or ventricular aneurysm, may also result

in cardiogenic shock. Regardless of the category of shock, three phases occur. (See *Stages of shock,* page 66.)

AGE ISSUE *Although cardiogenic shock is uncommon in children, it may occur after cardiac surgery. It can also occur in children with acute arrhythmias, heart failure, or cardiomyopathy.*

Regardless of the cause, left ventricular dysfunction initiates a series of compensatory mechanisms that increase heart rate, strengthen myocardial contractions, promote sodium and water retention, and cause selective vasoconstriction. These mechanisms attempt to increase CO and maintain vital organ function. However, these mechanisms also increase myocardial workload and oxygen consumption, thus reducing the heart's ability to pump blood, especially if the patient has myocardial ischemia. As CO falls, aortic and carotid baroreceptors activate sympathetic nervous responses. These compensatory responses increase heart rate, left ventricular filling pressure, and peripheral resistance to flow in order to enhance venous return to the heart. The action initially stabilizes the patient but later causes deterioration with rising oxygen demands on the compromised myocardium. These events constitute a vicious circle of low CO, sympathetic compensation, myocardial ischemia, and even lower CO. Consequently, blood backs up, resulting in pulmonary edema. Eventually, CO falls and multisystem organ failure develops as the compensatory mechanisms fail to maintain perfusion.

Stages of shock

Three basic stages are common to shock, regardless of the category: compensatory, progressive, and irreversible or refractory.

Compensatory stage
When arterial pressure and tissue perfusion are reduced, compensatory mechanisms are activated to maintain perfusion to the heart and brain. As the baroreceptors in the carotid sinus and aortic arch sense a drop in blood pressure, epinephrine and norepinephrine are secreted to increase peripheral resistance, blood pressure, and myocardial contractility. Reduced blood flow to the kidney activates the renin-angiotensin-aldosterone system, causing vasoconstriction and sodium and water retention, leading to increased blood volume and venous return. As a result of these compensatory mechanisms, cardiac output (CO) and tissue perfusion are maintained.

Progressive stage
The progressive stage of shock begins as compensatory mechanisms fail to maintain CO. Tissues become hypoxic because of poor perfusion. As cells switch to anaerobic metabolism, lactic acid builds up, producing metabolic acidosis. This acidotic state depresses myocardial function. Tissue hypoxia also promotes the release of endothelial mediators, which produce vasodilation and endothelial abnormalities, leading to venous pooling and increased capillary permeability. Sluggish blood flow increases the risk of disseminated intravascular coagulation.

Irreversible (refractory) stage
As the shock syndrome progresses, permanent organ damage occurs as compensatory mechanisms can no longer maintain CO. Reduced perfusion damages cell membranes, lysosomal enzymes are released, and energy stores are depleted, possibly leading to cell death. As cells use anaerobic metabolism, lactic acid accumulates, increasing capillary permeability and the movement of fluid out of the vascular space. This loss of intravascular fluid further contributes to hypotension. Perfusion to the coronary arteries is reduced, causing myocardial depression and a further reduction in CO. Eventually, circulatory and respiratory failure occur. Death is inevitable.

Comprehensive assessment
Typically, the patient's history includes a disorder (such as MI or cardiomyopathy) that severely decreases left ventricular function. A patient with underlying cardiac disease may complain of anginal pain because of decreased myocardial perfusion and oxygenation. Urine output is usually less than 20 ml/hour. Inspection usually reveals pale skin, decreased sensorium, and rapid, shallow respirations. Palpation of peripheral pulses may detect a rapid, thready pulse. The skin feels cold and clammy.

Auscultation of blood pressure usually discloses a mean arterial pressure of less than 60 mm Hg and a narrowing pulse pressure. In a patient with chronic hypotension, the mean pressure may fall below 50 mm Hg before the patient exhibits signs of shock. Auscultation of the heart detects gallop rhythm, faint heart sounds and, possibly (if shock results from rupture of the ventricular septum or papillary muscles), a holosystolic murmur.

Although many of these clinical features also occur in heart failure and other shock syndromes, they're usually more profound in cardiogenic shock. Patients with pericardial tamponade may have distant heart sounds.

The patient's signs and symptoms may also provide clues to the stage of shock. For example, in the compensatory stage of shock, signs and symptoms may include:

- tachycardia and bounding pulse due to sympathetic stimulation
- restlessness and irritability related to cerebral hypoxia
- tachypnea to compensate for hypoxia
- reduced urine output secondary to vasoconstriction
- cool, pale skin associated with vasoconstriction; warm, dry skin in septic shock due to vasodilation.

In the progressive stage of shock, signs and symptoms may include:

- hypotension as compensatory mechanisms begin to fail
- narrowed pulse pressure associated with reduced stroke volume
- weak, rapid, thready pulse caused by decreased CO
- shallow respirations as the patient weakens
- reduced urine output as poor renal perfusion continues
- cold, clammy skin caused by vasoconstriction
- cyanosis related to hypoxia.

In the irreversible stage, clinical findings may include:

- unconsciousness and absent reflexes caused by reduced cerebral perfusion, acid-base imbalance, or electrolyte abnormalities
- rapidly falling blood pressure as decompensation occurs

- weak pulse caused by reduced CO
- slow, shallow or Cheyne-Stokes respirations secondary to respiratory center depression
- anuria related to renal failure.

Diagnosis

- Pulmonary artery pressure monitoring reveals increased pulmonary artery pressure (PAP) and pulmonary artery wedge pressure (PAWP), reflecting a rise in left ventricular end-diastolic pressure (preload) and heightened resistance to left ventricular emptying (afterload) caused by ineffective pumping and increased peripheral vascular resistance. Thermodilution catheterization reveals a reduced cardiac index.
- Invasive arterial pressure monitoring shows systolic arterial pressure less than 80 mm Hg caused by impaired ventricular ejection.
- Arterial blood gas (ABG) analysis may show metabolic and respiratory acidosis and hypoxia.
- Electrocardiography (ECG) demonstrates possible evidence of acute MI, ischemia, or ventricular aneurysm.
- Echocardiography determines left ventricular function and reveals valvular abnormalities.
- Serum enzyme measurements display elevated levels of creatine kinase (CK), lactate dehydrogenase (LD), aspartate aminotransferase, and alanine aminotransferase, which indicate MI or ischemia and suggest heart failure or shock. CK-MB (an isoenzyme of CK that occurs in cardiac tissue) and LD isoenzyme levels may confirm acute MI.
- Cardiac catheterization and echocardiography may reveal other conditions that can lead to pump dysfunc-

tion and failure, such as cardiac tamponade, papillary muscle infarct or rupture, ventricular septal rupture, pulmonary emboli, venous pooling (associated with venodilators and continuous or intermittent positive-pressure breathing), and hypovolemia.

Collaborations

Treatment of cardiogenic shock usually begins with emergency care. Emergency medical services (EMS) personnel must focus on maintaining adequate tissue perfusion to sustain life. Because shock is a progressive state requiring treatment within an hour after an injury that could cause death, EMS personnel initiate treatment on the scene of an accident and continue care as they transport the patient to an acute-care facility. After that, medical and surgical management may be required, and various specialists may be consulted.

Treatment and care

Treatment aims to enhance cardiovascular status by increasing CO, improving myocardial perfusion, and decreasing cardiac workload with combinations of cardiovascular drugs and mechanical-assist techniques. These goals are accomplished by optimizing preload, decreasing afterload, increasing contractility, and optimizing heart rate.

The following measures are appropriate for any category of shock:
■ identification and treatment of the underlying cause, if possible
■ maintaining a patent airway and preparing for intubation and mechanical ventilation if the patient develops respiratory distress
■ supplemental oxygen to increase oxygenation

■ continuous cardiac monitoring to detect changes in heart rate and rhythm and administration of antiarrhythmics, as necessary
■ initiating and maintaining at least two I.V. lines with large-gauge needles for fluid and drug administration
■ I.V. fluids, crystalloids, colloids, or blood products, as necessary, to maintain intravascular volume.

For the patient with cardiogenic shock, I.V. drugs may include dopamine (a vasopressor that increases CO, blood pressure, and renal blood flow), dopamine, amrinone, or dobutamine (inotropic agents that increase myocardial contractility and increase CO), and norepinephrine (when a more potent vasoconstrictor is necessary). Nitroglycerin or nitroprusside (vasodilators) may be used with a vasopressor to further improve CO by decreasing afterload and reducing preload. However, the patient's blood pressure must be adequate to support nitroprusside therapy and must be monitored closely. Diuretics may also be used to reduce preload in the patient with fluid volume overload.

Treatment may also include an intra-aortic balloon pump (IABP), a mechanical-assist device that attempts to improve coronary artery perfusion and decrease cardiac workload. The inflatable balloon pump is inserted through the femoral artery into the descending thoracic aorta. The balloon inflates during diastole to increase coronary artery perfusion pressure and deflates before systole (before the aortic valve opens) to reduce resistance to ejection (afterload), thereby lessening cardiac workload. Improved ventricular ejection, which significantly improves CO, and a subsequent vasodilation in the peripheral vessels lead to lower pre-load volume. IABP therapy reduces the work of the left ventricle by decreasing systemic vascular resistance. Diastolic pressure is increased, resulting in improved coronary artery perfusion.

When drug therapy and IABP insertion fail, a ventricular-assist pump may be inserted to assist the pumping action of the heart. When all other medical and surgical therapies fail, cardiac transplantation may be considered.

Additional treatment measures for cardiogenic shock may include:
■ thrombolytic therapy or coronary artery revascularization to restore coronary artery blood flow, if cardiogenic shock is due to acute MI
■ emergency surgery to repair papillary muscle rupture or ventricular septal defect, if either is the cause of cardiogenic shock.

Complications
Death usually ensues because the vital organs can't overcome the deleterious effects of extended hypoperfusion. Despite advances in treatment, mortality from cardiogenic shock remains greater than 80%.

Nursing considerations
■ Begin I.V. infusions of normal saline solution or lactated Ringer's solution, using a large-bore (14G to 18G) catheter, which allows easier administration of later blood transfusions.
■ Administer oxygen by face mask or artificial airway to ensure adequate oxygenation of tissues. Adjust the oxygen flow rate to a higher or lower level, as blood gas measurements indicate. Many patients will need 100% oxygen, and some will require 5 to 15 cm H_2O of positive end-expiratory

or continuous positive airway pressure ventilation.
■ Monitor and record blood pressure, pulse, respiratory rate, and peripheral pulses every 1 to 5 minutes until the patient stabilizes. Monitor cardiac rhythm continuously. Systolic blood pressure less than 80 mm Hg usually results in inadequate coronary artery blood flow, cardiac ischemia, arrhythmias, and further complications of low CO. If blood pressure drops below 80 mm Hg, increase the oxygen flow rate and notify the physician immediately. A progressive drop in blood pressure accompanied by a thready pulse generally signals inadequate CO from reduced intravascular volume.
■ Using a pulmonary artery catheter, closely monitor PAP, PAWP and, if equipment is available, CO. Record hemodynamic pressure readings every 15 minutes. A high PAWP indicates heart failure, increased systemic vascular resistance, decreased CO, and decreased cardiac index and should be reported immediately. (See *Interpreting hemodynamic parameters in cardiogenic shock,* page 70.)
■ Determine how much fluid to give by checking blood pressure, urine output, central venous pressure (CVP), or PAWP. (To increase accuracy, measure CVP at the level of the right atrium, using the same reference point on the chest each time.) Whenever the fluid infusion rate is increased, watch for signs of fluid overload such as an increase in PAWP.

ALERT *If the patient is hypovolemic, preload may need to be increased, typically accomplished with I.V. fluids. However, I.V. fluids must be given cautiously, being increased gradually while hemodynamic parameters*

Interpreting hemodynamic parameters in cardiogenic shock

Parameter	Values associated with cardiogenic shock
Right atrial pressure	6 to 10 mm Hg
Right ventricular pressure	40 to 50/6 to 15 mm Hg
Pulmonary artery pressure	50/25 to 30 mm Hg
Pulmonary artery wedge pressure	25 to 40 mm Hg
Systemic vascular resistance	> 1200 dynes/sec/cm^5
Mixed venous oxygen saturation	≤ 50%
Cardiac output	< 4 L/minute
Cardiac index	< 1.5 L/minute/m^2

are closely monitored. In this situation, diuretics aren't given.

■ Insert an indwelling urinary catheter if necessary to measure hourly urine output. If output is less than 30 ml/hour in adults, increase the fluid infusion rate but watch for signs of fluid overload such as an increase in PAWP. Notify the physician if urine output doesn't improve.

■ Administer a diuretic, such as furosemide or bumetanide, as ordered to decrease preload and improve stroke volume and CO.

■ Monitor ABG values, complete blood count, and electrolyte levels. Expect to administer sodium bicarbonate by I.V. push if the patient is acidotic. Administer electrolyte replacement therapy as ordered and indicated by laboratory results.

■ During therapy, assess skin color and temperature and note changes. Cold, clammy skin may be a sign of continuing peripheral vascular constriction, indicating progressive shock.

■ When a patient is on the IABP, move him as little as possible. Never flex the patient's "ballooned" leg at the hip because this may displace or fracture the catheter. Never place the patient in a sitting position for any reason (including chest X-rays) while the balloon is inflated; the balloon will tear through the aorta and result in immediate death.

■ During use of the IABP, assess pedal pulses and skin temperature and color to ensure adequate peripheral circulation. Check the dressing over the insertion site frequently for bleeding, and change it according to your facility's protocol. Also, check the site for hematoma or signs of infection, and culture any drainage.

■ If the patient becomes hemodynamically stable, gradually reduce the frequency of balloon inflation to wean him from the IABP.

■ When weaning the patient from the IABP, watch for ECG changes, chest pain, and other signs of recurring cardiac ischemia as well as for shock.

■ Prepare the patient for possible emergency cardiac catheterization to determine eligibility for percutaneous transluminal coronary angioplasty or coronary artery bypass graft as means to reperfuse areas with reversible injury patterns.

■ To ease emotional stress, plan care to allow frequent rest periods and provide as much privacy as possible. Allow family members to visit and comfort the patient as much as possible.

■ Allow the family to express their anger, anxiety, and fear.

Patient teaching

■ Because the patient and his family may be anxious about the critical care unit and about the IABP and other devices, offer explanations and reassurance.

■ Prepare the patient and his family for a probable fatal outcome, and help them find effective coping strategies.

Cardiomyopathy

Cardiomyopathy generally applies to disease of the heart muscle fibers, and it occurs in three main forms: dilated, hypertrophic, and restrictive (extremely rare). Cardiomyopathy is the second most common direct cause of sudden death; coronary artery disease is first. Approximately 5 to 8 Americans per 100,000 have *dilated cardiomyopathy,* the most common type. At greatest risk of cardiomyopathy are males and blacks; other risk factors include hypertension, pregnancy, viral infections, and alcohol use. Because dilated cardiomyopathy usually isn't diagnosed until its advanced stages, the prognosis is generally poor. There are two types of *hypertrophic cardiomyopathy.* The more common form is caused by pressure overload–hypertension or aortic valve stenosis. Hypertrophic obstructive cardiomyopathy (HOCM) is due

to a genetic abnormality. The course of hypertrophic cardiomyopathy is variable. Some patients progressively deteriorate, whereas others remain stable for years. An estimated 50% of sudden deaths in competitive athletes age 35 or younger are due to HOCM. If severe, *restrictive cardiomyopathy* is irreversible.

Pathophysiology

Most patients with cardiomyopathy have idiopathic, or primary, disease, but some are secondary to identifiable causes. (See *Comparing cardiomyopathies,* pages 72 and 73.) HOCM is almost always inherited as a non–sex-linked autosomal dominant trait.

Dilated cardiomyopathy results from extensively damaged myocardial muscle fibers with accompanying reduced contractility in the left ventricle. As systolic function declines, stroke volume, ejection fraction, and cardiac output (CO) fall. As end-diastolic volumes rise, pulmonary congestion may occur. The elevated end-diastolic volume is a compensatory response to preserve stroke volume despite a reduced ejection fraction. The sympathetic nervous system is also stimulated to increase heart rate and contractility. The kidneys are stimulated to retain sodium and water to maintain CO, and vasoconstriction also occurs as the renin-angiotensin system is stimulated. When these compensatory mechanisms can no longer maintain CO, the heart begins to fail. Left ventricular dilation occurs as venous return and systemic vascular resistance rise. Eventually, the atria also dilate as more work is required to pump blood into the full ventricles. Cardiomegaly occurs as a consequence of dilation of
(Text continues on page 74.)

Comparing cardiomyopathies

Cardiomyopathies include various structural or functional abnormalities of the ventricles. They are grouped into three main pathophysiologic types—dilated, hypertrophic, and restrictive. These conditions may lead to heart failure by impairing myocardial structure and function.

Normal heart	**Dilated cardiomyopathy**
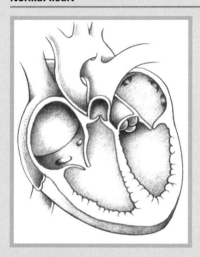	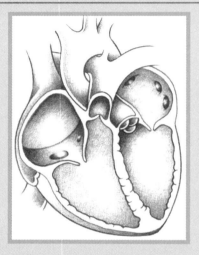

Ventricles	• Greatly increased chamber size • Thinning of left ventricular muscle
Atrial chamber size	• Increased
Myocardial mass	• Increased
Ventricular inflow resistance	• Normal
Contractility	• Decreased
Possible causes	• Viral or bacterial infection • Hypertension • Peripartum syndrome related to toxemia • Ischemic heart disease • Valvular disease • Drug hypersensitivity • Chemotherapy • Cardiotoxic effects of drugs or alcohol

Hypertrophic cardiomyopathy	**Restrictive cardiomyopathy**
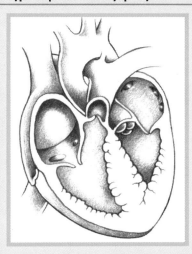	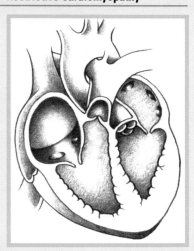
• Normal or decreased chamber size • Left ventricular hypertrophy • Thickened interventricular septum	• Decreased ventricular chamber size • Left ventricular hypertrophy
• Increased	• Increased
• Increased	• Normal
• Increased	• Increased
• Increased or decreased	• Normal or decreased
• Autosomal dominant trait • Hypertension • Obstructive valvular disease • Thyroid disease	• Amyloidosis • Sarcoidosis • Hemochromatosis • Infiltrative neoplastic disease

the atria and ventricles. Blood pooling in the ventricles increases the risk of emboli.

AGE ISSUE *Barth syndrome is a rare genetic disorder that can cause dilated cardiomyopathy in boys. This syndrome may be associated with skeletal muscle changes, short stature, neutropenia, and increased susceptibility to bacterial infections. Evidence of dilated cardiomyopathy may appear as early as the first few days or months of life.*

Unlike dilated cardiomyopathy, which affects systolic function, hypertrophic cardiomyopathy primarily affects diastolic function. The hypertrophied ventricle becomes stiff and noncompliant, and can't relax during ventricular filling. Consequently, ventricular filling is reduced and left ventricular filling pressure rises, causing a rise in left atrial and pulmonary venous pressures and leading to venous congestion and dyspnea. Ventricular filling time is further reduced as a compensatory response to tachycardia, leading to low CO. If papillary muscles become hypertrophied and don't close completely during contraction, mitral insufficiency occurs. The features of HOCM include asymmetrical left ventricular hypertrophy; hypertrophy of the intraventricular septum; rapid, forceful contractions of the left ventricle; impaired relaxation; and obstruction to left ventricular outflow. The forceful ejection of blood draws the anterior leaflet of the mitral valve to the intraventricular septum. This causes early closure of the outflow tract, decreasing ejection fraction. Moreover, intramural coronary arteries are abnormally small and may not be sufficient to supply the hypertrophied muscle with enough blood and oxygen to

meet the increased needs of the hyperdynamic muscle.

Restrictive cardiomyopathy is characterized by stiffness of the ventricle caused by left ventricular hypertrophy and endocardial fibrosis and thickening, thus reducing the ability of the ventricle to relax and fill during diastole. Moreover, the rigid myocardium fails to contract completely during systole. As a result, CO falls.

Comprehensive assessment

Generally, for patients with dilated or restrictive cardiomyopathy, the onset is insidious. As the disease progresses, exacerbations and hospitalizations are frequent regardless of the type of cardiomyopathy.

For the patient with dilated cardiomyopathy, signs and symptoms may be overlooked until left-sided heart failure occurs. Be sure to evaluate the patient's current condition and then compare it with that over the past 6 to 12 months. Signs and symptoms of dilated cardiomyopathy may include:

■ shortness of breath, orthopnea, dyspnea on exertion, paroxysmal nocturnal dyspnea, fatigue, and a dry cough at night due to left-sided heart failure
■ peripheral edema, hepatomegaly, jugular vein distention, and weight gain caused by right-sided heart failure
■ peripheral cyanosis associated with a low CO
■ tachycardia as a compensatory response to low CO
■ pansystolic murmur associated with mitral and tricuspid insufficiency secondary to cardiomegaly and weak papillary muscles
■ S_3 and S_4 gallop rhythms associated with heart failure
■ irregular pulse (if atrial fibrillation exists).

For the patient with hypertrophic cardiomyopathy, signs and symptoms may include:

■ angina caused by the inability of the intramural coronary arteries to supply enough blood to meet the increased oxygen demands of the hypertrophied heart

■ dyspnea due to elevated left ventricular filling pressure

■ fatigue associated with a reduced CO

■ peripheral pulse with a characteristic double impulse (pulsus bisferiens) caused by powerful left ventricular contractions and rapid ejection of blood during systole

■ abrupt arterial pulse secondary to vigorous left ventricular contractions

■ irregular pulse if an enlarged atrium causes atrial fibrillation.

Clinical manifestations of HOCM may include:

■ syncope resulting from arrhythmias or reduced ventricular filling leading to a reduced CO

■ systolic ejection murmur along the left sternal border and at the apex caused by mitral insufficiency

■ angina caused by the inability of the intramural coronary arteries to supply enough blood to meet the increased oxygen demands of the hypertrophied heart

■ activity intolerance due to worsening of outflow tract obstruction from exercise-induced catecholamine release

■ abrupt arterial pulse secondary to vigorous left ventricular contractions and early termination of left ventricular ejection

■ irregular pulse if an enlarged atrium causes atrial fibrillation.

The patient with restrictive cardiomyopathy presents with signs of heart failure. Signs and symptoms of restrictive cardiomyopathy may include:

■ fatigue, dyspnea, orthopnea, chest pain, edema, liver engorgement, peripheral cyanosis, pallor, and S_3 or S_4 gallop rhythms due to heart failure

■ systolic murmurs caused by mitral and tricuspid insufficiency.

Diagnosis
The following tests help diagnose cardiomyopathy:

■ Echocardiography confirms dilated cardiomyopathy.

■ Chest X-ray may reveal cardiomegaly associated with any of the cardiomyopathies.

■ Cardiac catheterization with possible heart biopsy can be definitive with hypertrophic cardiomyopathy.

■ Diagnosis requires elimination of other possible causes of heart failure and arrhythmias. (See *Comparing diagnostic tests in cardiomyopathy,* pages 76 and 77.)

Collaborations
A multidisciplinary approach to the patient's care is needed. Medical and nursing health care providers focus on maintaining and reestablishing CO and hemodynamic stability with the administration of medications, pacemakers, implantable cardioverter-defibrillator or intra-aortic balloon pump, and reducing myocardial oxygen demand with rest and limitation of activity. Surgical health care providers are usually consulted if the patient is considered a candidate for cardiac transplantation. Nutritional consultation may be necessary to help with dietary measures. Physical and occupational therapy may be necessary to help with activity limitations and energy conservation.

Comparing diagnostic tests in cardiomyopathy

Test	Dilated cardiomyopathy	Hypertrophic cardiomyopathy
Electrocardiography	Biventricular hypertrophy, sinus tachycardia, atrial enlargement, atrial and ventricular arrhythmias, bundle-branch block, and ST-segment and T-wave abnormalities	Left ventricular hypertrophy, ST-segment and T-wave abnormalities, left anterior hemiblock, Q waves in precordial and inferior leads, ventricular arrhythmias and, possibly, atrial fibrillation
Echocardiography	Left ventricular thrombi, global hypokinesia, enlarged atria, left ventricular dilation and, possibly, valvular abnormalities	Symmetrical thickening of the left ventricular wall and intraventricular septum and left atrial dilation
Chest X-ray	Cardiomegaly, pulmonary congestion, pulmonary venous hypertension, and pleural or pericardial effusions	Cardiomegaly
Cardiac catheterization	Elevated left atrial and left ventricular end-diastolic pressures, left ventricular enlargement, and mitral and tricuspid incompetence; may identify coronary artery disease as a cause	Elevated ventricular end-diastolic pressure and, possibly, mitral insufficiency, hyperdynamic systolic function, and aortic valve pressure gradient if aortic valve is stenotic
Radionuclide studies	Left ventricular dilation and hypokinesis, reduced ejection fraction	Reduced left ventricular volume, increased muscle mass, and ischemia

Treatment and care

No known cure exists for cardiomyopathy. Treatment is individualized based on the type of cardiomyopathy and the patient's condition.

For the patient with dilated cardiomyopathy, treatment may involve:
■ treatment of the underlying cause if identifiable
■ angiotensin-converting enzyme (ACE) inhibitors, as first-line therapy, to reduce afterload through vasodilation
■ diuretics, taken with ACE inhibitors, to reduce fluid retention

■ digoxin, for patients not responding to ACE inhibitor and diuretic therapy, to improve myocardial contractility
■ hydralazine and isosorbide dinitrate, in combination, to produce vasodilation
■ beta-adrenergic blockers for patients with mild or moderate heart failure
■ antiarrhythmics such as amiodarone, used cautiously, to control arrhythmias
■ an implantable cardioverter-defibrillator (ICD) to treat ventricular arrhythmias and for prophylaxis (due to high incidence of sudden death)
■ cardioversion to convert atrial fibrillation to sinus rhythm
■ pacemaker insertion to correct arrhythmias

Hypertrophic obstructive cardiomyopathy	Restrictive cardiomyopathy
Left ventricular hypertrophy with QRS complexes tallest across mid-precordium, ST-segment and T-wave abnormalities, left axis deviation, left atrial abnormality, supraventricular tachycardia, and ventricular tachycardia	Low voltage, hypertrophy, atrioventricular conduction defects, and arrhythmias
Asymmetrical septal hypertrophy; anterior movement of the anterior mitral leaflet during systole, early termination of left ventricular ejection that worsens with dobutamine or nitrate provocation, mitral insufficiency, and atrial dilation	Increased left ventricular muscle mass, normal or reduced left ventricular cavity size, and normal systolic function; rules out constrictive pericarditis
Normal or mild cardiomegaly	Cardiomegaly, pericardial effusion, and pulmonary congestion; increased left ventricular end-diastolic pressure; rules out constrictive pericarditis
Asymmetrical septal hypertrophy, early termination of systole with decreased ejection fraction, outflow tract pressure gradient increasing from the apex to just below the aortic valve, and mitral insufficiency	Normal or reduced systolic function and myocardial infiltration
Reduced left ventricular volume, increased septal muscle mass, and septal ischemia	Left ventricular hypertrophy with restricted ventricular filling

■ biventricular pacemaker for cardiac resynchronization therapy if symptoms continue despite optimal drug therapy, the patient has advanced heart failure, QRS duration is 0.13 second or more, or ejection fraction is 35% or less
■ anticoagulants (controversial) to reduce the risk of emboli
■ revascularization, such as coronary artery bypass graft surgery, if dilated cardiomyopathy is due to ischemia
■ valvular repair or replacement, if dilated cardiomyopathy is due to valve dysfunction
■ heart transplantation in patients refractory to medical therapy

■ lifestyle modifications, such as smoking cessation; low-fat, low-sodium diet; physical activity; and abstinence from alcohol.

Management of hypertrophic cardiomyopathy may involve:
■ optimal control of hypertension
■ aortic valve replacement if valve is stenotic
■ verapamil or diltiazem to reduce ventricular stiffness and elevated diastolic pressures
■ cardioversion to treat atrial fibrillation
■ anticoagulation to reduce the risk of systemic embolism with atrial fibrillation.

Treatment of HOCM may involve:
■ beta-adrenergic blockers to slow the heart rate, reduce myocardial oxygen demands, and increase ventricular filling by relaxing the obstructing muscle, thereby increasing CO
■ antiarrhythmic drugs, such as amiodarone, to reduce arrhythmias
■ cardioversion to treat atrial fibrillation
■ anticoagulation to reduce risk of systemic embolism with atrial fibrillation
■ verapamil and diltiazem to reduce ventricular stiffness and elevated diastolic pressures
■ ablation of the atrioventricular node and implantation of a dual-chamber pacemaker (controversial), in patients with HOCM and ventricular tachycardias, to reduce the outflow gradient by altering the pattern of ventricular contraction
■ ICD to treat ventricular arrhythmias
■ ventricular myotomy or myectomy (resection of the hypertrophied septum) to ease outflow tract obstruction and relieve symptoms
■ mitral valve replacement to treat mitral insufficiency
■ cardiac transplantation for intractable symptoms.

For the patient with restrictive cardiomyopathy, treatment may involve:
■ treatment of the underlying cause, such as administering deferoxamine to bind iron in restrictive cardiomyopathy due to hemochromatosis
■ digoxin, diuretics, and a restricted sodium diet to ease the symptoms of heart failure (no therapy exists for restricted ventricular filling)
■ oral vasodilators to decrease afterload and facilitate ventricular ejection.

Complications

Complications may include:
■ heart failure
■ arrhythmias
■ systemic or pulmonary embolization
■ sudden death.

Nursing considerations

■ Administer pharmacologic agents, as ordered, to promote adequate heart function.
■ Assess hemodynamic status approximately every 2 hours, or more frequently depending on the patient's condition.

ALERT *Keep in mind that right-atrial pressure, pulmonary artery pressure, and pulmonary wedge pressure are increased, and CO and cardiac index are decreased in a patient with cardiomyopathy. Although CO should be approximately 4 to 7 L/minute and a cardiac index of 2.5 to 4 L/minute/m², a patient may require a CO and cardiac index slightly below normal values.*

■ Monitor intake and output closely and obtain daily weight; institute fluid restrictions as ordered.
■ Institute continuous cardiac monitoring to evaluate for arrhythmias and, should any occur, begin expected treatment.
■ Assess the patient for possible adverse effects of pharmacologic agents administered, such as orthostatic hypotension with vasodilators, diuretics, or ACE inhibitors. Urge the patient to change positions slowly.
■ Auscultate heart and breath sounds, being alert for S_3 heart sounds or murmurs, or crackles, rhonchi, and wheezes indicative of heart failure; monitor vital signs for changes, especially a heart rate greater than 100 beats/minute, respiratory rate greater than 20 breaths/minute,

a systolic blood pressure less than 90 mm Hg, and an elevated temperature, all of which suggest heart failure.

■ Assist the patient with activities of daily living to decrease oxygen demand. Assess patient's response to activity, such as complaints of shortness of breath, increases in heart rate or systolic blood pressure over resting rate, or changes in cardiac rhythm.

■ Administer supplemental oxygen as ordered; assess level of consciousness for changes, such as restlessness or decreased responsiveness, indicating diminished cerebral perfusion. If the patient has a pulmonary artery catheter in place, evaluate mixed venous oxygen saturation levels; if not, monitor oxygen saturation levels via pulse oximetry.

■ Organize care to promote periods of rest for the patient.

■ Prepare the patient, as indicated for insertion of pacemaker, ICD, intra-aortic balloon pump, or cardiac transplantation.

Patient teaching

■ Explain the underlying disorder and rationales for treatment; teach the patient how to monitor intake, output and weights, with specific instructions for when to notify the physician.

■ Instruct the patient and his family in lifestyle changes and restrictions including occupation, sports, and physical or strenuous activities.

■ Teach the patient about care following insertion of ICD or pacemaker, as appropriate.

■ Educate the patient about required drug therapy, including the reason for drug, dosage and schedule, possible adverse effects, and signs and symptoms to report to the physician.

■ Urge the patient to continue medications even if asymptomatic.

■ Advise the patient about the need for follow-up, such as physician visits and laboratory testing for monitoring of medication levels.

Continuous cardiac monitoring

Because it allows continuous observation of the heart's electrical activity, cardiac monitoring is used for the patient with conduction disturbances and for a patient at risk for life-threatening arrhythmias. Like other forms of electrocardiography (ECG), continuous cardiac monitoring uses electrodes placed on the patient's chest to transmit electrical signals that are converted into a tracing of cardiac rhythm on an oscilloscope.

Two types of monitoring may be performed: hardwire or telemetry. In hardwire monitoring, the patient is connected to a monitor at the bedside. The rhythm display appears at bedside, but it may also be transmitted to a console at a remote location. Telemetry uses a small transmitter connected to the ambulatory patient to send electrical signals to another location where they're displayed on a monitor screen. Battery-powered and portable, telemetry frees the patient from cumbersome wires and cables and lets him be comfortably mobile and safely isolated from the electrical leakage and accidental shock occasionally associated with hardwire monitoring. Telemetry is especially useful for monitoring arrhythmias that occur during sleep, rest, exercise, or stressful situations. However, unlike hardwire monitoring, telemetry can monitor only heart rate and rhythm.

Regardless of the type, cardiac monitors can display the patient's heart rate and rhythm, produce a printed record of cardiac rhythm, and sound an alarm if the heart rate exceeds or falls below specified limits. Monitors also recognize and count abnormal heartbeats as well as changes. For example, ST-segment monitoring helps detect myocardial ischemia, electrolyte imbalance, coronary artery spasm, and hypoxic events. The ST segment represents early ventricular repolarization, and any changes in this waveform component reflect alterations in myocardial oxygenation.

Equipment

Cardiac monitor ▪ leadwires ▪ patient cable ▪ disposable pregelled electrodes (number of electrodes varies from three to five, depending on patient's needs) ▪ alcohol pads ▪ 4″ × 4″ gauze pads ▪ washcloth ▪ optional: clippers

For telemetry monitoring

Transmitter ▪ transmitter pouch ▪ telemetry battery pack, leads, and electrodes

Essential steps

▪ Plug the cardiac monitor into an electrical outlet and turn it on to warm up the unit while the patient and equipment is prepared.
▪ Insert the cable into the appropriate socket in the monitor. Connect the leadwires to the cable (*Note*: In some systems, the leadwires are permanently secured to the cable). Each leadwire should indicate the location for attachment to the patient: right arm (RA), left arm (LA), right leg (RL), left leg (LL),

and ground (C or V). This should appear on the leadwire — if it's permanently connected — or at the connection of the leadwires and cable to the patient. Connect an electrode to each of the leadwires, carefully checking that each leadwire is in its correct outlet.
▪ For telemetry monitoring, insert a new battery into the transmitter. Be sure to match the poles on the battery with the polar markings on the transmitter case.
▪ Press the button at the top of the unit to test the battery charge and test the unit to ensure that the battery is operational. If the leadwires aren't permanently affixed to the telemetry unit, attach them securely. If they must be attached individually, be sure to connect each one to the correct outlet.
▪ Explain the procedure to the patient, provide privacy, and ask the patient to expose his chest. Wash your hands.
▪ Determine electrode positions on the patient's chest based on which system and lead you're using. (See *Positioning monitoring leads*.)
▪ If the leadwires and patient cable aren't permanently attached, verify that the electrode placement corresponds to the label on the patient cable.
▪ If necessary, clip the hair from an area about 4″ (10 cm) in diameter around each electrode site. Clean the area with an alcohol pad and dry it completely to remove skin secretions that may interfere with electrode function. Gently abrade the dried area by rubbing it briskly until it reddens to remove dead skin cells and to promote better electrical contact with living cells. (Some electrodes have a small, rough patch for abrading the skin; otherwise, use a dry washcloth or a dry gauze pad.)

Positioning monitoring leads

This chart shows the correct electrode positions for some of the monitoring leads you'll use most often—a five-leadwire system, a three-leadwire system, and a telemetry system.

In the three- and five- leadwire systems, the electrode positions for one lead may be identical to those for another lead. When that happens, change the lead selector switch to the setting that corresponds to the lead you want. In some cases, you'll need to reposition the electrodes.

In the telemetry monitoring system, you can create the same leads as the other system with just two electrodes and a ground wire.

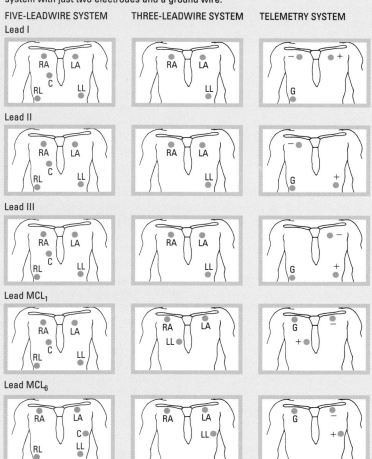

FIVE-LEADWIRE SYSTEM   THREE-LEADWIRE SYSTEM   TELEMETRY SYSTEM

Lead I

Lead II

Lead III

Lead MCL_1

Lead MCL_6

Key: C, chest; G, ground; LA, left arm; LL, left leg; RA, right arm; and RL, right leg.

■ Remove the backing from the pregelled electrode. Check the gel for moistness. If it's dry, discard the electrode and replace it with a fresh one.

■ Apply the electrode to the site and press firmly to ensure a tight seal. Repeat with the remaining electrodes.

■ After all the electrodes are in place, check for a tracing on the cardiac monitor. Assess the quality of the ECG. Then verify that the monitor is detecting each beat by comparing the digital heart rate display with your count of the patient's apical heart rate.

■ If necessary, use the gain control to adjust the size of the rhythm tracing and use the position control to adjust the waveform position on the recording paper.

■ Set the upper and lower limits of the heart rate alarm, based on unit policy. Turn the alarm on.

For telemetry monitoring

■ Prepare the patient and equipment as you would for hardwire monitoring.

■ Apply the electrode to the appropriate site by pressing one side of the electrode against the patient's skin, pulling gently, and then pressing the other side against the skin. Press your fingers in a circular motion around the electrode to fix the gel and stabilize the electrode. Repeat for each electrode, attaching each to the end of each leadwire.

■ Place the transmitter in the pouch. Tie the pouch strings around the patient's neck and waist, making sure that the pouch fits snugly without causing him discomfort. If no pouch is available, place the transmitter in the patient's bathrobe pocket.

■ Check the patient's waveform for clarity, position, and size. Adjust the gain and baseline as needed. (If necessary, ask the patient to remain resting or sitting in his room while you locate his telemetry monitor at the central station.)

■ Obtain a rhythm strip by pressing the RECORD key at the central station. Label the strip with the patient's name and room number, date, and time. Also, identify the rhythm. Place the rhythm strip in the appropriate location in the patient's chart.

Complications

Skin irritation due to electrode placement may occur. Electrodes should be repositioned every 24 hours or as necessary.

Nursing considerations

■ Evaluate the waveform on the monitor frequently, noting the quality of the ECG. (See *Troubleshooting cardiac monitor problems.*) Note any evidence of problems and report immediately. As ordered, obtain a rhythm strip and evaluate for changes.

ALERT *Be aware that some types of artifacts resemble arrhythmias and the monitor will interpret them as such. For example, the monitor may sense a small movement as a potentially lethal ventricular arrhythmia. Therefore, always remember to treat the patient, not the monitor.*

■ Ensure that all electrical equipment and outlets are grounded to avoid electric shock and interference (artifacts). Also, ensure that the patient is clean and dry to prevent electric shock.

■ Open the electrode packages just before using to prevent the gel from drying out.

■ Avoid placing the electrodes on bony prominences, hairy locations,

Troubleshooting cardiac monitor problems

Problem	Possible cause	Interventions
Artifact (waveform interference)	● Patient experiencing seizures, chills, or anxiety	● If the patient is having a seizure, notify the physician and intervene as ordered. ● Keep the patient warm and encourage him to relax.
	● Dirty or corroded connections	● Replace dirty or corroded wires.
	● Improper electrode applications	● Check the electrodes and reapply if necessary. Clean the patient's skin well because skin oils and dead skin cells inhibit conduction. ● Check the electrode gel. If the gel is dry, apply new electrodes.
	● Short circuit in leadwires or cable	● Replace broken equipment.
	● Electrical interference from other equipment in the room	● Make sure all electrical equipment is attached to a common ground. Check all three-pronged plugs to ensure that none are loose. Notify the biomedical department.
	● Static electricity interference from inadequate room humidity	● Regulate room humidity to 40% if possible.
False-high-rate alarm	● Gain setting too high, particularly with MCL_1 setting	● Assess patient for signs and symptoms of hyperkalemia. ● Reset gain.
	● HIGH alarm set too low or LOW alarm set too high	● Set alarm limits according to patient's heart rate.
Weak signals	● Improper electrode application	● Reapply the electrodes.
	● QRS complex too small to register	● Reset gain so that height of complex is greater than 1 mV. ● Try monitoring the patient on another lead.
	● Wire or cable failure	● Replace any faulty wires or cables.

(continued)

Troubleshooting cardiac monitor problems *(continued)*

Problem	Possible cause	Interventions
Wandering baseline	• Patient restlessness	• Encourage the patient to relax.
	• Chest wall movement during respiration	• Make sure tension on cable isn't pulling the electrode away from the patient's body.
	• Improper electrode application; electrode positioned over a bone	• Reposition improperly placed electrodes.
Fuzzy baseline (electrical interference)	• Electrical interference from other equipment in the room	• Ensure that all electrical equipment is attached to a common ground. • Check all three-pronged plugs to ensure that none are loose.
	• Improper grounding of the patient's bed	• Ensure that the bed ground is attached to the room's common ground.
	• Electrode malfunction	• Replace electrodes.
Baseline (no waveform)	• Improper electrode placement (perpendicular to axis of heart)	• Reposition improperly positioned electrodes.
	• Electrode disconnection	• Check if electrodes are disconnected.
	• Dry electrode gel	• Check electrode gel. If dry, apply new electrodes.
	• Wire or cable failure	• Replace any faulty wires or cables.

areas where defibrillator pads will be placed, or areas for chest compression.
■ If the patient's skin is very oily, scaly, or diaphoretic, rub the electrode site with a dry 4″ × 4″ gauze pad before applying the electrode to help reduce interference in the tracing. Have the patient breathe normally during the procedure. If his respirations distort the recording, ask him to hold his breath briefly to reduce baseline wander in the tracing.
■ Assess skin integrity and reposition the electrodes every 24 hours or as necessary.

■ If the patient is being monitored by telemetry, show him how the transmitter works. If applicable, show him the button that will produce a recording of his ECG at the central station. Teach him how to push the button whenever he has symptoms. This causes the central console to print a rhythm strip. Tell the patient to remove the transmitter if he takes a shower or bath, but stress that he should tell you before removing the unit.

■ Document in the patient's medical record and the facility's flowchart, the date and time that monitoring begins and the monitoring lead used.

■ Obtain a rhythm strip at least every 8 hours and with any changes in the patient's condition (or as stated by your facility's policy). Label the rhythm strip with the patient's name and room number, the date, and the time and place in the patient's chart.

Cardiac output monitoring

Measuring cardiac output (CO) — the amount of blood ejected by the heart — helps evaluate cardiac function. The most widely used method for monitoring CO is the bolus thermodilution technique. Performed at the bedside, the thermodilution technique is the most practical method of evaluating the cardiac status of critically ill patients and those suspected of having cardiac disease. Other methods include the Fick method and the dye dilution test. (See *Other methods of measuring cardiac output,* page 86.)

To measure CO, a quantity of solution colder than the patient's blood is injected into the right atrium via a port on a pulmonary artery (PA) catheter. This indicator solution mixes with the blood as it travels through the right ventricle into the pulmonary artery, and a thermistor on the catheter registers the change in temperature of the flowing blood. A computer then plots the temperature change over time as a curve and calculates flow based on the area under the curve.

Iced or room-temperature injectant may be used. The choice should be based on facility policy as well as the patient's status. The accuracy of the bolus thermodilution technique depends on the computer being able to differentiate the temperature change caused by the injectant in the pulmonary artery and the temperature changes in the pulmonary artery. Because iced injectant is colder than room-temperature injectant, it provides a stronger signal to be detected.

Typically, however, room-temperature injectant is more convenient and provides equally accurate measurements. Iced injectant may be more accurate in patients with high or low COs, hypothermic patients, or when smaller volumes of injectant must be used (3 to 5 ml), as in patients with volume restrictions or in children.

Some PA catheters contain a filament that permits continuous CO monitoring. With these catheters, an average in CO value is determined over a span of 3 minutes and updated every 30 to 60 seconds. This type of monitoring allows for close scrutiny of the patient's hemodynamic status and prompt intervention should problems arise.

Other methods of measuring cardiac output

In the Fick method (especially useful in detecting low cardiac output [CO] levels), the blood oxygen content is measured before and after it passes through the lungs. First, blood is removed from the pulmonary and brachial arteries and analyzed for oxygen content. Next, a spirometer measures oxygen consumption—the amount of air entering the lungs each minute. Finally, CO is calculated using this formula:

$$CO \text{ (L/minute)} = \frac{\text{oxygen consumption (ml/minute)}}{\text{arterial oxygen content} - \text{venous oxygen content (ml/minute)}}$$

In the dye dilution test, a known volume and concentration of dye is injected into the pulmonary artery; at the same time, the amount of dye in the brachial artery is measured. To calculate CO, these values are entered into a formula or plotted into a time and dilution-concentration curve. A computer similar to one used for the thermodilution test performs the computation. Dye dilution measurements are particularly helpful in detecting intracardiac shunts and valvular insufficiency.

Equipment

For the thermodilution method

Thermodilution PA catheter in position ▪ output computer and cables (or a module for the bedside cardiac monitor) ▪ closed or open injectant delivery system ▪ 10-ml syringe ▪ 500-ml bag of dextrose 5% in water or normal saline solution ▪ crushed ice and water (if iced injectant is used)

The newer bedside cardiac monitors measure CO continuously, using either an invasive or a noninvasive method. If your bedside monitor doesn't have this capability, you'll need a freestanding CO computer.

Essential steps

▪ Wash your hands thoroughly, and assemble the equipment at the patient's bedside. Insert the closed injectant system tubing into the 500-ml bag of I.V. solution. Connect the 10-ml syringe to the system tubing and prime the tubing with I.V. solution until it's free from air. Then clamp the tubing. The steps that follow differ, depending on the temperature of the injectant.

For room-temperature injectant, closed delivery system

▪ After clamping the tubing, connect the primed system to the stopcock of the proximal injectant lumen of the PA catheter.

▪ Connect the temperature probe from the CO computer to the closed injectant system's flow-through housing device.

▪ Connect the CO computer cable to the thermistor connector on the PA catheter and verify the blood temperature reading.

▪ Turn on the CO computer and enter the correct computation constant as provided by the catheter's manufacturer. The constant is determined by the volume and temperature of the injectant as well as the size and type of catheter.

AGE ISSUE *For children, you'll need to adjust the computation constant to reflect a smaller volume and a smaller catheter size.*

▪ Unclamp the I.V. tubing and withdraw 5 ml of solution into the syringe.

AGE ISSUE *For children, use 3 ml or less of solution.*

■ Inject the solution to flow past the temperature sensor, verifying that the injectant temperature registers between 43° and 54° F (6.1° and 12.2° C) on the computer.

■ Verify presence of a pulmonary artery waveform on the cardiac monitor.

■ Withdraw exactly 10 ml of cooled solution before reclamping the tubing.

■ Turn the stopcock at the catheter injectant hub to open a fluid path between the injectant lumen of the PA catheter and syringe.

■ Press the START button on the CO computer or wait for the INJECT message to flash. Then inject the solution smoothly within 4 seconds, making sure it doesn't leak at the connectors.

■ If available, analyze the contour of the thermodilution washout curve on a strip chart recorder for a rapid upstroke and a gradual, smooth return to baseline.

■ Wait 1 minute between injections and repeat the procedure until three values are within 10% and 15% of the median value. Compute the average and record the patient's CO.

■ Return the stopcock to its original position, and make sure the injectant delivery system tubing is clamped.

■ Verify presence of a pulmonary artery waveform on the cardiac monitor.

For iced-injectant, closed delivery system

■ After clamping the tubing, place the coiled segment into the Styrofoam container and add crushed ice and water to cover the entire coil.

■ Let the solution cool for 15 to 20 minutes.

■ Proceed as for the room-temperature injectant, closed delivery system detailed above.

Complications

Potential complications include carotid artery puncture, air embolism, hemorrhage, pneumothorax, cardiac tamponade, and cardiac arrhythmias secondary to insertion of PA catheter.

Nursing considerations

■ Make sure the patient is in a comfortable position. Tell him not to move during the procedure because movement can cause an error in measurement.

■ Explain to the patient that the procedure will help determine how well his heart is pumping and that he'll feel no discomfort.

■ Perform CO measurements and monitoring at least every 1 to 2 hours, especially if the patient is receiving vasoactive or inotropic agents, or fluids are being added or restricted.

■ Discontinue CO measurements when the patient is hemodynamically stable and weaned from his vasoactive and inotropic medications. You can leave the PA catheter inserted for pressure measurements.

■ Disconnect and discard the injectant delivery system and the I.V. bag. Cover any exposed stopcocks with air-occlusive caps.

■ Monitor the patient for signs and symptoms of inadequate perfusion, including restlessness, fatigue, changes in level of consciousness, prolonged capillary refill time, diminished peripheral pulses, oliguria, and pale, cool skin.

■ Remember that the normal range for CO is 4 to 8 L/minute. You can better assess the adequacy of your patient's CO by calculating his cardiac index (CI), adjusted for his body size.

■ To calculate the patient's CI, divide his CO by his body surface area (BSA), a function of height and weight. For example, a CO of 4 L/minute might be adequate for a 65″, 120-lb (165.1-cm, 54.4-kg) patient (normally a BSA of 1.59 and a CI of 2.5) but would be inadequate for a 74″, 230-lb (188-cm, 104.3-kg) patient (normally a BSA of 2.26 and a CI of 1.8). The normal CI for adults ranges from 2.5 to 4.2 L/minute/m^2; for pregnant women, 3.5 to 6.5 L/minute/m^2.

■ **AGE ISSUE** *Normal CI for infants and children is 3.5 to 4 L/minute/m^2. Normal CI for elderly adults is 2 to 2.5 L/minute/m^2.*

■ Add the fluid volume injected for CO determinations to the patient's total intake. Injectant delivery of 30 ml/hour will contribute 720 ml to the patient's 24-hour intake.

■ After CO measurement, make sure the clamp on the injectant bag is secured to prevent inadvertent delivery of the injectant.

■ Record the patient's CO, CI, and other hemodynamic values and vital signs at the time of measurement. Note the patient's position during measurement and any other unusual occurrences, such as bradycardia or neurologic changes.

Coronary artery bypass graft

Coronary artery bypass graft (CABG) circumvents an occluded coronary artery with an autogenous graft (usually a segment of the saphenous vein from the leg or internal mammarian artery), thereby restoring blood flow to the myocardium. Performed to prevent a myocardial infarction (MI) in a patient with acute or chronic myocardial ischemia, CABG is one of the most commonly performed surgeries today in the United States. The need for CABG is determined from the results of cardiac catheterization and patient symptomology.

Prime candidates for CABG include patients who have any of the following:

■ medically uncontrolled angina interfering with the patient's lifestyle
■ left main coronary artery stenosis
■ severe proximal left anterior descending coronary artery stenosis
■ three-vessel disease with proximal stenoses or left ventricular dysfunction
■ three-vessel disease with normal left ventricular function at rest but with inducible ischemia and poor exercise capacity.

If successful, CABG can relieve anginal pain, improve cardiac function and, possibly, enhance the patient's quality of life. CABG techniques vary according to the patient's condition and the number of arteries being bypassed. Newer surgical techniques, such as the mini-CABG and direct coronary artery bypass, are being used to reduce the risk of cerebral complications and accelerate recovery for a patient requiring grafts of only one or two arteries. (See *Minimally invasive direct coronary artery bypass.*)

Procedure

After the patient has received general anesthesia, surgery begins with graft harvesting by making a series of inci-

Minimally invasive direct coronary artery bypass

Minimally invasive direct coronary artery bypass (MIDCAB) is a newer procedure available for performing CABG, It's used primarily in patients who have disease in their left anterior descending or right coronary artery. It isn't used for those patients who have CAD in multiple vessels. In a traditional CABG, a 12" (30.5 cm) incision is made into the chest (see below right) and the sternum is divided to provide access to the heart. The patient is then placed on the heart-lung bypass machine. With a MIDCAB, a small incision is made in the chest, directly over the heart (see below left). A MIDCAB does not require a heart lung bypass but only requires the heart rate to be slowed down with the use of medications.

Other variations of MIDCAB include port access bypass surgery, off-pump bypass surgery, keyhole or buttonhole surgery or laparoscopic bypass, and robotic visualization techniques.

MIDCAB

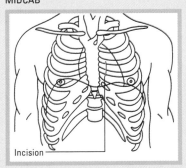

Incision

TRADITIONAL CABG

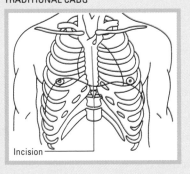

Incision

sions in the patient's thigh or calf and removing a saphenous vein segment for grafting. Most surgeons prefer using a segment of the internal mammarian artery because this provides an artery doing the job of an artery, as opposed to using a vein to do the work of an artery.

After the autografts are obtained, the surgeon performs a medial sternotomy and exposes the heart. He then initiates cardiopulmonary bypass. To reduce myocardial oxygen demands during surgery and to protect the heart, he induces cardiac hypothermia and standstill by injecting a cold cardioplegic solution (potassium-enriched saline solution) into the aortic root.

After the patient is fully prepared, the surgeon sutures one end of the venous graft to the ascending aorta and the other end to a patent coronary artery distal to the occlusion. He sutures the graft in a reversed position to promote proper blood flow. He repeats this procedure for each artery he bypasses.

When the grafts are in place, he flushes the cardioplegic solution from the heart and discontinues cardiopulmonary bypass. He then implants epicardial pacing electrodes, inserts a chest tube, closes the incision, and applies a sterile dressing.

Complications

CABG can cause many postoperative complications, including arrhythmias, hypertension or hypotension, cardiac tamponade, thromboembolism, hemorrhage, postpericardiotomy syndrome, and MI. Noncardiac complications include stroke, postoperative depression or emotional instability, pulmonary embolism, decreased renal function, and infection. Also, such problems as graft rupture or closure or the development of atherosclerosis in other coronary arteries may require repeat surgery.

Nursing considerations

When caring for a CABG patient, your major roles include patient instruction and caring for the patient's changing cardiovascular needs.

Before CABG

■ Reinforce the physician's explanation of the surgery.

■ Explain the complex equipment and procedures that will be used on the critical care unit or postanesthesia care unit.

■ Inform him that he'll awaken from surgery with an endotracheal (ET) tube in place and be connected to a mechanical ventilator. He'll also be connected to a cardiac monitor and have in place a nasogastric tube, a chest tube, an indwelling urinary catheter, arterial lines, epicardial pacing wires and, possibly, a pulmonary artery catheter. Tell him that discomfort will be minimal and the equipment will be removed as soon as possible.

■ Review techniques of incentive spirometry and range of motion with the patient.

■ Make sure the patient or a responsible family member has signed a consent form.

■ Before the surgery, prepare the patient's skin as ordered.

■ Immediately before surgery, assist with pulmonary artery catheterization and insertion of arterial lines. Begin cardiac monitoring.

After CABG

■ Following CABG, look for signs of hemodynamic compromise, such as severe hypotension, decreased cardiac output, and shock.

■ Institute warming procedures as per the facility's policy.

■ Check and record vital signs and hemodynamic parameters every 5 to 15 minutes until the patient's condition stabilizes. Administer medications and titrate according to patient's response as ordered

■ Monitor the electrocardiogram (ECG) continuously for disturbances in heart rate and rhythm. If you detect serious abnormalities, notify the physician and be prepared to assist with epicardial pacing or, if necessary, cardioversion or defibrillation.

■ To ensure adequate myocardial perfusion, keep arterial pressure within the limits set by the physician. Usually, mean arterial pressure (MAP) below 70 mm Hg results in inadequate tissue perfusion; pressure above 110 mm Hg can cause hemorrhage and graft rupture. Monitor pulmonary artery, central venous, and left atrial pressures as ordered.

■ Frequently evaluate the patient's peripheral pulses, capillary refill time, and skin temperature and color, and auscultate for heart sounds; report any abnormalities.

■ Evaluate tissue oxygenation by assessing breath sounds, chest excursion, and symmetry of chest expansion. Check arterial blood gas (ABG) analysis results every 2 to 4 hours, and adjust ventilator settings to keep ABG values within ordered limits.

■ Maintain chest tube drainage at the ordered negative pressure (usually –10 to –40 cm H_2O), and assess regularly for hemorrhage, excessive drainage (greater than 200 ml/hour), and sudden decrease or cessation of drainage.

■ Monitor the patient's intake and output, and assess for electrolyte imbalance, especially hypokalemia. Assess urine output at least hourly during the immediate postoperative period and then less frequently as the patient's condition stabilizes.

■ As the patient's incisional pain increases, give an analgesic as ordered. Give other drugs as ordered.

■ Throughout the recovery period, assess for symptoms of stroke, pulmonary embolism, and impaired renal perfusion.

■ After weaning the patient from the ventilator and removing the ET tube, provide chest physiotherapy. Start him on incentive spirometry, and encourage him to cough, turn frequently, and deep-breathe. Assist him with range-of-motion exercises, as ordered, to enhance peripheral circulation and prevent thrombus formation.

■ Monitor the elderly patient closely for complications.

AGE ISSUE *Older adult patients are at high risk for developing complications after CABG because they have a smaller margin of physiologic reserve and a decreased ability to compensate or adapt to change. Infection, hemorrhage, blood pressure changes, and fluid and electrolyte imbalances are more problematic in the older adult. Inelasticity of blood vessels, poor nutritional status, increased risk of infection, and decreased cardiac, respiratory, and renal reserves can cause complications to occur more often. Watch for pneumonia, delayed wound healing or wound infection, MI, arrhythmias, intestinal obstruction, confusion, and adverse drug reactions.*

■ Explain that postpericardiotomy syndrome commonly develops after open-heart surgery. Inform the patient about the signs and symptoms, such as fever, muscle and joint pain, weakness, or chest discomfort.

■ Prepare the patient for the possibility of postoperative depression, which may not develop until weeks after discharge. Reassure him that this depression is normal and should pass quickly.

■ Maintain nothing-by-mouth status until bowel sounds return. Then begin clear liquids and advance diet as tolerated and as ordered. Expect sodium and cholesterol restrictions. Explain that this diet can help reduce the risk of recurrent arterial occlusion.

Patient teaching

■ Teach the patient about dose, frequency of administration, and possible adverse effects of prescribed medications.

■ Advise female patients who have had a midline sternotomy that the scar tissue may be sensitive for up to a year.

■ Encourage the patient to follow his prescribed diet; enlist the aid of a dietitian for proper food choices.

■ Instruct the patient to maintain a balance between activity and rest. Tell him to try to sleep at least 8 hours per night, to schedule a short rest period for each afternoon, and to rest frequently when engaging in tiring physical activity. As appropriate, tell him he can climb stairs, engage in sexual activity, take baths and showers, and do light chores. Tell him to avoid lifting heavy objects (more than 20 lb [9.1 kg]), driving a car, or doing strenuous work (such as lawn mowing and vacuuming) until his physician grants permission. If the physician has prescribed an exercise program, encourage the patient to follow it.

■ Refer the patient to a local chapter of the Mended Hearts Club and the American Heart Association for information and support.

■ Advise the patient to become involved in a smoking-cessation program and to avoid smoking.

Defibrillation

Defibrillation involves the use of electrode paddles to direct an electric current through the patient's heart. The current causes the myocardium to depolarize, which in turn encourages the sinoatrial node to resume control of the heart's electrical activity. The electrode paddles delivering the current may be placed on the patient's chest or, during cardiac surgery, directly on the myocardium.

Because specific arrhythmias can lead to death if not corrected, the success of defibrillation depends on early recognition and quick treatment (see algorithms earlier in this chapter).

Ventricular fibrillation (VF) is one such arrhythmia. In addition to treating VF, defibrillation may also be used to treat ventricular tachycardia (VT) that doesn't produce a pulse. Recently, a new type of defibrillation has been introduced in hospitals. Biphasic defibrillation uses lower energy levels and fewer shocks, thus reducing damage to the myocardial muscle. For more information on this new technology, see *Biphasic defibrillators*.

Equipment

Defibrillator ■ external paddles ■ internal paddles (sterilized for cardiac surgery) ■ conductive medium pads ■ electrocardiogram (ECG) monitor with recorder ■ oxygen therapy equipment ■ handheld resuscitation bag ■ airway equipment ■ emergency pacing equipment ■ emergency cardiac medications

Essential steps

■ Assess the patient to determine whether he lacks a pulse. Call for help and perform cardiopulmonary resuscitation (CPR) until the defibrillator and other emergency equipment arrive.

■ If the defibrillator has "quick-look" capability, place the paddles on the patient's chest to quickly view his cardiac rhythm. Otherwise, connect the monitoring leads of the defibrillator to the patient and assess his cardiac rhythm.

■ Expose the patient's chest and apply conductive pads at the paddle placement positions.

– For anterolateral placement, place one paddle to the right of the upper sternum, just below the right clavicle, and the other over the fifth or sixth intercostal space at the left anterior axillary line.

Biphasic defibrillators

With biphasic defibrillation, pad or paddle placement is the same as with the monophasic defibrillator; however, the electrical current discharged from the pads or paddles travels in a positive direction for a specified duration and then reverses and flows in a negative direction for the remaining time of the electrical discharge. It delivers two currents of electricity and lowers the defibrillation threshold of the heart muscle, making it possible to successfully defibrillate ventricular fibrillation (VF) with smaller amounts of energy. Instead of using 200 joules, an initial shock of 150 joules is often effective. The biphasic defibrillator is able to adjust for differences in impedance or the resistance of the current through the chest. This helps reduce the number of shocks needed to terminate VF. Biphasic defibrillators, when used at the clinically appropriate energy level, may be used for defibrillation and, when placed in the synchronized mode, may be used for synchronized cardioversion.

– For anteroposterior placement, place the anterior paddle directly over the heart at the precordium, to the left of the lower sternal border. Place the flat posterior paddle under the patient's body beneath the heart and immediately below the scapulae (but not under the vertebral column).

■ Turn on the defibrillator and, if performing external defibrillation, set the energy level for 200 joules for an adult patient; initially 2 joules/kg then 4 joules/kg for a child.

■ Charge the paddles by pressing the charge buttons, which are located either on the machine or on the paddles themselves.

■ Place the paddles over the conductive pads and press firmly against the patient's chest, using 25 lb (11.3 kg) of pressure.

ALERT *Keep in mind that a conducting gel or paste may be used instead of conductive pads. In this case, be sure to use only the gel or paste specified for use with the paddles.*

■ Reassess the patient's cardiac rhythm.

■ If the patient remains in VF or pulseless VT, instruct all personnel to stand clear of the patient and the bed.

■ Discharge the current by pressing both paddle charge buttons simultaneously.

ALERT *When discharging the current, make sure that no one is touching the patient or the bed because the electric current could be conducted through the patient or the bed and passed to the person in contact with the patient or bed.*

■ Leaving the paddles in position on the patient's chest, reassess the patient's cardiac rhythm and have someone else assess the pulse.

■ If necessary, prepare to defibrillate a second time. Instruct someone to reset the energy level on the defibrillator to 200 to 300 joules. Announce that you're preparing to defibrillate and follow the procedure described above.

■ Reassess the patient. If defibrillation is again necessary, instruct someone to reset the energy level to 360 joules. Then follow the same procedure as before.

■ Perform the three countershocks in rapid succession, reassessing the patient's rhythm before each defibrillation.

■ If the patient still has no pulse after three initial defibrillations, resume CPR, give supplemental oxygen, and begin administering appropriate medications such as epinephrine. Also, consider possible causes for failure of the patient's rhythm to convert, such as acidosis and hypoxia.

■ If defibrillation restores a normal rhythm, check the patient's central and peripheral pulses and obtain a blood pressure reading, heart rate, and respiratory rate. Assess the patient's level of consciousness, cardiac rhythm, breath sounds, skin color, and urine output. Obtain baseline arterial blood gas levels and a 12-lead ECG. Provide supplemental oxygen, ventilation, and medications as needed. Check the patient's chest for electrical burns and treat them as ordered with corticosteroid or lanolin-based creams. Also, prepare the defibrillator for immediate reuse.

Complications

Defibrillation can cause accidental electric shock to those providing care. Use of an insufficient amount of conductive medium can lead to skin burns.

Nursing considerations

■ Familiarize yourself with your facility's equipment because defibrillators vary from one manufacturer to the next.

■ Be sure to check defibrillator operation at least every 8 hours and after each use.

■ Continue to monitor the patient frequently for changes after defibrillation, including vital signs and heart rate. If not already being done, institute continuous cardiac monitoring as ordered.

■ Keep in mind that defibrillation can be affected by several factors, including paddle size and placement, condition of the patient's myocardium, duration of the arrhythmia, chest resistance, and the number of countershocks.

■ Document the procedure, including the patient's ECG rhythms before and after defibrillation, the number of times defibrillation was performed, the voltage used during each attempt, whether a pulse returned, whether CPR was used, how the airway was maintained, the dosage, route, and time of any drugs administered, and the patient's outcome.

Electrophysiologic study

Electrophysiologic study (EPS), an invasive test, is a specialized form of cardiac catheterization specifically done to identify arrhythmias, determine their specific characteristics such as origin, and identify appropriate management strategies for treatment. This test can be used to provide information about the underlying cause of syncope, for example, bradycardia. It's also helpful in evaluating patients with tachyarrhythmias, specifically those due to reentry.

Procedure

With the patient under conscious sedation, the physician inserts multielectrode catheters into a major vein, guiding the catheters to various locations within the heart. The femoral vein is typically the site for catheter insertion; however, if the patient has deep vein thrombosis or a vena caval filter in place, a superior vein is used for insertion. For a complete study, three catheters are used. One catheter is placed high in the right atrium; a second one is placed at the apex of the right ventricle; and a third one is placed at the tricuspid valve. When the catheters are in place, a baseline electrocardiogram (ECG) using leads I, aV_F, V_1, and V_6 is obtained. Electrodes are also placed on the patient's body to obtain simultaneous recordings. The physician uses the electrodes on the catheters to stimulate the patient's heart; for example, to induce an arrhythmia. These same electrodes can also be used to defibrillate the heart internally should an arrhythmia occur spontaneously. During this programmed stimulation, external and intracardiac ECGs are being continuously monitored so that when an event occurs, it can be evaluated and treated as necessary.

During EPS, various medications, such as isoproterenol, procainamide, atropine, and adenosine may be used for diagnostic and treatment purposes. For example, if an arrhythmia is induced by the stimulation, medications and other strategies such as electrical therapies may be used to end the arrhythmia. The study is repeated after each medication or strategy is used to evaluate which therapies or combinations are most effective in controlling the arrhythmia. In addition, if a patient has been receiving antiarrhythmic therapy and the physician can't induce the arrhythmia to occur, then drug treatment is assumed to be effective.

Complications

Complications may include:

- bleeding at the catheter insertion site
- hematoma at the catheter insertion site
- pneumothorax
- deep vein thrombosis
- stroke
- sudden death.

Nursing considerations

Before EPS

- Make sure an informed consent has been signed and that the patient demonstrates understanding of the procedure, reasons for it, and potential complications. Also, review any post-study measures that may be necessary, such as bed rest and keeping the extremity straight.
- Maintain nothing-by-mouth status for at least 8 hours before the procedure and withhold antiarrhythmic agents for 24 hours before the study as ordered.

ALERT *Keep in mind that the patient should be clinically stable before undergoing this test because the risk of complications is greater in a clinically unstable patient.*

- Continue to monitor the patient's cardiac rate and rhythm, especially when antiarrhythmic agents are being withheld.
- Inform the patient that he'll receive a mild sedative before the procedure to help relax him. Let him know that he'll probably be sleepy but able to respond

to the physician. Typically, the patient won't remember the events.

■ Obtain serum electrolyte and digoxin levels, and coagulation studies as ordered.

■ Make sure that continuous ECG and blood pressure monitoring are in place before the study.

After EPS

■ Assess vital signs frequently — at least every hour until stable.

■ Monitor ECG continuously for changes in rate or rhythm.

■ Auscultate heart sounds and report any pericardial friction rub, which indicates bleeding into the pericardial sac.

■ Maintain bed rest, keeping the extremity used for catheter insertion as straight as possible, as per facility's policy, usually for 4 to 6 hours. Elevate the head of the bed no more than 30 degrees.

■ Inspect the catheter insertion site frequently, at least every 2 hours initially, and then at least every 4 hours for signs of redness, irritation, bleeding or hematoma formation.

■ Resume oral intake as soon as the patient is alert and the gag reflex is present.

Endocarditis

An infection of the endocardium (the innermost heart layer), heart valves, or cardiac prosthesis, endocarditis results from bacterial, viral, fungal, or rickettsial invasion. If untreated, endocarditis is usually fatal. With proper treatment, however, about 70% of patients recover. The prognosis is worst

when endocarditis causes severe valvular damage — leading to insufficiency and left-sided heart failure — or when it involves a prosthetic valve. Recurrent infection occurs in approximately 10% to 20% of patients.

Pathophysiology

Four mechanisms are involved with the development of infective endocarditis:

■ a congenital or acquired defect in the heart valve or septum, with blood flowing from an area of high to low pressure through this narrowed opening, that allows an optimal area of growth for any organism

■ formation of a sterile platelet fibrin clot that leads to vegetation

■ bacteremia secondary to colonization at the site of vegetation

■ antibody agglutination promoting vegetation growth.

Organisms enter via the mouth and GI tract, upper airway, skin or external genitourinary tract and travel to the heart. In infective endocarditis, fibrin and platelets cluster on valve tissue and engulf circulating organisms. This produces friable verrucous vegetation. The vegetation may cover the valve surfaces, causing deformities and destruction of valvular tissue. It may also extend to the chordae tendineae, causing them to rupture and leading to valvular insufficiency.

Sometimes vegetation forms on the endocardium, usually in areas altered by rheumatic, congenital, or syphilitic heart disease. It may also form on normal surfaces. Vegetative growth on the heart valves, endocardial lining of a heart chamber, or endothelium of a blood vessel may embolize to the spleen, kidneys, central nervous system, and lungs. (See *Recognizing infarction sites in endocarditis*.)

The most common causative organisms are group A nonhemolytic streptococci, staphylococci, and enterococci. However, almost any organism can cause endocarditis, including *Neisseria gonorrhoeae*, *Pseudomonas*, *Salmonella*, *Streptobacillus*, *Serratia marcescens*, bacteroids, *Haemophilus*, *Brucella*, *Mycobacterium*, *N. meningitidis*, *Listeria*, *Legionella*, diphtheroids, enteric gramnegative bacilli, spirochetes, rickettsiae, chlamydiae, and the fungi *Candida* and *Aspergillus*.

Subacute infective endocarditis typically occurs in people with acquired valvular or congenital cardiac lesions. It can also follow dental, genitourinary (GU), gynecologic, and GI procedures. The most common infecting organisms are *Streptococcus viridans*, which usually inhabits the upper respiratory tract, and *Enterococcus faecalis*, found in GI and perineal flora.

Preexisting conditions, including rheumatic valvular disease, congenital heart disease, mitral valve prolapse, degenerative heart disease, calcific aortic stenosis (in elderly people), asymmetrical septal hypertrophy, Marfan syndrome, syphilitic aortic valve, I.V. drug abuse, and long-term hemodialysis with an arteriovenous shunt or fistula, can predispose a person to endocarditis. However, up to 40% of affected patients have no underlying heart disease.

Comprehensive assessment

The patient may have a history of an underlying predisposing condition.

ALERT *Investigate for history of recent invasive procedures, such as temporary pacemaker or pulmonary*

> # Recognizing infarction sites in endocarditis
>
> Embolization from vegetating lesions or diseased valvular tissue may produce typical characteristics of splenic, renal, cerebral, or pulmonary infarction or peripheral vascular occlusion.
>
> **Splenic infarction**
> - Abdominal rigidity
> - Pain in the left upper quadrant, radiating to the left shoulder
>
> **Renal infarction**
> - Decreased urine output
> - Flank pain
> - Hematuria
> - Pyuria
>
> **Cerebral infarction**
> - Aphasia
> - Hemiparesis
> - Neurologic deficits
>
> **Pulmonary infarction**
> - Cough
> - Dyspnea
> - Hemoptysis
> - Pleural friction rub
> - Pleuritic pain
>
> **Peripheral vascular occlusion**
> - Impending peripheral gangrene
> - Numbness and tingling in an extremity

or central venous catheter insertion, endoscopy, surgery, or dental work, especially in patients with a history of a preexisting valve disorder. Together, these greatly increase the risk of infective endocarditis.

The patient may complain of nonspecific signs and symptoms, such as weakness, fatigue, weight loss, anorexia, arthralgia, night sweats, and an intermittent fever that may recur for weeks. Inspection may reveal petechiae of the skin (especially common on the upper anterior trunk) and the buccal, pharyngeal, or conjunctival mucosa, and splinter hemorrhages under the nails. Rarely, you may see Osler's nodes (tender, raised, subcutaneous lesions on the fingers or toes), Roth's spots (hemorrhagic areas with white centers on the retina), and Janeway lesions (purplish macules on the palms or soles). Clubbing of the fingers may be present in the patient with long-standing disease.

Auscultation may reveal a murmur in all patients except those with early acute endocarditis and I.V. drug users with tricuspid valve infection. The murmur is usually loud and regurgitant, which is typical of the underlying rheumatic or congenital heart disease.

ALERT *A murmur that changes suddenly and a new murmur that develops in the presence of fever are classic physical signs of endocarditis.*

Percussion and palpation may reveal splenomegaly in long-standing disease. In patients who have developed left-sided heart failure, assessment may reveal dyspnea, tachycardia, bilateral basilar crackles, and neck vein distention.

Diagnosis

Three or more blood cultures taken during a 24- to 48-hour period identify the causative organism in up to 90% of patients. The remaining 10% may have negative blood cultures, possibly suggesting fungal or difficult-to-diagnose infections, such as *Haemophilus parainfluenzae*. Other abnormal but nonspecific laboratory results include:

■ normal or elevated white blood cell count and differential
■ abnormal histiocytes (macrophages)
■ normocytic, normochromic anemia (in subacute infective endocarditis)
■ elevated erythrocyte sedimentation rate and serum creatinine levels
■ positive serum rheumatoid factor in about one-half of patients with endocarditis after the disease is present for 6 weeks
■ proteinuria and microscopic hematuria.

Echocardiography may identify valvular damage in up to 80% of patients with native valve disease. It may also show atrial fibrillation and other arrhythmias that accompany valvular disease.

Electrocardiogram, although not specific to infective endocarditis, usually is done to identify conduction defects due to the spread of the infection. The atrioventricular node and bundle of His are common sites affected. Atrial arrhythmias may occur as the atria enlarge from volume overload.

Additional studies, such as site-specific arteriograms or computed tomography scans may be done to identify possible embolization sites.

Collaborations

The patient with endocarditis can be acutely ill and require the attention of a cardiologist and a skilled team to stabilize and manage his condition. Other specialists (surgeons, nephrologists, and cardiac and stroke rehabilitation teams) may be consulted if complications arise.

Treatment and care

The goal of treatment is to eradicate the infecting organisms from the vegetation. Therapy should start promptly and continue over several weeks. Selection of an anti-infective drug is based on identification of the infecting organism and sensitivity studies. If blood cultures are negative, the physician may want to determine the probable infecting organism. I.V. antibiotic therapy usually lasts about 4 to 6 weeks.

In addition, diuretics and vasodilators may be used to decrease the signs and symptoms of heart failure. Positive inotropic agents such as digoxin and dobutamine may be useful in increasing cardiac contractility and output. Nitroprusside or nitroglycerin may be used to reduce afterload.

Supportive treatment includes bed rest, analgesics, and sufficient fluid intake. Supplemental oxygen may be necessary to maintain oxygen saturation (SaO_2) levels at greater than 95%. Severe valvular damage, especially aortic insufficiency or infection of a cardiac prosthesis, may require corrective surgery if refractory heart failure develops, an infected prosthetic valve must be replaced, hemodynamic function deteriorates, or the infection doesn't respond to medications.

Complications

Typically, the heart compensates for the malfunctioning valves for years until left-sided heart failure, valve stenosis or insufficiency, or myocardial erosion sets in. Also, vegetative growth on the valves can cause embolic debris to lodge in the small vasculature of the visceral tissue.

Nursing considerations

■ Before giving antibiotics, obtain the patient's history of allergies and take blood cultures. Administer antibiotics on time to maintain consistent drug levels in the blood. Monitor therapeutic levels.

■ Observe for signs of infiltration or inflammation at the venipuncture site, a possible complication of long-term I.V. therapy. To reduce the risk of infiltration or inflammation at the I.V. site, rotate venous access sites.

■ Assess cardiovascular status frequently, and watch for signs of left-sided heart failure, such as dyspnea, hypotension, tachycardia, tachypnea, crackles, neck vein distention and signs of right-sided heart failure, such as distended neck veins, edema, and ascites. Auscultate heart sounds at least every 2 hours and report murmurs or abnormal heart sounds.

ALERT *The appearance of a new S_3 or S_4 might suggest heart failure.*

■ Institute continuous cardiac monitoring and check for changes in cardiac rhythm or conduction; report evidence of arrhythmias to the physician.

■ If indicated, monitor hemodynamic status looking for increased pulmonary artery wedge pressure and decreased cardiac output (suggests left-sided heart failure) or increased central venous pressure (suggests right-sided heart failure).

■ Administer diuretics and vasodilators as ordered and limit fluid and sodium intake to decrease preload if right-atrial pressure is elevated; if afterload is low, administer vasopressors as ordered; give positive inotropic agents as ordered to increase contractility.

■ Monitor for signs and symptoms of embolization (such as hematuria, pleuritic chest pain, left upper quadrant pain, and paresis). Tell the patient to watch for and report these signs and symptoms because they may indicate impending peripheral vascular occlusion or splenic, renal, cerebral, or pulmonary infarction.

■ Assess patient's respiratory status, auscultating lungs at least every 2 hours, and report evidence of abnormal breath sounds; if hemodynamic monitoring is in place, assess mixed venous oxygen saturation levels.

■ Evaluate arterial blood gas (ABG) values as needed to ensure adequate oxygenation.

ALERT *Be alert for signs of hypoxemia as evidenced by partial pressure of arterial oxygen less than 80 mm Hg; for respiratory acidosis as evidenced by a partial pressure of arterial carbon dioxide ($PaCO_2$) greater than 45 mm Hg and pH less than 7.35; or for respiratory alkalosis as evidenced by a $PaCO_2$ less than 35 mm Hg and a pH greater than 7.45.*

■ Administer supplemental oxygen as necessary based on ABG results and mixed venous oxygen saturation or SaO_2 levels; elevate the head of the bed unless contraindicated.

■ Monitor the patient's renal status (including blood urea nitrogen levels, creatinine clearance levels, and urine output) to check for signs of renal emboli and drug toxicity. Assess urine output hourly. Obtain daily weights, notifying physician of a weight gain greater than 2 lb (1 kg) in one day. If patient has an indwelling urinary catheter, assess urine color and clarity; clean perineal area from front to back daily.

■ Stress the importance of bed rest. Assist the patient with bathing if necessary. Provide a bedside commode be-

cause this method puts less stress on the heart than using a bedpan. Offer physically undemanding diversional activities.

■ Adhere to strict sterile technique when caring for any invasive devices or when performing invasive procedures or techniques. Change tubing, collection devices, and peripheral sites every 48 to 72 hours or as per facility policy.

■ Monitor complete blood count frequently.

■ Provide supportive care as indicated.

■ To reduce anxiety, allow the patient to express his concerns about the effects of activity restrictions on his responsibilities and routines. Reassure him that the restrictions are temporary.

Patient teaching

■ Teach the patient about the anti-infective drugs he'll need to continue to take. Stress the importance of taking the medication and restricting his activities for as long as the physician orders.

■ Tell the patient to watch closely for fever, anorexia, and other signs of relapse for about 2 weeks after treatment stops.

■ Make sure the susceptible patient understands the need for prophylactic antibiotics before, during, and after dental work, childbirth, and GU, GI, or gynecologic procedures.

■ Teach the patient how to recognize symptoms of endocarditis, and tell him to notify the physician immediately if such symptoms occur.

■ Stress the importance of dental hygiene to prevent caries and possible recurrent endocarditis.

Heart failure

A syndrome rather than a disease, heart failure occurs when the heart can't pump enough blood to meet the body's metabolic needs. Heart failure results in intravascular and interstitial volume overload and poor tissue perfusion. An individual with heart failure experiences reduced exercise tolerance, a reduced quality of life, and a shortened life span.

Although the most common cause of heart failure is coronary artery disease (CAD), it also occurs in infants, children, and adults with congenital and acquired heart defects.

AGE ISSUE *The incidence of heart failure rises with age. Approximately 1% of people over age 50 experience heart failure; it occurs in 10% of people over age 80. In ambulatory individuals, the majority with heart failure are over age 60. About 700,000 Americans die of heart failure each year, nearly one-half dying within 5 years of being diagnosed with heart failure. Mortality from heart failure is greater for males, blacks, and elderly people.*

For many patients, the symptoms of heart failure restrict the ability to perform activities of daily living, severely affecting quality of life. Advances in diagnostic and therapeutic techniques have greatly improved the outlook for these patients, but the prognosis still depends on the underlying cause and its response to treatment.

Pathophysiology

Causes of heart failure may be divided into four general categories. (See *Causes of heart failure,* page 102.)

Heart failure may be classified according to the side of the heart affected (left- or right-sided heart failure) or by the cardiac cycle involved (systolic or diastolic dysfunction).

Left-sided heart failure occurs as a result of ineffective left ventricular contractile function. As the left ventricle's pumping ability fails, cardiac output (CO) falls. Blood is no longer effectively pumped out into the body; it backs up into the left atrium and then into the lungs, causing pulmonary congestion, dyspnea, and activity intolerance. If the condition persists, pulmonary edema and right-sided heart failure may result. Common causes include left ventricular infarction, hypertension, and aortic and mitral valve stenosis.

Right-sided heart failure results from ineffective right ventricular contractile function. Consequently, blood isn't pumped effectively through the right ventricle to the lungs, causing blood to back up into the right atrium and into the peripheral circulation. The patient gains weight and develops peripheral edema and engorgement of the kidney and other organs. Right-sided heart failure may be due to an acute right ventricular infarction or a pulmonary embolus. However, the most common cause is profound backward flow due to left-sided heart failure.

Systolic dysfunction occurs when the left ventricle can't pump enough blood out to the systemic circulation during systole and the ejection fraction falls. Consequently, blood backs up

Causes of heart failure

Cause	Examples
Abnormal cardiac muscle function	• Cardiomyopathy • Myocardial infarction
Abnormal left ventricular volume	• High-output states: – Arteriovenous fistula – Beriberi – Chronic anemia – Infusion of large volume of I.V. fluids in a short time – Pregnancy – Septicemia – Thyrotoxicosis • Valvular insufficiency
Abnormal left ventricular pressure	• Aortic or pulmonic valve stenosis • Chronic obstructive pulmonary disease • Hypertension • Pulmonary hypertension
Abnormal left ventricular filling	• Atrial myxoma • Atrial fibrillation • Constrictive pericarditis • Impaired ventricular relaxation: – Hypertension – Myocardial hibernation – Myocardial stunning • Mitral valve stenosis • Tricuspid valve stenosis

into the pulmonary circulation and pressure rises in the pulmonary venous system. CO falls; weakness, fatigue, and shortness of breath may occur. Causes of systolic dysfunction include myocardial infarction and dilated cardiomyopathy.

Diastolic dysfunction occurs when the ability of the left ventricle to relax and fill during diastole is reduced and the stroke volume falls, necessitating higher volumes in the ventricles to maintain CO. Consequently, pulmonary congestion and peripheral edema develop. Diastolic dysfunction may occur as a result of left ventricular hypertrophy, hypertension, or restrictive cardiomyopathy. This type of heart failure is less common than systolic dysfunction, and its treatment isn't as clear.

All causes of heart failure eventually lead to reduced CO that triggers compensatory mechanisms, such as increased sympathetic activity, activation of the renin-angiotensin-aldosterone system, ventricular dilation, and hypertrophy. These mechanisms improve CO at the expense of increased ventricular work.

Increased sympathetic activity — a response to decreased CO and blood pressure — enhances peripheral vascular resistance, contractility, heart rate, and venous return. Signs of increased sympathetic activity, such as cool extremities and clamminess, may indicate impending heart failure.

Increased sympathetic activity also restricts blood flow to the kidneys, causing them to secrete renin which, in turn, converts angiotensinogen to angiotensin I, which then becomes angiotensin II — a potent vasoconstrictor. Angiotensin causes the adrenal cortex to release aldosterone, leading to sodium and water retention and an increase in circulating blood volume. This renal mechanism is helpful; however, if it persists unchecked, it can aggravate heart failure as the heart struggles to pump against the increased volume.

In ventricular dilation, an increase in end-diastolic ventricular volume (preload) causes increased stroke work and stroke volume during contraction, stretching cardiac muscle fibers so that the ventricle can accept the increased intravascular volume. Eventually, the muscle becomes stretched beyond optimum limits and contractility declines.

In ventricular hypertrophy, an increase in ventricular muscle mass allows the heart to pump against increased resistance to the outflow of blood, improving CO. However, this increased muscle mass also increases the myocardial oxygen requirements. An increase in the ventricular diastolic pressure necessary to fill the enlarged ventricle may compromise diastolic coronary blood flow, limiting the oxygen supply to the ventricle, and causing ischemia and impaired muscle contractility.

In heart failure, counterregulatory substances — prostaglandins and atrial natriuretic factor — are produced in an attempt to reduce the negative effects of volume overload and vasoconstriction caused by the compensatory mechanisms.

The kidneys release the prostaglandins, prostacyclin and prostaglandin E_2, which are potent vasodilators. These vasodilators also act to reduce volume overload produced by the renin-angiotensin-aldosterone system by inhibiting sodium and water reabsorption by the kidneys.

Atrial natriuretic factor is a hormone that's secreted mainly by the atria in response to stimulation of the stretch receptors in the atria caused by excess fluid volume. Atrial natriuretic factor works to counteract the negative effects of sympathetic nervous system stimulation and the renin-angiotensin-aldosterone system by producing vasodilation and diuresis.

Comprehensive assessment

The patient's history reveals a disorder or condition that can precipitate heart failure. Manifestations exhibited by the patient vary depending on the type of heart failure. However, failure in one ventricle commonly leads to decreased function in the other ventricle.

Early manifestations of left-sided heart failure include:
■ dyspnea caused by pulmonary congestion
■ orthopnea as blood is redistributed from the legs to the central circulation when the patient lies down at night
■ paroxysmal nocturnal dyspnea due to the reabsorption of interstitial fluid when lying down and reduced sympathetic stimulation while sleeping
■ fatigue associated with reduced oxygenation and a lack of activity

■ nonproductive cough associated with pulmonary congestion.

Later clinical manifestations of left-sided heart failure may include:

■ crackles due to pulmonary congestion

■ hemoptysis resulting from bleeding veins in the bronchial system caused by venous distention

■ point of maximal impulse displaced toward the left anterior axillary line caused by left ventricular hypertrophy

■ tachycardia due to sympathetic stimulation

■ S_3 caused by rapid ventricular filling

■ S_4 resulting from atrial contraction against a noncompliant ventricle

■ cool, pale skin resulting from peripheral vasoconstriction

■ restlessness and confusion due to reduced CO.

Clinical manifestations of right-sided heart failure include:

■ elevated jugular vein distention due to venous congestion

■ positive hepatojugular reflux and hepatomegaly secondary to venous congestion

■ right upper quadrant pain caused by liver engorgement

■ anorexia, fullness, and nausea caused by congestion of the liver and intestines

■ nocturia as fluid is redistributed at night and reabsorbed

■ weight gain due to the retention of sodium and water

■ edema associated with fluid volume excess

■ ascites or anasarca caused by fluid retention.

Diagnosis

The following tests help diagnose heart failure:

■ Chest X-rays show increased pulmonary vascular markings, interstitial edema, or pleural effusion and cardiomegaly.

■ Electrocardiogram (ECG) may indicate hypertrophy, ischemic changes, or infarction, and may also reveal tachycardia and extrasystoles.

■ Laboratory testing may reveal abnormal liver function tests and elevated blood urea nitrogen (BUN) and creatinine levels.

■ Arterial blood gas (ABGs) analysis may reveal hypoxemia from impaired gas exchange and respiratory alkalosis secondary to patient's blowing off more carbon dioxide as respiratory rate rises in compensation.

■ Echocardiography may reveal left ventricular hypertrophy, dilation, and abnormal contractility.

■ Pulmonary artery monitoring typically demonstrates elevated pulmonary artery and pulmonary artery wedge pressures, left ventricular end-diastolic pressure in left-sided heart failure, and elevated right atrial pressure or central venous pressure in right-sided heart failure.

■ Radionuclide ventriculography may reveal an ejection fraction less than 40%; in diastolic dysfunction, the ejection fraction may be normal.

Collaborations

The patient with heart failure requires multidisciplinary care to determine the underlying cause and precipitating factors. Various health care personnel are involved in the patient's care. Treatments including medications, oxygen therapy, diet therapy, and activity restrictions require input from medical and nursing care personnel, and respiratory, nutritional or dietary, and physical therapies. Surgery may be indicated for the patient with CAD or one experiencing severe limitations or recurrent hospitalizations despite maximal medical treatment. Social service consultation may be necessary to aid the patient's transition to home after the acute situation is resolved.

Treatment and care

The aim of therapy is to improve pump function. Correction of heart failure may involve:

- treatment of the underlying cause, if known

AGE ISSUE *Heart failure in children occurs mainly as a result of congenital heart defects. Therefore, treatment guidelines are directed toward the specific cause.*

- angiotensin-converting enzyme (ACE) inhibitors for patients with left ventricular dysfunction to reduce production of angiotensin II, resulting in preload and afterload reduction

AGE ISSUE *Older adults may require lower doses of ACE inhibitors because of impaired renal clearance. Monitor for severe hypotension, signifying a toxic effect.*

- digoxin for patients with heart failure due to left ventricular systolic dysfunction to increase myocardial contractility, improve CO, reduce the volume of the ventricle, and decrease ventricular stretch
- diuretics to reduce fluid volume overload, venous return, and preload
- beta-adrenergic blockers in patients with mild to moderate heart failure caused by left ventricular systolic dysfunction to prevent remodeling

- diuretics, nitrates, morphine, and oxygen to treat pulmonary edema
- lifestyle modifications (to reduce symptoms of heart failure) such as weight loss (if obese), limited sodium (to 3 g/day) and alcohol intake, reduced fat intake, smoking cessation, reduced stress, and development of an exercise program (Heart failure is no longer a contraindication to exercise and cardiac rehabilitation.)
- coronary artery bypass surgery or angioplasty for heart failure due to CAD
- cardiac transplantation in patients receiving aggressive medical treatment but still experiencing limitations or repeated hospitalizations.

Other surgery or invasive procedures may be recommended for patients with severe limitations or repeated hospitalizations despite maximal medical therapy. Some are controversial and may include cardiomyoplasty, insertion of an intra-aortic balloon pump (IABP), partial left ventriculectomy, use of a mechanical ventricular assist device, cardiac resynchronization therapy, and implanting an implantable cardioverter-defibrillator (ICD).

Complications

Patients with heart failure can experience acute and chronic complications. Acute complications of heart failure include:

- pulmonary edema
- acute renal failure
- arrhythmias.
  Chronic complications include:
- activity intolerance
- renal impairment
- cardiac cachexia
- metabolic impairment
- thromboembolism.

Nursing considerations

- Place the patient in Fowler's position to maximize chest expansion and give supplemental oxygen, as ordered, to ease his breathing. Monitor oxygen saturation levels and ABGs as indicated. If respiratory status deteriorates, anticipate the need for endotracheal intubation and mechanical ventilation.
- Institute continuous cardiac monitoring and notify the physician of changes in rhythm and rate. If the patient develops tachycardia, administer beta-adrenergic blockers as ordered and follow the tachycardia algorithm (see *Tachycardia algorithm,* pages 38 and 39); if atrial fibrillation is present, expect to administer anticoagulants or antiplatelet agents as ordered to prevent thrombus formation.
- If the patient develops a new arrhythmia, obtain a 12-lead ECG immediately.
- Monitor hemodynamic status, including CO, cardiac index, pulmonary and systemic vascular pressures closely, at least hourly, noting trends. If available, institute continuous CO monitoring. Evaluate parameters for effectiveness of therapy or for indications that more aggressive therapy is needed.
- Administer pharmacotherapy as ordered. Check apical heart rate before administering digoxin.
- Avoid taking rectal temperatures to prevent bradycardia.
- Assess respiratory status frequently, at least every 1 to 2 hours. Auscultate lungs for abnormal breath sounds, such as crackles, wheezes, and rhonchi. Encourage coughing and deep breathing.
- Obtain daily weight to help detect fluid retention and observe for peripheral edema. Note amount of pitting.
- Assess hourly urine output, especially when the patient is receiving diuretics and ACE inhibitors. Also, monitor fluid intake, including I.V. fluids.

ALERT *For the patient receiving ACE inhibitors, be alert for signs and symptoms of renal insufficiency. If any occur, notify the physician; anticipate the need to stop ACE therapy and administer diuretics or institute hemodialysis.*

- Frequently monitor BUN and serum creatinine levels, liver function studies, and serum potassium, sodium, chloride, and magnesium levels daily.
- Organize activities to provide maximum rest periods. Assess for signs of activity intolerance, such as increased shortness of breath, chest pain, increased arrhythmias, heart rate above 120 beats/minute, and ST-segment changes. If any of these signs are present, have the patient stop activity.
- To prevent deep vein thrombosis due to vascular congestion, assist the patient with range-of-motion exercises. Enforce bed rest and apply antiembolism stockings or intermittent compression devices.
- Prepare the patient for surgical intervention or insertion of IABP or ICD if indicated.

Patient teaching

- Teach the patient to avoid foods high in sodium content, such as canned and commercially prepared foods and dairy products, to curb fluid overload.
- Instruct the patient how to replace the potassium lost through diuretic

therapy by taking a prescribed potassium supplement and eating potassium-rich foods, such as bananas and apricots, and drinking orange juice.

■ Encourage the patient to weigh himself daily and to maintain a record of his weight. Advise the patient to report a weight gain or loss of 2 lb (1 kg) or more in 3 or 4 days.

■ Stress the need for regular medical checkups and periodic blood tests to monitor drug levels.

■ Stress the importance of taking medication exactly as prescribed. Tell the patient to watch for and immediately report signs of toxicity, such as anorexia, vomiting, confusion, slow or irregular pulse rate and, in elderly patients, flulike symptoms.

■ Tell the patient to notify the physician if his pulse rate is unusually irregular or less than 60 beats/minute; if he experiences dizziness, blurred vision, shortness of breath, persistent dry cough, palpitations, increased fatigue, paroxysmal nocturnal dyspnea, swollen ankles, or decreased urine output; or if he gains 3 to 5 lb (1.4 to 2.3 kg) in 1 week.

 MULTISYSTEM DISORDER

Hypertensive crisis

Hypertensive crisis refers to the abrupt, acute, and marked increase in blood pressure from the patient's baseline that ultimately leads to acute and rapidly progressing end-organ damage. Typically, the diastolic blood pressure is greater than 120 mm Hg. The increased blood pressure value, although important, is probably less important

than how rapidly the blood pressure is rising.

Hypertensive crisis is seen in approximately 1% of the population. Most patients who develop this condition have a long history of chronic, poorly controlled or untreated primary hypertension. However, conditions responsible for secondary hypertension, such as pheochromocytoma or Cushing's syndrome may also be responsible. Regardless, prompt recognition and intervention are crucial to prevent further end-organ damage. If untreated, this condition is fatal in more than 75% of those affected within 1 year. With treatment, the mortality rate after 1 year is approximately 30%; at 5 years, the rate is approximately 50%.

Pathophysiology

Arterial blood pressure is a product of total peripheral resistance and cardiac output (CO). CO is increased by conditions that increase heart rate or stroke volume, or both. Peripheral resistance is increased by factors that increase blood viscosity or reduce the lumen size of vessels, especially the arterioles. Hypertension may result from a disturbance in one of the intrinsic mechanisms: renin-angiotensin-aldosterone system, autoregulation, sympathetic nervous system, or antidiuretic hormone.

The renin-angiotensin-aldosterone system acts to increase blood pressure through the following mechanisms:

■ Sodium depletion, reduced blood pressure, and dehydration stimulate renin release.

■ Renin reacts with angiotensin, a liver enzyme, and converts it to angiotensin I, which increases preload and afterload.

- Angiotensin I converts to angiotensin II in the lungs; angiotensin II is a potent vasoconstrictor that targets the arterioles.
- Circulating angiotensin II works to increase preload and afterload by stimulating the adrenal cortex to secrete aldosterone, which increases blood volume by conserving sodium and water.

With autoregulation, several intrinsic mechanisms work to change an artery's diameter to maintain tissue and organ perfusion despite fluctuations in systemic blood pressure. These mechanisms include stress relaxation and capillary fluid shifts:

- In stress relaxation, blood vessels gradually dilate when blood pressure rises to reduce peripheral resistance.
- In capillary fluid shift, plasma moves between vessels and extravascular spaces to maintain intravascular volume.

The sympathetic nervous system mechanism controls blood pressure. When blood pressure drops, baroreceptors in the aortic arch and carotid sinuses decrease their inhibition of the medulla's vasomotor center. The consequent increases in sympathetic stimulation of the heart by norepinephrine increase CO by strengthening the contractile force, raising the heart rate, and augmenting peripheral resistance by vasoconstriction. Stress can also stimulate the sympathetic nervous system to increase CO and peripheral vascular resistance.

The release of antidiuretic hormone can regulate hypotension by increasing reabsorption of water by the kidney. With reabsorption, blood plasma volume increases, thus raising blood pressure. In hypertensive crisis, one or more of these regulating mechanisms is disrupted. (See *What happens in hypertensive crisis*.)

Hypertensive crisis can result in hypertensive encephalopathy resulting from cerebral vasodilation from an inability to maintain autoregulation. Blood flow increases, causing an increase in pressure and subsequent cerebral edema. This increase in pressure damages the intimal and medial lining of the arterioles.

Comprehensive assessment

Assessment of a patient with hypertensive crisis almost always reveals a history of hypertension that's poorly controlled or has gone untreated. The most common complaint is a severe, throbbing headache in the back of the head. The patient may also complain of nausea, vomiting, or anorexia.

Other signs and symptoms may include:
- irritability
- confusion, somnolence, stupor
- vision loss, blurred vision, or diplopia
- dizziness
- dyspnea on exertion, orthopnea, paroxysmal nocturnal dyspnea, and edema secondary to heart failure
- angina secondary to coronary artery disease.

If the patient has hypertensive encephalopathy, the following may be noted:
- decreased level of consciousness
- disorientation
- seizures
- focal neurologic deficits, such as hemiparesis, and unilateral sensory deficits.

If the hypertensive crisis has affected the kidneys, the following may be noted:

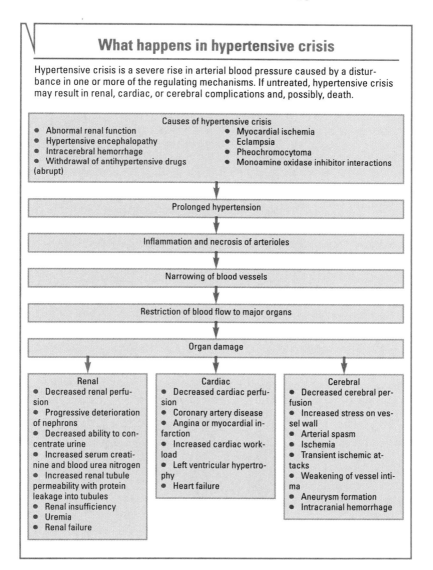

What happens in hypertensive crisis

Hypertensive crisis is a severe rise in arterial blood pressure caused by a disturbance in one or more of the regulating mechanisms. If untreated, hypertensive crisis
may result in renal, cardiac, or cerebral complications and, possibly, death.

Causes of hypertensive crisis
- Abnormal renal function
- Hypertensive encephalopathy
- Intracerebral hemorrhage
- Withdrawal of antihypertensive drugs (abrupt)
- Myocardial ischemia
- Eclampsia
- Pheochromocytoma
- Monoamine oxidase inhibitor interactions

Prolonged hypertension

Inflammation and necrosis of arterioles

Narrowing of blood vessels

Restriction of blood flow to major organs

Organ damage

Renal
- Decreased renal perfusion
- Progressive deterioration of nephrons
- Decreased ability to concentrate urine
- Increased serum creatinine and blood urea nitrogen
- Increased renal tubule permeability with protein leakage into tubules
- Renal insufficiency
- Uremia
- Renal failure

Cardiac
- Decreased cardiac perfusion
- Coronary artery disease
- Angina or myocardial infarction
- Increased cardiac workload
- Left ventricular hypertrophy
- Heart failure

Cerebral
- Decreased cerebral perfusion
- Increased stress on vessel wall
- Arterial spasm
- Ischemia
- Transient ischemic attacks
- Weakening of vessel intima
- Aneurysm formation
- Intracranial hemorrhage

- reduced urine output
- elevated blood urea nitrogen (BUN) and creatinine levels.

On examination, a left ventricular heave may be palpated at the mitral valve area along with auscultation of an S_4. These suggest left ventricular hypertrophy. If heart failure is present, the point of maximum impulse is felt closer to the anterior axillary line rather than at the midclavicular line. Crackles may also be heard on lung auscultation. Tachycardia or other arrhythmias, narrowed pulse pressure, and distended neck veins may be found.

Examination of the eye may reveal acute retinopathy and hemorrhage, retinal exudates, and papilledema. Arterial-venous nicking may also be seen.

Blood pressure measurement, obtained several times at an interval of at least 2 minutes, reveals an elevated diastolic pressure above 120 mm Hg.

Diagnosis

Blood pressure measurement confirms the diagnosis of hypertensive crisis. After hypertension is confirmed, additional tests may be done to determine further problems. However, because of the emergency nature of the condition, time is limited. Additional tests may include:

■ Complete blood count to identify azotemia. If renal involvement is present, the red blood cell count may be decreased secondary to hematuria.

■ BUN and creatinine levels to determine extent of renal involvement evidenced by a BUN may be greater than 20 mg/dl and a serum creatinine level greater than 1.3 mg/dl.

■ Electrocardiogram (ECG) may reveal ischemic changes or left ventricular hypertrophy; ST-segment depression, and T-wave inversion, suggesting repolarization problems from endocardial fibrosis associated with left ventricular hypertrophy.

■ Echocardiography may reveal increased wall thickness with or without an increase in left ventricular size.

■ Chest X-ray may reveal enlargement of the cardiac silhouette with left ventricular dilation; pulmonary congestion and pleural effusions with heart failure.

■ Urinalysis may be normal unless renal impairment is present; then specific gravity will be low (less than 1.010); hematuria, casts, and proteinuria may also be found. If the patient's condition is due to a disease condition such as pheochromocytoma, a 24-hour urine specimen will reveal increases in vanillylmandelic acid and urinary catecholamines.

Collaborations

Because hypertensive crisis is a multisystem problem, a multidisciplinary approach to care is necessary. Immediate and rapid reduction of blood pressure is crucial. Medical and nursing health care providers focus on administering medications to treat hypertension and prevent potential complications. Surgical health care providers may be needed to correct the underlying problem associated with secondary hypertension, such as removal of tumor in pheochromocytoma. Nutritional consultation may be necessary to help with lifestyle changes involving diet. If the patient experiences end-organ damage, additional specialists may be needed to address these problems.

Treatment and care

Treatment focuses on immediately reducing the patient's blood pressure with I.V. antihypertensive therapy. However, care must be taken not to reduce the patient's blood pressure too rapidly, because the patient's autoregulatory control is impaired. The current recommendation is to reduce the blood pressure by no more than 25% of the mean arterial pressure over the first 2 hours. Further reductions should occur over the next several days.

The drug of choice for treating hypertensive crisis is sodium nitroprusside, given as an I.V. infusion and titrated according to the patient's response. It has a rapid onset of action and its effects cease within 1 to 5 minutes of stopping the drug. Thus, if the patient's blood pressure dropped too low, stopping the drug would almost immediately allow the blood pressure to rise.

Other agents that may be used include labetalol, nitroglycerin (the drug of choice for treating hypertensive crisis when myocardial ischemia, acute myocardial infarction [MI], or pulmonary edema are present), and hydralazine (specifically indicated for treating hypertension in pregnant women with preeclampsia).

Treatment also involves lifestyle changes, such as weight reduction, smoking cessation, exercise, and dietary changes. After the acute episode is controlled, maintenance pharmacotherapy to control blood pressure plays a key role.

Complications

Numerous complications may occur, including:
- stroke
- subarachnoid hemorrhage
- dissecting aortic aneurysm
- MI
- lethal arrhythmias
- sudden death
- retinopathy
- renal failure.

Nursing considerations

- Immediately obtain the patient's blood pressure to confirm your suspicions, and ensure that the patient's airway is patent.
- If not already in place, institute continuous cardiac and arterial pressure monitoring to assess blood pressure directly; determine the patient's mean arterial pressure.
- Assess arterial blood gas levels. Monitor the patient's oxygen saturation level via pulse oximetry; if the patient is being hemodynamically monitored, assess the patient's mixed venous oxygen saturation; administer supplemental oxygen as ordered based on findings.
- Administer I.V. antihypertensive therapy as ordered; if using nitroprusside, wrap the container in foil to protect it from the light and titrate dose based on specified target ranges for systolic and diastolic pressures. Immediately stop the drug if the patient's blood pressure drops below the target ranges.

 ALERT *Remember that nitroprusside is metabolized to thiocyanate, which is excreted by the kidneys. Be alert for signs and symptoms of thiocyanate toxicity, such as fatigue, nausea, tinnitus, blurred vision, and delirium. If the patient exhibits any of these, obtain a serum thiocyanate level. If the level is greater than 10 mg/dl, toxicity is present, you should notify the physician because he'll most likely stop the drug.*

- Monitor blood pressure every 1 to 5 minutes while titrating drug therapy, then every 15 minutes to 1 hour as the patient's condition stabilizes.

AGE ISSUE *Older adults are at an increased risk for adverse ef-*

fects of antihypertensives, especially orthostatic hypotension. Lower doses may be necessary.

■ Continuously monitor ECG and institute treatment as indicated should arrhythmias occur; auscultate heart, noting signs of heart failure such as the presence of an S_3 or S_4.

■ Assess the patient's neurologic status every hour initially and then every 4 hours as the patient's condition stabilizes.

■ Monitor urine output every hour and notify the physician if output is less than 0.5 ml/kg/hour. Evaluate BUN and serum creatinine levels for changes, and monitor daily weight.

■ Obtain serum thiocyanate levels after 48 hours of therapy and then regularly thereafter while the patient is receiving nitroprusside.

■ Administer other antihypertensives as ordered. As the patient's condition stabilizes, expect to begin oral antihypertensive therapy while gradually weaning I.V. agents to prevent hypotension. If the patient is experiencing fluid overload, administer diuretics as ordered.

■ Assess the patient's visual ability and report such changes as increased blurred vision, diplopia, or loss of vision.

■ Administer analgesics as ordered for headache; keep environment quiet, with low lighting.

Patient teaching

■ Teach the patient about all aspects of blood pressure control, including the need for medication adherence and frequent follow-ups.

■ Instruct the patient in specific drug therapy regimen, including dosage,

frequency, adverse effects, and when to notify the physician.

■ Reinforce necessary lifestyle changes including smoking cessation and the need for regular exercise.

■ Inform the patient about the signs and symptoms associated with complications, such as changes in level of alertness, vision, urine output, or weight gain and the need to notify the physician if any occur.

Implantable cardioverter-defibrillator

An implantable cardioverter-defibrillator (ICD) is an electronic device implanted in the body to provide continuous monitoring of the heart for bradycardia, ventricular tachycardia, and ventricular fibrillation (VF). The device then administers either shocks or paced beats to treat the dangerous arrhythmia. In general, ICDs are indicated for patients for whom drug therapy, surgery, or catheter ablation has failed to prevent the arrhythmia.

The system consists of a programmable pulse generator and one or more leadwires. The pulse generator is a small computer powered by a battery. The generator is responsible for monitoring the heart's electrical signals and delivering electrical therapy when it identifies an abnormal rhythm. It also stores information about the heart's activity before, during, and after an arrhythmia, along with tracking the treatment delivered and the outcome of the treatment. Many devices also store electrograms (electrical tracings

Types of ICD therapies

Implantable cardioverter-defibrillators (ICDs) can deliver a range of therapies depending on the arrhythmia detected and how the device is programmed. Therapies include antitachycardia pacing, cardioversion, defibrillation, and bradycardia pacing.

Therapy	Description
Antitachycardia pacing	A series of small, rapid, electrical pacing pulses are used to interrupt ventricular tachycardia (VT) and return the heart to its normal rhythm. Antitachycardia pacing isn't appropriate for all patients; it will be ordered by the patient's physician after appropriate evaluation of electrophysiologic studies.
Cardioversion	A low- or high-energy shock (up to 34 joules) is timed to the R wave to terminate VT and return the heart to its normal rhythm.
Defibrillation	A high-energy shock (up to 34 joules) to the heart is used to terminate ventricular fibrillation and return the heart to its normal rhythm.
Bradycardia pacing	Electrical pacing pulses are used when the heart's natural electrical signals are too slow. Most ICD systems can pace one chamber (VVI pacing) of the heart at a preset rate. Some systems will sense and pace both chambers (DDD pacing).

similar to electrocardiograms [ECGs]). With an interrogation device, a physician can retrieve this information to evaluate ICD function and battery status and to adjust ICD system settings. The leads are insulated wires that carry the heart signal to the pulse generator and deliver the electrical energy from the pulse generator to the heart.

Today's advanced devices can detect a wide range of arrhythmias and automatically respond with the appropriate therapy, such as bradycardia pacing (both single- and dual-chamber), antitachycardia pacing, cardioversion, and defibrillation. ICDs that provide therapy for atrial arrhythmias, such as atrial fibrillation, are under evaluation. (See *Types of ICD therapies.*)

Procedure

Insertion of an ICD is most commonly performed in the cardiac catheterization laboratory by a specially trained cardiologist. Occasionally, a patient who requires other surgery, such as coronary artery bypass, may have the device implanted in the operating room.

To insert an ICD, the cardiologist makes a small incision near the clavicle to gain access to the subclavian vein. The leadwires are inserted through the subclavian vein, threaded into the heart, and placed in contact with the endocardium. The leads are then connected to the pulse generator, which is inserted under the skin in a specially prepared pocket in the right or left upper chest, similar to that used for a pacemaker. The incision is then closed and the device is programmed.

Complications

Complications of ICD implantation include serous or bloody drainage from the insertion site, swelling, ecchymosis, incisional pain, and impaired mobility. Other complications include venous thrombosis, embolism, infection, pneumothorax, pectoral or diaphragmatic muscle stimulation from the ICD, arrhythmias, cardiac tamponade, heart failure, and abnormal ICD operation with lead dislodgment. Late complications include failure to function, resulting in untreated VF and cardiac arrest

Nursing considerations

The care of a patient with an ICD includes monitoring device function, providing emergency care if indicated, observing precautions, and recognizing complications.

Before ICD implantation

■ If the patient is scheduled for ICD implantation, ensure that he and his family understand the physician's explanation of the need for the device, the potential complications, and the alternatives. Make sure they also understand ICD terminology and functioning.
■ Obtain baseline vital signs and record a 12-lead ECG or rhythm strip. Evaluate radial and pedal pulses and assess the patient's mental status.
■ Restrict food and fluids for 12 hours before the procedure.
■ Explain to the patient that he may receive a sedative before the procedure and will probably have his upper chest shaved and scrubbed with an antiseptic solution. Inform him that when he arrives in the cardiac catheterization laboratory, his hands may be restrained so that they don't inadvertently touch the sterile area and that his chest or abdomen will be draped with sterile towels.
■ Make sure the patient or a responsible family member has signed an informed consent form.
■ Document any arrhythmias in a monitored patient.
■ Notify the physician if a change in pulse pattern or rate occurs in an unmonitored patient or if a monitored patient exhibits an arrhythmia.
■ Be prepared to initiate cardiopulmonary resuscitation (CPR), if indicated, when a life-threatening arrhythmia occurs.
■ Administer medications as ordered, and prepare to assist with medical procedures (such as defibrillation) if indicated.

After ICD implantation

When caring for a patient with an ICD, knowing how the device is programmed is important. This information is available through a status report that can be obtained and printed when the physician or specially trained technician interrogates the device, which involves placing a specialized piece of equipment over the implanted pulse generator to retrieve pacing function. Program information includes:
■ type and model of ICD
■ status of the device (on or off)
■ detection rates
■ therapies that will be delivered: pacing, antitachycardia pacing, cardioversion, and defibrillation.

    If the patient experiences an arrhythmia or the device delivers a therapy, the information recorded helps to evaluate the functioning of the device. (See *Analyzing ICD function.*)

Analyzing ICD function

To analyze the function of an implantable cardioverter-defibrillator (ICD), compare the monitor strips with the device status report. The example shown below demonstrates proper device function for ventricular tachycardia (VT) according to the programmed parameters. When VT occurs, the device is programmed to deliver antitachycardia pacing consisting of eight pacing stimuli six separate times. If the arrhythmia doesn't terminate or deteriorates to ventricular fibrillation, the device is programmed to deliver a cardioversion shock. This episode of VT converts to normal sinus rhythm with the first cardioversion.

STATUS REPORT

VT therapy	1	2	3	4
Therapy status	On	On	On	On
Therapy type	ATP	CV	CV	CV
Initial number of pulses	8	—	—	—
Number of sequences	6	—	—	—
Energy (joules)	—	10	34	34
Waveform	—	Biphasic	Biphasic	Biphasic

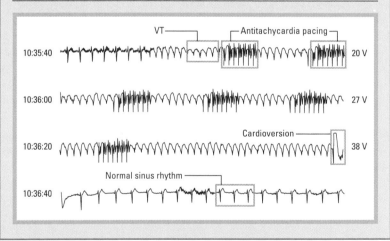

■ If the patient experiences cardiac arrest, initiate CPR and advanced cardiac life support.
■ Be aware that the ICD delivers a shock to the patient. While you're performing chest compressions, you may also feel a slight shock. Prevent shock by wearing latex gloves.
■ Externally defibrillating the patient is safe as long as the paddles aren't placed directly over the pulse generator. The anteroposterior paddle position is preferred.

■ Watch for signs of a perforated ventricle, with resultant cardiac tamponade. Ominous signs include persistent hiccups, distant heart sounds, pulsus paradoxus, hypotension accompanied by narrow pulse pressure, increased venous pressure, bulging neck veins, cyanosis, decreased urine output, restlessness, and complaints of fullness in the chest. Report any of these signs immediately and prepare the patient for emergency surgery.

■ Assess the area around the incision for swelling, tenderness, and hematoma, but don't remove the occlusive dressing for the first 24 hours without a physician's order. When you remove the dressing, check the wound for drainage, redness, and unusual warmth or tenderness.

■ After the first 24 hours, begin passive range-of-motion exercises if ordered and progress as tolerated.

Patient teaching

■ Advise the patient to wear a medical identification bracelet indicating ICD placement and to educate family members in emergency techniques (such as dialing 911 and performing CPR) in case the device fails. Explain that electrical or electronic devices may cause disruption of the device.

■ Warn the patient to avoid placing excessive pressure over the insertion site or moving or jerking the area until the postoperative visit. Tell the patient to follow normal routines as allowed by the physician and to increase exercise as tolerated.

■ Remind the patient to carry information regarding his ICD at all times and to inform airline clerks when he travels as well as individuals performing diagnostic functions (such as computed tomography scans and magnetic resonance imaging). Stress the importance of follow-up care and checkups.

Intra-aortic balloon pump

Providing temporary support for the heart's left ventricle, intra-aortic balloon pump (IABP) mechanically displaces blood within the aorta by means of an intra-aortic balloon attached to an external pump console. The balloon is usually inserted through the common femoral artery and positioned with its tip just distal to the left subclavian artery. It monitors myocardial perfusion and the effects of drugs on myocardial function and perfusion. When used correctly, IABP improves two key aspects of myocardial physiology: It increases the supply of oxygen-rich blood to the myocardium and decreases myocardial oxygen demand.

The intra-aortic balloon, made of polyurethane, is attached to an external pump console by means of a large-lumen catheter. The balloon inflates as the aortic valve closes and diastole begins. Diastole increases perfusion to the coronary arteries. The balloon deflates before ventricular ejection, when the aortic valve opens. This permits ejection of blood from the left ventricle against a lowered resistance. As a result, aortic end-diastolic pressure and afterload decrease and cardiac output (CO) increases.

IABP is recommended for patients with a wide range of low-CO disorders or cardiac instability, including refractory anginas, ventricular arrhythmias associated with ischemia, and pump failure caused by cardiogenic shock, intraoperative myocardial infarction (MI), or low CO after bypass surgery. IABP is also indicated for patients with low CO secondary to acute mechanical defects after MI (such as ventricular septal defect, papillary muscle rupture, or left ventricular aneurysm).

Preoperatively, the technique is used to support and stabilize patients with a suspected high-grade lesion who are undergoing such procedures as angioplasty, thrombolytic therapy, cardiac surgery, and cardiac catheterization. IABP is contraindicated in patients with severe aortic insufficiency, aortic aneurysm, or severe peripheral vascular disease.

Procedure

Under strict asepsis, the physician may insert the balloon percutaneously through the femoral artery into the descending thoracic aorta by accessing the vessel with an 18G angiography needle, removing the inner stylet, then passing the guide wire through the needle and removing the needle. Next, the physician passes an introducer (dilator and sheath assembly) over the guide wire into the vessel until about 1″ (2.5 cm) remains above the insertion site. He then removes the inner dilator, leaving the introducer sheath and guide wire in place. After passing the balloon over the guide wire into the introducer sheath, the physician advances the catheter into position, ³⁄₈″ to ³⁄₄″ (1 to 2 cm) distal to the left subclavian artery under fluoroscopic guidance. He attaches the balloon to the control system to initiate counterpulsation. The balloon catheter then unfurls.

If the physician chooses not to insert the catheter percutaneously, he usually inserts it by femoral arteriotomy in which the physician passes the balloon through a Dacron graft that has been sewn to the artery. Using fluoroscopic guidance as necessary, he advances the catheter up the descending thoracic aorta and places the catheter tip between the left subclavian artery and the renal arteries. Then the physician sews the Dacron graft around the catheter at the insertion point and connects the other end of the catheter to the pump console.

If the balloon can't be inserted through the femoral artery, the physician inserts it in an antegrade direction through the anterior wall of the ascending aorta. He positions it ³⁄₈″ to ³⁄₄″ beyond the left subclavian artery and brings the catheter out through the chest wall. After the balloon has been inserted, the physician will clean the site and cover it with a sterile dressing.

Complications

IABP may cause numerous complications. The most common, arterial embolism, stems from clot formation on the balloon surface. Other potential complications include extension or rupture of an aortic aneurysm, femoral or iliac artery perforation, femoral artery occlusion, and sepsis. Bleeding at the insertion site may become aggravated by pump-induced thrombocytopenia, which is caused by platelet aggregation around the balloon.

Nursing considerations
Before IABP insertion
■ Depending on your facility's policy, you or a perfusionist must balance the

pressure transducer in the external pump console and calibrate the oscilloscope monitor to ensure accuracy.

■ Explain to the patient that the physician will place a special balloon catheter in his aorta to help his heart pump more easily. Briefly explain the insertion procedure, and mention that the catheter will be connected to a large console next to his bed. Tell him that the balloon will temporarily reduce his heart's workload to promote rapid healing of the ventricular muscle. Let him know that it will be removed after his heart can resume an adequate workload.

■ Make sure the patient or a family member understands and signs a consent form. Verify that the form is attached to his chart.

■ Obtain the patient's baseline vital signs, including pulmonary artery pressure (PAP). (A pulmonary artery [PA] line should be in place.) Attach the patient to an electrocardiograph (ECG) machine for continuous monitoring. Apply chest electrodes in a standard lead II position — or in whatever position produces the largest R wave — because the R wave triggers balloon inflation and deflation. Obtain a baseline ECG.

■ Attach another set of ECG electrodes to the patient unless the ECG pattern is being transmitted from the patient's bedside monitor to the balloon pump monitor through a phone cable. Administer oxygen as ordered and as necessary.

■ Make sure the patient has an arterial line, a PA line, and a peripheral I.V. line in place. The arterial line is used for withdrawing blood samples, monitoring blood pressure, and assessing the therapy's timing and effectiveness.

The PA line allows measurement of PAP, aspiration of blood samples, and CO studies. Increased PAP indicates increased myocardial workload and ineffective balloon pumping. CO studies are usually performed with and without the balloon to check the patient's progress. The central lumen of the intra-aortic balloon, which is used to monitor central aortic pressure, produces an augmented pressure waveform that allows you to check for proper timing of the inflation-deflation cycle and demonstrates the effects of counterpulsation, elevated diastolic pressure, and reduced end-diastolic and systolic pressures.

■ Insert an indwelling urinary catheter with a urinometer so you can measure the patient's urine output and assess his fluid balance and renal function. To reduce the risk of infection, prepare the patient's skin bilaterally from the lower abdomen to the lower thigh, including the pubic area according to the facility's policy.

■ Observe and record the patient's peripheral leg pulse and document sensation, movement, color, and temperature of the legs.

■ Administer a sedative as ordered.

■ Have the defibrillator, suction setup, temporary pacemaker setup, and emergency medications readily available in case the patient develops complications during insertion such as an arrhythmia.

After IABP insertion

■ Obtain a chest X-ray to verify correct balloon placement.

■ Monitor the function of the system and proper balloon function. (See *Interpreting IABP waveforms,* pages 120 and 121.)

ALERT *If the control system malfunctions or becomes inoperable, don't let the balloon catheter remain dormant for more than 30 minutes. Get another control system and attach it to the balloon; then resume pumping. In the meantime, inflate the balloon manually, using a 60-ml syringe and room air a minimum of once every 5 minutes, to prevent thrombus formation in the catheter.*

■ Assess and record pedal and posterior tibial pulses as well as color, sensation, and temperature in the affected limb every 15 minutes for 1 hour, then hourly. Notify the physician immediately if you detect circulatory changes because the balloon may need to be removed.

■ Observe and record the patient's baseline arm pulses, arm sensation and movement, and arm color and temperature every 15 minutes for 1 hour after balloon insertion, then every 2 hours while the balloon is in place. Loss of left-arm pulses may indicate upward balloon displacement. Notify the physician of any changes.

■ Monitor the patient's urine output every hour. Note baseline blood urea nitrogen (BUN) and serum creatinine levels, and monitor these levels daily. Changes in urine output, BUN, and serum creatinine levels may signal reduced renal perfusion from downward balloon displacement.

■ Auscultate and record bowel sounds every 4 hours. Check for abdominal distention and tenderness as well as changes in the patient's elimination patterns.

■ Measure the patient's temperature every 1 to 4 hours. If it's elevated, obtain blood samples for a culture, send them to the laboratory immediately,

and notify the physician. Culture any drainage at the insertion site.

■ Monitor the patient's hematologic status. Observe for bleeding gums, blood in the urine or stools, petechiae, and bleeding at the insertion site. Monitor his platelet count, hemoglobin level, and hematocrit daily. Expect to administer blood products to maintain hematocrit at 30%. If the platelet count drops, expect to administer platelets.

■ Monitor partial thromboplastin time (PTT) every 6 hours while the heparin dose is adjusted to maintain PTT at $1\frac{1}{2}$ to 2 times the normal value, then every 12 to 24 hours while the balloon remains in place.

■ Measure PAP and pulmonary artery wedge pressure (PAWP) every 1 to 2 hours as ordered. A rising PAWP reflects preload, signaling increased ventricular pressure and workload; notify the physician if this occurs. Some patients require I.V. nitroprusside during IABP to reduce preload and afterload.

■ Obtain samples for arterial blood gas analysis as ordered.

■ Monitor serum electrolyte levels — especially sodium and potassium — to assess the patient's fluid and electrolyte balance and help prevent arrhythmias.

■ Watch for signs and symptoms of a dissecting aortic aneurysm, such as a blood pressure differential between the left and right arms, elevated blood pressure, syncope, pallor, diaphoresis, dyspnea, a throbbing abdominal mass, a reduced red blood cell count with an elevated white blood cell count, and pain in the chest, abdomen, or back. Notify the physician immediately if you detect any of these complications.

(Text continues on page 122.)

Interpreting IABP waveforms

During intra-aortic balloon pump therapy, the electrocardiogram and arterial pressure waveforms can be used to determine whether the balloon pump is functioning properly.

Normal inflation-deflation timing

Balloon inflation occurs after aortic valve closure; deflation occurs during isovolumetric contraction, just before the aortic valve opens. In a properly timed waveform, as shown, the inflation point lies at or slightly above the dicrotic notch. Both inflation and deflation cause a sharp V. Peak diastolic pressure exceeds peak systolic pressure; peak systolic pressure exceeds assisted peak systolic pressure.

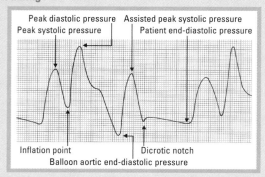

Peak diastolic pressure   Assisted peak systolic pressure
Peak systolic pressure   Patient end-diastolic pressure

Inflation point   Dicrotic notch
Balloon aortic end-diastolic pressure

Early inflation

The inflation point lies before the dicrotic notch in early inflation, which dangerously increases myocardial stress and decreases cardiac output.

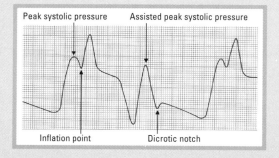

Peak systolic pressure   Assisted peak systolic pressure

Inflation point   Dicrotic notch

Early deflation
With early deflation, a U shape appears and peak systolic pressure is less than or equal to assisted peak systolic pressure. This won't decrease afterload or myocardial oxygen consumption.

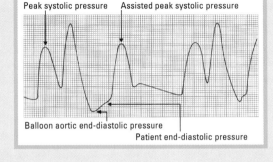

Peak systolic pressure   Assisted peak systolic pressure

Balloon aortic end-diastolic pressure

Patient end-diastolic pressure

Late inflation
With late inflation, the dicrotic notch precedes the inflation point, and the notch and the inflation point create a W shape. This can lead to a reduction in peak diastolic pressure, coronary and systemic perfusion augmentation time, and augmented coronary perfusion pressure.

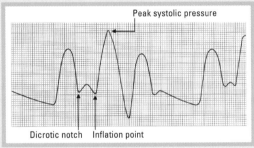

Peak systolic pressure

Dicrotic notch   Inflation point

Late deflation
With late deflation, peak systolic pressure exceeds assisted peak systolic pressure. This threatens the patient by increasing afterload, myocardial oxygen consumption, cardiac workload, and preload. It occurs when the balloon has been inflated too long.

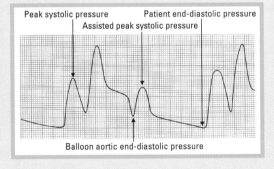

Peak systolic pressure   Patient end-diastolic pressure

Assisted peak systolic pressure

Balloon aortic end-diastolic pressure

■ Assess the cardiac index, systemic blood pressure, and PAWP to help the physician evaluate the patient's readiness for weaning — usually about 24 hours after balloon insertion. The patient's hemodynamic status should be stable on minimal doses of inotropic agents such as dobutamine.

■ Change the dressing at the balloon insertion site every 24 hours or as needed, using strict sterile technique.

■ Make sure the head of the bed is elevated no more than 30 degrees.

■ Watch for pump interruptions, which may result from loose ECG electrodes or leadwires, static or 60-cycle interference, catheter kinking, or improper body alignment.

■ Make sure PTT is within normal limits before the balloon is removed to prevent hemorrhage at insertion site.

■ To begin weaning, gradually decrease the frequency of balloon augmentation to 1:2 and 1:4, as ordered. Although each facility has its own weaning protocol, be aware that assist frequency is usually maintained for an hour or longer. If the patient's hemodynamic indices remain stable during this time, weaning may continue.

■ Avoid leaving the patient on a low augmentation setting for more than 2 hours to prevent embolus formation.

■ Assess the patient's tolerance of weaning. Signs and symptoms of poor tolerance include confusion and disorientation, urine output below 30 ml/hour, cold and clammy skin, chest pain, arrhythmias, ischemic ECG changes, and elevated PAP. If the patient develops any of these problems, notify the physician at once.

■ When the patient's hemodynamic status remains stable after the frequency of balloon augmentation is de-

creased, anticipate removal of the IABP.

■ After the physician has removed the IABP catheter, apply direct pressure to the site for 30 minutes or until bleeding stops. (In some facilities, this is the physician's responsibility.)

■ Provide wound care according to your facility's policy. Record the patient's pedal and posterior tibial pulses, and the color, temperature, and sensation of the affected limb. Enforce bed rest as appropriate (usually for 24 hours).

■ Record all aspects of patient assessment and management, including the patient's response to therapy. If you're responsible for the IABP device, document all routine checks, problems, and troubleshooting measures. If a technician is responsible for the IABP device, record only when and why the technician was notified and the result of his actions on the patient. Also, document teaching of the patient, family, or close friends as well as their responses.

Pacemakers

A pacemaker is an artificial device consisting of a battery-powered pulse generator and a lead and electrode system that electrically stimulates the myocardium to depolarize, initiating mechanical contractions. The devices generate an impulse from a power source and transmit that impulse to the heart muscle. The impulse flows throughout the heart and causes the heart muscle to depolarize.

The capabilities of pacemakers are described by a five-letter coding system, although three letters are more commonly used.

■ The first letter of the code identifies the heart chamber being paced — V (ventricle), A (atrium), D (dual, ventricle and atrium), or O (none).

■ The second letter of the code identifies the heart chamber where the pacemaker senses the intrinsic activity — V (ventricle), A (atrium), D (dual, ventricle and atrium), or O (none).

■ The third letter of the code indicates the pacemaker's mode of response to the intrinsic activity that it senses in the atrium or ventricle — T (triggered), I (inhibited), D (dual, triggered or inhibited), or O (none).

■ The fourth letter of the code indicates the pacemaker's programmability — P (basic function programmability), M (multiprogrammable), C (communicating functions such as telemetry), R (rate responsiveness or modulation), or O (none).

■ The fifth letter of the code denotes special tachyarrhythmia functions and identifies how the pacemaker will respond to a tachyarrhythmia — P (pacing ability), S (shock), D (dual, can shock and pace), or O (none).

A permanent pacemaker is used to treat chronic heart conditions such as atrioventricular (AV) block; it's surgically implanted, usually under local anesthesia.

A biventricular pacemaker is also available for patients with heart failure. This device differs from a standard pacemaker in that it has three leads instead of one or two. One lead is placed in the right atrium and the others are placed in each of the ventricles, where they simultaneously stimulate the right and left ventricle. This allows the ventricles to coordinate their pumping ac-

tion and makes the heart more efficient.

Usually inserted in an emergency, a temporary pacemaker supports the patient until the emergency resolves. It can also serve as a bridge until a permanent pacemaker is inserted. A temporary pacemaker is used for the patient with high-grade heart block, bradycardia, or low CO. Several types of temporary pacemakers are available including transvenous, epicardial, transcutaneous, and transthoracic.

Procedure

Permanent pacemaker

Under fluoroscopy and using the transvenous approach, the physician inserts a catheter percutaneously or by venous cutdown and then threads the catheter through the cephalic or external jugular vein until the tip reaches the endocardium. For lead placement in the atrium, the tip must lodge in the right atrium or coronary sinus. For lead placement in the ventricle, the tip must lodge within the right ventricular apex in one of the interior muscular ridges or trabeculae.

When the lead is in the proper position, the pulse generator is secured in a subcutaneous pocket of tissue just below the clavicle. Changing the generator's battery or microchip circuitry requires only a shallow incision over the site and a quick component change.

Temporary pacemaker

The procedure for insertion of a temporary pacemaker varies depending on the type of pacemaker. (See *Temporary pacemakers,* pages 124 and 125.)

Temporary pacemakers

Four types of temporary pacemakers exist: transvenous, epicardial, transcutaneous, and transthoracic. Settings are similar for all four types.

Transvenous pacemakers

Physicians usually use the transvenous approach—inserting the pacemaker through a vein, such as the subclavian or internal jugular vein—when inserting a temporary pacemaker. The transvenous pacemaker is probably the most common and reliable type of temporary pacemaker. It's usually inserted at the bedside or in a fluoroscopy suite. The leadwires are advanced through a catheter into the right ventricle or atrium and connected to the pulse generator.

Epicardial pacemakers

Epicardial pacemakers are commonly used for patients undergoing cardiac surgery. The tips of the leadwires are attached to the heart's surface and then the wires are brought through the chest wall, below the incision. They're then at-

tached to the pulse generator. The lead-wires are usually removed several days after surgery or when the patient no longer requires them.

Transcutaneous pacemakers

Use of an external, or transcutaneous, pacemaker has become commonplace. In this noninvasive method, one electrode is placed on the patient's anterior chest wall to the right of the upper sternum but below the clavicle, and a second electrode is applied to his back (anterior-posterior electrodes), as shown below. One may also be placed to the left of the left nipple with the center of the electrode in the midaxillary line (also called the anterior-apex position). An external pulse generator then emits pacing impulses that travel through the skin to the heart muscle.

TRANSCUTANEOUS PACEMAKER

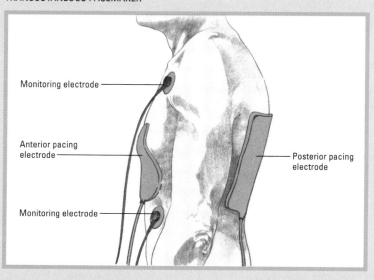

Monitoring electrode

Anterior pacing electrode

Posterior pacing electrode

Monitoring electrode

Temporary pacemakers *(continued)*

Transcutaneous pacing is a quick, effective method of pacing heart rhythm and is commonly used in emergencies until a transvenous pacemaker can be inserted. However, some patients can't tolerate the irritating sensations produced from prolonged pacing at the levels needed to pace the heart externally. If hemodynamically stable, these patients may require sedation.

Transthoracic pacemakers
A transthoracic pacemaker is a type of temporary ventricular pacemaker only used during cardiac emergencies as a last resort. Transthoracic pacing requires insertion of a long needle into the right ventricle using a subxyphoid approach. A pacing wire is then guided directly into the endocardium.

Temporary pacemaker settings
A temporary pacemaker has several types of settings on the pulse generator.

The rate control regulates how many impulses are generated in 1 minute and is measured in pulses per minute (ppm). The rate is usually set at 60 to 80 ppm. The pacemaker fires if the patient's heart rate falls below the preset rate. The rate may be set higher if the patient has a tachyarrhythmia being treated with overdrive pacing. The energy output of a pacemaker is measured in milliamperes (mA), a measurement that represents the stimulation threshold, or how much energy is required to stimulate the cardiac muscle to depolarize. The stimulation threshold is sometimes referred to as the energy required for capture.

You can also program the pacemaker's sensitivity, which is measured in millivolts (mV). Most pacemakers allow the heart to function naturally and assist only when necessary. The sensing threshold allows the pacemaker to do this by sensing the heart's normal activity.

Complications

Insertion of a permanent pacemaker places the patient at risk for infection, lead displacement, ventricle perforation, cardiac tamponade, or lead fracture and disconnection. Complications associated with a temporary pacemaker include microshock, equipment failure, and competitive or fatal arrhythmias.

Transcutaneous pacemakers may also cause skin breakdown, and muscle pain and twitching with firing. Transvenous pacemakers may cause such complications as pneumothorax or hemothorax, cardiac perforation and tamponade, diaphragmatic stimulation, pulmonary embolism, thrombophlebitis, and infection. Also, if the

physician threads the electrode through the antecubital or femoral vein, venous spasm, thrombophlebitis, or lead displacement may occur.

Complications associated with transthoracic pacemakers include pneumothorax, cardiac tamponade, emboli, sepsis, lacerations of the myocardium or coronary artery, and perforations of a cardiac chamber. Epicardial pacemakers carry a risk of infection, cardiac arrest, and diaphragmatic stimulation.

Nursing considerations
Before pacemaker insertion
■ Explain the procedure to the patient. If time permits, provide and review literature to help the patient un-

derstand how the device works. Emphasize that the pacemaker merely augments his natural heart rate.

■ Make sure the patient or a responsible family member signs a consent form, and ask the patient if he's allergic to anesthetics or iodine.

■ Complete skin preparation as per facility policy.

■ Establish an I.V. line at a keep-vein-open rate if not already inserted so that you can administer emergency drugs if the patient experiences ventricular arrhythmia.

■ Obtain baseline vital signs and a baseline electrocardiogram (ECG).

■ Administer sedation as ordered.

■ For a temporary pacemaker, insert a new battery into the external generator and test it to make sure that it has a strong charge.

After pacemaker insertion

Regardless of the type of pacemaker inserted or implanted, assess pacemaker function and watch for signs of pacemaker malfunction. (See *Assessing pacemaker function*.)

■ Record the date and time of pacemaker insertion, the type of pacemaker, the reason for insertion, and the patient's response. Note the pacemaker settings. Document any complications and the interventions taken.

If the patient has had a permanent pacemaker inserted, then complete the following:

■ Monitor the patient's ECG continuously to check for arrhythmias and to ensure correct pacemaker functioning.

■ Maintain I.V. flow rate; the I.V. line is usually kept in place for 24 to 48 hours postoperatively to allow for possible emergency treatment of arrhythmias.

■ Check the dressing for signs of bleeding and infection (swelling, redness, or exudate). The physician may order prophylactic antibiotics for up to 7 days after the implantation.

■ Change the dressing as per facility policy.

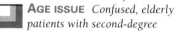 **ALERT** *If the dressing becomes soiled or the site is exposed to air, change the dressing immediately, regardless of when it was changed last.*

■ Check vital signs and level of consciousness (LOC) every 15 minutes for the first hour, every hour for the next 4 hours, every 4 hours for the next 48 hours, and then once every shift.

AGE ISSUE *Confused, elderly patients with second-degree heart block won't show immediate improvement in LOC.*

■ Assess cardiac status frequently, including vital signs, heart and breath sounds, hemodynamic parameters as indicated, and complaints of chest pain.

ALERT *Watch for signs and symptoms of a perforated ventricle, with resultant cardiac tamponade: persistent hiccups, distant heart sounds, pulsus paradoxus, hypotension with narrow pulse pressure, increased venous pressure, cyanosis, distended neck veins, decreased urine output, restlessness, or complaints of fullness in the chest. If the patient develops any of these, notify the physician immediately.*

■ Provide the patient with an identification card that lists the pacemaker type and manufacturer, serial number, pacemaker rate setting, date implanted, and physician's name. Also instruct the patient in measures for daily care, safety and activity guidelines, and special precautions.

Assessing pacemaker function

After a pacemaker has been inserted, follow these steps to assess its function:

1. Determine the pacemaker's mode and settings.
2. Review the patient's 12-lead electrocardiogram (ECG).
3. Select a monitoring lead that clearly shows the pacemaker spikes.
4. Consider the pacemaker mode and whether symptoms of decreased cardiac output are present when evaluating the ECG.
5. Look for information that tells you which chamber is paced. Ask:
  – Is there capture?
  – Is there a P wave or QRS complex after each atrial or ventricular spike?
  – Do P waves and QRS complexes stem from intrinsic activity?
  – If intrinsic activity is present, what's the pacemaker's response?
6. Determine the rate by quickly counting the number of complexes in a 6-second ECG strip or, more accurately, by counting the number of small boxes between complexes and dividing by 1,500.

Pacemaker impulses are visible on an ECG tracing as spikes. Large or small, pacemaker spikes appear above or below the isoelectric line. The illustration below shows an atrial and ventricular pacemaker spike.

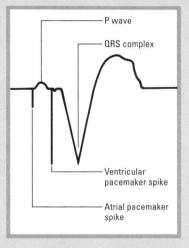

If the patient has had a temporary pacemaker inserted, complete the following:

■ After insertion of a temporary pacemaker, assess the patient's vital signs, skin color, LOC, and peripheral pulses to determine the effectiveness of the paced rhythm.

■ Perform a 12-lead ECG to serve as a baseline, and then perform additional 12-lead ECGs daily or with clinical changes. Also, if possible, obtain a rhythm strip before, during, and after pacemaker placement; any time pacemaker settings are changed; and whenever the patient receives treatment because of a complication due to the pacemaker.

■ Continuously monitor the ECG reading, noting capture, sensing, rate, intrinsic beats, and competition of paced and intrinsic rhythms. If the pacemaker is sensing correctly, the sense indicator on the pulse generator should flash with each beat. (See *Recognizing a malfunctioning pacemaker,* pages 128 and 129.)

■ Watch for oversensing. If the pacemaker is too sensitive, it can misinterpret muscle movements or other events in the cardiac cycle as intrinsic cardiac electrical activity. Pacing won't

Recognizing a malfunctioning pacemaker

When a pacemaker fails to function properly, you'll need to take immediate action to correct the problem. The rhythm strips below show examples of problems that can occur with a temporary pacemaker.

Failure to capture

- If the patient's condition has changed, notify the physician and request new settings.
- If the pacemaker settings have been altered by anyone not authorized to do so, return them to their correct positions. Make sure the pacemaker's face is covered with its plastic shield. Remind the patient not to touch the dials.

- If the heart still doesn't respond, carefully check all connections. You can also increase the milliampere setting slowly (according to your facility's policy or the physician's orders), turn the patient from side to side, change the battery, and reverse the cables in the pulse generator so the positive wire is in the negative terminal and vice versa. Keep in mind that chest X-rays may be needed to determine electrode position.

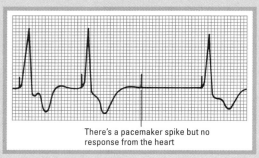

There's a pacemaker spike but no response from the heart

Failure to pace

- If the pacing or indicator light flashes, check the connections to the cable and the position of the pacing electrode in the patient (performed by X-ray).

- If the pulse generator is turned on but the indicators aren't flashing, change the battery. If the battery is functioning properly, use a different pulse generator.

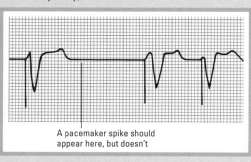

A pacemaker spike should appear here, but doesn't

Recognizing a malfunctioning pacemaker *(continued)*

Failure to sense intrinsic beats

● If the pacemaker is undersensing (it fires but at the wrong times or for the wrong reasons), turn the sensitivity control completely to the right. If the pacemaker is oversensing (it incorrectly senses depolarization and refuses to fire when it should), turn the sensitivity control slightly to the left.

● Change the battery or pulse generator.

● Remove items in the room that might be causing electromechanical interfer-ence. Ensure that the bed is grounded. Unplug each piece of equipment in turn, checking to see whether the interfer-ence stops.

● If the pacemaker is still firing on the T wave and all corrective actions have failed, turn off the pacemaker per the physician's order. Make sure atropine is available in case the patient's heart rate drops, and be prepared to initiate car-diopulmonary resuscitation if necessary.

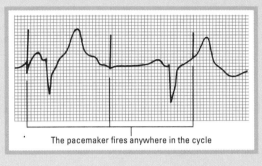

The pacemaker fires anywhere in the cycle

---

occur when it's needed, and the heart rate and AV synchrony won't be main-tained.

■ When using a transcutaneous pace-maker, don't place the electrodes over a bony area because bone conducts current poorly. With a female patient, place the anterior electrode under the patient's breast but not over her di-aphragm. If the physician inserts the electrode through the brachial or femoral vein, immobilize the patient's arm or leg to avoid putting stress on the pacing wires.

■ If the patient has epicardial pacing wires in place, clean the insertion site as per facility policy and change dress-ing daily. At the same time, monitor the site for signs of infection. Always keep the pulse generator nearby in case pacing becomes necessary.

■ Institute precautions to prevent mi-croshock. This includes warning the patient not to use any electrical equip-ment that isn't grounded, such as tele-phones, electric shavers, televisions, or lamps.

■ Place a plastic cover supplied by the manufacturer over the pacemaker con-trols to avoid an accidental setting change. Also, insulate the pacemaker by covering exposed metal parts, such as electrode connections and pacemak-er terminals, with nonconducting tape, or place the pacing unit in a dry, rub-ber surgical glove.

■ If the patient is disoriented or unco-operative, use restraints as necessary to prevent accidental removal of pace-maker wires. If the patient needs emer-gency defibrillation, make sure the pacemaker can withstand the proce-dure. If unsure, disconnect the pulse generator to prevent damage.

Percutaneous transluminal coronary angioplasty

A nonsurgical approach to opening coronary vessels narrowed by arte-riosclerosis, percutaneous transluminal coronary angioplasty (PTCA) uses a balloon-tipped catheter that's inserted into a narrowed coronary artery. This procedure, performed in the cardiac catheterization laboratory under local anesthesia, relieves pain due to angina and myocardial ischemia.

PTCA provides an alternative for patients who are poor surgical risks because of chronic medical problems. It's also useful for patients who have total coronary occlusion, unstable angina, and plaque buildup in several areas and for those with poor left ven-tricular function. The ideal candidate for PTCA has single- or double-vessel disease excluding the left main coro-nary artery with at least 50% proximal stenosis. The lesion should be discrete, uncalcified, concentric, and not locat-ed near a bifurcation. Laser-enhanced angioplasty is showing promising re-sults in vaporizing occlusions in ather-osclerosis.

Procedure

Cardiac catheterization usually accom-panies PTCA to assess the stenosis and the angioplasty's efficacy. Catheteriza-tion is used as a visual tool to direct the balloon-tipped catheter through the vessel's area of stenosis. After coro-nary angiography confirms the occlu-sion's presence and location, the physi-cian threads a guide catheter through the patient's femoral artery and into the coronary artery under fluoroscopic guidance.

When the guide catheter's position at the occlusion site is confirmed by angiography, the physician carefully introduces a double-lumen balloon (the lumen is smaller than that of the catheter) into the catheter. He then di-rects the balloon through the lesion where a marked pressure gradient is obvious. The physician alternately in-flates and deflates the balloon until ar-teriography verifies successful arterial dilation and decrease in the pressure gradient. With balloon inflation, the plaque is compressed against the ves-sel wall, allowing coronary blood to flow more freely.

Complications

The most common complication of PTCA is prolonged angina. Others in-clude coronary artery perforation, bal-loon rupture, reocclusion (necessitat-ing a coronary artery bypass graft), myocardial infarction, pericardial tam-ponade, hematoma, hemorrhage, reperfusion arrhythmias, and closure of the vessel. Vascular stents may be inserted to prevent vessel closure.

Nursing considerations

Before PTCA

■ Explain the procedure to the patient and his family to reduce fear and promote cooperation.

■ Inform the patient that the procedure lasts from 1 to 4 hours and that he may feel some discomfort from lying on a hard table for that long.

■ Tell him that a catheter will be inserted into an artery or a vein in his groin and that he may feel pressure as the catheter moves along the vessel.

■ Reassure him that although he'll be awake during the procedure, he'll be given a sedative. Explain that the physician or nurse may ask him how he's feeling and that he should tell them if he experiences angina.

■ Explain that the physician will inject a contrast medium to outline the lesion's location. Warn the patient that he may feel a hot, flushing sensation or transient nausea during the injection.

■ Check the patient's history for allergies; if he's had allergic reactions to shellfish, iodine, or contrast media, notify the physician.

■ Give 650 mg of aspirin the evening before the procedure, as ordered, to prevent platelet aggregation.

■ Make sure the patient or a responsible family member has signed a consent form.

■ Restrict food and fluids for at least 6 hours before the procedure or as ordered.

■ Ensure that the results of coagulation studies, complete blood count, serum electrolyte studies, and blood typing and crossmatching are available; obtain baseline vital signs and assess peripheral pulses.

■ Apply electrocardiogram (ECG) electrodes and insert an I.V. line if not already in place to provide continuous monitoring and administer emergency medications if necessary; ensure I.V. line patency.

■ Administer oxygen through a nasal cannula.

■ Perform skin preparation as per facility policy.

■ Give the patient a sedative as ordered.

After PTCA

Care of the patient following PTCA is similar to that for the patient following a cardiac catheterization (see discussion earlier in this chapter). Be sure to include the following:

■ Assess the patient's vital signs every 15 minutes for the first hour, then every 30 minutes for 4 hours, unless his condition warrants more frequent checking. Monitor I.V. infusions, such as heparin or nitroglycerin, as indicated.

■ Assess peripheral pulses distal to the catheter insertion site as well as the color, sensation, temperature, and capillary refill of the affected extremity.

■ Monitor ECG rhythm continuously; assess hemodynamic parameters closely for changes.

ALERT *Because coronary spasm may occur during or after PTCA, monitor the patient's ECG for ST-segment and T-wave changes, and take vital signs frequently. Coronary artery dissection may occur with no early symptoms, but it can cause restenosis of the vessel. Be alert for symptoms of ischemia, which requires emergency coronary revascularization.*

■ Instruct the patient to remain in bed for 8 hours and to keep the affected extremity straight; if the patient is restless and moving his extremities, apply soft restraints if necessary. Maintain sandbags in position if used to apply pressure to catheter site. Elevate the head of the bed 15 to 30 degrees. If a hemostatic device was used to close the catheter insertion site, anticipate that the patient may be allowed out of bed in only a few hours.

■ Assess the catheter site for hematoma, ecchymosis, and hemorrhage. If an area of expanding hematoma appears, mark the site and alert the physician. If bleeding occurs, locate the artery and apply manual pressure; then notify the physician.

■ Administer I.V. fluids as ordered (usually 100 ml/hour) to promote excretion of the contrast medium. Be sure to assess for signs of fluid overload (distended neck veins, atrial and ventricular gallops, dyspnea, pulmonary congestion, tachycardia, hypertension, and hypoxemia).

■ After the physician removes the catheter, apply direct pressure for at least 10 minutes and monitor the site often.

■ Keep in mind that PTCA is contraindicated in patients with left main coronary artery disease, especially when the patient is a poor surgical risk; in patients with variant angina or critical valvular disease; and in patients with vessels that are occluded at the aortic wall orifice.

■ Document the patient's tolerance of the procedure and status after it, including vital signs, hemodynamic parameters, appearance of catheter site, ECG findings, the condition of the extremity distal to the insertion site and any complications and interventions necessary.

Pericarditis

Pericarditis is an inflammation of the pericardium — the fibroserous sac that envelops, supports, and protects the heart. It occurs in acute and chronic forms. Acute pericarditis can be fibrinous or effusive, with purulent, serous, or hemorrhagic exudate. Chronic constrictive pericarditis is characterized by dense fibrous pericardial thickening. The prognosis depends on the underlying cause but is generally good in acute pericarditis, unless constriction occurs.

Pericarditis may result from the following:

■ bacterial, fungal, or viral infection (infectious pericarditis)

■ neoplasms (primary, or metastasis from lungs, breasts, or other organs)

■ high-dose radiation to the chest

■ uremia

■ hypersensitivity or autoimmune disease, such as acute rheumatic fever (most common cause of pericarditis in children), systemic lupus erythematosus, and rheumatoid arthritis

■ previous cardiac injury, such as myocardial infarction (MI) (Dressler's syndrome), trauma, or surgery (postcardiotomy syndrome), that leaves the pericardium intact but causes blood to leak into the pericardial cavity

■ drugs, such as hydralazine or procainamide

■ idiopathic factors (most common in acute pericarditis)

■ aortic aneurysm with pericardial leakage (less common)

■ myxedema with cholesterol deposits in the pericardium (less common).

Pathophysiology

Pericardial tissue damaged by bacteria or other substances results in the release of chemical mediators of inflammation (prostaglandins, histamines, bradykinins, and serotonin) into the surrounding tissue, thereby initiating the inflammatory process. Friction occurs as the inflamed pericardial layers rub against each other. Histamines and other chemical mediators dilate vessels and increase vessel permeability. Vessel walls then leak fluids and protein (including fibrinogen) into tissues, causing extracellular edema. Macrophages already present in the tissue begin to phagocytize the invading bacteria and are joined by neutrophils and monocytes. After several days, the area fills with an exudate composed of necrotic tissue and dead and dying bacteria, neutrophils, and macrophages. Eventually, the cavity's contents autolyze and are gradually reabsorbed into healthy tissue.

A pericardial effusion develops if fluid accumulates in the pericardial cavity. Cardiac tamponade results when fluid accumulates rapidly in the pericardial space, compressing the heart and preventing it from filling during diastole, and resulting in a drop in cardiac output (CO). (See "Cardiac tamponade," page 51.)

Chronic constrictive pericarditis develops if the pericardium becomes thick and stiff from chronic or recurrent pericarditis, encasing the heart in a stiff shell and preventing the heart from properly filling during diastole. This causes an increase in both left- and right-sided filling pressures, leading to a drop in stroke volume and CO.

Comprehensive assessment

The patient with acute pericarditis typically complains of sharp, sudden pain, usually starting over the sternum and radiating to the neck, shoulders, back, and arms. The pain is usually pleuritic, increasing with deep inspiration and decreasing when the patient sits up and leans forward. This decrease occurs because leaning forward pulls the heart away from the diaphragmatic pleurae of the lungs. The patient may complain of dyspnea. His history may include an event or disease that can cause pericarditis, such as chest trauma, MI, or recent bacterial infection.

Pericarditis can mimic the pain of MI. However, the patient may have no pain if he has slowly developing tuberculous pericarditis or postirradiation, neoplastic, or uremic pericarditis.

Auscultation may reveal muffled and distant heart sounds. It almost always reveals a pericardial friction rub, which is a grating sound heard as the heart moves. You can hear it best during forced expiration, while the patient leans forward or is on his hands and knees in bed. The rub may have up to three components that correspond to atrial systole, ventricular systole, and the rapid-filling phase of ventricular diastole. Occasionally, the friction rub is heard only briefly or not at all. If acute pericarditis has caused very large pericardial effusions, heart sounds may be distant.

Palpation may reveal a diminished or an absent apical impulse. Constrictive pericarditis causes the membrane to calcify and become rigid. It also causes a gradual increase in systemic venous pressure and symptoms similar to those of chronic right-sided heart failure (fluid retention, ascites, hepato-megaly).

Tachycardia, an ill-defined substernal chest pain, and a feeling of fullness in the chest may indicate pericardial effusion. Pallor, clammy skin, hypotension, pulsus paradoxus (drop in systolic blood pressure of 15 mm Hg or greater during slow inspiration), neck vein distention, and dyspnea indicate cardiac tamponade.

Additional signs and symptoms may include:
■ mild fever caused by the inflammatory process
■ pericardial knock in early diastole along the left sternal border produced by restricted ventricular filling
■ Kussmaul's sign, increased jugular vein distention on inspiration, due to restricted right-sided filling.

Diagnosis

■ Electrocardiogram (ECG) may reveal diffuse ST-segment elevation in the limb leads and most precordial leads that reflects the inflammatory process. Upright T waves are present in most leads. QRS segments may be diminished when pericardial effusion exists. Arrhythmias, such as atrial fibrillation and sinus arrhythmias, may occur. In chronic constrictive pericarditis, there may be low-voltage QRS complexes, T-wave inversion or flattening, and P mitrale (wide P waves) in leads I, II, and V_6.
■ Laboratory testing may reveal an elevated erythrocyte sedimentation rate as a result of the inflammatory process or a normal or elevated white blood cell count, especially in infectious pericarditis; blood urea nitrogen may detect uremia as a cause of pericarditis.

■ Blood cultures may identify an infectious cause.
■ Antistreptolysin-O titers may be positive if pericarditis is due to rheumatic fever.
■ Reaction to purified protein derivative skin test may be positive if pericarditis is due to tuberculosis.
■ Echocardiography may show an echo-free space between the ventricular wall and the pericardium, and reduced pumping action of the heart.
■ Chest X-rays may be normal with acute pericarditis. The cardiac silhouette may be enlarged with a water bottle shape caused by fluid accumulation, if pleural effusion is present.

Collaborations

The patient with pericarditis can be acutely ill and require the attention of a cardiologist and a skilled team to stabilize and manage the patient. Disciplines, such as respiratory therapy and physical therapy for rehabilitation, may be consulted.

Treatment and care

Appropriate treatment aims to relieve symptoms, manage underlying systemic disease, and prevent or treat pericardial effusion and cardiac tamponade. In idiopathic pericarditis, postmyocardial infarction pericarditis, and postthoracotomy pericarditis, treatment consists of bed rest as long as fever and pain persist and the administration of nonsteroidal drugs, such as aspirin and indomethacin, to relieve pain and reduce inflammation. If symptoms continue, the physician may prescribe corticosteroids. Although they provide rapid and effective relief, corticosteroids must be used cautiously because the disorder may recur when drug therapy stops.

When infectious pericarditis results from disease of the left pleural space, mediastinal abscesses, or septicemia, the patient will require antibiotics, surgical drainage, or both. If cardiac tamponade develops, the physician may perform emergency pericardiocentesis and may inject antibiotics directly into the pericardial sac. (See *Understanding pericardiocentesis*, pages 136 and 137.)

Recurrent pericarditis may require partial pericardectomy, which creates a window that allows fluid to drain into the pleural space. In constrictive pericarditis, total pericardectomy may be necessary to permit the heart to fill and contract adequately. Treatment must also include management of rheumatic fever, uremia, tuberculosis, and other underlying disorders.

Complications

Pericardial effusion is the major complication of acute pericarditis. If fluid accumulates rapidly, cardiac tamponade may occur, resulting in shock, cardiovascular collapse, and eventually death.

Nursing considerations

■ Maintain the patient on bed rest until fever and pain have diminished. Assist the patient with bathing if necessary. Provide a bedside commode to reduce myocardial oxygen demand. Offer physically undemanding diversional activities.
■ Place the patient in an upright position to relieve dyspnea and chest pain. Auscultate breath sounds at least every 4 hours or more frequently if indicated. Administer supplemental oxygen as needed based on oxygen saturation or mixed venous oxygen saturation levels.
■ Administer analgesics to relieve pain and nonsteroidal anti-inflammatory drugs (NSAIDs) as ordered to reduce inflammation. Evaluate patient's response to NSAIDs. Expect to administer steroids such as prednisone if the patient fails to respond to NSAIDs.
■ If a pulmonary artery catheter is present, monitor the patient's hemodynamic status.

ALERT   *Keep in mind that central venous pressure, pulmonary artery pressure, and pulmonary artery wedge pressure will be elevated with pericarditis. Be alert for decreases in CO, which suggest increasing effusion.*

■ Assess the patient's cardiovascular status frequently, watching for signs of cardiac tamponade.
■ Before giving antibiotics, obtain a patient history of allergies. Administer antibiotics on time to maintain consistent drug levels in the blood.
■ Institute continuous cardiac monitoring to evaluate for changes in ECG; look for return of ST segments to baseline with T-wave flattening by the end of the first 7 days.
■ Keep a pericardiocentesis set readily available if pericardial effusion is suspected and prepare the patient for pericardiocentesis, as indicated.
■ To reduce anxiety, allow the patient to express his concerns about the effects of activity restrictions on his responsibilities and routines. Reassure him that the restrictions are temporary.
■ Provide appropriate postoperative care, similar to that given after cardiothoracic surgery.

Understanding pericardiocentesis

Typically performed at bedside in a critical care unit, pericardiocentesis involves the needle aspiration of excess fluid from the pericardial sac. It may be the treatment of choice for life-threatening cardiac tamponade (except when fluid accumulates rapidly, in which case immediate surgery is usually preferred). Pericardiocentesis may also be used to aspirate fluid in subacute conditions, such as viral or bacterial infections and pericarditis. What's more, it provides a sample for laboratory analysis to confirm diagnosis and identify the cause of pericardial effusion.

Procedure

After starting continuous electrocardiogram (ECG) monitoring and administering a local anesthetic at the puncture site, the physician inserts the aspiration needle in one of three areas. He'll probably choose the xiphocostal approach, with needle insertion in the angle between the left costal margin and the xiphoid process, to avoid needle contact with the pleura and the coronary vessels, thus decreasing the risk of damage to these structures.

As an alternative, he may use the parasternal approach, inserting the needle into the fifth or sixth intercostal space next to the left side of the sternum, where the pericardium normally isn't covered by lung tissue; however, this method poses a risk of puncture of the left anterior descending coronary artery or the internal mammary artery.

He may opt for a third method, the apical approach, in which he inserts the needle at the cardiac apex; however, because this method poses the greatest risk of complications, such as pneumothorax, he'll need to proceed cautiously.

After inserting the needle tip, the physician slowly advances it into the pericardial sac to a depth of 1″ to 2″ (2.5 to 5 cm), or until he can aspirate fluid. He then clamps a hemostat to the needle at the chest wall to prevent needle movement.

The physician then slowly aspirates pericardial fluid. If he finds large amounts of fluid, he may place an indwelling catheter into the pericardial sac to allow continuous, slow drainage. After the physician has removed the fluid, he withdraws the needle and places a dressing over the puncture site.

Complications

Pericardiocentesis carries some risk of potentially fatal complications, such as inadvertent puncture of internal organs (particularly the heart, lung, stomach, or liver) or laceration of the myocardium or of a coronary artery. Therefore, keep emergency equipment readily available during the procedure.

Nursing considerations
Before the procedure

● Help the patient comply by clearly explaining the procedure. Briefly discuss possible complications, such as arrhythmias and organ or artery puncture, but reassure him that such complications rarely occur. Tell him he'll have an I.V. line inserted to provide access for medications, if needed.

● Make sure the patient (or a family member, if appropriate) has signed a consent form.

● Place the patient in a supine position in his bed, with his upper torso raised 60 degrees and his arms supported by pillows. Shave the needle insertion site on his chest if necessary, and clean the area with an antiseptic solution. Next, apply 12-lead ECG electrodes. If ordered, assist the physician in attaching the pericardial needle to the precordial lead (V) of the ECG and also to a three-way stopcock.

Understanding pericardiocentesis *(continued)*

During the procedure
● Closely monitor the patient's blood pressure and hemodynamic parameters. Check the ECG pattern continuously for premature ventricular contractions and elevated ST segments, which may indicate that the needle has touched the ventricle; for elevated PR segments, which may indicate that the needle has touched the atrium; and for large, erratic QRS complexes, which may indicate that the needle has penetrated the heart. Also watch for signs of organ puncture, such as hypotension, decreased breath sounds, chest pain, dyspnea, hematoma, and tachycardia.
● Note and record the volume and character of any aspirated fluid. Blood that has accumulated slowly in the patient's pericardial sac usually doesn't clot after it has been aspirated; blood

from a sudden hemorrhage, however, will clot.

After the procedure
● Check the patient's vital signs at least hourly and maintain continuous ECG monitoring.
● Expect the patient's blood pressure to rise as the pressure from the fluid is relieved. Be alert for the development of recurring fluid collection; watch for decreased blood pressure, narrowing pulse pressure, increased central venous pressure, tachycardia, muffled heart sounds, tachypnea, pleural friction rub, distended neck veins, anxiety, and chest pain. Notify the physician of these signs; he may need to repeat pericardiocentesis or surgically drain the pericardium in the operating room.

Patient teaching
■ Explain tests and treatments to the patient.
■ If surgery will be necessary, teach the patient how to perform deep-breathing and coughing exercises before he undergoes the procedure.
■ Instruct the patient in energy conservation measures, with gradual resumption of activities as tolerated with frequent rest periods.

Pulmonary artery pressure monitoring

Continuous pulmonary artery pressure (PAP) and intermittent pulmonary artery wedge pressure (PAWP) measurements provide important informa-

tion about left ventricular function and preload. You can use this information not only for monitoring but also for aiding diagnosis, refining assessment, guiding interventions, and projecting patient outcomes.

Nearly all acutely ill patients are candidates for PAP monitoring — especially those who are hemodynamically unstable, who need fluid management or continuous cardiopulmonary assessment, or who are receiving multiple or frequently administered cardioactive drugs. PAP monitoring is also crucial for patients with shock, trauma, pulmonary or cardiac disease, or multisystem disease.

The original PAP monitoring catheter, called Swan-Ganz catheter or more commonly a pulmonary artery (PA) catheter, had two lumens. Current versions have up to six lumens, allowing more hemodynamic information to be gathered. In addition to distal and proximal lumens used to measure pressures, a PA catheter has a balloon inflation lumen that inflates the balloon for PAWP measurement and a thermistor connector lumen that allows cardiac output measurement. Some catheters also have a pacemaker wire lumen that provides a port for pacemaker electrodes and measures continuous mixed venous oxygen saturation.

Fluoroscopy usually isn't required during catheter insertion because the catheter is flow-directed, following venous blood flow from the right-heart chambers into the pulmonary artery. Also, the pulmonary artery, right atrium, and right ventricle produce characteristic pressures and waveforms that can be observed on the monitor to help track catheter-tip location. Marks on the catheter shaft, with 10-cm graduations, assist tracking by showing how far the catheter is inserted.

The PA catheter is inserted into the heart's right side with the distal tip lying in the pulmonary artery. Left-sided pressures can be assessed indirectly. No specific contraindications for PAP monitoring exist. However, some patients, such as elderly patients with pulmonary hypertension, those with left bundle-branch heart block, and those for whom a systemic infection would be life-threatening, require special precautions during insertion and use.

Equipment

Balloon-tipped, flow-directed PA catheter ▪ prepared pressure transducer system ▪ I.V. solutions ▪ sterile syringes ▪ alcohol pads ▪ medication-added label ▪ monitor and monitor cable ▪ I.V. pole with transducer mount ▪ emergency resuscitation equipment ▪ electrocardiogram (ECG) monitor ▪ ECG electrodes ▪ arm board (for antecubital insertion) ▪ lead aprons (if fluoroscope is necessary) ▪ sutures ▪ sterile $4'' \times 4''$ gauze pads or other dry, occlusive dressing material ▪ prepackaged introducer kit ▪ optional: dextrose 5% in water, shaving materials (for femoral insertion site), small sterile basin, and sterile water

If a prepackaged introducer kit is unavailable, obtain the following: an introducer (one size larger than the catheter) ▪ sterile tray containing instruments for procedure ▪ masks ▪ sterile gowns ▪ sterile gloves ▪ sterile drapes ▪ povidone-iodine ointment and solution ▪ sutures ▪ two 10-ml syringes ▪ local anesthetic (1% to 2% lidocaine) ▪ one 5-ml syringe ▪ 25G $1^{1}/_{2}''$ needle ▪ 1″ and 3″ tape

Essential steps
Before insertion

▪ To obtain reliable pressure values and clear waveforms, make sure that the pressure monitoring system and bedside monitor are properly calibrated and zeroed. Make sure the monitor has the correct pressure modules; then calibrate it according to the manufacturer's instructions.
▪ Turn the monitor on before gathering the equipment to give it time to warm up. Be sure to check the operations manual for the monitor you're using; some older monitors may need 20 minutes to warm up.
▪ Prepare the pressure monitoring system according to policy. Check your facility's guidelines, which may also specify whether to mount the

transducer on the I.V. pole or tape it to the patient and whether to add heparin to the flush.

🖐 **ALERT** *To manage complications from catheter insertion, be sure to have emergency resuscitation equipment on hand (defibrillator, oxygen, and supplies for intubation and emergency drug administration).*

■ Prepare a sterile field for insertion of the introducer and catheter. A bedside tray, placed on the same side as the insertion site for easier access, may be sufficient.

■ Check the patient's chart for heparin sensitivity, which contraindicates adding heparin to the flush solution. If the patient is alert, explain the procedure to him to reduce his anxiety. Mention that the catheter will monitor pressures from the pulmonary artery and heart. Reassure him that the catheter poses little danger and rarely causes pain. Tell him that if he feels pain at the introducer insertion site, the physician will order an analgesic or a sedative.

■ Be sure to tell the patient and his family not to be alarmed if they see the pressure waveform on the monitor "move around." Explain that the cause usually is artifact.

Positioning the patient for catheter placement

■ Position the patient at the proper height and angle. If the physician will use a superior approach for percutaneous insertion (most commonly using the internal jugular or subclavian vein), place the patient flat or in a slight Trendelenburg position. Remove the patient's pillow to help engorge the vessel and prevent air embolism. Turn his head to the side opposite the insertion site.

■ If the physician will use an inferior approach to access a femoral vein, position the patient flat. Be aware that with this approach, certain catheters are harder to insert and may require more manipulation.

■ Adhere to standard precautions throughout catheter preparation and insertion and assist the physician with catheter insertion, being sure to maintain strict sterile technique throughout.

■ To remove air from the catheter and verify its patency, flush the catheter. In the more common flushing method, connect the I.V. solutions using sterile technique to the appropriate pressure lines, and then flush them before insertion. This method makes pressure waveforms easier to identify on the monitor during insertion. Alternatively, flush the lumens with sterile I.V. solution from sterile syringes attached to the lumens. Leave the filled syringes on during insertion.

■ If the system has multiple pressure lines (such as a distal line to monitor PAP and a proximal line to monitor right atrial pressure), make sure the distal PA lumen hub is attached to the pressure line that will be observed on the monitor.

🖐 **ALERT** *Inadvertently attaching the distal PA line to the proximal lumen hub will prevent the proper waveform from appearing during insertion.*

■ Observe the diastolic values carefully during insertion. Make sure the scale is appropriate for lower pressures. A scale of 0 to 25 mm Hg or 0 to 50 mm Hg (more common) is preferred. (With a higher scale, such as 0 to 100 or 0 to 250 mm Hg, waveforms appear too small and the location of the catheter tip will be hard to identify.)

■ After the physician verifies the integrity of the balloon (usually with 1.5 cc of air), attach the lumens to the pressure monitoring system. He then observes the balloon for symmetrical shape. He may also submerge it in a small, sterile basin filled with sterile water and observe it for bubbles, which indicate a leak.

Inserting the catheter

■ Assist the physician as he inserts the introducer to access the vessel. He may perform a cutdown or (more commonly) insert the catheter percutaneously.

■ After the introducer is placed, and the catheter lumens are flushed, observe as the physician inserts the catheter through the introducer. In the internal jugular or subclavian approach, he inserts the catheter into the end of the introducer sheath with the balloon deflated, directing the curl of the catheter toward the patient's midline.

■ As insertion begins, observe the bedside monitor for waveform variations. (See *Normal PA waveforms*.)

■ When the catheter exits the end of the introducer sheath and reaches the junction of the superior vena cava and right atrium (at the 15- to 20-cm mark on the catheter shaft), watch the monitor for oscillations that correspond to the patient's respirations. The balloon is then inflated with the recommended volume of air to allow normal blood flow and aid catheter insertion. Using a gentle, smooth motion, the physician advances the catheter through the heart chambers, moving rapidly to the pulmonary artery because prolonged manipulation here may reduce catheter stiffness.

■ When the mark on the catheter shaft reaches 15 to 20 cm (the catheter is entering the right atrium), watch the waveform for two small, upright waves; pressure is low (between 4 and 6 mm Hg). Read pressure values in the mean mode because systolic and diastolic values are similar. This is the right atrial pressure, essentially the same as the central venous pressure.

■ As the physician advances the catheter into the right ventricle, working quickly to minimize irritation, look for the waveform to show sharp systolic upstrokes and lower diastolic dips. Depending on the size of the patient's heart, the catheter should reach the 30- to 35-cm mark. (The smaller the heart, the shorter the catheter length needed to reach the right ventricle.) Record systolic and diastolic pressures. Systolic pressure normally ranges from 15 to 25 mm Hg; diastolic pressure, from 0 to 8 mm Hg.

■ As the catheter floats into the pulmonary artery, note that the upstroke from right ventricular systole is smoother, and systolic pressure is nearly the same as right ventricular systolic pressure. Record systolic, diastolic, and mean pressures (typically ranging from 8 to 15 mm Hg). A dicrotic notch on the diastolic portion of the waveform indicates pulmonic valve closure.

Wedging the catheter

■ Obtain a wedge tracing. The physician lets the inflated balloon float downstream with venous blood flow to a smaller, more distal branch of the pulmonary artery. Here, the catheter

Normal PA waveforms

During pulmonary artery (PA) catheter insertion, the monitor shows various waveforms as the catheter advances through the heart's chambers.

Right atrium

When the catheter tip enters the right atrium, a waveform like the one shown appears on the monitor. Note the two small upright waves. The a waves represent left atrial contraction; the v waves, increased pressure or volume in the left atrium during left ventricular systole.

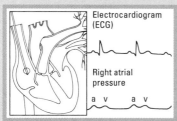

Electrocardiogram (ECG)

Right atrial pressure

a v a v

Right ventricle

As the catheter tip enters the right ventricle, you'll see a waveform with sharp systolic upstrokes and lower diastolic dips.

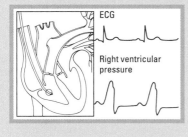

ECG

Right ventricular pressure

Pulmonary artery

The catheter then floats into the pulmonary artery causing a waveform as shown. Note that the upstroke is smoother than on the right ventricular waveform. The dicrotic notch indicates pulmonic valve closure.

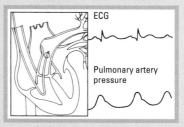

ECG

Pulmonary artery pressure

PAWP

Floating into a distal branch of the pulmonary artery, the balloon wedges where the vessel becomes too narrow for it to pass. The monitor now shows a pulmonary artery wedge pressure (PAWP) waveform with two small uprises from left atrial systole and diastole. The balloon is then deflated and the catheter is left in the pulmonary artery.

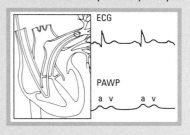

ECG

PAWP

a v a v

lodges, or wedges, causing occlusion of right ventricular and pulmonary artery diastolic pressures. The tracing resembles the right atrial tracing because the catheter tip is recording left atrial pressure.

■ Observe the waveform, which should show two small uprises. Record

PAWP in the mean mode (usually between 6 and 12 mm Hg). A PAWP waveform, or wedge tracing, appears when the catheter has been inserted 45 to 50 cm. (In a large heart, a longer catheter length — up to 55 cm — typically is required. However, a catheter should never be inserted more than 60 cm.) Usually, 30 to 45 seconds elapse from the time the physician inserts the introducer until the wedge tracing appears. Then the physician deflates the balloon, and the catheter drifts out of the wedge position and into the pulmonary artery, its normal resting place.

■ If the appropriate waveforms don't appear at the expected times during catheter insertion, be aware that the catheter may be coiled in the right atrium and ventricle. To correct this problem, deflate the balloon. To do this, unlock the gate valve or turn the stopcock to the ON position and then detach the syringe from the balloon inflation port. Back pressure in the pulmonary artery causes the balloon to deflate on its own. (Active air withdrawal may compromise balloon integrity.) To verify balloon deflation, observe the monitor for return of the pulmonary artery tracing.

■ Obtain a portable chest X-ray as ordered to confirm catheter position.

■ Apply a sterile occlusive dressing to the insertion site.

Obtaining intermittent PAP values

■ After inserting the catheter and recording initial pressure readings, record subsequent PAP values and monitor waveforms. These values will be used to calculate other important hemodynamic indices. To ensure accurate values, make sure the transducer is properly leveled and zeroed.

■ If possible, obtain PAP values at end expiration (when the patient completely exhales). At this time, intrathoracic pressure approaches atmospheric pressure and has the least effect on PAP. If you obtain a reading during other phases of the respiratory cycle, respiratory interference may occur. For instance, during inspiration, when intrathoracic pressure drops, PAP may be false-low because the negative pressure is transmitted to the catheter. During expiration, when intrathoracic pressure rises, PAP may be false-high.

■ Use the average of the digital readings obtained over time for patients with a rapid respiratory rate and subsequent variations. If possible, obtain a printout. Use the averaged values obtained through the full respiratory cycle. To analyze trends accurately, be sure to record values at consistent times during the respiratory cycle.

Taking a PAWP reading

By inflating the balloon and letting it float in a distal artery, you can record PAWP. Some facilities allow only physicians or specially trained nurses to take a PAWP reading because of the risk of pulmonary artery rupture — a rare but life-threatening complication. If your facility permits you to perform this procedure, do so with extreme caution and make sure you're thoroughly familiar with intracardiac waveform interpretation.

■ To begin, verify that the transducer is properly leveled and zeroed. Detach the syringe from the balloon inflation hub. Draw 1.5 cc of air into the syringe, and then reattach the syringe to the hub. Watching the monitor, inject the air through the hub slowly and smoothly. When you see a wedge tracing on the monitor, immediately stop inflating the balloon.

ALERT *Never inflate the balloon beyond the volume needed to obtain a wedge tracing. Otherwise the pulmonary artery could rupture.*

■ Take the pressure reading at end expiration.

■ Note the amount of air needed to change the pulmonary artery tracing to a wedge tracing (normally, 1.25 to 1.5 cc). If the wedge tracing appeared with injection of less than 1.25 cc, suspect that the catheter has migrated into a more distal branch and requires repositioning. If the balloon is in a more distal branch, the tracings may move up the oscilloscope, indicating that the catheter tip is recording balloon pressure rather than PAWP. This may lead to pulmonary artery rupture.

Removing the catheter

To assist the physician, inspect the chest X-ray for signs of catheter kinking or knotting. (In some states, you may be permitted to remove a PA catheter yourself under an advanced collaborative standard of practice.)

■ Obtain the patient's baseline vital signs, and note the ECG pattern.

■ Explain the procedure to the patient. Place the head of the bed flat, unless ordered otherwise. If the catheter was inserted using a superior approach, turn the patient's head to the side opposite the insertion site. Gently remove the dressing.

■ Prepare for the physician to remove any sutures securing the catheter. However, if he wants to leave the introducer in place after catheter re-

moval, he won't remove the sutures used to secure it.

■ Turn all stopcocks off to the patient. (You may turn stopcocks on to the distal port if you wish to observe waveforms. However, use caution because this may cause an air embolism.)

■ After putting on sterile gloves and verifying that the balloon is deflated, assist as necessary as the physician withdraws the catheter slowly and smoothly. If he feels any resistance, he'll stop immediately.

■ Watch the ECG monitor for arrhythmias.

■ If the introducer was removed, apply pressure to the site and check it frequently for signs of bleeding. Dress the site again as necessary. If the introducer is left in place, observe the diaphragm for any blood backflow, which verifies the integrity of the hemostasis valve.

■ Return equipment to the appropriate location. Turn off the bedside pressure modules but leave the ECG module on.

■ Reassure the patient and his family that he'll be observed closely. Make sure he understands that the catheter was removed because his condition has improved and he no longer needs it.

Complications

Complications of PA catheter insertion include pulmonary artery perforation, pulmonary infarction, catheter knotting, local or systemic infection, cardiac arrhythmias, and heparin-induced thrombocytopenia.

Nursing considerations

■ Advise the patient to use caution when moving about in bed to avoid dislodging the catheter.

■ Never leave the balloon inflated because this may cause pulmonary infarction. To determine if the balloon is inflated, check the monitor for a wedge tracing, which indicates inflation. (A PA tracing confirms balloon deflation.)

■ Never inflate the balloon with more than the recommended air volume (specified on the catheter shaft) because this may cause loss of elasticity or balloon rupture. With appropriate inflation volume, the balloon floats easily through the heart chambers and rests in the main branch of the pulmonary artery, producing accurate waveforms.

■ If the patient has a suspected left-to-right shunt, use carbon dioxide to inflate the balloon, as ordered, because it diffuses more quickly than air. Never inflate the balloon with fluids because they may not be able to be retrieved from inside the balloon, preventing deflation.

■ Be aware that the catheter may slip back into the right ventricle. Because the tip may irritate the ventricle, check the monitor for a right ventricular waveform to detect this problem promptly.

■ To minimize valvular trauma, make sure the balloon is deflated whenever the catheter is withdrawn from the pulmonary artery to the right ventricle or from the right ventricle to the right atrium.

■ Adhere to your facility's policy for dressing, tubing, catheter, and flush changes.

■ Document the date and time of catheter insertion, the physician who performed the procedure, the catheter insertion site, pressure waveforms and values for the various heart chambers, balloon inflation volume required to obtain a wedge tracing, any arrhythmias occurring during or after the procedure, type of flush solution used and its heparin concentration (if any), type of dressing applied, and the patient's tolerance of the procedure.

■ Remember to initial and date the dressing.

■ After catheter removal, document the patient's tolerance for the removal procedure, and note any problems encountered during removal.

ST-segment monitoring

A sensitive indicator of myocardial damage, the ST segment is normally flat or isoelectric. A depressed ST segment may result from cardiac glycosides, myocardial ischemia, or a subendocardial infarction. An elevated ST segment suggests myocardial infarction.

Continuous ST-segment monitoring is helpful for patients who have received thrombolytic therapy or have undergone coronary angioplasty. ST-segment monitoring allows early detection of reocclusion, always a possibility with these two procedures. It's also useful for patients who have had previous episodes of cardiac ischemia without chest pain, those who have difficulty distinguishing cardiac pain and pain from other sources, and for those who have difficulty communicating.

Because ischemia typically occurs in only one portion of the heart muscle, not all electrocardiogram (ECG) leads detect it. Select the most appropriate lead by examining ECG tracings obtained during an ischemic episode. The leads showing ischemia are the same leads to use for ST-segment monitoring.

Equipment

ECG electrodes ▪ gauze pads ▪ ECG monitor cable ▪ leadwires ▪ alcohol pads ▪ cardiac monitor programmed for ST-segment monitoring

Essential steps

▪ Bring the equipment to the patient's bedside and explain the procedure to the patient. Wash your hands. If the patient isn't already on a monitor, turn on the device and attach the cable.

▪ Select the sites for electrode placement and prepare the patient's skin for attachment as you would for continuous cardiac monitoring or a 12-lead ECG. Attach the leadwire the electrodes and position the electrodes on the patient's skin appropriately.

▪ Activate ST-segment monitoring by pressing the "monitoring procedures" key and then the ST key. Activate individual ST parameters by pressing the ON/OFF Parameter key.

▪ Select the appropriate ECG for each ST channel to be monitored by pressing the "parameters" key and then the key labeled "ECG."

▪ Press the key labeled, "change lead" to select the appropriate lead. Repeat this for all three channels.

▪ Adjust the ST-segment measurement points if necessary; adjust base-

line for ST segment by pressing the "iso point" to move the cursor to the PQ or TP interval.

▪ Adjust the J point by pressing the key labeled "J point" to move the cursor to the appropriate location.

▪ Adjust the ST point to 80 milliseconds after the J point.

▪ Set the alarm limits for each ST-segment parameter by manipulating the high- and low-limit keys.

▪ Press the key labeled "standard display" to return to the display screen.

▪ Assess the waveform shown on the monitor.

Complications

None

Nursing considerations

▪ Be sure to abrade the patient's skin gently to ensure electrode adhesion and promote electrical conductivity.

▪ If monitoring only one lead, choose the lead most likely to show arrhythmias and ST-segment changes.

ALERT *Always give precedence to the lead that shows arrhythmias.*

▪ Check the facility's policy for the measurement of the ST point. Some facilities recommend using 60 milliseconds instead of 80.

▪ Verify limit parameters for the patient with the physician. Commonly, when a limit is surpassed for more than 1 minute, visual and audible alarms are activated.

▪ If the patient isn't being monitored continuously, remove the electrodes, clean the skin, and disconnect the leadwires from the electrodes.

▪ Evaluate the monitor for ST-segment depression or elevation. (See

Understanding ST-segment elevation and depression

Closely monitoring the ST segment can help detect ischemia or injury before infarction develops.

ST-segment elevation

An ST segment is considered elevated when it's 1 mm or more above the baseline. An elevated ST segment may indicate myocardial injury.

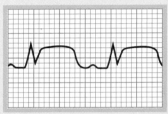

ST-segment depression

An ST segment is considered depressed when it's 0.5 mm or more below the baseline. A depressed ST segment may indicate myocardial ischemia or digoxin toxicity.

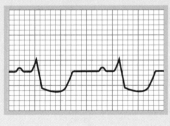

Synchronized cardioversion

Cardioversion (synchronized countershock) is an elective or emergency procedure used to treat tachyarrhythmias (such as atrial tachycardia, atrial flutter, atrial fibrillation, and symptomatic ventricular tachycardia [VT]). It's also the treatment of choice for arrhythmias that don't respond to drug therapy or vagal massage. Cardioversion delivers electric current to the heart to correct an arrhythmia but unlike defibrillation, it uses much lower energy levels.

Cardioversion delivers an electric charge to the myocardium at the peak of the R wave, causing immediate depolarization, interrupting reentry circuits and allowing the sinoatrial node to resume control. Synchronizing the electric charge with the R wave ensures that the current won't be delivered on the vulnerable T wave and disrupt repolarization. Thus, it reduces the risk that the current will strike during the relative refractory period of a cardiac cycle and induce ventricular fibrillation (VF).

Equipment

Cardioverter-defibrillator ▪ electrocardiograph (ECG) ▪ conductive gel or defibrillation pads

Essential steps

▪ Obtain a 12-lead ECG to serve as a baseline.
▪ Connect the patient to a pulse oximeter and blood pressure cuff if available.
▪ If the patient is awake and time permits, administer a sedative as ordered.

Understanding ST-segment elevation and depression.)
▪ Document the leads being monitored and the ST measurement points in the patient's medical record.

■ Place the leads on the patient's chest and assess his cardiac rhythm to see if cardioversion is appropriate.

■ Apply conductive material (gel to the paddles or defibrillation pads to the chest wall); position the pads so that one pad is to the right of the sternum, just below the clavicle, and the other is at the fifth or sixth intercostal space in the left anterior axillary line.

■ Turn on the defibrillator and select the appropriate energy level — usually between 50 and 100 joules.

■ Activate the synchronized mode by depressing the synchronizer switch.

■ Check that the machine is sensing the R wave correctly.

■ Place the paddles on the chest and apply firm pressure.

■ Charge the paddles.

■ Instruct other personnel to stand clear of the patient and the bed to avoid the risk of an electric shock.

■ Discharge the current by pushing both paddles' DISCHARGE buttons simultaneously.

ALERT *Don't remove the paddles from the chest until the device discharges. (Unlike in defibrillation, the discharge won't occur immediately; you'll notice a slight delay while the defibrillator synchronizes with the R wave.)*

■ If cardioversion is unsuccessful, repeat the procedure two or three times, as ordered, gradually increasing the energy with each additional countershock.

■ If normal rhythm is restored, continue to monitor the patient and provide supplemental ventilation as long as needed.

■ If the patient's cardiac rhythm changes to VF, switch the mode to defibrillate (change it from the synchronized mode) and defibrillate the patient immediately after charging the machine.

Complications

Complications of synchronized cardioversion include induced VF if the machine isn't synchronized to occur on the R wave and lethal arrhythmias when used in patients with digoxin toxicity.

Nursing considerations

■ Explain to the patient that synchronized cardioversion is an elective procedure and make sure that he, or a responsible family member, has signed a consent form.

■ Withhold all food and fluids for 6 to 12 hours before the procedure. If cardioversion is urgent, withhold food beginning as soon as possible.

■ When using handheld paddles, continue to hold the paddles on the patient's chest until the energy is delivered.

■ Use the following amperage sequences for cardioversion:
  – unstable VT with a pulse: 100, 200, 300, 360 joules
  – unstable paroxysmal supraventricular tachycardia: 50, 100, 200, 300, 360 joules
  – atrial fibrillation with a rapid ventricular response and an unstable patient: 100, 200, 300, 360 joules
  – atrial flutter with a rapid ventricular response and an unstable patient: 50, 100, 200, 300, 360 joules.

■ Remember to reset the "sync mode" on the defibrillator after each synchronized cardioversion. Resetting this switch is necessary because most defibrillators will automatically reset to an unsynchronized mode.

■ Document the use of synchronized cardioversion, rhythm before and after cardioversion, amperage used, and how the patient tolerated the procedure.

12-lead electrocardiogram

The 12-lead electrocardiogram (ECG) is used to help identify pathologic conditions, especially angina and acute myocardial infarction. It provides a more complete view of the heart's electrical activity than a rhythm strip and can be used to assess left ventricular function more effectively. Patients with conditions that affect the heart's electrical system may also benefit from a 12-lead ECG, including those with:

■ cardiac arrhythmias
■ heart chamber enlargement or hypertrophy
■ digoxin or other drug toxicity
■ electrolyte imbalances
■ pulmonary embolism
■ pericarditis
■ pacemakers
■ hypothermia.

Like other diagnostic tests, a 12-lead ECG must be viewed in conjunction with other clinical data. Therefore, always correlate the patient's ECG results with his history, physical assessment findings, drug regimen, and results of laboratory and other diagnostic studies.

The 12-lead ECG records the heart's electrical activity using a series of electrodes placed on the patient's extremities and chest wall. The 12 leads include three bipolar limb leads (I, II, III), three unipolar augmented limb leads (aV_R, aV_L, and aV_F), and six unipolar precordial, or chest, leads (V_1, V_2, V_3, V_4, V_5, and V_6). These leads provide 12 different views of the heart's electrical activity. (See *ECG leads.*) The six limb leads record electrical activity in the heart's frontal plane, a view through the middle of the heart from top to bottom. Electrical activity is recorded from the anterior to the posterior axes. The six precordial leads provide information on electrical activity in the heart's horizontal plane, a transverse view through the middle of the heart, dividing it into upper and lower portions. Electrical activity is recorded from either a superior or an inferior approach.

Scanning up, down, and across, each lead transmits information about a different area of the heart. The waveforms obtained from each lead vary, depending on the location of the lead in relation to the wave of depolarization passing through the myocardium.

In addition to assessing 12 different leads, a 12-lead ECG records the heart's electrical axis (the direction of depolarization as it spreads through the heart). As impulses travel through the heart, they generate small electrical forces called instantaneous vectors. The mean of these vectors represents the force and direction of the wave of depolarization through the heart — the electrical axis. The electrical axis is also called the mean instantaneous vector and the mean QRS vector.

In a healthy heart, impulses originate in the sinoatrial node, travel

ECG leads

Each of the leads on a 12-lead electrocardiogram (ECG) views the heart from a different angle. The following illustrations show the direction of electrical activity (depolarization) monitored by each lead and the 12 views of the heart.

Views reflected on a 12-lead ECG

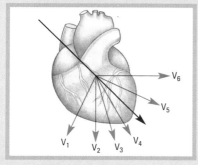

Lead	View of the heart
Standard limb leads (bipolar)	
I	lateral wall
II	inferior wall
III	inferior wall
Augmented limb leads (unipolar)	
aV_R	no specific view
aV_L	lateral wall
aV_F	inferior wall
Precordial, or chest, leads (unipolar)	
V_1	anteroseptal wall
V_2	anteroseptal wall
V_3	anterior and anteroseptal walls
V_4	anterior wall
V_5	lateral wall
V_6	lateral wall

through the atria to the atrioventricular node, and then to the ventricles. Most of the movement of the impulses is downward and to the left, the direction of a normal axis. However, when the heart is unhealthy, axis direction varies because the direction of electrical activity travels away from areas of damage or necrosis and toward areas of hypertrophy. Knowing the normal deflection of each lead will help you evaluate whether the electrical axis is normal or abnormal.

Equipment
ECG machine ▪ recording paper

Essential steps
After you have obtained the ECG recording, prepare to interpret it using a systematic approach. (See *Obtaining a 12-lead ECG,* pages 150 and 151.) Compare the patient's previous ECG

(Text continues on page 152.)

Obtaining a 12-lead ECG

● Gather all necessary supplies, including the electrocardiogram (ECG) machine, recording paper, electrodes, and gauze pads. Explain the procedure to the patient, emphasizing that the test takes about 10 minutes and is a safe and painless way to evaluate the heart's electrical activity. Answer the patient's questions, and offer reassurance.

● Place the patient in a supine position in the center of the bed with his arms at his sides. If he can't tolerate lying flat, raise the head of the bed to semi-Fowler's position. Ensure privacy, and expose the patient's arms, legs, and chest, draping for comfort.

● Select the areas where you'll apply the electrodes. Choose areas that are flat and fleshy — not muscular or bony. Clip the hair in the area if it's excessively hairy. Remove excess oil and other substances from the skin to enhance electrode contact. Remember, the better the electrode contact, the better the recording. Be sure to apply the electrodes correctly; inaccurate placement of an electrode by greater than ⅜″ (1.5 cm) from its standardized position may lead to inaccurate waveforms and an incorrect

ECG interpretation.

● Place electrodes on the patient's arms and legs, and position the chest electrodes (shown below) as follows:

V_1: Fourth intercostal space at right sternal border
V_2: Fourth intercostal space at left sternal border
V_3: Halfway between V_2 and V_4
V_4: Fifth intercostal space at midclavicular line
V_5: Fifth intercostal space at anterior axillary line (halfway between V_4 and V_6
V_6: Fifth intercostal space at midaxillary line, level with V_4

Recording the ECG

To record an ECG, follow these steps:

● Plug the cord of the ECG machine into a grounded outlet. (If the machine operates on a charged battery, it may not need to be plugged in.)

● If necessary, enter the patient's identification data.

● Ensure that all leads are securely attached, and then turn on the machine.

● Instruct the patient to relax, lie still, and breathe normally. Ask him not to talk

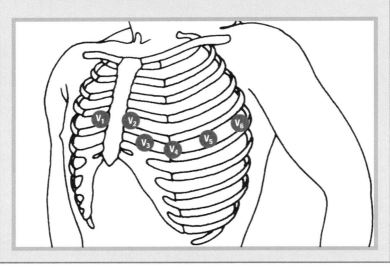

Obtaining a 12-lead ECG *(continued)*

during the recording, to prevent distortion of the ECG tracing.
- Press the AUTO button and record the ECG.
- Observe the quality of the tracing.

When the machine finishes the recording, turn it off.
- Remove the electrodes, and clean the patient's skin.

NORMAL ECG WAVEFORMS

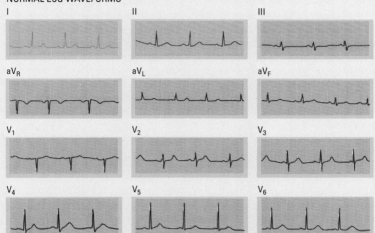

I   II   III

aV_R aV_L aV_F

V_1 V_2 V_3

V_4 V_5 V_6

Posterior-lead ECG

Because of lung and muscle barriers, the usual chest leads can't "see" the heart's posterior surface to record myocardial damage there. So some practitioners add three posterior leads to the 12-lead ECG: leads V_7, V_8, and V_9. These leads are placed opposite anterior leads V_4, V_5, and V_6, on the left side of the patient's back, following the same horizontal line, as shown below.

Right chest lead ECG

The standard 12-lead ECG evaluates only the left ventricle. If the right ventricle needs to be assessed for damage or dysfunction, the practitioner may order a right chest lead ECG.

With this type of ECG, the six leads are placed on the right side of the chest in a mirror image of the standard precordial lead placement, as shown below. Electrodes start at the left sternal border and swing down under the right breast area.

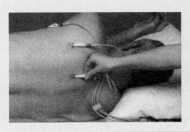

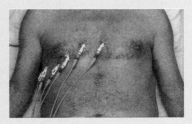

with the current one, if available. This will help you identify changes.

■ Check the ECG tracing to see if it's technically correct. Make sure that the baseline is free from electrical interference and drift.

■ Scan the limb leads I, II, and III. The R-wave voltage in lead II should equal the sum of the R-wave voltage in leads I and III. Lead aV_R is typically negative. If these rules aren't met, the tracing may be recorded incorrectly.

■ Locate the lead markers on the waveform. Lead markers are the points where one lead changes to another.

■ Check the standardization markings to make sure all leads were recorded with the ECG machine's amplitude at the same setting. Standardization markings are usually located at the beginning of the strip.

■ Assess the heart's rate and rhythm.

■ Determine the heart's electrical axis using either the quadrant method or the degree method. (See *Determining the electrical axis.*)

■ Examine limb leads I, II, and III. The R wave in lead II should be taller than in lead I. The R wave in lead III should be a smaller version of the R wave in lead I. The P wave or QRS complex may be inverted. Each lead should have flat ST segments and upright T waves. Pathologic Q waves should be absent.

■ Examine limb leads aV_L, aV_F, and aV_R. The tracings from leads aV_L and aV_F should be similar, but lead aV_F should have taller P and R waves. Lead aV_R has little diagnostic value. Its P wave, QRS complex, and T wave should be deflected downward.

■ Examine the R wave in the precordial leads. Normally, the R wave — the

first positive deflection of the QRS complex — gets progressively taller from lead V_1 to V_5. It gets slightly smaller in lead V_6. (See *R-wave progression,* page 155.)

■ Examine the S wave (the negative deflection after an R wave) in the precordial leads. It should appear extremely deep in lead V_1 and become progressively more shallow, usually disappearing by lead V_5.

Complications

None

Nursing considerations

The printout will show the patient's name and room number and, possibly, his medical record number. At the top of the printout, you'll see the patient's heart rate and wave durations, measured in seconds. (See *Multichannel ECG recording,* page 156.)

In addition, some machines can record ST-segment elevation and depression. The name of the lead will appear next to each 6-second strip.

When interpreting the recording, pay particular attention to each lead, noting where changes occur so you can identify the area of the heart affected. Keep in mind the following:

■ P waves should be upright; however, they may be inverted in lead aV_R or biphasic or inverted in leads III, aV_L, and V_1.

■ PR intervals should always be constant, just like QRS-complex durations.

■ QRS-complex deflections will vary in different leads. Observe for pathologic Q waves.

■ ST segments should be isoelectric or have minimal deviation.

Determining the electrical axis

Determine your patient's electrical axis by examining the waveforms recorded from the six frontal plane leads: I, II, III, aV_R, aV_L, and aV_F. Imaginary lines drawn from each of the leads intersect the center of the heart and form a diagram known as the hexaxial reference system (shown at right).

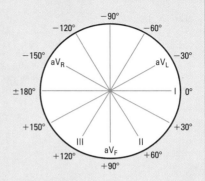

An axis that falls between 0 and 90 degrees is considered normal. An axis between 90 and 180 degrees indicates right axis deviation, and one between 0 and −90 degrees indicates left axis deviation. An axis between −180 and −90 degrees indicates extreme axis deviation and is called an indeterminate axis.

To determine your patient's electrical axis, use the quadrant method or the degree method.

Quadrant method

The quadrant method — a fast, easy way to plot the heart's axis — involves observing the main deflection of the QRS complex in leads I and aV_F. Lead I indicates whether impulses are moving to the right or left, and lead aV_F indicates whether they're moving up or down.

If the QRS-complex deflection is positive or upright in both leads, the electrical axis is normal. If lead I is upright and lead aV_F points down, left axis deviation exists.

When lead I points down and lead aV_F is upright, right axis deviation exists. Both waves pointing down signal extreme axis deviation.

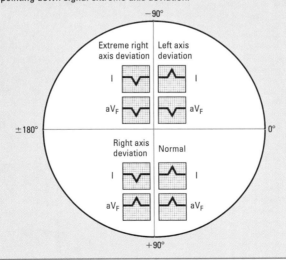

(continued)

Determining the electrical axis *(continued)*

Degree method

The degree method is more precise because it provides an exact measurement of the electrical axis. It also allows you to determine the axis even if the QRS complex isn't clearly positive or negative in leads I and aV$_F$. To use this method, follow these steps:

1. Review all six leads, and identify the one that contains either the smallest QRS complex or the complex with an equal deflection above and below the baseline. (In the example shown it's lead III.)

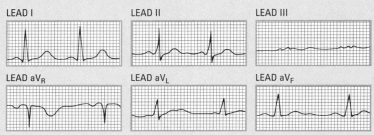

LEAD I　　　　　　LEAD II　　　　　　LEAD III

LEAD aV$_R$　　　　LEAD aV$_L$　　　　LEAD aV$_F$

2. Use the hexaxial diagram to identify the lead perpendicular to this lead. For example, if lead I has the smallest QRS complex, then the lead perpendicular to the line representing lead I would be lead aV$_F$. (In this example, the lead perpendicular to lead III is lead aV$_R$.)

3. After you've identified the perpendicular lead, examine its QRS complex. If the electrical activity is moving toward the positive pole of a lead, the QRS complex deflects upward. If it's moving away from the positive pole of a lead, the QRS complex deflects downward.

4. Plot this information on the hexaxial diagram to determine the direction of the electrical axis. (In this example, the QRS complex for this lead is negative, indicating that the current is moving toward the negative pole of aV$_R$, which is the right lower quadrant at +30 degrees on the hexaxial diagram. So the electrical axis here is normal at +30 degrees.)

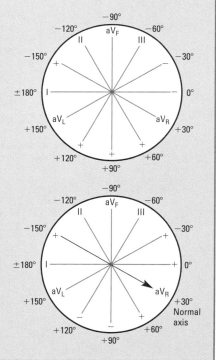

- ST-segment elevation greater than 1 mm above the baseline and ST-segment depression greater than 0.5 mm below the baseline are considered abnormal. Leads facing an injured area will have ST-segment elevations, and leads facing away will show ST-segment depressions.
- The T wave normally deflects upward in leads I, II, and V_3 through V_6. It's inverted in lead aV_R and variable in the other leads. T-wave changes have many causes and aren't always a reason for alarm. Excessively tall, flat, or inverted T waves occurring with symptoms such as chest pain may indicate ischemia.
- A normal Q wave generally has a duration of under 0.04 second. An abnormal Q wave has either a duration of 0.04 second or more, a depth greater than 4 mm, or a height one-fourth of the R wave. Abnormal Q waves indicate myocardial necrosis, developing when depolarization can't follow its normal path due to damaged tissue in the area.
- Remember that lead aV_R normally has a large Q wave, so disregard this lead when searching for abnormal Q waves.

Finding a patient's electrical axis can help confirm a diagnosis or narrow the range of possible diagnoses. However, axis deviation isn't always clinically significant, and it isn't always cardiac in origin. For example, infants and children usually have right axis deviation. Pregnant women normally have left axis deviation. Factors that affect the location of the axis include the heart's position in the chest, the heart's size, the patient's body size or type, the conduction pathways, and the force of the electrical impulses being generat-

R-wave progression

R waves should progress normally through the precordial leads. Note that the R wave in the illustration is the first positive deflection in the QRS complex. Also note that the S wave gets smaller, or regresses, from lead V_1 to V_6, until it finally disappears.

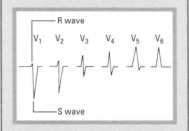

ed. Remember that electrical activity in the heart swings away from areas of damage or necrosis, so the damaged part of the heart will be the last area depolarized. For example, in right bundle-branch block, the impulse travels quickly down the normal left side and then moves slowly down the right side. This shifts the electrical forces to the right, causing right axis deviation.

Be sure to write the following pieces of information on the printout: date, time, physician's name, and special circumstances. For example, you might record an episode of chest pain, abnormal electrolyte levels, related drug treatment, abnormal placement of the electrodes, or the presence of an artificial pacemaker and whether a magnet was used while the ECG was obtained. Remember, ECGs are legal documents. They belong in the patient's medical record and must be

Multichannel ECG recording

The top of a 12-lead electrocardiogram (ECG) recording usually shows patient identification information along with an interpretation by the machine. A rhythm strip is commonly included at the bottom of the recording.

Standardization

Look for standardization marks on the recording, usually 10 small squares high. If the patient has high-voltage complexes, the marks will be one-half as high. You'll also notice that lead markers separate the lead recordings on the paper and that each lead is labeled.

Familiarize yourself with the order in which the leads are arranged on an ECG tracing. Getting accustomed to the tracing's layout will help you interpret the ECG more quickly and accurately.

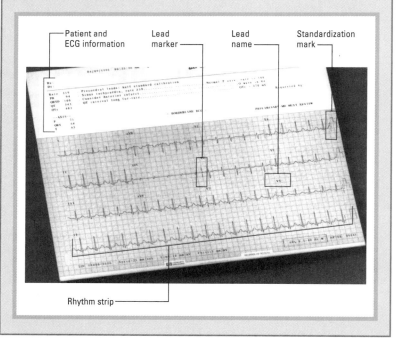

Patient and ECG information — Lead marker — Lead name — Standardization mark —

Rhythm strip —

saved for future reference and comparison with baseline strips.

Valvular heart disease

In valvular heart disease, three types of mechanical disruption can occur: stenosis, or narrowing, of the valve opening; incomplete closure of the valve; or prolapse of the valve. Valvular disorders in children and adolescents most commonly occur as a result of congenital heart defects, whereas in adults, rheumatic heart disease is a common cause.

Pathophysiology

Valvular heart disease may be the result of numerous conditions, which vary and are different for each type of valve disorder. (See *Types of valvular heart disease,* pages 158 and 159.) Pathophysiology of valvular heart disease varies according to the valve and the disorder.

Mitral insufficiency

Any abnormality of the mitral leaflets, mitral annulus, chordae tendineae, papillary muscles, left atrium, or left ventricle can lead to mitral insufficiency. Blood from the left ventricle flows back into the left atrium during systole, causing the atrium to enlarge to accommodate the backflow. As a result, the left ventricle also dilates to accommodate the increased volume of blood from the atrium and to compensate for diminishing cardiac output (CO). Ventricular hypertrophy and increased end-diastolic pressure result in increased pulmonary artery pressure, eventually leading to left-sided and right-sided heart failure.

Mitral stenosis

Narrowing of the valve by valvular abnormalities, fibrosis, or calcification obstructs blood flow from the left atrium to the left ventricle. Consequently, left atrial volume and pressure rise and the chamber dilates. Greater resistance to blood flow causes pulmonary hy-

pertension, right ventricular hypertrophy, and right-sided heart failure. Also, inadequate filling of the left ventricle produces low CO.

Aortic insufficiency

Blood flows back into the left ventricle during diastole, causing fluid overload in the ventricle, which dilates and hypertrophies. The excess volume causes fluid overload in the left atrium and, finally, the pulmonary system. Left-sided heart failure and pulmonary edema eventually result.

Aortic stenosis

Increased left ventricular pressure tries to overcome the resistance of the narrowed valvular opening. The added workload increases the demand for oxygen, and diminished CO causes poor coronary artery perfusion, ischemia of the left ventricle, and left-sided heart failure.

Pulmonic stenosis

Obstructed right ventricular outflow causes right ventricular hypertrophy, eventually resulting in right-sided heart failure.

Comprehensive assessment

The history and physical examination findings vary according to the type of valvular defects. Be especially alert for atrial fibrillation in patients with longstanding valvular disease that results in atrial enlargement.

Diagnosis

The diagnosis of valvular heart disease can be made through cardiac catheterization, chest X-rays, echocardiography, or electrocardiography (ECG).

(Text continues on page 160.)

Types of valvular heart disease

Causes and incidence	Clinical findings
Mitral stenosis • Results from rheumatic fever (most common cause) • Most common in females • May be associated with other congenital anomalies	• Dyspnea on exertion, paroxysmal nocturnal dyspnea, orthopnea, weakness, fatigue, and palpitations • Peripheral edema, jugular vein distention, ascites, and hepatomegaly (right-sided heart failure) • Crackles, atrial fibrillation, and signs of systemic emboli • Auscultation reveals a loud S_1 or opening snap and a diastolic murmur at the apex
Mitral insufficiency • Results from rheumatic fever, hypertrophic cardiomyopathy, mitral valve prolapse, myocardial infarction, severe left-sided heart failure, or ruptured chordae tendineae • Associated with other congenital anomalies such as transposition of the great arteries • Rare in children without other congenital anomalies	• Orthopnea, dyspnea, fatigue, angina, and palpitations • Peripheral edema, jugular vein distention, and hepatomegaly (right-sided heart failure) • Tachycardia, crackles, and pulmonary edema • Auscultation reveals a holosystolic murmur at apex, a possible split S_2, and an S_3
Aortic insufficiency • Results from rheumatic fever, syphilis, hypertension, or endocarditis, or may be idiopathic • Associated with Marfan syndrome • Most common in males • Associated with ventricular septal defect, even after surgical closure	• Dyspnea, cough, fatigue, palpitations, angina, and syncope • Pulmonary congestion, left-sided heart failure, and "pulsating" nail beds (Quincke's sign) • Rapidly rising and collapsing pulses (pulsus bisferiens), cardiac arrhythmias, and widened pulse pressure • Auscultation reveals an S_3 and a diastolic blowing murmur at left sternal border • Palpation and visualization of apical impulse in chronic disease
Aortic stenosis • Results from congenital aortic bicuspid valve (associated with coarctation of the aorta), congenital stenosis of valve cusps, rheumatic fever, or atherosclerosis in the elderly • Most common in males	• Dyspnea on exertion, paroxysmal nocturnal dyspnea, fatigue, syncope, angina, and palpitations • Pulmonary congestion, and left-sided heart failure • Diminished carotid pulses, decreased cardiac output (CO), and cardiac arrhythmias; may have pulsus alternans • Auscultation reveals systolic murmur heard at base or in carotids and, possibly, an S_4
Pulmonic stenosis • Results from congenital stenosis of valve cusp or rheumatic heart disease (infrequent) • Associated with tetralogy of Fallot	• Asymptomatic or symptomatic with dyspnea on exertion, fatigue, chest pain, and syncope • May cause jugular vein distention and right-sided heart failure • Auscultation reveals a systolic murmur at the left sternal border and a split S_2 with a delayed or absent pulmonic component

Diagnostic measures

- Cardiac catheterization: diastolic pressure gradient across valve; elevated left atrial and pulmonary artery wedge pressures (PAWP) > 15 mm Hg with severe pulmonary hypertension; elevated right-sided heart pressure with decreased CO; and abnormal contraction of the left ventricle
- Chest X-rays: left atrial and ventricular enlargement, enlarged pulmonary arteries, and mitral valve calcification
- Echocardiography: thickened mitral valve leaflets and left atrial enlargement
- Electrocardiography: left atrial hypertrophy, atrial fibrillation, right ventricular hypertrophy, and right axis deviation

- Cardiac catheterization: mitral insufficiency with increased left ventricular end-diastolic volume and pressure, increased atrial pressure and PAWP, and decreased CO
- Chest X-rays: left atrial and ventricular enlargement and pulmonary venous congestion
- Echocardiography: abnormal valve leaflet motion, and left atrial enlargement
- Electrocardiography: may show left atrial and ventricular hypertrophy, sinus tachycardia, and atrial fibrillation

- Cardiac catheterization: reduction in arterial diastolic pressures, aortic insufficiency, other valvular abnormalities, and increased left ventricular end-diastolic pressure
- Chest X-rays: left ventricular enlargement and pulmonary venous congestion
- Echocardiography: left ventricular enlargement, alterations in mitral valve movement (indirect indication of aortic valve disease), and mitral thickening
- Electrocardiography: sinus tachycardia, left ventricular hypertrophy, and left atrial hypertrophy in severe disease

- Cardiac catheterization: pressure gradient across valve (indicating obstruction), and increased left ventricular end-diastolic pressures
- Chest X-rays: valvular calcification, left ventricular enlargement, and pulmonary vein congestion
- Echocardiography: thickened aortic valve and left ventricular wall, possibly coexistent with mitral valve stenosis
- Electrocardiography: left ventricular hypertrophy

- Cardiac catheterization: increased right ventricular pressure, decreased pulmonary artery pressure, and abnormal valve orifice
- Electrocardiography: may show right ventricular hypertrophy, right axis deviation, right atrial hypertrophy, and atrial fibrillation

Collaborations

A multidisciplinary approach to care is key. Medical and nursing care focus on maximizing cardiac function, maintaining the patient's hemodynamic stability, and adequate tissue perfusion. Nutritional therapy may be required to assist the patient with appropriate low-sodium food selections. Surgery including commissurotomy, balloon valvuloplasty, and valve replacement may be necessary. Postoperatively, additional therapies such as physical and occupational therapies may be needed to assist the patient to regain maximum level of function.

Treatment and care

Treatment of valvular disorders commonly includes:

■ digoxin, a low-sodium diet, diuretics, vasodilators, and especially angiotensin-converting enzyme inhibitors to treat left-sided heart failure

■ oxygen in acute situations, to increase oxygenation

■ anticoagulants to prevent thrombus formation around diseased or replaced valves

■ prophylactic antibiotics before and after surgery or dental care to prevent endocarditis

■ nitroglycerin to relieve angina in conditions such as aortic stenosis

■ beta-adrenergic blockers or digoxin to slow the ventricular rate in atrial fibrillation or atrial flutter

■ cardioversion to convert atrial fibrillation to sinus rhythm

■ open or closed commissurotomy to separate thick or adherent mitral valve leaflets

■ balloon valvuloplasty to enlarge the orifice of a stenotic mitral, aortic, or pulmonic valve

■ annuloplasty or valvuloplasty to reconstruct or repair the valve in mitral insufficiency

■ valve replacement with a prosthetic valve for mitral and aortic valve disease.

AGE ISSUE *In a child who doesn't have calcified valves, simple commissurotomy under direct visualization is usually effective. If the child has a valve replacement, long-term anticoagulant therapy may be indicated. Sometimes valve replacement surgery in a child is postponed (if possible) until the child can receive an adult-size valve. Adults with calcified valves will need valve replacement when they become symptomatic or are at risk for developing left-sided heart failure. Percutaneous balloon aortic valvuloplasty is useful in the child or young adult who has congenital aortic stenosis and in the older adult patient with severe calcifications. This procedure may improve left ventricular function so that the patient can tolerate valve replacement surgery.*

Complications

Possible complications of valvular heart disease include:
■ heart failure
■ pulmonary edema
■ thromboembolism
■ hemorrhage
■ endocarditis.

Although valve replacement surgery carries a low mortality, it can cause serious complications. Hemorrhage may result from unligated vessels, anticoagulant therapy (with mechanical prosthetic valve replacement), or coagulopathy resulting from cardiopulmonary bypass during surgery. Stroke may result from thrombus formation due to turbulent blood flow through the prosthetic valve or from poor cerebral perfusion during cardiopulmonary bypass. Bacterial endocarditis can develop within days of implantation or months later. Valve dysfunction or failure may occur as the prosthetic device wears out. (This may occur 5 to 10 years after insertion of a biological prosthetic valve and 15 to 20 years after insertion of a mechanical prosthetic valve.)

Balloon valvuloplasty can worsen valvular insufficiency by misshaping the valve so that it doesn't close completely. Another serious complication is embolism caused by pieces of the calcified valve breaking off and traveling to the brain or lungs. In addition, valvuloplasty can cause severe damage to the delicate valve leaflets, requiring immediate surgery to replace the valve. Other complications include bleeding and hematoma at the arterial puncture site, arrhythmias, myocardial ischemia, myocardial infarction (MI), and circulatory insufficiency distal to the catheter entry site.

AGE ISSUE *Older adult patients with aortic disease frequently experience restenosis 1 to 2 years after undergoing valvuloplasty.* Fortunately, the most serious complications of valvuloplasty — valvular destruction, MI, and calcium emboli — rarely occur.

Nursing considerations

■ Assess the patient's vital signs, arterial blood gas (ABG) values, pulse oximetry, intake and output, daily weights, blood chemistry studies, chest X-rays, and ECG.
■ If the patient needs bed rest, stress its importance. Assist with bathing as

necessary. Provide a bedside commode to reduce myocardial oxygen demands. Offer diversional, physically undemanding activities.
■ Place the patient in an upright position to relieve dyspnea if needed. Administer oxygen to prevent tissue hypoxia, as needed and indicated by ABG levels and pulse oximetry.
■ Institute continuous cardiac monitoring to evaluate for arrhythmias; if any occur, administer appropriate therapy as per facility policy and physician's order.
■ For the patient with aortic insufficiency, observe ECG for arrhythmias, which can increase the risk of pulmonary edema, fever, and infection.
■ If the patient has mitral stenosis, watch closely for signs of pulmonary dysfunction caused by pulmonary hypertension, tissue ischemia caused by emboli, and adverse reactions to drug therapy.
■ For the patient with mitral insufficiency, observe for signs and symptoms of left-sided heart failure, pulmonary edema, and adverse reactions to drug therapy.

After valve replacement surgery
■ Closely monitor the patient's hemodynamic status for signs of compromise. Watch especially for severe hypotension, decreased CO, and shock. Check and record vital signs every 15 minutes until his condition stabilizes. Frequently assess heart sounds; report distant heart sounds or new murmurs, which may indicate prosthetic valve failure.
■ Monitor the ECG continuously for disturbances in heart rate and rhythm, such as bradycardia, ventricular tachycardia, and heart block. Such distur-

bances may signal injury of the conduction system, which may occur during valve replacement from proximity of the atrial and mitral valves to the atrioventricular node. Arrhythmias may also result from myocardial irritability or ischemia, fluid and electrolyte imbalance, hypoxemia, or hypothermia. If you detect serious abnormalities, notify the physician and be prepared to assist with temporary epicardial pacing.

■ To ensure adequate myocardial perfusion, maintain the patient's mean arterial pressure within the guidelines set by the physician (for adults, usually between 70 and 100 mm Hg). Also monitor pulmonary artery and left atrial pressures as ordered.

■ Frequently assess the patient's peripheral pulses, capillary refill time, and skin temperature and color, and auscultate for heart sounds. Evaluate tissue oxygenation by assessing breath sounds, chest excursion, and symmetry of chest expansion. Report any abnormalities.

■ Check ABG values every 2 to 4 hours, and adjust ventilator settings as needed.

■ Maintain chest tube drainage at the prescribed negative pressure (usually −10 to −40 cm H_2O for adults). Assess chest tubes every hour for signs of hemorrhage, excessive drainage (greater than 200 ml/hour), and a sudden decrease or cessation of drainage.

■ As ordered, administer analgesic, anticoagulant, antibiotic, antiarrhythmic, inotropic, and pressor medications as well as I.V. fluids and blood products. Monitor intake and output and assess for electrolyte imbalances, especially hypokalemia. When anticoagulant therapy begins, evaluate its effectiveness by monitoring prothrombin time daily.

■ Throughout the patient's recovery period, observe him carefully for complications. Watch especially for symptoms of stroke (such as altered level of consciousness, pupillary changes, weakness and loss of movement in the extremities, ataxia, aphasia, dysphagia, and sensory disturbances), pulmonary embolism (such as dyspnea, cough, hemoptysis, chest pain, pleural friction rub, cyanosis, and hypoxemia), and impaired renal perfusion (such as decreased urine output and elevated blood urea nitrogen and serum creatinine levels).

■ After weaning the patient from the ventilator and removing the endotracheal tube, promote chest physiotherapy. Start him on incentive spirometry and encourage him to cough, turn frequently, and deep-breathe. Gradually increase his activities as tolerated.

After a balloon valvuloplasty

■ Remember that the patient will probably be receiving I.V. heparin or nitroglycerin. He may also have a sandbag placed over the cannulation site to minimize bleeding.

■ To prevent excessive hip flexion and catheter migration, keep the affected leg straight and elevate the head of the bed no more than 15 degrees (at mealtimes, 15 to 30 degrees). For the first hour, monitor vital signs every 15 minutes, then every 30 minutes for 2 hours, and then hourly for the next 5 hours. If vital signs are unstable, notify the physician and continue to check them every 5 minutes.

■ In conjunction with monitoring vital signs, also assess peripheral pulses distal to the insertion site and the color, temperature, and capillary refill time of the extremity. If pulses are difficult to palpate because of the size of the arterial catheter, use an ultrasound stethoscope. Notify the physician immediately if pulses are absent.

■ Observe the catheter insertion site for hematoma formation, ecchymosis, or hemorrhage. If an expanding ecchymotic area appears, mark the area to help determine the pace of expansion. If bleeding occurs, apply direct pressure and notify the physician.

■ Auscultate regularly for murmurs, which may indicate worsening valvular insufficiency. Report any new or worsening murmurs.

■ Administer I.V. fluids at a rate of at least 100 ml/hour, or as ordered, to help the kidneys excrete the contrast medium.

ALERT *Be sure to assess for signs of fluid overload: distended neck veins, atrial and ventricular gallops, dyspnea, pulmonary congestion, tachycardia, hypertension, and hypoxemia. If any of these signs are present, notify the physician immediately,*

■ Prepare for catheter removal by the physician in approximately 6 to 12 hours after valvuloplasty. Afterward, apply a pressure dressing and assess vital signs according to the same schedule you used when the patient first returned to the unit. Also, monitor the insertion site and peripheral pulses distal to the site.

Patient teaching
■ Advise the patient to plan for periodic rest in his daily routine to prevent undue fatigue.

■ Teach the patient about diet and activity restrictions, medications, symptoms that should be reported, and the importance of consistent follow-up care.

■ Advise the patient to carry medical identification with information and instructions on his anticoagulant and antibiotic therapy.

■ Make sure the patient and his family understand the need to comply with prolonged antibiotic therapy and follow-up care and the possible need for prophylactic antibiotics during dental surgery or other invasive procedures.

Ventricular assist device

A ventricular assist device (VAD) is implanted to provide support to a failing heart. The device consists of a blood pump, cannulas, and a pneumatic or electrical drive console. VAD can provide systemic and pulmonary support. A right VAD (RVAD) provides pulmonary support by diverting blood from the failing right ventricle to the VAD, which then pumps the blood to the pulmonary circulation via the VAD connection to the pulmonary artery. With a left VAD (LVAD), blood flows from the left ventricle to the VAD, which then pumps blood back to the body via the VAD connection to the aorta. (See *Left VAD,* page 164.) When RVAD and LVAD are used, biventricular (BiVaD) support is being provided.

VADs are designed to decrease the heart's workload and increase cardiac output (CO) in patients with ventricular failure. They are commonly used as a bridge to cardiac transplantation. In addition, VADs also are indicated for use in patients with:

Left VAD

Ventricular assist devices (VADs) are commonly used as a bridge to heart transplantation. A completely implanted left VAD is shown here.

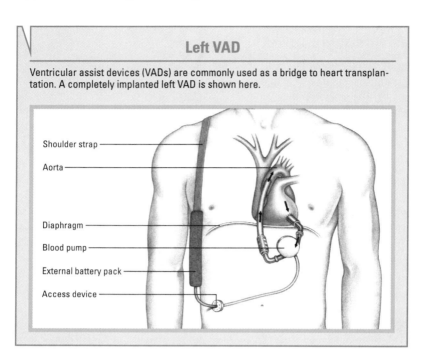

- Shoulder strap
- Aorta
- Diaphragm
- Blood pump
- External battery pack
- Access device

cardiogenic shock that's refractory to maximum pharmacologic therapy and intra-aortic balloon pump support
inability to be weaned from cardiopulmonary bypass.

Procedure

In a surgical procedure, blood is diverted from a ventricle to an artificial pump. This pump, which is synchronized to the patient's electrocardiogram (ECG), then functions as the ventricle.

Complications

Complications may include:
- hemorrhage
- air embolus
- thrombus
- infection
- lethal arrhythmias.

Nursing considerations

Before VAD insertion
- Prepare the patient and his family for insertion, reinforcing explanations of device, purpose, and what to expect after insertion.
- Make sure the patient or a responsible family member has signed an informed consent form.
- Provide emotional support to the patient and his family; allow the patient to verbalize fears and feelings of powerlessness.
- Continue close patient monitoring including continuous ECG monitoring, pulmonary artery and hemodynamic status monitoring, and intake and output.

After VAD insertion

■ Assess cardiovascular status at least every 15 minutes until stable, and then hourly. Monitor blood pressure, hemodynamic parameters including CO and cardiac index, ECG, and peripheral pulses.

■ Inspect incision and dressing at least every hour initially, and then every 2 to 4 hours as indicated by the patient's condition.

■ Monitor urine output hourly and maintain I.V. fluid therapy as ordered; watch for signs of fluid overload or decreasing urine output.

■ Assess chest tube drainage and function. Notify the physician if drainage is greater than 150 ml over 2 hours. Auscultate lungs for evidence of abnormal breath sounds. Evaluate oxygen saturation or mixed venous oxygen saturation levels and administer oxygen as needed and ordered.

■ Obtain hemoglobin level, hematocrit, and coagulation studies as ordered. Administer blood component therapy as indicated and ordered.

■ Assess for signs and symptoms of bleeding; keep in mind that a continuous heparin infusion may be needed.

■ When the patient is stable, turn him every 2 hours and begin range-of-motion exercises.

■ Administer antibiotics prophylactically if ordered.

■ Inspect tubing for tension or kinks.

ALERT *Keeping tubing free from kinks aids in preventing thrombus formation.*

2 | *Respiratory system challenges*

Imagine you have a patient who presents with tachypnea and shortness of breath. Do these symptoms signal an acute upper respiratory infection — or some other, more acute disorder such as adult respiratory distress syndrome or pulmonary embolism? What assessment would you do first to help confirm a diagnosis? Another patient requires mechanical ventilation. Do you know the difference between continuous positive airway pressure and positive end-expiratory pressure ventilation? For what type of pneumothorax would you monitor the patient? What if the patient required end-tidal carbon dioxide monitoring? Would you know what to do and how to interpret the results? Imagine that the patient's ventilator alarm sounded. Could you troubleshoot to determine whether the patient was experiencing a problem or the equipment was malfunctioning? Would you be able to analyze a patient's ventilatory parameters to help determine whether he's ready to be weaned from mechanical ventilation? If lung transplantation was indicated, would you know how to care for the patient after the surgery? Another patient needs a chest tube inserted. How would you prepare the patient prior to insertion — and how would you care for him after insertion? Do you know how to assess for the presence of an air leak with a chest tube? Answers to these questions, and more, are presented in this chapter to provide you with the essential information to address the major challenges involving the respiratory system commonly encountered by critical care nurses.

 MULTISYSTEM DISORDER

Acute respiratory failure

Acute respiratory failure occurs when the lungs can't adequately maintain arterial oxygenation or eliminate carbon dioxide (CO_2). Acute respiratory failure can lead to tissue hypoxia. In patients with normal lung tissue, respiratory failure is indicated by partial pressure of arterial CO_2 ($PaCO_2$) above 50 mm Hg and partial pressure of arterial oxygen (PaO_2) below 50 mm Hg. However, for patients with chronic obstructive pulmonary disease (COPD), these same parameters don't apply. That's because patients with COPD have a consistently high $PaCO_2$ (hypercapnia) and a low PaO_2 (hypoxemia). Therefore, acute deterioration in arterial blood gas (ABG) values for these patients and corresponding clinical deterioration signify acute respiratory failure.

Rapid diagnosis and intervention are necessary to stop progression of acute respiratory failure. Depending on the patient's age and the cause, acute respiratory failure can progress rapidly, resulting in a poor outcome because the ongoing lack of O_2 and build up of CO_2 eventually lead to hypoxia and cellular death.

Pathophysiology

Respiratory failure results from impaired gas exchange. Any condition associated with alveolar hypoventilation, ventilation-perfusion ($\dot{V}/\dot{Q}$) mismatch, and intrapulmonary (right-to-left) shunting can cause acute respiratory failure if left untreated. Examples include pneumonia, bronchospasm, ventilatory failure, pneumothorax, atelectasis, cor pulmonale, and pulmonary edema.

Decreased O_2 saturation may result from alveolar hypoventilation, in which chronic airway obstruction reduces alveolar minute ventilation. PaO_2 levels fall and $PaCO_2$ levels rise, resulting in hypoxemia. Hypoventilation can occur from a decrease in the rate or duration of inspiratory signal from the respiratory center, such as with central nervous system (CNS) conditions or trauma or CNS depressant drugs such as anesthetics, sedation, and hypnotics. Neuromuscular diseases, such as poliomyelitis or amyotrophic lateral sclerosis, can result in alveolar hypoventilation if the condition affects normal respiratory muscle contraction. The most common cause of alveolar hypoventilation is airway obstruction, often seen with COPD (emphysema or bronchitis).

Most commonly, hypoxemia — $\dot{V}/\dot{Q}$ imbalance — occurs when such condi-

tions as pulmonary embolism or adult respiratory distress syndrome (ARDS) interrupt normal gas exchange in a specific lung region. Too little ventilation with normal blood flow or too little blood flow with normal ventilation may cause the imbalance, resulting in decreased PaO_2 levels and, thus, hypoxemia.

Although uncommon, decreased fraction of inspired oxygen (FIO_2) may also lead to respiratory failure. Here, inspired air doesn't contain adequate O_2 to establish an adequate gradient for diffusion into the blood — for example, at high altitudes or in confined, enclosed spaces. As a result, hypoxemia occurs.

The hypoxemia and hypercapnia characteristic of respiratory failure stimulate strong compensatory responses by all of the body systems, including the respiratory and cardiovascular systems and the CNS. In response to hypoxemia, for example, the sympathetic nervous system triggers vasoconstriction, increases peripheral resistance, and increases the heart rate. Untreated $\dot{V}/\dot{Q}$ imbalances can lead to right-to-left shunting, in which blood passes from the right side to the left side of the heart without being oxygenated.

Tissue hypoxia occurs, resulting in anaerobic metabolism and lactic acidosis. Respiratory acidosis occurs from hypercapnia. Heart rate increases, stroke volume increases, and heart failure may occur. Cyanosis occurs due to increased amounts of unoxygenated blood. Hypoxia of the kidneys results in release of erythropoietin from renal cells, causing the bone marrow to increase production of red blood cells—

an attempt by the body to increase the blood's oxygen-carrying capacity.

The body responds to hypercapnia with cerebral depression, hypotension, circulatory failure, and an increased heart rate and cardiac output (CO). Hypoxemia or hypercapnia (or both) cause the brain's respiratory control center to increase respiratory depth (tidal volume), and then to increase the respiratory rate. As respiratory failure worsens, intercostal, supraclavicular, and suprasternal retractions may also occur.

Comprehensive assessment

The patient's history may reveal an underlying respiratory condition or an acute process leading to respiratory failure (such as asphyxia, drug overdose, or trauma). However, because acute respiratory failure is life-threatening, time to conduct an in-depth patient interview is severely limited. Rely on family members or the patient's medical records to discover the precipitating incident.

The patient may have nasal flaring (secondary to hypoxia), ashen skin, and cyanosis of the oral mucosa, lips, and nail beds (due to hypoxemia). He may yawn and use accessory muscles to breathe. The patient may appear restless, anxious, depressed, lethargic, agitated, or confused due to cerebral hypoxia. He may exhibit tachypnea due to hypoxia, which signals impending respiratory failure.

Palpation may reveal cold, clammy skin (due to vasoconstriction) and asymmetrical chest movement, which suggests pneumothorax. If tactile fremitus is present, it typically decreases over obstructed bronchi or pleural

effusion areas but increases over consolidated lung tissue.

Percussion reveals hyperresonance, especially in patients with COPD. If acute respiratory failure results from atelectasis or pneumonia, percussion usually produces a dull or flat sound.

Auscultation typically discloses diminished breath sounds indicating areas of hypoventilation. In patients with pneumothorax, breath sounds may be absent. In other cases of respiratory failure, adventitious breath sounds such as wheezes (in asthma) and rhonchi (in bronchitis) may be heard.

ALERT *If crackles are present, pulmonary edema may be the cause of respiratory failure.*

Diagnosis

These tests help diagnose acute respiratory failure:

- ABG analysis indicates respiratory failure by deteriorating values (typically PaO_2 less than 60 mm Hg and $PaCO_2$ greater than 45 mm Hg) and a pH below 7.35. Patients with COPD may have a lower-than-normal pH compared with their previous levels.
- Chest X-ray identifies pulmonary diseases or conditions, such as emphysema, atelectasis, lesions, pneumothorax, infiltrates, and effusions.
- Electrocardiography can show arrhythmias, which are commonly found with cor pulmonale and myocardial hypoxia.
- Pulse oximetry reveals a decreasing arterial oxygen saturation (SaO_2); mixed venous oxygen saturation ($S\bar{v}O_2$) level of less than 50% indicates impaired tissue oxygenation.
- White blood cell count aids in detecting an underlying infection as the cause.

■ Abnormally low hemoglobin and hematocrit levels signal blood loss, indicating a decreased oxygen-carrying capacity.

■ Hypokalemia may result from compensatory hyperventilation, the body's attempt to correct acidosis.

■ Hypochloremia may occur if the patient develops metabolic alkalosis.

■ Blood cultures, sputum culture, and Gram stain may identify pathogens.

■ Pulmonary artery catheterization helps to distinguish pulmonary and cardiovascular causes of acute respiratory failure and monitors hemodynamic pressures.

Collaborations

Because acute respiratory failure can affect multiple systems, a multidisciplinary approach to care is needed. A pulmonary specialist can help evaluate, treat, and manage the patient's respiratory system. If infectious agents may be involved, an infectious disease specialist may be consulted; likewise, if cardiac involvement is suspected, consultation with a cardiologist is indicated. Initially, the patient may require total parenteral nutrition, depending on the severity of the condition and the status of the patient. As his condition improves, however, he may require nutritional support to maintain and improve overall nutrition, strengthen the immune system, and meet metabolic needs. If he's able to eat, a registered dietitian can help you plan to meet his dietary needs. A respiratory therapist may be needed to assist with O_2 therapy and ventilatory support. Other therapies, such as physical and occupational therapy, may be necessary to help with energy conservation and rehabilitation depending on the patient's

condition and length of stay. If a prolonged hospital stay is expected and the patient requires long-term care, consult social services early on in the patient's care.

Treatment and care

Treatment of acute respiratory failure typically focuses on restoring adequate gas exchange to provide O_2 to the organs, tissues, and cells, and on correcting the underlying causative condition. Treatment includes:

■ O_2 therapy to promote oxygenation and raise PaO_2

■ mechanical ventilation with an endotracheal (ET) or a tracheostomy tube, if needed, to provide adequate oxygenation and to reverse acidosis

■ high-frequency ventilation if patient doesn't respond to treatment, to force the airways open, promoting oxygenation and preventing collapse of alveoli

■ reversal agents such as naloxone (Narcan) if drug overdose is suspected

■ antibiotics to treat infection

■ bronchodilators to maintain patency of the airways

■ corticosteroids to decrease inflammation

■ fluid restrictions (in cor pulmonale) to reduce volume and cardiac workload

■ positive inotropic agents to increase CO

■ vasopressors to maintain blood pressure

■ diuretics to reduce edema and fluid overload

■ deep breathing with pursed lips to prevent alveolar collapse if patient isn't intubated and mechanically ventilated

■ incentive spirometry to increase lung volume; chest physiotherapy or nasotracheal suction to maintain airway clearance.

Complications

Possible complications of acute respiratory failure may include:
- tissue hypoxia
- metabolic acidosis
- lactic acidosis
- multiple organ dysfunction syndrome
- cardiac arrhythmias
- cardiac arrest.

Nursing considerations

- To reverse hypoxemia, administer O_2 as ordered at appropriate concentrations to maintain PaO_2 at a minimum pressure range of 50 to 60 mm Hg.

ALERT *Keep in mind that the patient with COPD usually requires only small amounts of supplemental O_2. Administering too high a concentration of O_2 depresses the patient's stimulus to breathe.*

- Assess the patient's respiratory status at least every 2 hours — or more frequently, as indicated. Observe for a positive response to O_2 therapy, such as improved breathing, color, and oximetry and ABG values.

ALERT *Remember that O_2 can be toxic and directly injure the lung if given too long or at excessive concentrations. Therefore, use the lowest FIO_2 necessary to maintain adequate oxygenation for the shortest time possible.*

- Maintain a patent airway. If the patient retains CO_2, encourage him to cough and breathe deeply with pursed lips. If he's alert, have him use an incentive spirometer at least every 2 hours. If he's intubated and lethargic, reposition him every 1 to 2 hours. Use postural drainage and chest physiotherapy to help clear secretions.

- Auscultate chest for changes in breath sounds. Report any changes in ABG values or SaO_2 or $S\bar{v}O_2$ saturation levels immediately.

- Assess vital signs frequently, at least every 2 hours or more often if indicated. Note and report an increasing pulse rate, rising or falling respiratory rate, declining blood pressure, or febrile state.

- Institute continuous cardiac monitoring if indicated and observe for arrhythmias.

- If indicated, assist with insertion of pulmonary artery catheter and monitor hemodynamic status, as ordered.

- Obtain serial serum electrolyte levels to monitor for trends and take steps to correct imbalances.

- Administer pharmacologic therapy, such as antibiotics, as ordered.

- Assess urine output hourly to evaluate renal function; record intake and output and daily weight.

- Maintain the patient in a normothermic state to reduce his body's demand for O_2.

- Position the patient for comfort and optimal gas exchange, such as semi-Fowler's to high Fowler's position. Place the call button within his reach.

- Provide opportunities for rest periods to minimize O_2 demands.

  If the patient requires mechanical ventilation:

- Check ventilator settings, cuff pressures, oximetry, and capnometry values frequently according to your facility's policy; evaluate ABG values as indicated to ensure correct FIO_2 settings.

- Monitor changes in oximetry or capnometry values after each change in the FIO_2 setting.

■ Suction the trachea as needed after hyperoxygenation. Provide humidification to liquefy secretions.

■ When suctioning the patient, check for any changes in sputum quality, consistency, odor, or color.

■ Use sterile technique while suctioning; change ventilator tubing every 24 hours or according to your facility's policy to reduce the risk of infection.

■ Routinely assess ET tube position and patency. Make sure the tube is placed properly and taped securely.

ALERT Immediately after intubation, auscultate the lung fields to check for accidental intubation of the esophagus or the mainstem bronchus, which may have occurred during ET tube insertion. Also, be alert for transtracheal or laryngeal perforation, aspiration, broken teeth, nosebleeds, and vagal reflexes, such as bradycardia, arrhythmias, and hypotension.

■ After tube placement, watch for complications, such as tube displacement, herniation of the tube's cuff, respiratory infection, and tracheal malacia and stenosis.

■ Prevent tracheal erosion that can result from an overinflated artificial airway cuff compressing the tracheal wall's vasculature. Use the minimal-leak technique and a cuffed tube with high residual volume (low-pressure cuff), a foam cuff, or a pressure-regulating valve on the cuff. Measure cuff pressure at least every 8 hours.

■ Implement measures to prevent nasal tissue necrosis. Position and maintain the nasotracheal tube midline within the nostrils, and provide meticulous care. Reposition the oral ET tube daily to prevent oral mucosal breakdown. Avoid excessive movement of any tubes, and make sure the ventilator tubing has adequate support.

■ Watch for complications of mechanical ventilation, such as reduced CO, pneumothorax or other barotrauma, increased pulmonary vascular resistance, diminished urine output, increased intracranial pressure, and GI bleeding.

■ To minimize the risk of GI bleeding, inspect gastric secretions for blood, especially if the patient has a nasogastric tube or reports epigastric tenderness, nausea, or vomiting. Monitor hemoglobin levels and hematocrit, and routinely check stools for blood.

Patient teaching

■ Orient the patient and his family to the unit and acquaint them with procedures, sounds, and sights to help minimize anxiety.

■ Describe all tests and procedures to the patient and his family. Discuss the reasons for suctioning, mechanical ventilation, and blood tests.

■ If the patient is intubated or has a tracheostomy, explain why he can't speak. Suggest alternative means of communication, such as using a writing pad.

ALERT Teach the patient and his family about signs and symptoms to report immediately, including increasing respiratory distress, progressive cyanosis, or continuing deterioration in neurologic status.

■ Emphasize the value of a pulmonary rehabilitation program.

MULTISYSTEM DISORDER

Adult respiratory distress syndrome

Adult respiratory distress syndrome (ARDS) is a form of noncardiogenic pulmonary edema that can quickly lead to acute respiratory failure. Also known as shock, stiff, white, wet, or DaNang lung, ARDS may follow direct or indirect lung injury.

Trauma is the most common cause of ARDS, possibly because trauma-related factors, such as fat emboli, sepsis, shock, pulmonary contusions, and multiple transfusions, increase the likelihood that microemboli will develop. Other common causes of ARDS include anaphylaxis, aspiration of gastric contents, diffuse pneumonia (especially viral), drug overdose (for example, heroin, aspirin, or ethchlorvynol), idiosyncratic drug reaction (to ampicillin or hydrochlorothiazide), inhalation of noxious gases (such as ammonia, chlorine, or nitrous oxide), near-drowning, and oxygen toxicity. Less common causes of ARDS include coronary artery bypass grafting, hemodialysis, leukemia, acute miliary tuberculosis, pancreatitis, thrombotic thrombocytopenic purpura, uremia, and venous air embolism.

The prognosis for the patient with ARDS varies depending on the cause, the patient's age, and presence of co-morbid conditions. Survival is high (over 90%) for patients who are young and relatively healthy prior to the event. However, if the patient is elderly, has other chronic disorders and multisystem organ dysfunction, the mortality rate ranges from 50% to 60%.

Pathophysiology

In ARDS, injury to the alveolar epithelium and the pulmonary capillary epithelium triggers a sequence of events resulting in the production of inflammatory mediators, including oxidants, proteases, kinins, growth factors, and neuropeptides, which initiate the complement cascade, intravascular coagulation, and fibrinolysis. The resulting increased vascular permeability ultimately affects the hydrostatic pressure gradient of the capillary. Elevated capillary pressure, which may result from insults of fluid overload or cardiac dysfunction in sepsis, greatly increases interstitial and alveolar edema. This edema is evident in dependent lung areas and can be visualized as whitened areas on chest X-rays. Alveolar closing pressure then exceeds pulmonary pressure, and alveolar closure and collapse begin.

Fluid accumulates in the lung interstitium, the alveolar spaces, and the small airways. The lungs then stiffen, impairing ventilation and reducing oxygenation of the pulmonary capillary blood, thereby reducing normal blood flow to the lungs. Damage can occur directly, by aspiration of gastric contents and inhalation of noxious gases, or indirectly, from chemical mediators released in response to systemic disease. The release of serotonin, bradykinin, and histamine attracts and activates neutrophils that inflame and damage the alveolar membrane and increase capillary permeability. Additional chemotactic factors are released, including endotoxins (such as those present in septic states), tumor necrosis factor, and interleukin-1. In the early stages of ARDS, signs and symptoms may be undetectable.

Histamines and other inflammatory substances further increase capillary permeability, allowing fluids to move into the interstitial space. At this stage, the patient experiences tachypnea, dyspnea, and tachycardia. As capillary permeability increases, proteins, blood cells, and more fluid leak out, increasing interstitial osmotic pressure and causing pulmonary edema. Tachycardia, dyspnea, and cyanosis may occur. Hypoxia (usually unresponsive to increasing the fraction of inspired oxygen [FIO_2]), decreased pulmonary compliance, crackles, and rhonchi develop. The resulting pulmonary edema and hemorrhage significantly reduce lung compliance and impair alveolar ventilation.

Decreased blood flow and fluid in the alveoli damage the surfactant in the alveoli and impair the ability of alveolar cells to produce more surfactant. Without surfactant, alveoli and bronchioles fill with fluid or collapse, gas exchange is impaired, and the lungs are much less compliant. Ventilation of the alveoli is further decreased. The burden of ventilation and gas exchange shifts to uninvolved areas of the lung, and pulmonary blood flow is shunted from right to left. The patient must labor to breathe and may develop thick frothy sputum and marked hypoxemia with increasing respiratory distress.

Mediators released by neutrophils and macrophages also cause varying degrees of pulmonary vasoconstriction, resulting in pulmonary hypertension and a ventilation-perfusion mismatch. Although the patient responds with an increased respiratory rate, sufficient oxygen (O_2) can't cross the alveolar capillary membrane, whereas carbon dioxide (CO_2) continues to cross easily and is lost with every exhalation. As both O_2 and CO_2 levels in the blood decrease, the patient develops increasing tachypnea, hypoxemia, and hypocapnia (low partial pressure of arterial CO_2 [$PaCO_2$]).

Pulmonary edema worsens and hyaline membranes form. Inflammation leads to fibrosis, further impeding gas exchange. Fibrosis progressively obliterates alveoli, respiratory bronchioles, and the interstitium. Functional residual capacity decreases and shunting becomes more serious. Hypoxemia leads to metabolic acidosis. At this stage, the patient develops increasing $PaCO_2$, decreasing pH and partial pressure of arterial O_2 (PaO_2), decreasing bicarbonate levels (HCO_3^-) and mental confusion. (See *Phases of adult respiratory distress syndrome,* page 174.)

The end result is respiratory failure. Systemically, neutrophils and inflammatory mediators cause generalized endothelial damage and increased capillary permeability throughout the body. Multisystem organ dysfunction syndrome (MODS) occurs as the cascade of mediators affects each system. Death may occur from the influence of both ARDS and MODS.

Comprehensive assessment

ARDS progresses in stages, from I to IV, each of which has typical signs and symptoms. In stage I, the patient may report dyspnea, especially on exertion. His respiratory and pulse rates are normal to high. Auscultation may reveal diminished breath sounds. Rapid, shallow breathing and dyspnea can occur hours to days after the initial injury in response to decreasing O_2 levels in the blood. The ventilatory rate

Phases of adult respiratory distress syndrome

The diagrams here show the process and progress of adult respiratory distress syndrome (ARDS).

In phase 1 of ARDS, injury reduces normal blood flow to the lungs. Platelets aggregate and release histamine (H), serotonin (S), and bradykinin (B).

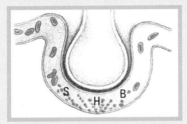

In phase 2, the released substances inflame and damage the alveolar capillary membrane, increasing capillary permeability. Fluids then shift into the interstitial space.

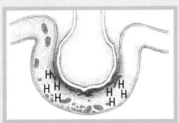

In phase 3, capillary permeability increases and proteins and fluids leak out, increasing interstitial osmotic pressure and causing pulmonary edema.

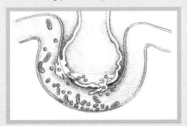

In phase 4, decreased blood flow and fluids in the alveoli damage surfactant and impair the cell's ability to produce more. The alveoli then collapse, thus impairing gas exchange.

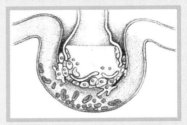

In phase 5, oxygenation is impaired, but carbon dioxide easily crosses the alveolar capillary membrane and is expired. Blood oxygen and carbon dioxide levels are low.

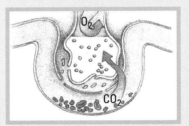

In phase 6, pulmonary edema worsens and inflammation leads to fibrosis. Gas exchange is further impeded.

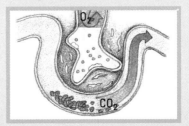

increases due to hypoxemia and its effects on the pneumotaxic center.

In stage II, respiratory distress becomes more apparent. The patient may use accessory muscles to breathe (intercostal and suprasternal retractions) due to the increased effort required to expand the stiff lung. He may appear restless, apprehensive, and mentally sluggish as the result of cerebral hypoxia. He may have a dry cough with thick, frothy sputum and bloody, sticky secretions. Blood pressure may be elevated and, possibly, accompanied by tachycardia and tachypnea. Palpation may disclose cool, clammy skin. Lung auscultation may detect basilar crackles.

ALERT *Be alert for stage II signs and symptoms because they are sometimes incorrectly attributed to other causes such as multiple trauma.*

In stage III, the patient may struggle to breathe. Vital signs reveal tachypnea (more than 30 breaths/minute), tachycardia with arrhythmias (usually premature ventricular contractions), and a labile blood pressure. Tachycardia signals the heart's effort to deliver more oxygen to the cells and vital organs. Inspection may reveal a productive cough and pale, cyanotic skin. Auscultation may disclose crackles and rhonchi resulting from fluid accumulation in the lungs. Endotracheal intubation and mechanical ventilation usually are necessary at this stage.

In stage IV, the patient has acute respiratory failure with severe hypoxemia. His mental status deteriorates and he may become comatose. Motor dysfunction occurs as hypoxia ensues. His skin appears pale and cyanotic. Spontaneous respirations are lacking. Bradycardia with arrhythmias accompanies hypotension. Metabolic and respiratory acidosis develop. Respiratory acidosis occurs as CO_2 accumulates in the blood and O_2 levels decrease. Metabolic acidosis eventually results from failure of compensatory mechanisms. When ARDS reaches this stage, the patient is at high risk for fibrosis. Pulmonary damage becomes life-threatening.

Diagnosis

These tests help diagnose ARDS:
- Arterial blood gas (ABG) analysis (with the patient breathing room air) initially shows reduced PaO_2 (less than 60 mm Hg), and decreased $PaCO_2$ (less than 35 mm Hg).

ALERT *Hypoxemia despite increased supplemental oxygen is the hallmark of ARDS.*

- The resulting blood pH usually reflects respiratory alkalosis. As ARDS worsens, ABG values show respiratory acidosis (increasing $PaCO_2$ [more than 45 mm Hg]), metabolic acidosis (decreasing HCO_3^- levels [less than 22 mEq/L]), and declining PaO_2 despite oxygen therapy.
- Pulmonary artery (PA) catheterization helps identify the cause of pulmonary edema by measuring pulmonary artery wedge pressure (PAWP). PAWP values in ARDS are 12 mm Hg or less.
- Serial chest X-rays in early stages may be normal initially, because bilateral infiltrates may not appear for up to 24 hours. In later stages, findings demonstrate lung fields with a ground-glass appearance and, eventually (with irreversible hypoxemia), "whiteouts" of both lung fields.

Differential diagnosis must rule out cardiogenic pulmonary edema, pulmonary vasculitis, and diffuse pulmonary hemorrhage. Tests to determine the causative agent may involve sputum analyses (including Gram stain and culture and sensitivity), blood cultures (to identify infectious organisms), toxicology tests (to screen for drug ingestion), and serum amylase tests (to rule out pancreatitis).

Collaborations

A pulmonary specialist can help evaluate, treat, and manage the respiratory system of a patient with ARDS. If infectious agents may be involved, an infectious disease specialist may be called in; likewise, if cardiac involvement is suspected, a consultation with a cardiologist is indicated. As other systems, such as the kidneys, become involved, the patient may require consults with other specialists. If a prolonged course of treatment is expected, a nutritional consult for total parenteral nutrition may be needed, as well as physical therapy to assist with rehabilitation.

If ARDS is arrested in the initial stages, the patient may be discharged to home with instructions to follow-up with his physician after discharge. If the patient progresses through later stages of ARDS, he may require an extended care facility that accepts ventilator-dependent patients, once he is stabilized. He may also need follow-up with the appropriate specialists and teams if he requires hemodialysis, physical rehabilitation, and occupational rehabilitation, depending on the extent of his illness and involved body systems. Social services should be consulted early on if a prolonged hospital stay is expected and the patient requires long-term care.

Treatment and care

Therapy focuses on correcting the cause of the syndrome, if possible, and preventing the progression of life-threatening hypoxemia and respiratory acidosis. Supportive care consists of administering humidified O_2 by a tight-fitting mask to facilitate the use of continuous positive airway pressure (CPAP). However, this therapy alone seldom fulfills the ARDS patient's ventilatory requirements. If his hypoxemia doesn't subside with this treatment, he may require intubation, mechanical ventilation, and positive end-expiratory pressure (PEEP). High-frequency jet ventilation may also be required. Suctioning, humidification, percussion, and vibration techniques help clear secretions.

When a patient with ARDS needs mechanical ventilation, sedatives, narcotics, or neuromuscular blocking agents (such as vecuronium) may be ordered to minimize restlessness (thereby minimizing O_2 consumption and CO_2 production) and facilitate ventilation. Neuromuscular blocking agents and sedation should be given at regular intervals for maximum effect. Such ventilatory modalities as pressure-controlled inverse ratio ventilation may be needed to reverse the conventional inspiration-to-expiration ratio and minimize the risk of barotrauma (mechanical breaths are pressure-limited to prevent increased damage to the alveoli). Permissive hypercapnia may be used to limit peak inspiratory pressure (although CO_2 removal is compromised, treatment isn't given for subsequent changes in blood hydrogen and O_2 concentration). When the patient is on a ventilator, tubing should be drained promptly to ensure maximum O_2 delivery. An alert patient will need to communicate by other means, such as writing or picture boards, to convey his needs and feelings.

Treatment is also individualized depending on assessment findings and diagnostic testing results. When ARDS results from fatty emboli or a chemical injury, a short course of high-dose corticosteroids may help if given early to optimize cellular membranes. Treatment with sodium bicarbonate may be necessary to reverse severe metabolic acidosis. Fluids may be used to treat hypovolemia and vasopressors may be needed to maintain blood pressure. Nonviral infections require treatment with antimicrobial drugs.

Diuretics may be needed to reduce interstitial and pulmonary edema. Electrolyte and acid-base imbalances should be corrected to maintain cellular integrity, particularly the sodium-potassium pump. Fluid restriction may be needed to prevent increase of interstitial and alveolar edema.

Complications

Rapid diagnosis and intervention is necessary to stop progression of ARDS through the various stages. Depending on the age of the patient and cause of respiratory distress, ARDS can progress rapidly, resulting in a downward spiral and poor outcome. Possible complications of ARDS include:
- hypotension
- decreased urine output
- metabolic acidosis
- respiratory acidosis
- MODS
- ventricular fibrillation
- ventricular standstill.

Nursing considerations

- Assess the patient's respiratory status at least every 2 hours — or more often, if indicated. Note respiratory rate, rhythm, and depth, reporting any dyspnea and accessory muscle use. Be alert for inspiratory retractions.
- Administer oxygen as ordered. Monitor FIO_2 levels frequently.
- Auscultate lungs bilaterally for adventitious or diminished breath sounds. Inspect the color and character of sputum, keeping in mind that clear, frothy sputum indicates pulmonary edema. To maintain PEEP, suction only as needed.
- Check ventilator settings frequently. Assess O_2 saturation continuously via pulse oximetry or mixed venous O_2 saturation ($S\bar{v}O_2$) via pulmonary artery (PA) catheter, if in place. Monitor serial ABG levels; document and report changes in arterial O_2 saturation (SaO_2) as well as metabolic and respiratory acidosis and PaO_2 changes.
- Closely monitor the patient's heart rate and blood pressure at least every 2 hours, or more frequently, as indicated by the patient's condition. Institute continuous cardiac monitoring and observe for arrhythmias that may result from hypoxemia, acid-base disturbances, or electrolyte imbalance.
- Note and record any changes in respiratory status, temperature, or hypotension that may indicate a deteriorating condition. Notify the physician should any such changes occur.

ALERT *If the patient has injuries that affect his lungs, watch for adverse respiratory changes, especially in the first few days after the injury, when his condition may appear to be improving.*

■ Monitor the patient's level of consciousness, noting confusion or mental sluggishness.

■ Be alert for signs of treatment-induced complications, including arrhythmias, disseminated intravascular coagulation, GI bleeding, infection, malnutrition, paralytic ileus, pneumothorax, pulmonary fibrosis, renal failure, thrombocytopenia, and tracheal stenosis.

■ Give sedatives as ordered to reduce restlessness. Administer sedatives and analgesics at regular intervals if the patient is receiving neuromuscular blocking agents. Monitor and record the patient's response to medication.

■ Administer anti-infective agents as ordered if the underlying cause is sepsis or an infection.

■ Place the patient in a comfortable position that maximizes air exchange, such as semi-Fowler's to high Fowler's position. Use SaO_2 levels as a guide to most effective position. Reposition the patient often. A high Fowler's position or a continuous rotation bed may be needed.

■ Allow for periods of rest to prevent fatigue and reduce O_2 demand.

■ If a PA catheter has been inserted, know the desired PAWP level; check readings as indicated and watch for decreasing $S\bar{v}O_2$. Because PEEP may lower cardiac output, check for hypotension, tachycardia, and decreased urine output. Change PA catheter dressings according to your facility's guidelines, using strict aseptic technique.

■ Evaluate the patient's serum electrolyte levels, as ordered, frequently. Monitor urine output hourly to ensure adequate renal function. Measure intake and output. Weigh the patient daily.

■ Record caloric intake. Administer tube feedings and parenteral nutrition as ordered.

■ Perform passive range-of-motion exercises to maintain joint mobility. If possible, help the patient perform active exercises. Monitor SaO_2 levels throughout any activity for changes indicating a deterioration in the patient's condition.

■ Provide meticulous skin care. To prevent skin breakdown, reposition the endotracheal tube from side to side every 24 hours.

■ Prepare the patient and his family for additional therapies such as extracorporeal membrane oxygenation or inhaled nitrous oxide.

■ Provide emotional support. Answer the patient's — and his family's — questions as fully as possible to allay their fears and concerns.

Patient teaching

■ Explain the disorder to the patient and his family. Explain the signs and symptoms that may occur and review the treatment that may be required.

■ Orient the patient and his family to the unit and surroundings. Provide them with simple explanations and demonstrations of treatments and procedures. Involve them in his care as much as reasonably possible.

■ Inform the patient that recovery will take some time and that weakness may be present for a while. Urge him to share his concerns with the staff.

Bronchoscopy

Bronchoscopy allows direct visualization of the larynx, trachea, and bronchi most commonly via a flexible fiber-optic bronchoscope in an ambulatory surgical area or at the bedside using local anesthesia and I.V. sedation. A rigid metal bronchoscope may be used when massive hemoptysis occurs or when a lesion is obstructing the airway. When this type of bronchoscope is used, however, general anesthesia is necessary.

Bronchoscopy is performed to:
■ examine the tracheobronchial tree for tumors, obstruction, foreign bodies, secretions, or bleeding
■ aid in diagnosis of bronchogenic carcinoma, tuberculosis, interstitial pulmonary disease, or fungal or parasitic pulmonary infection
■ remove foreign bodies, malignant or benign tumors, mucus plugs, or excessive secretions from the tracheobronchial trees.

Procedure

Approximately 30 minutes to 1 hour before the procedure, the patient is typically premedicated with atropine to dry secretions and a mild anti-anxiety agent or sedative to help him relax. Prior to insertion of the bronchoscope, a topical anesthetic is applied to the oropharynx or nasopharynx, larynx, vocal cords, and trachea.

With the patient in the supine or sitting position, the physician inserts the fiber-optic bronchoscope through the mouth or nose into the pharynx and trachea. If the patient has an endotracheal tube in place or a tracheostomy, the bronchoscope may be in-

Inserting a fiber-optic bronchoscope

In the illustration below, a flexible fiber-optic bronchoscope is inserted via an endotracheal tube and is passed through the tracheobronchial tree.

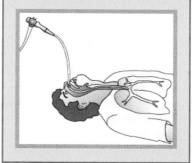

serted through it. The physician typically examines the right lung first, and then the left lung, obtaining specimens for analysis as appropriate. (See *Inserting a fiber-optic bronchoscope*.)

Various ports on the bronchoscope allow for suctioning, oxygen (O_2) administration, and biopsies during the procedure. O_2 saturation levels are monitored continuously throughout the procedure and arterial blood gas (ABG) values are usually obtained during and after the bronchoscopy.

Complications

The most common complication associated with bronchoscopy is hypercarbia resulting from inadequate ventilation. If this occurs, ventricular arrhythmias can develop. Another common complication is hypoxemia, resulting from intermittent and erratic ventilation. Other complications may include:

- damage to the teeth or larynx from intubation
- airway rupture
- laryngospasm or bronchospasm
- pneumothorax
- hemorrhage
- airway obstruction
- allergic reaction to anesthetic or sedation
- respiratory distress and failure.

Nursing considerations

Before bronchoscopy

- Explain the purpose, procedure, and reason for the procedure to the patient and his family; ensure that a signed informed consent is in the patient's medical record.
- Check to make sure the necessary information is available in the patient's medical record, including a recent history and physical examination, appropriate blood studies and urinalysis, chest X-ray, and ABG results; if the patient is older than age 40, make sure that an electrocardiogram is also in the patient's medical record.
- Keep the patient on nothing by mouth (NPO) status for at least 6 hours prior to the procedure, if possible.
- Remove, or ask the patient to remove, any dentures or oral prostheses to reduce the risk of inadvertent injury.
- Inform the patient that he may experience feeling something at the back of his throat and a thick tongue after administration of the topical anesthetic.
- Administer preprocedural medications, such as atropine and a sedative.

ALERT *Morphine is contraindicated in patients with a history of bronchospasm or asthma because it can lead to bronchospasm. If the patient*

has respiratory insufficiency, assess him closely for possible respiratory arrest that may be precipitated by the use of sedatives.

- If the bronchoscopy is to be performed at the bedside, assemble the necessary equipment.

AGE ISSUE *Children's airways are smaller in diameter than those of adults, so be sure that an appropriately sized bronchoscope is available. Instruments used for bronchoscopy can precipitate inflammation and edema, narrowing an already smaller airway, predisposing a child to an increased risk for oxygen desaturation and hypoxemia. Be sure that emergency equipment is readily available.*

- Obtain baseline O_2 saturation levels to use for comparison during and after the procedure.

After bronchoscopy

- Monitor the patient's vital signs at least every 15 minutes for the first hour, every 30 minutes for the second hour, and then hourly until he's stable. Assess respiratory status closely, including rate and ease of breathing and O_2 saturation levels. Note any signs and symptoms of respiratory distress, such as dyspnea or hypoxemia.

ALERT *Palpate for evidence of subcutaneous crepitus around the patient's face, neck, and chest area, which suggests rupture of the trachea or major bronchi or a severe pneumothorax.*

- Inspect sputum for color and evidence of bleeding. Report excessive bleeding immediately.
- Obtain ABG values as ordered.

ALERT *Keep in mind that arterial O_2 concentration may be altered for several hours after a bron-*

choscopy. *Anticipate the need for additional O_2 therapy or controlled ventilation with 100% O_2.*

■ Monitor cardiac status frequently for changes in heart rate or rhythm. Report any tachycardia or evidence of arrhythmias.

■ Obtain a chest X-ray as ordered to detect pneumothorax or evaluate lung status.

■ If the patient isn't intubated, assess for return of gag, cough, and swallowing reflexes. Keep him NPO until these reflexes return.

■ Position the patient in semi-Fowler's position (if conscious) or a side-lying position with the head of the bed slightly elevated (if unconscious) to reduce the risk of aspiration.

■ Ensure that specimens obtained during the procedure are properly labeled and immediately taken to the laboratory for analysis.

Chest drainage

Chest, or thoracic, drainage uses gravity (and occasionally suction) to restore negative pressure and remove any material that collects in the pleural cavity. The disposable drainage system combines drainage collection, a water seal, and suction control into a single unit. The underwater seal in the drainage system allows air and fluid to escape from the pleural cavity but doesn't allow air to reenter.

An alternative to an underwater seal drainage system is the use of a one-way flutter valve such as the Heimlich valve. As the name implies, this one-way valve is connected to the end of the chest tube and allows accumulated air to escape, but not enter. Suction also can be used with this valve. A one-way flutter valve may be used for the patient being discharged with a chest tube or being transferred to another health care facility. It allows portability for patients who require a chest tube for a longer period of time.

Thoracic drainage may be ordered to restore negative pressure in the pleural cavity, to reexpand a partially or totally collapsed lung, or to remove accumulated air, fluids (blood, pus, chyle, and serous fluids), or solids (blood clots) from the pleural cavity.

Equipment
Thoracic drainage system (Pleur-Evac or Thora-Klex system, which can function as gravity draining systems or be connected to suction to enhance chest drainage) ■ sterile distilled water (usually 1 L) ■ tape ■ sterile clear plastic tubing ■ two rubber-tipped Kelly clamps ■ sterile 50-ml catheter-tip syringe ■ suction source, if ordered ■ rubber band or safety pin

Essential steps
■ Check the physician's order to determine the type of drainage system to be used and specific procedural details. Gather the appropriate equipment and take it to the patient's bedside.

■ Explain the procedure to the patient and wash your hands.

■ Set up a commercially prepared disposable system and connect to the patient:

– Open the packaged system and place it on the floor in the rack supplied by the manufacturer to avoid accidentally knocking it over or dislodging the components. After the

Commercial chest drainage system

The illustration here depicts a commercial, disposable chest drainage system that combines drainage collection, water seal, and suction control in one unit.

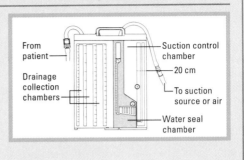

system is prepared, it may be hung from the side of the patient's bed.
− Remove the plastic connector from the short tube that's attached to the water-seal chamber. Using a 50-ml catheter-tip syringe, instill sterile distilled water into the water-seal chamber until it reaches the 2-cm mark or the mark specified by the manufacturer. The Ohio and Thora-Klex systems are ready to use, but with the Thora-Klex system, 15 ml of sterile water may be added to help detect air leaks. Replace the plastic connector.
− If suction is ordered, remove the cap (also called the muffler or atmosphere vent cover) on the suction-control chamber to open the vent. Next, instill sterile distilled water until it reaches the 20-cm mark or the ordered level and recap the suction-control chamber.
− Using the long tube, connect the patient's chest tube to the closed drainage collection chamber. Secure the connection with tape.
− Connect the short tube on the drainage system to the suction source and turn on the suction.

Gentle bubbling should begin in the suction chamber, indicating that the correct suction level has been reached. (See *Commercial chest drainage system.*)
■ Once attached, note the character, consistency, and amount of drainage in the collection chamber every hour initially, and then every 2 to 4 hours or according to your facility's policy.

ALERT *Notify the physician immediately if the amount of drainage is greater than 200 ml in 1 hour, which indicates bleeding.*
■ Mark the drainage level in the drainage collection chamber by noting the time and date at the drainage level on the chamber at least every 8 hours, or more frequently if there's a large amount of drainage.
■ Check the water level in the water-seal chamber at least every 8 hours. If necessary, carefully add sterile distilled water until the level reaches the 2-cm mark indicated on the water-seal chamber of the commercial system.
■ Check for fluctuation in the water-seal chamber as the patient breathes. Normal fluctuations of 2″ to 4″ (5 to 10 cm) reflect pressure changes in the

pleural space during respiration. To check for fluctuation when a suction system is being used, momentarily disconnect the suction system so the air vent is opened and observe for fluctuation.

ALERT *Fluid in the water-seal chamber typically rises on inspiration and falls on expiration; however, if the patient is receiving positive-pressure ventilation, the opposite is normal.*

■ Check for intermittent bubbling in the water-seal chamber, which occurs when the system is removing air from the pleural cavity (during expiration). If bubbling isn't readily apparent during quiet breathing, have the patient take a deep breath or cough. Absence of bubbling indicates that the lung has reexpanded or there's a kink or obstruction in the chest tube. Continuous bubbling during inspiration and expiration indicates a leak in the system.

■ Check the water level in the suction-control chamber. Detach the chamber or bottle from the suction source; when bubbling ceases, observe the water level. If necessary, add sterile distilled water to bring the level to −20 cm, or as ordered.

■ Check for gentle bubbling in the suction-control chamber because it indicates that the proper suction level has been reached. Vigorous bubbling in this chamber increases the rate of water evaporation.

■ Periodically confirm that the air vent in the system is working properly. Occlusion of the air vent results in a buildup of pressure in the system that could cause the patient to develop a tension pneumothorax.

■ Coil the system's tubing and secure it to the edge of the bed with a rubber band or tape and a safety pin.

ALERT *Avoid creating dependent loops, kinks, or pressure in the tubing. Don't lift the drainage system above the patient's chest, because fluid may flow back into the pleural space. Keep two rubber-tipped clamps at the bedside to clamp the chest tube if the system cracks, or to locate an air leak in the system.*

■ Assist the patient into an upright sitting position to promote optimal lung expansion.

■ Encourage the patient to cough frequently and breathe deeply to help drain the pleural space and expand the lungs, as appropriate. Splint, or assist with splinting, the insertion site to minimize pain when the patient coughs.

■ Assess the patient's hemodynamic and respiratory status at least every 2 to 4 hours, or more frequently, if indicated. Check the rate and quality of the patient's respirations and auscultate his lungs periodically to assess air exchange in the affected lung. Diminished or absent breath sounds may indicate that the lung hasn't reexpanded.

■ Tell the patient to report any breathing difficulty immediately.

ALERT *Notify the physician immediately if the patient develops cyanosis, rapid or shallow breathing, subcutaneous emphysema, chest pain, or excessive bleeding.*

■ Inspect the chest tube dressing at least every 8 hours. Palpate the area surrounding the dressing for crepitus or subcutaneous emphysema, which indicates that air is leaking into the subcutaneous tissue surrounding the insertion site. Change the dressing if

Checking for leaks

When attempting to locate a leak, try:
* clamping the tube momentarily at various points along its length, beginning at the tube's proximal end and working down toward the drainage system
* paying special attention to the seal around the connections
* pushing any loose connections back together and taping them securely.

The bubbling will stop when a clamp is placed between the air leak and the water seal. If you clamp along the tube's entire length and the bubbling doesn't stop, you'll probably need to replace the drainage unit because it may be cracked.

necessary or according to your facility's policy.

■ Encourage active or passive range-of-motion (ROM) exercises for the patient's arm or the affected side if his arm is splinted. (Usually, the thoracotomy patient's arm is splinted to decrease his discomfort.)

■ Administer analgesics, as ordered and needed, for comfort and to help with deep-breathing, coughing, and ROM exercises.

■ When getting the patient out of bed, keep the drainage system below chest level and be careful not to disconnect the tubing to maintain the water seal. With a suction system, keep the patient within range of the length of tubing attached to a wall outlet or portable pump.

Complications

Tension pneumothorax may result from excessive accumulation of air, drainage, or both and eventually may

exert pressure on the heart and aorta, causing a precipitous fall in cardiac output. Bleeding is another complication that can occur.

Nursing considerations

■ Instruct staff and visitors to avoid touching the equipment to prevent inadvertent disconnection and subsequent complications.

■ If excessive continuous bubbling is present in the water-seal chamber, especially if suction is being used, rule out a leak in the drainage system. (See *Checking for leaks.*)

■ If the drainage collection chamber fills, replace it. To do this, double-clamp the tube close to the insertion site (use two clamps facing in opposite directions), exchange the system, remove the clamps, and retape the connection.

ALERT *To prevent a tension pneumothorax (which may occur when clamping stops air and fluid from escaping), never leave the tubes clamped for more than a minute.*

■ If the system cracks, clamp the chest tube momentarily with the two rubber-tipped clamps at the bedside (placed there at the time of tube insertion). Place the clamps close to each other near the insertion site, facing in opposite directions to provide a more complete seal. Observe the patient for altered respirations while the tube is clamped. Then replace the damaged equipment. (Prepare the new unit before clamping the tube.)

■ Alternatively, instead of clamping the tube, submerge the distal end of the tube in a container of normal saline solution to create a temporary water seal while you replace the drainage system. Check your facility's policy for the proper procedure.

■ Document the date and time that chest drainage began, type of system used, amount of suction applied to the pleural cavity, presence or absence of bubbling or fluctuation in the water-seal chamber, initial amount and type of drainage, and the patient's respiratory status.

■ Record the frequency of system inspection, noting the patient's respiratory status, pain medication (if given), condition of the chest dressings, amount, color, and consistency of drainage, presence or absence of bubbling or fluctuation in the water-seal chamber, any complications, and the nursing actions taken.

 MULTISYSTEM DISORDER

Chest trauma

Chest trauma accounts for almost one-half of all trauma occurrences and almost one-fourth of all trauma-related deaths. Chest trauma is commonly classified as penetrating or blunt, depending on the type of injury. *Penetrating* chest trauma involves an injury by a foreign object, such as a knife (most common stabbing injury), bullet (most common missile injury), pitchfork, or other pointed object that penetrates the thorax. These are considered open injuries because the thoracic cavity is exposed to pressure from the outside atmosphere. *Blunt* chest trauma, which is considered a closed injury, results from sudden compression or positive pressure inflicted by a direct blow to the organ and surrounding tissue. Blunt chest trauma commonly occurs in motor vehicle acci-

dents (when the chest strikes the steering wheel), falls, or crushing injury.

Typically, penetrating chest trauma is fairly limited, usually involving isolated organs and lacerated tissues. In some cases, however, extensive tissue damage can occur if a bullet explodes in the chest cavity. Blunt chest trauma can cause extensive injury to the chest wall, lung, pleural space, and great vessels. Injuries resulting from blunt chest trauma include pulmonary contusion, rib fractures, pneumothorax, hemothorax, and rupture of the diaphragm or great vessels. (See *Injuries associated with chest trauma,* pages 186 to 189.) Blunt injuries are associated with multisystem organ injuries and carry a higher mortality rate than penetrating injuries.

Pathophysiology

Injuries to the chest usually involve one or more of these conditions:

■ hypoxemia resulting from airway alteration, damage to the chest muscles, lung parenchyma or ribs, severe hemorrhage, collapse of the lungs, or pneumothorax

■ hypovolemia resulting from massive fluid loss

■ cardiac failure resulting from an increase in intrathoracic pressure or subsequent cardiac injury such as cardiac tamponade or contusion. (See also "Cardiac trauma" in chapter 1, page 60.)

Tissue damage caused by penetrating trauma, such as an impaled object or foreign body, is related to the object size as well as the depth and velocity of penetration. For example, penetrating chest trauma by a bullet has many variables. The extent of injury depends

(*Text continues on page 188.*)

Injuries associated with chest trauma

Injury	Pathophysiologic mechanism of injury
Pneumothorax	Blunt or penetrating injury allowing air to accumulate in the pleural space
Tension pneumothorax	Blunt or penetrating injury allowing air to accumulate in the pleural space without a way to escape, leading to complete lung collapse
Hemothorax	Blunt or penetrating trauma allowing blood to accumulate in the pleural space
Chylothorax	Blunt or penetrating trauma usually to the thoracic duct or lymphatics allowing lymphatic fluid to drain and accumulate in pleural space
Pneumomediastinum	Blunt or penetrating trauma allowing air to accumulate in the mediastinum
Flail chest	Blunt trauma resulting in rib or sternal fractures leading to instability of the chest
Pulmonary contusion	Blunt trauma injuring lung tissue with the potential to cause respiratory failure

Assessment findings	Treatment considerations
• Dyspnea • Chest pain • Decreased or absent breath sounds • Chest X-ray positive for air between visceral and parietal pleura	• Chest tube insertion
• Severe dyspnea • Restlessness • Cyanosis • Tracheal shift to unaffected side • Distended neck veins • Absence of breath sounds on affected side • Tachycardia • Hypotension • Distant heart sounds • Hypoxemia	• Emergency lung reexpansion; possible thoracotomy for penetrating injury • Chest tube insertion
• Dyspnea • Tachycardia • Tachypnea • Cool clammy skin • Hypotension • Diminished capillary refill • Absent breath sounds on affected side • Chest X-ray positive for blood accumulation	• Chest tube insertion with possible autotransfusion
• Chest X-ray positive for pleural effusion (although may not be evident for 2 to 4 weeks) after injury	• Chest tube insertion • Possible thoracotomy to ligate thoracic duct
• Dyspnea • Chest pain	• Chest tube placement with repair of underlying injury
• Dyspnea • Labored shallow respirations • Chest wall pain • Crepitus from body fragments (subcutaneous emphysema) • Asymmetrical (paradoxical) chest movements • Chest X-ray positive for fractures	• Symptomatic and supportive care • Prevention of hemothorax and pneumothorax
• Dyspnea • Restlessness • Hemoptysis • Tachycardia • Crackles • Decreased lung compliance • Atelectasis • Arterial blood gas analysis revealing hypoxemia and hypercarbia • Chest X-ray revealing local or diffuse patchy, poorly outlined densities or irregular linear infiltrates	• Intubation and mechanical ventilation • Hemodynamic monitoring • Possible thoracotomy if massive hemorrhage suspected

(continued)

Injuries associated with chest trauma *(continued)*

Injury	Pathophysiologic mechanism of injury
Tracheobronchial tear	Blunt trauma causing injury to the tracheobronchial tree, possibly leading to airway obstruction and tension pneumothorax
Diaphragmatic rupture	Blunt trauma causing a tear in the diaphragm, possibly allowing abdominal contents to herniate into the thorax
Cardiac contusion	Blunt trauma resulting in bruising of the cardiac muscle
Cardiac tamponade	Blunt or penetrating trauma allowing blood to accumulate in the pericardial sac, ultimately impairing venous return and cardiac output
Great vessel rupture	Blunt trauma resulting in injury to major blood vessels such as the aorta

on the distance at which the weapon was fired, the type of ammunition, the velocity of the ammunition, and the entrance and (if present) exit wounds. Additional factors to be considered when assessing the extent of a penetrating chest injury include the type of weapon; for example, the caliber, barrel, and length of a gun and the powder composition. An intact bullet causes less damage than a bullet that explodes on impact. A bullet that explodes within the chest may break up and scatter fragments, burn tissue, fracture bone, disrupt vascular structures, or cause a bullet embolism. Other weapons that can cause penetrating trauma include knives and arrows.

Injury resulting from blunt chest trauma is related to the amount of

Assessment findings	Treatment considerations
• Dyspnea • Palpable fracture, hoarseness, and subcutaneous edema (laryngeal fracture) • Noisy breathing, labored respirations, and altered level of consciousness (tracheal injury) • Hemoptysis, subcutaneous emphysema, and possible tension pneumothorax (bronchial injury)	• Emergency surgical repair of injury
• Chest pain referred to the shoulder • Dyspnea • Diminished breath sounds • Bowels sounds audible in chest • Tachypnea • Chest X-ray positive for tear	• Surgical repair
• Chest discomfort • Electrocardiogram abnormalities (unexplained sinus tachycardia, atrial fibrillation, bundle branch block, ST segment changed) • Serial creatine kinase levels revealing possible muscle damage	• Supportive and symptomatic care
• Dyspnea • Midthoracic pain • Tachycardia • Tachypnea • Hypotension, distended neck veins, and muffled heart sounds (Beck's triad) • Paradoxical pulse	• Pericardiocentesis
• Dyspnea • Hoarseness • Stridor • Absent femoral pulses • Retrosternal or interscapular pain • Widening mediastinum	• Transfusion • Surgical repair

force, compression, and cavitation. Blunt force that strikes the chest wall at high velocity fractures the ribs and transfers that force to underlying organ and lung tissue. The direct impact of force is transmitted internally and the energy is dissipated to internal structures. The flexibility or elasticity of the chest wall directly affects the degree of injury. The first and second ribs take an enormous amount of blunt force to fracture and therefore are associated with significant intrathoracic injuries.

AGE ISSUE *Because the chest of a frail older person is inflexible and fragile, injury and mortality, even from minor chest trauma, are more probable.*

Comprehensive assessment

A patient who has experienced chest trauma undergoes an initial or primary assessment focusing on airway, breathing, and circulation and cervical spinal immobilization in the emergency department. Life-threatening injuries are diagnosed and treated immediately.

A secondary assessment involves obtaining information about the mechanism of injury and incorporating this information into a head-to-toe assessment. Signs and symptoms, although possibly subtle, can provide important clues to serious problems. A key aspect is inspection and palpation of the anterior and posterior chest.

Signs and symptoms may include:
- dyspnea and shortness of breath
- agitation and restlessness
- anxiety
- chest pain.

ALERT *In blunt injury, chest pain is severe and occurs during respirations with the patient able to locate the site of the pain; in penetrating injury, chest pain is moderate.*

On inspection, the patient may exhibit elevated respiratory rate, hyperpnea, accessory muscle use, nasal flaring, and respiratory distress. Hemoptysis may be present with blunt chest trauma. Chest-wall motion may be asymmetric or paradoxic (seen in blunt chest trauma indicating flail chest). The patient's skin, lips, and nail beds may be pale or cyanotic. Ecchymosis suggests injury to surrounding underlying organs. Jugular venous distention may be seen with blunt chest trauma. The penetrating object may be visible.

ALERT *Never remove an object that has penetrated the chest or other body part. The object may pro-vide a sealing effect to the surrounding tissues or organ and its removal could result in massive hemorrhage.*

Palpation typically reveals tracheal deviation, subcutaneous emphysema, weak or irregular pulses, and cool, clammy skin. For the patient with blunt chest trauma, tenderness may be noted at fracture sites and bony fragments may protrude. On percussion, dullness over the lung fields suggests a hemothorax or atelectasis, whereas hyperresonance suggests a pneumothorax.

Auscultation typically reveals diminished breath sounds, muffled heart sounds, respiratory stridor, and apical tachycardia. If the diaphragm has been torn or ruptured from the chest trauma, bowel sounds may be heard in the chest area. In addition, a paradoxical pulse may be noted if the patient has developed cardiac tamponade. If the patient has a blunt chest injury, bony crepitus may be heard at fracture sites.

Diagnosis

These tests help diagnose chest trauma:
- Chest X-ray identifies air or fluid in the pleural space (evidence of hemothorax or pneumothorax), and reveals evidence or absence of fractures and mediastinal shift.
- Arterial blood gas (ABG) analysis reveals degree of hypoxemia and possible acid-base imbalances with results showing partial pressure of arterial oxygen less than 80 mm Hg, partial pressure of arterial carbon dioxide greater than 45 mm Hg, and a pH of less than 7.35.
- Electrocardiogram (ECG) reveals possible arrhythmias.

■ Hemoglobin level and hematocrit reveal possible anemia secondary to blood loss.

Collaborations

Chest trauma is a multisystem problem requiring a multidisciplinary approach to care with a focus on maximizing the patient's respiratory and cardiac function and maintaining hemodynamic stability. The patient requires careful monitoring in a critical care unit. Emergency medical personnel at the scene of the trauma or in the emergency department are the first persons to intervene. Medical management and, if necessary, surgical intervention, are key components of care. In addition, other services may be necessary:

■ respiratory therapy to assist with pulmonary function
■ nutritional therapy for nutritional support and recommendations
■ physical or occupational therapy to assist with rehabilitation needs
■ social service to aid in facilitating care for specific trauma-related causes and financial needs.

Treatment and care

Treatment of the patient with chest trauma focuses on minimizing the patient's acute state of respiratory distress while managing the underlying pathophysiologic mechanisms of injury associated with the trauma. Close monitoring for signs and symptoms of cardiopulmonary compromise is important because chest trauma is associated with both pulmonary and cardiac injuries. Chest-tube insertion is commonly performed to reexpand the lung. Supplemental oxygen administration and assessment of oxygen saturation are important. If the degree of associated pulmonary trauma is great, endotracheal intubation and mechanical ventilation may be warranted to maintain adequate oxygenation.

Maintaining hemodynamic stability is crucial to the patient's care. Penetrating trauma may be associated with massive hemorrhage, leading to acute hypotension and shock. I.V. fluid therapy, including blood component therapy, may be necessary, especially in cases of severe bleeding.

In addition, cardiac output (CO) is affected if the patient develops cardiac tamponade or arrhythmias occurring with cardiac contusion. Hemodynamic monitoring is key to evaluating the patient's status and maintaining cardiopulmonary adequacy. Continuous ECG monitoring is important to detect possible arrhythmias.

If the patient is experiencing severe pain, I.V. morphine is administered in small amounts unless the patient is hypotensive. In addition, surgery may be indicated to repair tears to the tracheobronchial tree, diaphragm, or great vessels and other penetrating injuries. Pericardiocentesis is used to treat cardiac tamponade.

Complications

Complications associated with chest trauma may include:
■ adult respiratory distress syndrome
■ bronchopleural fistula
■ ventilator-induced lung injury
■ pneumonia
■ infection
■ pulmonary emboli.

Nursing considerations

Nursing care of the patient with chest trauma focuses on maintaining gas exchange, minimizing oxygen demands, and preventing complications.

■ Assess the patient's cardiopulmonary status at least every 2 hours — or more frequently, if indicated — to detect signs and symptoms of possible injury. Auscultate breath sounds at least every 2 hours, reporting any decrease in or absence of breath sounds or signs of congestion or fluid accumulation.

■ Palpate for crepitus. Evaluate peripheral pulses and capillary refill to detect decreased peripheral tissue perfusion.

■ Continuously monitor oxygen saturation levels and obtain ABGs as ordered; administer supplemental oxygen at the ordered flow rate.

■ Assist with insertion of chest tubes and monitor drainage closely, at least every hour for the first 4 hours, then every 2 hours for the next 24 hours. Notify the physician if the drainage is greater than 100 ml in 1 hour or if the drainage is bright red.

■ Assess dressings over penetrating chest trauma sites frequently, at least every 2 to 4 hours for the first 24 to 48 hours.

ALERT *Notify the physician if dressings become saturated, require changing more frequently than twice in 24 hours, or drainage appears bright red in color.*

■ Anticipate the need for endotracheal intubation and mechanical ventilation if the patient's respiratory status deteriorates or if the patient has difficulty maintaining a patent airway and adequate breathing.

■ Monitor heart rate and rhythm, heart sounds, and blood pressure every hour for changes; institute hemodynamic monitoring, including central venous pressure, pulmonary capillary wedge pressure, and CO, as indicated, at least every 1 to 2 hours.

■ Institute continuous cardiac monitoring to detect possible arrhythmias. If arrhythmias occur, administer antiarrhythmic agents as ordered.

■ Administer fluid replacement therapy, including blood component therapy as prescribed, typically to maintain systolic blood pressure above 90 mm Hg.

■ Monitor urinary output every hour. Notify the physician if output is less than 30 ml/hour.

■ Evaluate such laboratory test results as hemoglobin and hematocrit for changes.

■ Assess the patient's degree of pain and administer analgesic therapy as ordered, monitoring the patient for effectiveness. Position the patient comfortably, usually with the head of the bed elevated 30 to 45 degrees.

■ Encourage coughing and deep breathing, splinting the chest as necessary, provide frequent rest periods to decrease oxygen demands, and assist the patient out of bed to chair and to ambulate as tolerated and determined by his condition.

■ If the patient has undergone surgery, monitor and assess chest tubes for patency, volume and color of drainage, and presence of air leak; assess vital signs postoperatively, especially temperature; and inspect surgical site for evidence of infection at least every 2 to 4 hours, noting any redness, drainage, warmth, edema, or localized pain at the site.

■ Arrange for possible social service consultation depending on the cause of the injury; for example, for patients whose chest trauma resulted from an alcohol-related automobile accident or gang-related gunshot injury.

Patient teaching

■ Provide brief explanations about the patient's condition and why it's occurring. Inform the patient and his family about how the condition will be treated, making sure to explain new procedures before beginning.

■ Review signs and symptoms of a worsening condition, such as increasing respiratory distress, increasing jugular venous distention, or decreasing level of consciousness. Stress the importance of reporting any such signs immediately.

■ Remind the patient about the need for follow-up care.

Endotracheal intubation

Endotracheal (ET) intubation involves the insertion — orally or nasally — of a flexible tube through the larynx into the trachea for the purpose of obtaining or maintaining a patent airway. It also provides a means for mechanically ventilating the patient. ET intubation is considered the gold standard of invasive airway control in unconscious patients.

Performed by a physician, anesthetist, respiratory therapist, or specially trained nurse, ET intubation is usually performed during emergency situations such as cardiopulmonary arrest, or with disorders that can lead to airway obstruction — for example, epiglottiditis. In addition, ET intubation may also be performed under more controlled circumstances such as just before surgery. In such instances, ET intubation requires patient teaching and preparation.

ET intubation is indicated in:
■ cardiopulmonary arrest
■ respiratory distress
■ persistent apnea
■ accidental extubation of a patient unable to maintain adequate spontaneous ventilation
■ obstructive angioedema
■ upper airway hemorrhage
■ risk of increased intracranial pressure
■ laryngeal and upper airway edema
■ absent swallowing or gag reflexes
■ conditions in which noninvasive ventilatory efforts are unsuccessful.

ET intubation aids in establishing and maintaining a patent airway. It also protects against aspiration by sealing off the trachea from the digestive tract, and permits removal of tracheobronchial secretions in patients who can't cough effectively. Moreover, ET intubation provides a route for mechanical ventilation. Unfortunately, ET intubation bypasses normal respiratory defenses against infection, reduces cough effectiveness, and prevents communication.

In emergencies, oral ET intubation (also called orotracheal intubation) is preferred over nasotracheal intubation because insertion is easier and faster. However, maintaining exact tube placement is more difficult in orotracheal intubation because the tube must be well-secured to avoid kinking and prevent bronchial obstruction or accidental extubation. Orotracheal intubation is poorly tolerated by conscious patients because it stimulates salivation, coughing, and retching. Oral ET intubation is contraindicated

Alternative forms of airway maintenance

Retrograde intubation
When a patient's airway can't be secured using conventional oral or nasal intubation, consider using retrograde intubation. In this technique, a wire is inserted through the trachea and out the mouth and is then used to guide the insertion of an endotracheal (ET) tube (as shown here).

Only physicians, nurses, and paramedics who have been specially trained may perform retrograde intubation. However, the procedure has numerous advantages: It requires little or no head movement, doesn't require direct visualization of the vocal cords, and is less invasive than cricothyrotomy or tracheotomy (and doesn't leave a permanent scar). Retrograde

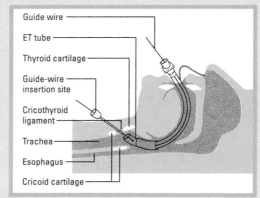

Guide wire
ET tube
Thyroid cartilage
Guide-wire insertion site
Cricothyroid ligament
Trachea
Esophagus
Cricoid cartilage

intubation is contraindicated in patients with complete airway obstruction, a thyroid tumor, an enlarged thyroid gland that overlies the cricothyroid ligament, or coagulopathy and in those whose mouths can't open wide enough to allow

the guide wire to be retrieved. Possible complications include minor bleeding and hematoma formation at the puncture site, subcutaneous emphysema, hoarseness, and bleeding into the trachea.

in patients with acute cervical spinal injury and degenerative spinal disorders, whereas nasal intubation is contraindicated in patients with apnea, bleeding disorders, chronic sinusitis, or nasal obstructions.

Nasotracheal intubation is preferred for elective insertion when the patient is capable of spontaneous ventilation for a short period. Blind intubation is typically used in conscious patients who are at risk for imminent respiratory arrest or who have cervical spinal injury. Although nasotracheal intubation is more comfortable than oral intubation, it's also more difficult to perform. Because the tube passes blindly through the nasal cavity, the

procedure causes greater tissue trauma, increases the risk of infection by nasal bacteria introduced into the trachea, and increases the risk for pressure necrosis of the nasal mucosa. However, exact tube placement is easier, and the risk of dislodgment is lower.

When neither method of ET intubation is possible, alternatives include retrograde intubation and esophageal-tracheal combitube. (See *Alternative forms of airway maintenance*.)

Equipment
Two ET tubes (one spare) of appropriate size and type ▪ 10-ml syringe ▪ stethoscope ▪ gloves ▪ lighted laryngo-

Esophageal-tracheal combitube

The esophageal-tracheal combitube (ETC), or esophageal-tracheal double-lumen airway, is a plastic tube with two patent lumens and an occlusion balloon at the distal end. One lumen acts as an ET tube and the other acts as an esophageal tube, venting the stomach and facilitating gastric decompression.

The tube may be inserted by those not trained in ET intubation and may be inserted blindly. It's typically used in cases in which ET intubation attempts have failed, or in cardiac arrest situations. If utilized properly, insertion in either the esophagus or trachea provides satisfactory oxygenation. In addition, if a spontaneously breathing patient has a tracheal placement, he can still breathe through multiple small holes in the unused lumen. The tube also allows gastric contents to be suctioned immediately upon insertion. ETC is used as a temporary measure because it doesn't control an airway or provide ventilation as well as ET intubation.

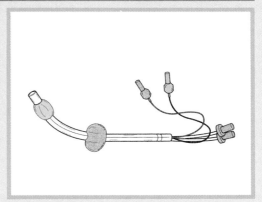

scope with a handle and blades of various sizes (curved and straight) ■ sedative ■ local anesthetic spray ■ mucosal vasoconstricting agent (optional, for nasal intubation) ■ water-soluble lubricant ■ adhesive or other strong tape or Velcro tube holder ■ transparent adhesive dressing (if necessary) ■ oral airway or bite block (for oral intubation) ■ suction equipment ■ handheld resuscitation bag with swivel adapter ■ humidified oxygen source ■ optional: prepackaged intubation tray, sterile gauze pad, stylet, Magill forceps, sterile water, and sterile basin

AGE ISSUE *Select an ET tube of the appropriate size — typically, 2.5 to 5.5 mm, uncuffed, for children and 6 to 10 mm, cuffed, for adults. The typical size of an oral tube is 7.5 mm for women and 8 mm for men. Select a slightly smaller tube for nasal intubation.*

Essential steps

■ Check the light in the laryngoscope by snapping the appropriately sized blade into place; if the bulb doesn't light, replace the batteries or the laryngoscope (whichever will be quicker).

■ Using sterile technique, open the package containing the ET tube and, if desired, open the other supplies on an overbed table. Pour the sterile water into the basin. To ease insertion, lubricate the first 1″ (2.5 cm) of the distal

Laryngoscope techniques

You may need to vary your laryngoscope technique during intubation depending on the type of blade used.

Curved blade
If you use a curved blade, apply upward traction with the tip of the blade in the vallecula. This displaces the epiglottis anteriorly.

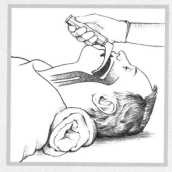

Straight blade
If you use a straight blade, elevate the epiglottis anteriorly, exposing the opening of the glottis.

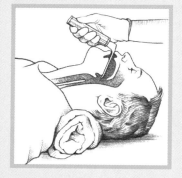

cant because it can be absorbed by mucous membranes.

■ Attach the syringe to the port on the tube's exterior pilot cuff and slowly inflate the cuff, observing for uniform inflation. If desired, submerge the tube in the sterile water and watch for air bubbles. Use the syringe to deflate the cuff.

■ Keep in mind that a stylet may be used for oral intubations to stiffen the tube. Lubricate the entire stylet. Insert the stylet into the tube so that its distal tip lies about ½" (1 cm) inside the distal end of the tube. Make sure that the stylet doesn't protrude from the tube to avoid vocal cord trauma.

■ Prepare the humidified oxygen source and the suction equipment for immediate use. If the patient is in bed, remove the headboard to provide easier access.

■ Administer medication as ordered to decrease respiratory secretions, induce amnesia or analgesia, and help calm and relax the conscious patient. Remove dentures and bridgework, if present.

■ Administer oxygen until the tube is inserted to prevent hypoxia.

■ Place the patient supine with the head and neck in the sniffing position to align the airway and visualize the larynx. For a blind intubation, place the patient's head and neck in a neutral position.

■ Put on gloves.

■ For oral intubation, spray a local anesthetic such as lidocaine deep into the posterior pharynx to diminish the gag reflex and reduce patient discomfort. For nasal intubation, spray a local anesthetic and a mucosal vasoconstrictor into the nasal passages to anes-

end of the ET tube with the water-soluble lubricant, using aseptic technique. Use only water-soluble lubri-

thetize the nasal turbinates and reduce the chance of bleeding.

■ Hyperventilate using a bag-valve mask and 100% oxygen. If necessary, suction the patient's pharynx just before tube insertion to improve visualization of the patient's pharynx and vocal cords.

ALERT *Time each intubation attempt, limiting attempts to less than 30 seconds to prevent hypoxemia.*

■ To intubate using direct visualization:

— Stand at the head of the patient's bed.

— Using your dominant hand, hold the patient's mouth open by crossing your index finger over your thumb, placing your thumb on the patient's upper teeth and your index finger on his lower teeth. This technique provides greater leverage.

— Grasp the laryngoscope handle in your nondominant hand and gently slide the lubricated blade into the right side of the patient's mouth. Center the blade, and push the patient's tongue to the left. Hold the patient's lower lip away from his teeth to prevent the lip from being traumatized. Advance the blade to expose the epiglottis. When using a straight blade, insert the tip under the epiglottis; when using a curved blade, insert the tip between the base of the tongue and the epiglottis. (See *Laryngoscope techniques.*)

— Lift the laryngoscope handle upward and away from your body at a 45-degree angle to reveal the vocal cords. Avoid pivoting the laryngoscope against the patient's teeth to avoid damaging them.

— If desired, have an assistant apply pressure to the cricoid ring to occlude the esophagus and minimize gastric regurgitation.

— When performing an oral intubation, insert the ET tube into the right side of the patient's mouth. When performing a nasotracheal intubation, insert the ET tube through the nostril and into the pharynx; use Magill forceps to guide the tube through the vocal cords.

— Guide the tube into the vertical openings of the larynx between the vocal cords, being careful not to mistake the horizontal opening of the esophagus for the larynx. If the vocal cords are closed because of a spasm, wait a few seconds for them to relax, and then gently guide the tube past them to avoid traumatic injury.

— Advance the tube until the cuff disappears beyond the vocal cords. Avoid advancing the tube further to avoid occluding a major bronchus and precipitating lung collapse.

— Holding the ET tube in place, quickly remove the stylet, if present.

■ To intubate blindly:

— Pass the ET tube along the floor of the nasal cavity. If necessary, use gentle force to pass the tube through the nasopharynx and into the pharynx.

— Listen and feel for air movement through the tube as it's advanced, to ensure that the tube is properly placed in the airway.

— Slip the tube between the vocal cords when the patient inhales because the vocal cords separate on inhalation. When the tube is past the vocal cords, the breath sounds should become louder.

ALERT *If, at any time during tube advancement, breath sounds disappear, withdraw the tube until they reappear.*

■ After the patient has been intubated, inflate the tube's cuff with 5 cc to 10 cc of air — until you feel resistance. When the patient is mechanically ventilated, you'll use the minimal leak technique or the minimal occlusive volume technique to establish correct inflation of the cuff. (See "Tracheal cuff-pressure measurement," page 251.)

■ Remove the laryngoscope. If the patient was intubated orally, insert an oral airway or bite block to prevent the patient from obstructing airflow or puncturing the tube with his teeth.

■ Observe for chest expansion and auscultate for bilateral breath sounds to ensure proper placement. If the patient is unconscious or uncooperative, use a handheld resuscitation bag while observing for upper chest movement and auscultating for breath sounds. Feel the tube's tip for warm exhalations and listen for air movement. Observe for condensation forming inside the tube. If you don't hear any breath sounds, auscultate over the stomach while ventilating with the resuscitation bag.

ALERT *Stomach distention, belching, or a gurgling sound indicates esophageal intubation. Immediately deflate the cuff and remove the tube. After reoxygenating the patient, to prevent hypoxemia, repeat insertion using a sterile tube to prevent contamination of the trachea.*

■ Auscultate bilaterally to exclude the possibility of endobronchial intubation.

ALERT *If you fail to hear breath sounds on both sides of the chest, you may have inserted the tube into one of the mainstem bronchi (usually the right one because of its wider angle at the bifurcation). Such insertion occludes the other bronchus and lungs and results in atelectasis on the obstructed side. Or, the tube may be resting on the carina, resulting in dry secretions that obstruct both bronchi. (The patient's coughing and fighting the ventilator will alert you to the problem.) To correct these situations, deflate the cuff, withdraw the tube 1 to 2 mm, auscultate for bilateral breath sounds, and reinflate the cuff.*

■ When tube placement is confirmed, administer oxygen or initiate mechanical ventilation, and suction as ordered.

■ Secure tube position, making sure that the patient's face is cleared of saliva or other secretions. (See *Securing an ET tube.*)

■ Clearly note the centimeter marking on the tube where it exits the patient's mouth or nose. Periodically monitor this mark to detect tube displacement.

■ Make sure that a chest X-ray is taken to verify tube position.

Complications

Potential complications of ET intubation include:

■ apnea caused by reflex breath-holding or interruption of oxygen delivery

■ bronchospasm

■ aspiration of blood, secretions, or gastric contents

■ tooth damage or loss; and injury to the lips, mouth, pharynx, or vocal cords

■ laryngeal edema and erosion

■ tracheal stenosis, erosion, and necrosis.

Potential complications of nasotracheal intubation include nasal bleeding, laceration, sinusitis, and otitis media.

Nursing considerations

■ Place a swivel adapter between the tube and the humidified oxygen source to allow for intermittent suctioning and to reduce tube tension.
■ Place the patient on his side with his head in a comfortable position to avoid tube kinking and airway obstruction.
■ Auscultate both sides of the chest, and watch chest movement as indicated by the patient's condition to ensure correct tube placement and full lung ventilation. After securing the ET tube, reconfirm tube placement every 5 to 10 minutes by noting bilateral breath sounds and continuing end-carbon dioxide readings.
■ Provide frequent oral care to the orally intubated patient and frequent nasal and oral care to the nasally intubated patient to prevent formation of pressure ulcers and drying of oral mucous membranes.
■ Position the ET tube to prevent the formation of pressure ulcers and avoid excessive pressure on the sides of the mouth.
■ Suction secretions through the ET tube as the patient's condition indicates to clear secretions and prevent mucus plugs from obstructing the tube.
■ Keep in mind that although low-pressure cuffs have significantly reduced the incidence of tracheal erosion and necrosis caused by cuff pressure on the tracheal wall, overinflation of a low-pressure cuff can negate the benefit. Use the minimal-leak tech-

Securing an ET tube

When securing an endotracheal (ET) tube, use either tape or ties and be sure that the tube is immobile.
 If you're using tape:
● Tear about 2′ (60 cm) of tape, split both ends in half about 4″ (10 cm), and place the tape adhesive-side up on a flat surface.
● Tear another piece of tape about 10″ (25 cm) long and place it adhesive-side down in the center of the 2′ piece.
● Slide the tape under the patient's neck and center it.
● Bring the right side of the tape up and wrap the top split end counterclockwise around the tube; secure the bottom split end beneath the patient's lower lip.
● Bring the left side of the tape up and wrap the bottom split piece clockwise around the tube; secure the top split about the patient's upper lip.
 If you're using ties:
● Cut about 2′ (60 cm) and place it under the patient's neck.
● Bring both ends up to the tube and cross them at the bottom of the tube near the patient's lips.
● Bring the ends to the top of the tube and tie them in an overhand knot.
● Bring the ends back to the bottom of the tube, tie another overhand knot, and then secure the ties with a square knot (right over left, left over right).

nique to avoid complications of tracheal erosion and necrosis from cuff pressure on the tracheal wall.
ALERT *Always record the volume of air needed to inflate the cuff.*
■ For the minimal-leak technique:
– Attach a 10-ml syringe to the port on the tube's exterior pilot cuff, and place a stethoscope on the side of the patient's neck.

– Inject small amounts of air with each breath until you hear no leak. Then aspirate 0.1 cc of air from the cuff to create a minimal air leak.

■ If the minimal leak technique isn't appropriate, inflate the cuff a bit more to make a complete seal with the least amount of air (considered the next most desirable method), called the minimal occlusive volume technique. For this technique:

– Follow the first two steps of the minimal-leak technique, but place the stethoscope over the trachea instead.

– Aspirate until you hear a small leak on inspiration, and add just enough air to stop the leak.

– Record the amount of air needed to inflate the cuff for subsequent monitoring of tracheal dilation or erosion.

■ When the cuff has been inflated, measure its pressure at least every 8 hours to avoid overinflation. Normal cuff pressure is about 18 mm Hg.

ALERT *A gradual increase in volume of cuff pressure indicates tracheal dilation or erosion. A sudden increase in volume indicates rupture of the cuff and requires immediate reintubation if the patient is being ventilated or if he requires continuous cuff inflation to maintain a high concentration of delivered oxygen.*

■ Record the date and time of the procedure, reason for insertion, and success or failure; also document tube type and size, cuff size, amount of inflation, and inflation technique, auscultation of breath sounds, chest X-ray results, and patient's tolerance of procedure.

■ Document the administration of medication and initiation of supplemental oxygen or ventilation therapy; also record any complications and necessary interventions.

■ Measure cuff pressure and record, including any abnormalities reported to the physician.

End-tidal carbon dioxide monitoring

Monitoring of end-tidal carbon dioxide ($ETCO_2$) determines the carbon dioxide (CO_2) concentration in exhaled gas. In this technique, a photodetector measures the amount of infrared light absorbed by airway gas during inspiration and expiration. (Light absorption increases along with the CO_2 concentration.) A monitor converts these data to a CO_2 value and a corresponding waveform, or capnogram, if capnography is used. (See *How $ETCO_2$ monitoring works.*)

$ETCO_2$ monitoring provides information about the patient's pulmonary, cardiac, and metabolic status that aids patient management and helps prevent clinical compromise. This technique has become standard during anesthesia administration and mechanical ventilation.

The sensor, which contains an infrared light source and a photodetector, is positioned at one of two sites in the monitoring setup. With a mainstream monitor, it's positioned directly at the patient's airway with an airway adapter, between the endotracheal

How ETco$_2$ monitoring works

The optical portion of an end-tidal carbon dioxide (ETco$_2$) monitor contains an infrared light source, a sample chamber, a special carbon dioxide (CO$_2$) filter, and a photodetector. The infrared light passes through the sample chamber and is absorbed in varying amounts, depending on the amount of CO$_2$ the patient has just exhaled. The photodetector measures CO$_2$ content and relays this information to the microprocessor in the monitor, which displays the CO$_2$ value and waveform.

The CO$_2$ waveform, or capnogram, produced in ETco$_2$ monitoring reflects the course of CO$_2$ elimination during exhalation. A normal capnogram (as shown below) consists of several segments, which reflect the various stages of exhalation and inhalation.

Normally, any gas eliminated from the airway during early exhalation is dead-space gas that hasn't undergone exchange at the alveolocapillary membrane. Measurements taken during this period contain no CO$_2$. As exhalation continues, CO$_2$ concentration rises sharply and rapidly. The sensor now detects gas that has undergone exchange producing measurable quantities of CO$_2$.

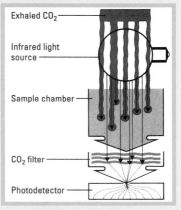

The final stages of alveolar emptying occur during late exhalation. During the alveolar plateau phase, CO$_2$ concentration rises more gradually because alveolar emptying is more constant.

The point at which ETco$_2$ value is derived is the end of exhalation, when CO$_2$ concentration peaks. Unless an alveolar plateau is present, this value doesn't accurately estimate alveolar CO$_2$. During inhalation, the CO$_2$ concentration declines sharply to zero.

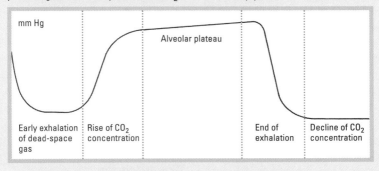

(ET) tube and the breathing circuit tubing. With a sidestream monitor, the airway adapter is positioned at the airway (regardless of whether the patient is intubated) to allow aspiration of gas from the patient's airway back to the sensor, which lies either within or close to the monitor.

Some CO_2 detection devices provide semiquantitative indications of CO_2 concentrations, supplying an approximate range rather than a specific value for $ETCO_2$. Other devices simply indicate whether CO_2 is present during exhalation (See *Analyzing CO_2 levels.*)

$ETCO_2$ monitoring may be used to help wean a patient with a stable acid-base balance from mechanical ventilation. It also reduces the need for frequent arterial blood gas (ABG) measurements, especially when combined with pulse oximetry. Other uses for $ETCO_2$ monitoring include assessing resuscitation efforts and identifying the return of spontaneous circulation. Because no CO_2 is exhaled when breathing stops, this technique also detects apnea.

When used during ET intubation, $ETCO_2$ monitoring can avert neurologic injury and even death by confirming correct ET tube placement and detecting accidental esophageal intubation because CO_2 isn't normally produced by the stomach. Ongoing $ETCO_2$ monitoring throughout intubation can also prove valuable because an ET tube may become dislodged during manipulation or patient movement or transport.

Equipment

Gloves ▪ mainstream or sidestream CO_2 monitor ▪ CO_2 sensor ▪ airway adapter as recommended by the manufacturer (a neonatal adapter may have a much smaller dead space, making it appropriate for a smaller patient)

Essential steps

▪ If the monitor you're using isn't self-calibrating, calibrate it as the manufacturer directs. (If you're using a sidestream CO_2 monitor, replace the water trap between patients, if directed.) The trap allows humidity from exhaled gases to be condensed into an attached container. Newer sidestream models don't require water traps.

▪ If the patient requires ET intubation, apply an $ETCO_2$ detector or monitor immediately after the tube is inserted. If he doesn't require intubation or is already intubated and alert, explain the purpose and expected duration of monitoring. Tell an intubated patient that the monitor will painlessly measure the amount of CO_2 he exhales. Inform a nonintubated patient that the monitor will track his CO_2 concentration to make sure his breathing is effective.

▪ Wash your hands. After turning on the monitor and calibrating it (if necessary), position the airway adapter and sensor as the manufacturer directs. For an intubated patient, position the adapter directly on the ET tube. For a nonintubated patient, place the adapter at or near the patient's airway. (An oxygen-delivery cannula may have a sample port through which gas can be aspirated for monitoring.)

▪ Turn on all alarms and adjust alarm settings as appropriate for your patient. Make sure the alarm volume is loud enough to hear.

Complications

Inaccurate measurements — from poor sampling technique, calibration drift, contamination of optics with moisture or secretions, or equipment malfunction — can lead to misdiagnosis and improper treatment. Other potential complications include:

■ altered findings from the effects of manual resuscitation or ingestion of alcohol or carbonated beverages

■ misleading color changes detected after fewer than six ventilations.

Nursing considerations

■ Wear gloves when handling the airway adapter to prevent cross-contamination. Make sure the adapter is changed with every breathing circuit and ET tube change.

■ Place the adapter on the ET tube to avoid contaminating exhaled gases with fresh gas flow from the ventilator. If you're using a heat and moisture exchanger, position the airway adapter between the exchanger and breathing circuit, if possible.

■ If your patient's $ETCO_2$ values differ from his partial pressure of arterial carbon dioxide ($PaCO_2$), assess him for factors that can influence $ETCO_2$ — especially when the differential between $PaCO_2$ and $ETCO_2$ values (the arterial absolute difference of carbon dioxide [$a\text{-}ADCO_2$]) is above normal. The $a\text{-}ADCO_2$ value, if correctly interpreted, provides useful information about your patient's status. For example, an increased $a\text{-}ADCO_2$ may mean that your patient has worsening dead space, especially if his tidal volume remains constant.

■ Remember that $ETCO_2$ monitoring doesn't replace ABG measurements because it doesn't assess oxygenation or blood pH. Supplementing $ETCO_2$ monitoring with pulse oximetry may provide more complete information. (See "Pulse oximetry," page 238.)

Analyzing CO₂ levels

Depending on which end-tidal carbon dioxide ($ETCO_2$) detector you use, the meaning of color changes within the detector dome may differ from the analysis for the Easy Cap detector described here.

● The rim of the Easy Cap is divided into four segments (clockwise from the top): CHECK, A, B, and C. The CHECK segment is solid purple, signifying the absence of CO_2.

● The numbers in the other sections range from 0.03 to 5, indicating the percentage of exhaled CO_2. The color should fluctuate during ventilation from purple (section A) during inspiration to yellow (section C) at the end of expiration. This indicates that the $ETCO_2$ levels are adequate (above 2%).

● An end-expiratory color change from C to the B range may be the first sign of hemodynamic instability.

● During cardiopulmonary resuscitation (CPR), an end-expiratory color change from the A or B range to the C range may mean the return of spontaneous ventilation.

● During prolonged cardiac arrest, inadequate pulmonary perfusion leads to inadequate gas exchange. The patient exhales little or no CO_2, so the color stays in the purple range even with proper intubation. Ineffective CPR also leads to inadequate pulmonary perfusion.

COLOR INDICATIONS ON DETECTOR DOME

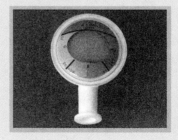

Disposable ETco$_2$ detector guidelines

When using a disposable end-tidal carbon dioxide (ETco$_2$) detector, check the instructions and ensure ideal working conditions for the device. In addition, follow the guidelines detailed here.

Humidity, moisture, and heat

• Watch for changes indicating that the ETco$_2$ detector's precision is decreasing — for example, sluggish color changes from breath to breath. A detector normally may be used for approximately 2 hours. However, using it with a ventilator that delivers high-humidity ventilation may shorten its lifespan to no more than 15 minutes.

• Don't use the detector with a heated humidifier or nebulizer.

• Keep the detector protected from secretions, which would render the device useless. If secretions enter the dome, remove and discard the detector.

• Use a heat and moisture exchanger to protect the detector. In some detectors, this filter fits between the endotracheal (ET) tube and the detector.

• If using a heat and moisture exchanger, remember that it will increase your patient's breathing effort. Be alert for increased resistance and breathing difficulties and remove the exchanger, if necessary.

Additional precautions

• Instilling epinephrine through the ET tube can damage the detector's indicator (color may stay yellow). If this happens, discard the device.

• Never reuse a disposable ETco$_2$ detector; it's intended for one-time, one-patient use only.

baseline, and shape to help evaluate gas exchange. Make sure you know how to recognize a normal waveform and can identify any abnormal waveforms and their possible causes. Describe the waveform's appearance (normal and abnormal waveforms) in the patient's medical record. If a printer is available, obtain a printout of the waveform for placement on the patient's medical record.

■ In a nonintubated patient, use ETco$_2$ values to establish trends. Be aware that in a nonintubated patient, exhaled gas is more likely to mix with ambient air, and exhaled CO_2 may be diluted by fresh gas flow from the nasal cannula.

■ Expect to discontinue ETco$_2$ monitoring when the patient has been weaned effectively from mechanical ventilation or when he's no longer at risk for respiratory compromise. Carefully assess your patient's tolerance for weaning. (See "Weaning from mechanical ventilation," page 267.) After extubation, continuous ETco$_2$ monitoring may detect the need for reintubation.

■ If you're using a disposable ETco$_2$ detector, always check its color under fluorescent or natural light because the dome looks pink under incandescent light. (See *Disposable ETco$_2$ detector guidelines*.)

AGE ISSUE *Take care when using an ETco$_2$ detector on a child who weighs less than 30 lb (13.6 kg). A small patient who rebreathes air from the dead space (about 38 cc) will inhale too much of his own CO_2.*

■ Document the initial ETco$_2$ value and all ventilator settings.

■ Obtain and record ETco$_2$ values at least as often as vital signs, whenever

■ If the CO_2 waveform is available, assess it for height, frequency, rhythm,

significant changes in waveform or patient status occur, and before and after weaning, respiratory, and other interventions. Periodically obtain samples for ABG analysis as the patient's condition dictates, and document the corresponding $ETCO_2$ values.

Extracorporeal membrane oxygenation

Extracorporeal membrane oxygenation (ECMO), one of a group of supportive therapies called extracorporeal life support, involves the oxygenation of blood outside the body. It exposes a patient's lungs to low pressures, allowing them to rest as well as providing a means for oxygen delivery and carbon dioxide removal. When ECMO is used, lower fraction of inspired oxygen (FIO_2) concentrations and volumes can be delivered via mechanical ventilation, thereby reducing the risk for oxygen toxicity and barotrauma; however, it doesn't cure the underlying disease. Historically, ECMO was used to treat neonates who experienced severe respiratory distress from meconium aspiration, persistent pulmonary hypertension, respiratory distress syndrome, congenital diaphragmatic hernia, and pneumonia. Today, ECMO is used to treat severe acute respiratory failure in patients of all ages.

AGE ISSUE *In neonates, ECMO is considered the standard treatment for severe respiratory distress. However, in adults, ECMO is used only after other modes of ventilation, such as low tidal volume ventilation, high-level positive end expiratory pressure (PEEP), and pharmacologic therapy, such as neuromuscular blocking agents, sedatives, and opiates to facilitate mechanical ventilation and minimize oxygen consumption, have been used without success.*

The primary indication for using ECMO is severe respiratory failure. It also may be indicated in other situations such as:

- adult respiratory distress syndrome (ARDS)
- perioperative cardiac failure
- primary myocardial failure
- bridge to transplantation.

There are two basic types of ECMO: veno-arterial ECMO (VA-ECMO) and veno-venous ECMO (VV-ECMO). VA-ECMO, the type commonly used for neonates, involves the insertion of a catheter into the internal jugular or femoral veins for blood removal. Blood is returned to the patient's arterial circulation via the carotid or femoral arteries. This type of ECMO provides partial to complete cardiopulmonary bypass and is used most commonly when the patient has severe cardiac failure in addition to pulmonary failure. VA-ECMO generally allows a higher PO_2 than VV-ECMO. Unfortunately, this type of ECMO increases the risk of air or blood being directly introduced into the arterial circulation, increasing the risk of emboli. In addition, neurological complications can occur with ligation of the carotid artery when therapy is discontinued and the arterial catheter is removed.

VV-ECMO involves the insertion of a catheter that removes and returns blood to the right atrium via the right internal jugular or femoral veins. Often a double lumen catheter is used. This type of ECMO is used for patients requiring only respiratory support, such as those with ARDS. It doesn't provide the cardiac support to assist systemic circulation. Pulmonary blood flow is maintained and the lungs are perfused with oxygenated blood.

The amount of ECMO support is decreased gradually as the patient's condition improves. He's removed from ECMO when lung function is adequate with low ventilatory support.

The mortality rate for adults undergoing ECMO averages around 50%. For neonates, approximately 50% of the deaths associated with ECMO are due to bleeding complications.

Procedure

At the patient's bedside in the critical care unit or in the operating room, the physician uses strict aseptic technique to insert a cannula (catheter; adult size ranging from 16F to 23F; neonate size commonly 14F) percutaneously into the appropriate vessel. The patient receives a loading dose of heparin I.V. to reduce the risk of clotting both in the ECMO circuit and the patient. The catheter is then connected to the ECMO circuit and therapy is initiated. A continuous heparin infusion is maintained throughout therapy.

As blood leaves the patient's body, it's pumped through a membrane oxygenator, which acts as an artificial lung, supplying oxygen to the blood. (See *ECMO setup*.) The circuit has numerous safety and pressure monitors located throughout. A roller pump regulates the blood flow to the oxygenator, turning off whenever the pump

flow is greater than blood return to the patient. In this way, excessive pressure on the right atrium or major vessels is averted. The pump automatically restarts when the flow rate balances.

AGE ISSUE *Typical blood flow rates for adults range from 70 to 90 ml/kg/minute; for children, 80 to 100 ml/kg/minute; for neonates, 120 to 170 ml/kg/minute.*

An in-line fiberoptic catheter is also used to monitor venous oxygen levels continuously. Before returning to the patient, the blood passes through a heat exchanger where it's warmed to prevent hypothermia. When ECMO is used, an ECMO specialist remains at the patient's bedside. The ECMO specialist can be an experienced critical care nurse or respiratory therapist who has received specialized training and education.

Complications

ECMO is associated with numerous complications, both mechanical or patient-related. (See *Complications of ECMO,* page 208.)

Nursing considerations

When caring for the patient receiving ECMO, nursing care focuses on preparing the patient and his family both physically and emotionally for the procedure, including instructing them about the procedure and events that follow as well as instituting measures to prevent complications.

Before ECMO

■ Instruct the patient and his family about the procedure and the rationale for treatment.
■ Reinforce the physician's explanation of the procedure, equipment, and

ECMO setup

Extracorporeal membrane oxygenation (ECMO) is managed by either a critical care nurse or respiratory therapist with special training in its operation. Illustrated and described here is a typical ECMO setup:

- *arterial filter*—removes air bubbles and clots from the blood as it travels through the ECMO circuit
- *cannula*—catheter through which blood travels to and from the patient
- *control desk module*—continuously monitors pressure throughout the circuit and regulates blood flow rate as needed in response to changing pressures in the system

- *heater*—generates heat needed to keep blood at a constant temperature
- *heat exchanger*—uses heat generated by a heater to maintain the temperature of the blood as it's oxygenated
- *hemochron*—monitors blood clotting
- *I.V. pump*—allows injection of medications such as antibiotics into the cannula of the ECMO circuit
- *membrane oxygenator*—serves as the artificial lung supplying oxygen to the blood
- *transonic blood flowmeter*—measures the amount of blood flowing through the cannula at various places along the ECMO circuit.

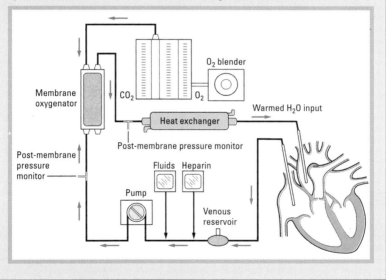

follow-up care. If one hasn't been inserted already, inform the patient that he will have an endotracheal (ET) tube in place and will be connected to a mechanical ventilator. Review other equipment, such as continuous cardiac monitoring, a nasogastric tube, an indwelling urinary catheter and, possibly, a pulmonary artery catheter.

■ Ensure that the patient or a responsible family member has signed a consent form.

■ Instruct family members in measures used to prevent complications.

Complications of ECMO

Extracorporeal membrane oxygenation (ECMO) is associated with numerous complications.

Mechanical complications
- Clots in the circuit (most common mechanical complication) leading to oxygenator failure, consumption coagulopathy, and pulmonary and systemic emboli
- Cannula placement leading to damage of internal jugular vein or dissection of the carotid arterial intima
- Air in the circuit
- Oxygenator failure
- Cracks in connectors and tube rupture
- Pump malfunction
- Heat exchanger malfunction
- Failure of entire circuit
- Failure of circuit monitoring equipment

Patient complications
- Seizures
- Intracranial bleeding
- Hemorrhage at catheter site, surgical site, or site of previous invasive procedures; intrathoracic, intra-abdominal, or retroperitoneal hemorrhage
- Thrombocytopenia
- Myocardial stun (decrease in left ventricular shortening fraction on initiation with return to normal after 48 hours of ECMO)
- Hypertension
- Pericardial tamponade
- Pneumothorax
- Pulmonary hemorrhage
- Oliguria
- Acute tubular necrosis
- Hemorrhage from stress, ischemia, or bleeding tendencies
- Hyperbilirubinemia
- Biliary calculi
- Infection; sepsis
- Metabolic acidosis or alkalosis
- Electrolyte imbalances (either high or low) involving potassium, sodium, and calcium
- Hyperglycemia or hypoglycemia

■ Provide emotional support to the patient and his family because this treatment is considered only after all other options have failed and it's associated with numerous complications.
■ Administer sedation as ordered to reduce pain and restrict movement during catheter insertion and treatment initiation.

After ECMO
■ Assess cardiopulmonary and hemodynamic status closely, including central venous pressure, pulmonary artery pressure, and cardiac output (CO), at least every 15 minutes immediately after the procedure and then hourly or more frequently as indicated by the patient's condition or your facility's policy.
■ If the patient becomes hemodynamically unstable, expect to administer dopamine (Intropin) to raise blood pressure and dobutamine (Dobutrex) to improve CO; titrate dosages to desired response.
■ Assess ET tube patency, position, and function, and mechanical ventilation. Monitor oxygen saturation levels and arterial blood gases as ordered. Administer supplemental oxygen as necessary. Suction as necessary. (See "Mechanical ventilation," page 213, "Endotracheal intubation," page 193, and "Tracheal suction," page 253.)

ALERT *After ECMO is initiated and the patient's gas exchange shows signs of improvement, expect to lower ventilator settings. Typically, settings are adjusted to provide FIO_2 less than 50%, peak inspiratory pressure less than 35 cm H_2O, PEEP less than 10 cm H_2O, and a respiratory rate of 4 to 10 breaths per minute at a tidal volume based on the patient's weight. Be alert to changes in tidal volumes, which should increase as the lungs improve.*

■ Perform chest physiotherapy and change the patient's position frequently. Ensure that the catheters don't become kinked or dislodged. Anticipate placing the patient with ARDS in the prone position, which helps to improve oxygenation. Support the extremities and head in proper body alignment. Ensure that the ECMO circuit is unimpaired.

■ Administer sedatives and analgesia as ordered to ease patient's tolerance of the procedure, enhance comfort, maximize oxygen delivery, and decrease risk of catheter dislodgement. If necessary, apply soft restraints as ordered to reduce the risk of the patient manipulating the catheter.

■ Monitor intake and output at least hourly and notify the physician if output is less than 30 ml/hour. Assess daily weights. Monitor blood urea nitrogen levels and serum creatinine levels closely for renal dysfunction. Administer diuretics as ordered to maintain fluid balance.

■ Assess for signs and symptoms of acute renal failure; anticipate the need for hemofiltration, which can be added to the ECMO circuit.

■ Monitor activated clotting times (ACT) as indicated and assist with adjustments to heparin infusion.

ALERT *The lowest possible dose of heparin is used to maintain the ACT at 180 to 200 seconds. Monitor the patient's neurologic status (including pupil size and reactivity) closely to assess for bleeding into the brain or an embolic event.*

■ Expect to administer blood transfusions, including packed red blood cells to increase the oxygen carrying capacity of the blood and help stabilize the patient's intravascular volume. Obtain hemoglobin and hematocrit and platelet counts every four hours and as needed. Anticipate platelet transfusion if the patient's platelet count drops below 100,000/mm^3.

ALERT *The patient is at risk for bleeding secondary to the continuous heparin infusion. This risk is further compounded because the patient is at risk for thrombocytopenia as platelets are lost in the ECMO circuit.*

■ Inspect catheter insertion sites for oozing or hematoma at least every four hours. Observe ECMO catheter insertion sites hourly; change dressings as needed to keep site clean and dry. If necessary, weigh saturated dressings to determine fluid volume loss.

■ If a hematoma develops, palpate and mark the borders to monitor for any increase in size.

■ Assess affected extremity distal to the ECMO catheter insertion site for pulses, color, and temperature at least every 2 hours.

ALERT *A thready or absent pulse, a pale, cyanotic, or cool extremity, and a decrease in sensation indicate the extremity isn't receiving adequate blood flow; this is an emergency situation that must be reported to the physician immediately.*

■ Monitor the results of chest X-rays obtained daily. Expect to begin weaning the patient when chest X-ray, arterial blood gases, tidal volume, and oxygen saturation levels show sustained improvement.

■ Monitor the patient's temperature and results of white blood cell count. The patient is at risk for severe blood infections that could lead to vital organ damage.

■ Explain all procedures and treatments, even if patient is sedated. Offer emotional support to the patient's family; encourage them to visit and interact with the patient.

Lung transplantation

Lung transplantation involves the replacement of one or both of a patient's lungs with those from a donor. In some cases, only a lobe of a lung may be transplanted. Single lung transplantation is considered for patients with end-stage restrictive or obstructive pulmonary disease. Typically the patient has a life expectancy of less than 2 years. Double lung transplantation may be considered for patients with cystic fibrosis (CF) or septic pulmonary diseases. One-year survival rates range from 75% to 85%; survival rate decreases to 50% after 5 years.

AGE ISSUE *CF is the most common reason for lung transplantation in children, adolescents, and young adults. Other common diseases affecting this age group that may require lung transplantation include bronchopulmonary dysplasia, pulmo-*

nary hypertension, and pulmonary fibrosis.

A patient must meet certain criteria to be a candidate for lung transplantation. These criteria include:

■ forced vital capacity of less than 40%

■ amount of air exhaled in 1st second of expiration less than 30% of predicted value

■ partial pressure of arterial oxygen less than 60 mm Hg on room air at rest

■ evidence of major pulmonary complications

■ demonstration of increased antibiotic resistance.

Lung transplantation is absolutely contraindicated in the following situations:

■ major organ dysfunction, especially involving the renal or cardiovascular system

■ positive human immunodeficiency virus status

■ active malignancy

■ positive for antigen to hepatitis B

■ hepatitis C with biopsy positive for liver damage

■ active infection

■ progressive neuromuscular disease.

Other conditions, such as symptomatic osteoporosis, or the need for invasive ventilation are relative contraindications for lung transplantation.

Procedure

The patient is placed under general anesthesia. If a single lung is to be transplanted, the patient is intubated with double lumen endotracheal (ET) tube to allow the other lung to be ventilated during the surgery. The surgeon makes a lateral thoracotomy incision and removes the patient's lung via a posterolateral approach. The donor lung is implanted and anastomosed to the patient's bronchus, pulmonary artery, and cuff of the left atrium. Typically, cardiopulmonary bypass isn't used unless the patient can't be supported with ventilation of a single lung.

For a double lung transplantation, the surgeon makes bilateral anterior thoracotomy incisions along with a transverse sternotomy incision. Intubation is accomplished with a double lumen ET tube. After removal of the patient's lungs, the donor lungs are implanted with anastomoses at the same sites as for a single lung transplant. Cardiopulmonary bypass is commonly used during a double lung transplant.

Complications

The major complication following lung transplantation is rejection, in which the patient's body detects the transplanted organ as a foreign body (antigen), triggering an immune response. This leads to fibrosis and scar formation on the transplanted lung. Because of immunosuppression to deter rejection, the patient is also at high risk for infection, most commonly bacterial pneumonia, thrush, and cytomegalovirus infection. Other complications include hemorrhage and reperfusion edema. Long-term complications (those typically occurring after 3 years) may include obliterative bronchiolitis and posttransplant lymphoproliferative disorder, both of which may lead to death.

Nursing considerations

When caring for the patient undergoing lung transplantation, nursing care focuses on preparing the patient and his family both physically and emotionally for the procedure, including instructing the patient about the procedure and events after it as well as instituting measures to prevent postoperative complications. Be ready to act rapidly once a donor lung becomes available.

Before lung transplantation
■ Instruct the patient and his family about the transplant procedure and necessary diagnostic tests such as antigen typing.
■ Reinforce the surgeon's and anesthesiologist's explanation of the surgery, equipment, and procedures used in the critical care or post-anesthesia care units. If one hasn't been inserted already, inform the patient that he'll awaken from surgery with an ET tube in place and be connected to a mechanical ventilator. Review the rationale for and function of other equipment, such as continuous cardiac monitoring, a nasogastric tube, a chest tube, an indwelling urinary catheter, arterial lines and, possibly, a pulmonary artery catheter. Tell him that discomfort will be minimal and the equipment will be removed as soon as possible.
■ Administer immunosuppressant agents as ordered.
■ Review techniques of incentive spirometry, coughing and deep breathing, and range-of-motion (ROM) exercises with the patient and his family.
■ Ensure that the patient or a responsible family member has signed a consent form.
■ Instruct family members in measures used to control infection and minimize rejection after transplant.

■ Provide emotional support to the patient and his family because waiting for a donor lung may be frustrating.

After lung transplantation

■ Assess cardiopulmonary and hemodynamic status closely at least every 15 minutes in the immediate postoperative period and then hourly or more frequently as indicated by the patient's condition.

ALERT Be alert for a cardiac index less than 2.2, increased pulmonary artery wedge pressure or central venous pressure, decreased hematocrit, hypotension, temperature above 99.5° F (37.5° C), increased white blood cell count, crackles or rhonchi, decreased oxygen saturation, shortness of breath, dyspnea, malaise, and increased sputum production. These signs and symptoms suggest acute rejection, infection, or bleeding. Notify the physician or transplant coordinator immediately.

■ If the patient becomes hemodynamically unstable, expect to administer vasoactive and inotropic agents as ordered and titrate to them until the desired response is achieved.

■ Assess ET tube placement, patency, and function, and mechanical ventilation; administer supplemental oxygen as necessary. Monitor oxygen saturation and arterial blood gases (ABGs) as ordered.

ALERT Remember that for patients undergoing a single lung transplant, the patient's newly implanted lung is denervated, but the patient's original lung continues to send messages to the brain indicating poor oxygenation. Be alert that the patient may complain of shortness of breath and dyspnea even with oxygen saturation levels above 90%.

■ Suction as necessary. (See "Mechanical ventilation," page 213, "Endotracheal intubation," page 193, and "Tracheal suction," page 253.)

■ Monitor chest tubes attached to suction (usually for the first 24 hours or until drainage is less than 100 ml in 8 hours). While chest tubes are in place, expect to administer antibiotics as ordered to prevent infection. Assess drainage amount, color, and characteristics. Assess for bleeding. Notify the physician if chest tube drainage is greater than 200 ml in 1 hour, appears increasingly bloody, a sudden stop in drainage occurs, or an air leak develops or increases. (See "Chest drainage," page 181.)

ALERT Encourage the patient to cough and deep breathe, splinting incision for comfort. Keep in mind that patients who have had lung transplants have difficulty with airway clearance due to denervation, loss of the cough reflex below the tracheal suture line, and slowing of the mucociliary clearance.

■ Institute continuous cardiac monitoring, evaluating waveforms frequently for arrhythmias that may result from hypoxemia, electrolyte imbalance, or hemorrhage.

■ Administer analgesics as ordered for pain relief.

■ In the immediate postoperative period, monitor laboratory test results including complete blood count, hemoglobin, hematocrit, platelets, serum chemistry, serum electrolyte levels, blood urea nitrogen (BUN) and creatinine levels, ABGs, and 12-lead electrocardiogram. Anticipate the following tests daily: serum electrolytes, liver and renal function studies, coagulation studies, chest X-ray, urine and sputum cultures, BUN and creatinine, cultures such as for cytomegalovirus (CMV) and toxoplasmosis, and immunosuppressant drug level.

■ Institute strict infection control precautions; perform meticulous handwashing.

ALERT *The postoperative transplant patient is continuously trying to balance the risk for infection with the risk of rejection. CMV is a major cause of morbidity and mortality with transplant patients. Expect to administer ganciclovir prophylactically and as treatment for CMV.*

■ Assist with extubating as soon as possible and administer supplemental oxygen as needed, based on mixed venous oxygen saturation or pulse oximetry levels. Encourage coughing and deep breathing and use of incentive spirometer after extubation, splinting and premedicating for pain as necessary.

■ Monitor hemodynamic parameters frequently. Assess intake and output at least hourly and notify physician if output is less than 30 ml/hour. Maintain fluids at 2,000 to 3,000 ml/day or as ordered to prevent fluid overload.

■ Administer postoperative drugs, such as corticosteroids (methylprednisolone [Solu-Medrol], prednisone) and immunosuppressants. Check blood glucose levels as ordered because corticosteroids may cause a transient or sustained hyperglycemia even in patients who aren't diabetic.

■ Maintain nothing-by-mouth status with nasogastric decompression to low intermittent suction until bowel sounds return. Administer histamine blockers to suppress gastric acid secretion. Begin clear liquids after patient is extubated, gag reflex is present, and bowel sounds are active. Consult with dietitian for adequate nutritional intake.

■ Change position at least every 2 hours, getting patient out of bed to the chair within 24 hours if condition is stable. Gradually increase patient's activity as tolerated.

■ Prepare the patient for transbronchial biopsy to rule out rejection and infection. Explain the procedure to the patient and his family.

■ Monitor pulmonary function tests to determine lung function; obtain sputum cultures as ordered to evaluate for infection.

■ Inspect incision site, chest tube insertion site, and other entry sites for signs and symptoms of infection or hematoma.

■ To ease emotional stress, plan care to allow frequent rest periods and provide as much privacy as possible. Allow family members to visit and comfort the patient as much as possible.

■ Allow the family to express their anger, anxiety, and fear.

■ Explain the need for close follow-up and instruct in danger signs and symptoms. Teach the patient and his family about infection control measures and explain the medication therapy regimen.

Mechanical ventilation

Mechanical ventilation refers to the use of a machine that moves air in and out of a patient's lungs. Although the equipment serves to ventilate a patient, it doesn't ensure adequate gas exchange. Mechanical ventilators may use either positive or negative pressure to ventilate patients.

Positive-pressure ventilators exert a positive pressure on the airway, which causes inspiration while increasing tidal volume (V_T). The inspiratory cycles of these ventilators may vary in volume, pressure, or time. For example, a volume-cycled ventilator, the type used most commonly, delivers a preset volume of air each time, regardless of the amount of lung resistance. A pressure-cycled ventilator generates flow until the machine reaches a preset pressure regardless of the volume delivered or the time required to achieve the pressure. A time-cycled ventilator generates flow for a preset amount of time. A high-frequency ventilator uses high respiratory rates and low V_T to maintain alveolar ventilation.

Negative-pressure ventilators act by creating negative pressure, which pulls the thorax outward and allows air to flow into the lungs. Examples of such ventilators include the iron lung, the cuirass (chest shell), and the body wrap. Negative-pressure ventilators are used primarily to treat neuromuscular disorders, such as Guillain-Barré syndrome, myasthenia gravis, and poliomyelitis.

Other indications for ventilator use include central nervous system disorders, such as cerebral hemorrhage and spinal cord transsection; adult respiratory distress syndrome; pulmonary edema; chronic obstructive pulmonary disease; flail chest; and acute hypoventilation.

Equipment

Oxygen source ■ air source that can supply 50 psi ■ mechanical ventilator ■ humidifier ■ ventilator circuit tubing, connectors, and adapters ■ condensation collection trap ■ in-line thermometer ■ gloves ■ handheld resuscitation bag with reservoir ■ suction equipment ■ sterile distilled water ■ equipment for arterial blood gas (ABG) analysis ■ optional: oximeter and soft restraints

Essential steps

■ Keep in mind that in most facilities, respiratory therapists assume responsibility for setting up the ventilator. If necessary, check the manufacturer's instructions for setting it up. In most cases, you'll need to add sterile distilled water to the humidifier and connect the ventilator to the appropriate gas source.

■ Verify the physician's order for ventilator support. If the patient isn't already intubated, prepare him for intubation. (See "Endotracheal intubation," page 193.)

■ When possible, explain the procedure to the patient and his family to help reduce anxiety and fear. Assure the patient and his family that staff members are nearby to provide care.

■ Perform a complete physical assessment and draw blood for ABG analysis to establish a baseline.

■ Suction the patient, if necessary.

■ Plug the ventilator into the electrical outlet and turn it on. Adjust the settings on the ventilator as ordered. Make sure that the ventilator's alarms are set as ordered and that the humidifier is filled with sterile distilled water.

■ Put on gloves, if you haven't already done so. Connect the endotracheal tube to the ventilator. Observe for chest expansion, and auscultate for bilateral breath sounds to verify that the patient is being ventilated.

■ Monitor the patient's ABG values after the initial ventilator setup (usually 20 to 30 minutes), after any changes in ventilator settings, and as the patient's clinical condition indicates to determine whether the patient is being adequately ventilated and to avoid oxygen toxicity. Be prepared to adjust ventilator settings based on ABG analysis.

■ Check the ventilator tubing frequently for condensation, which can cause resistance to airflow and may also be aspirated by the patient. As needed, drain the condensate into a collection trap or briefly disconnect the patient from the ventilator (ventilating him with a handheld resuscitation bag, if necessary; see *Manual ventilation,* page 216), and empty the water into a receptacle.

■ **AGE ISSUE** *For infants and children, use a pediatric handheld resuscitation bag. For a child, deliver 15 breaths/minute, or one compression of the bag every 4 seconds; for an infant, 20 breaths/minute, or one compression every 3 seconds. Infants and children should receive 250 to 500 cc of air with each bag compression.*

■ **ALERT** *Don't drain the condensate into the humidifier because the condensate may be contaminated with the patient's secretions.*

■ Check the in-line thermometer to make sure that the temperature of the air delivered to the patient is close to body temperature.

■ When monitoring the patient's vital signs, count spontaneous breaths as well as ventilator-delivered breaths.

■ Change, clean, or dispose of the ventilator tubing and equipment according to your facility's policy to reduce the risk of bacterial contamination. Typically, ventilator tubing should be changed every 48 to 72 hours and sometimes more often.

■ When ordered, begin to wean the patient from the ventilator. (See "Weaning from mechanical ventilation," page 267.)

Complications

Mechanical ventilation can cause these complications:

■ tension pneumothorax
■ decreased cardiac output (CO)
■ oxygen toxicity
■ fluid volume excess caused by humidification
■ infection
■ GI distention or bleeding from stress ulcers.

Nursing considerations

■ Provide emotional support to the patient during all phases of mechanical ventilation to reduce his anxiety and promote successful treatment. Even if the patient is unresponsive, continue to explain all procedures and treatments to him.

■ Make sure that the ventilator alarms are on at all times. These alarms alert the nursing staff to potentially hazardous conditions and changes in patient status. If an alarm sounds and the problem can't be identified easily, disconnect the patient from the ventilator and use a handheld resuscitation bag to ventilate him. (See "Troubleshooting ventilator alarms," pages 697 to 699.)

■ Assess cardiopulmonary status frequently, at least every 2 to 4 hours or more frequently, if indicated. Assess vi-

Manual ventilation

A handheld resuscitation bag is an inflatable device that can be attached to a face mask or directly to tracheostomy or endotracheal (ET) tube to allow manual delivery of oxygen or room air to the lungs of a patient who can't breathe by himself. Although usually used in an emergency, manual ventilation can also be performed while the patient is disconnected temporarily from a mechanical ventilator, such as during a tubing change, during transport, or before suctioning. In such instances, the use of the handheld resuscitation bag maintains ventilation. Oxygen administration with a resuscitation bag can help improve a compromised cardiorespiratory system.

To manually ventilate the patient with an ET or tracheostomy tube, follow these guidelines:
● If oxygen is readily available, connect the handheld resuscitation bag to the oxygen. Attach one end of the tubing to the bottom of the bag and the other end to the nipple adapter on the flowmeter of the oxygen source.
● Turn on the oxygen and adjust the flow rate according to the patient's condition.
● Before attaching the handheld resuscitation bag, suction the ET or tracheostomy tube to remove any secretions that may obstruct the airway.
● Remove the mask from the ventilation bag and attach the handheld resuscitation bag directly to the tube.

● Keeping your nondominant hand on the connection of the bag to the tube, exert downward pressure to seal the mask against his face. For an adult patient, use your dominant hand to compress the bag every 5 seconds to deliver approximately 1 L of air.
● Deliver breaths with the patient's own inspiratory effort, if any is present. Don't attempt to deliver a breath as the patient exhales.
● Observe the patient's chest to ensure that it rises and falls with each compression. If ventilation fails to occur, check the connection and the patency of the patient's airway; if necessary, reposition his head and suction.
● Be alert for possible underventilation, which commonly occurs because the handheld resuscitation bag is difficult to keep positioned while ensuring an open airway. In addition, the volume of air delivered to the patient varies with the type of bag used and the hand size of the person compressing the bag. An adult with a small- or medium-sized hand may not consistently deliver 1 L of air. For these reasons, have someone assist with the procedure, if possible.
● Keep in mind that air is forced into the patient's stomach with manual ventilation, placing the patient at risk for aspiration of vomitus (possibly resulting in pneumonia) and gastric distention.
● Record the date and time of the procedure, reason and length of time the patient was disconnected from mechanical ventilation and received manual ventilation, any complications and the nursing action taken, and the patient's tolerance of the procedure.

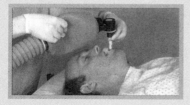

tal signs and auscultate breath sounds. Monitor pulse oximetry or end-tidal carbon dioxide levels and hemodynamic parameters as ordered.

■ Unless contraindicated, turn the patient from side to side every 1 to 2 hours to facilitate lung expansion and removal of secretions. Perform active or passive ROM exercises for all extremities to reduce the hazards of immobility. If the patient's condition permits, position him upright at regular intervals to increase lung expansion. When moving the patient or the ventilator tubing, be careful to prevent condensation in the tubing from flowing into the lungs because aspiration of this contaminated moisture can cause infection. Provide care for the patient's artificial airway as needed.

■ Assess the patient's peripheral circulation and monitor his urine output for signs of decreased CO. Watch for signs and symptoms of fluid volume excess or dehydration.

■ Place the call light within the patient's reach and establish a method of communication (such as a communication board) because intubation and mechanical ventilation impair the patient's ability to speak. An artificial airway may help the patient to speak by allowing air to pass through his vocal cords.

■ Administer a sedative or neuromuscular blocking agent as ordered to relax the patient or eliminate spontaneous breathing efforts that can interfere with the ventilator's action.

ALERT *Remember that the patient receiving a neuromuscular blocking drug requires close observation because of his inability to breathe or communicate. In addition, if the patient is receiving a neuromuscular blocking agent, make sure that he also receives a sedative. Neuromuscular blocking agents cause paralysis without altering the patient's level of consciousness. Reassure the patient and his family that the paralysis is temporary.*

■ Ensure that emergency equipment is readily available in case the ventilator malfunctions or the patient is extubated accidentally.

■ Continue to explain all procedures to the patient and take additional steps to ensure his safety, such as raising the side rails of his bed while turning him and covering and lubricating his eyes.

■ Ensure that the patient gets adequate rest and sleep because fatigue can delay weaning from the ventilator. Provide subdued lighting, safely muffle equipment noises, and restrict staff access to the area to promote quiet during rest periods.

■ When weaning the patient, continue to observe for signs of hypoxemia. Schedule weaning to fit comfortably and realistically with the patient's daily regimen, avoiding such times as after meals, baths, or lengthy therapeutic or diagnostic procedures. Have the patient help you set up the schedule to give him some sense of control over a frightening procedure. As the patient's tolerance for weaning increases, help him sit up and get out of bed to improve his breathing and sense of well-being. Suggest diversionary activities to take his mind off breathing.

■ If the patient will be discharged on a ventilator, evaluate the family's or the caregiver's ability and motivation to provide such care. Well before discharge, develop a teaching plan that will address the patient's needs, including ventilator care and settings, artificial airway care, suctioning, respiratory therapy, communication, nutrition, therapeutic exercise, the signs and symptoms of infection, ways to troubleshoot minor equipment malfunctions, adaptive equipment, and demonstration of all aspects of care.

■ Document the date and time of initiation of mechanical ventilation, including type of ventilator used for the patient and its settings.

■ Record the patient's subjective and objective response to mechanical ventilation, including vital signs, breath sounds, use of accessory muscles, intake and output, and weight. List any complications and nursing actions taken. Record all pertinent laboratory data, including ABG analysis results and oxygen saturation levels.

■ Document all teaching provided to patient and his family.

Pneumonia

An acute infection of the lung parenchyma that often impairs gas exchange, pneumonia can be classified in several ways. Based on microbiological etiology, it may be viral, bacterial, fungal, protozoal, mycobacterial, mycoplasmal, or rickettsial in origin. Based on location, pneumonia may be classified as bronchopneumonia, lobular pneumonia, or lobar pneumonia. Bronchopneumonia involves distal airways and alveoli; lobular pneumonia, part of a lobe; and lobar pneumonia, an entire lobe.

Infection is also classified as one of three types — primary, secondary, or aspiration pneumonia. Primary pneumonia results directly from inhalation or aspiration of a pathogen, such as bacteria or a virus; it includes pneumococcal and viral pneumonia. Secondary pneumonia may follow initial lung damage from a noxious chemical or other insult (superinfection) or may result from hematogenous spread of bacteria from a distant area. Aspiration pneumonia results from inhalation of foreign matter, such as vomitus or food particles, into the bronchi. It's more likely to occur in elderly or debilitated patients, those receiving nasogastric tube feedings, and those with an impaired gag reflex, poor oral hygiene, or a decreased level of consciousness.

Another classification categorizes the various types of pneumonia as community acquired, hospital acquired (or nosocomial), and aspiration. As the name implies, community-acquired pneumonia occurs in the community setting or within the first 48 hours after admission to a health care facility (due to community exposure). Nosocomial pneumonia refers to the development of pneumonia following 48 hours after admission to a health care facility. For example, development of pneumonia after endotracheal (ET) intubation and placement on a ventilator can be a type of nosocomial pneumonia. Aspiration pneumonia can occur in the community or health care facility setting. (See *Types of pneumonia*.)

Pneumonia occurs in both sexes and at all ages. More than 3 million cases of pneumonia occur annually in the United States. The infection carries a good prognosis for patients with normal lungs and adequate immune systems. In debilitated patients, however, bacterial pneumonia ranks as the leading cause of death. Pneumonia is also the leading cause of death from infectious disease in the United States.

Types of pneumonia

Type	Causative agent	Assessment findings
Aspiration pneumonia	Aspiration of gastric or oropharyngeal contents into trachea or lungs	• Fever • Crackles • Dyspnea • Hypotension • Tachycardia • Cyanosis • Chest X-ray with infiltrates
Community-acquired pneumonias		
Streptococcal pneumonia (pneumococcal pneumonia)	*Streptococcus pneumoniae*	• Sudden onset of single shaking chill • Fever 102° to 104° F (38.9° to 40° C) • History of previous upper respiratory infection • Pleuritic chest pain • Severe cough • Rust-colored sputum • Areas of consolidation on chest X-ray (usually lobar) • Elevated white blood cell (WBC) count • Sputum culture possibly positive for gram-positive *S. pneumoniae*
Hemophilus influenza	*Haemophilus influenzae*	• Insidious onset • History of upper respiratory tract infection 2 to 6 weeks earlier • Fever • Chills • Dyspnea • Productive cough • Nausea and vomiting • Chest X-ray with infiltrates in one or more lobes
Mycoplasma pneumonia	*Mycoplasma pneumoniae*	• Insidious onset • Sore throat • Nasal congestion • Ear pain • Headache • Low-grade fever • Pleuritic pain • Erythema rash • Pharyngitis

(continued)

Types of pneumonia *(continued)*

Type	Causative agent	Assessment findings
Community-acquired pneumonias *(continued)*		
Viral pneumonia	Influenza virus, type A	• Initially beginning as upper respiratory infection • Cough (initially nonproductive; later purulent sputum) • High fever • Chills • Malaise • Dyspnea • Substernal pain • Moist crackles • Cyanosis • Frontal headache • Chest X-ray with diffuse bilateral bronchopneumonia radiating from hilus • Normal to slightly elevated WBC
Legionnaires' disease	*Legionella pneumophila*	• Flulike symptoms • Malaise • Headache within 24 hours • Fever • Shaking chills • Progressive dyspnea • Mental confusion • Anorexia • Nausea, vomiting • Myalgia • Chest X-ray with patchy infiltrates, consolidation, and possible effusion
Hospital-acquired pneumonias		
Klebsiella pneumonia	*Klebsiella pneumoniae*	• Fever • Recurrent chills • Rusty, bloody viscous (currant jelly) sputum • Cyanosis of lips and nail beds • Shallow grunting respirations • Severe pleuritic chest pain • Chest X-ray typically with consolidation in upper lobe • Elevated WBC • Sputum culture and Gram stain possibly positive for gram-negative cocci, *Klebsiella*
Pseudomonas pneumonia	*Pseudomonas aeruginosa*	• Fever • Chills • Confusion • Delirium • Green foul-smelling sputum • Chest X-ray with diffuse consolidation

Types of pneumonia *(continued)*

Type	Causative agent	Assessment findings
Hospital-acquired pneumonias *(continued)*		
Staphylococcal pneumonia (may also be community acquired)	*Staphylococcus aureus*	• Cough • Chills • High fever 102° to 104° F (38.9° to 40° C) • Pleuritic pain • Progressive dyspnea • Bloody sputum • Tachypnea • Hypoxemia • Chest X-ray with multiple abscesses and infiltrate; empyema • Elevated WBC • Sputum culture and Gram stain possibly positive for gram-positive staphylocci

Pathophysiology

In bacterial pneumonia, which can occur in any part of the lungs, an infection initially triggers alveolar inflammation and edema. Capillaries become engorged with blood, causing stasis. As the alveolocapillary membrane breaks down, alveoli fill with blood and exudate, resulting in atelectasis. In severe bacterial infections, the lungs assume a heavy, liverlike appearance, as in adult respiratory distress syndrome (ARDS.)

Viral infection, which typically causes diffuse pneumonia, first attacks bronchiolar epithelial cells, causing interstitial inflammation and desquamation. It then spreads to the alveoli, which fill with blood and fluid. In advanced infection, a hyaline membrane may form. As with bacterial infection, severe viral infection may clinically resemble ARDS.

In aspiration pneumonia, aspiration of gastric juices or hydrocarbons triggers similar inflammatory changes and also inactivates surfactant over a large area. Decreased surfactant leads to alveolar collapse. Acidic gastric juices may directly damage the airways and alveoli. Particles in the aspirated gastric juices may obstruct the airways and reduce airflow, which in turn leads to secondary bacterial pneumonia.

Certain predisposing factors increase the risk of pneumonia. For bacterial and viral pneumonia, these include chronic illness and debilitation, cancer (particularly lung cancer), abdominal and thoracic surgery, atelectasis, common colds or other viral respiratory infections, chronic respiratory disease (chronic obstructive pulmonary disease, asthma, bronchiectasis, cystic fibrosis), influenza, smoking, malnutrition, alcoholism, sickle cell disease, tracheostomy, exposure to noxious gases, aspiration, and immunosuppressant therapy.

Aspiration pneumonia is more likely to occur in elderly or debilitated patients, those receiving nasogastric tube feedings, and those with an impaired gag reflex, poor oral hygiene, or a decreased level of consciousness.

Comprehensive assessment

The assessment findings may vary depending on the type of pneumonia that occurs. For example, the patient with bacterial pneumonia may report pleuritic chest pain, a cough, excessive sputum production, and chills. On assessment, fever may be noted. Inspection may reveal shaking and a productive cough. Creamy yellow sputum suggests staphylococcal pneumonia; green sputum denotes pneumonia caused by *Pseudomonas* organisms; sputum that looks like currant jelly indicates pneumonia caused by *Klebsiella*. (Clear sputum means that the patient doesn't have an infective process.)

In advanced cases of all types of pneumonia, percussion reveals dullness over the areas of consolidation. Auscultation may disclose crackles, wheezing, or rhonchi over the affected lung area as well as decreased breath sounds and decreased tactile fremitus.

Diagnosis

These tests will help confirm the diagnosis and type of pneumonia:
■ Chest X-rays disclose infiltrates, confirming the diagnosis.
■ Sputum specimen for Gram stain and culture and sensitivity tests shows acute inflammatory cells and identifies organism.
■ White blood cell count indicates leukocytosis in bacterial pneumonia and a normal or low count in viral or mycoplasmal pneumonia.
■ Blood cultures reflect bacteremia and help determine the causative organism.

■ Arterial blood gas (ABG) levels vary, depending on the severity of pneumonia and the underlying lung state.
■ Bronchoscopy or transtracheal aspiration allows the collection of material for culture to identify the causative organism; pleural fluid culture may also be obtained.
■ Pulse oximetry may show a reduced arterial oxygen saturation level.

Collaborations

Multidisciplinary care is needed for the patient with pneumonia. Medical and nursing care focuses on the use of oxygen therapy, possibly ET intubation and mechanical ventilation, pharmacotherapy, and hydration. Respiratory therapy may be consulted for chest physiotherapy and nebulized bronchodilator therapy if ordered. Nutritional therapy may be required to ensure an adequate diet. Depending on the causative organism, infectious disease personnel may be contacted for assistance. If the patient's stay is prolonged, physical therapy may be necessary for range-of-motion exercises and strengthening. Assistance from social services may be needed to assist the patient with the transition to home and with financial concerns should additional care be necessary.

Treatment and care

Typically, the patient needs antimicrobial therapy based on the causative agent. Therapy is then reevaluated early in the course of treatment to determine its effectiveness. Additionally, supportive treatment includes humidified oxygen therapy for hypoxemia, bronchodilator therapy, antitussives, mechanical ventilation for acute respiratory failure, a high-calorie diet and adequate fluid intake, bed rest, and an analgesic to relieve pleuritic chest pain. A patient with severe pneumonia who's receiving mechanical ventilation may require positive end-expiratory pressure or pressure support ventilation to maintain adequate oxygenation.

Complications

Without proper treatment, pneumonia can lead to these life-threatening complications:
- septic shock
- hypoxemia
- respiratory failure.

If the infection spreads within the patient's lungs, empyema or lung abscess, pleurisy, or pleural effusions may occur. If the infection spreads by way of the bloodstream or by cross-contamination to other parts of the body, bacteremia, endocarditis, pericarditis, or meningitis may result.

Nursing considerations

- Maintain a patent airway and adequate oxygenation.
- Place the patient in Fowler's position to maximize chest expansion and give supplemental oxygen, as ordered, to ease his breathing. Monitor oxygen saturation levels and ABGs as indicated. If the patient has an underlying chronic lung disease or is known to retain carbon dioxide, administer oxygen cautiously.

AGE ISSUE *If an older adult patient with pneumonia requires oxygen therapy, administer it cautiously. High oxygen levels can depress the respiratory stimulus in the brain, reducing respiration and promoting car-*

bon dioxide retention. Older adult patients typically have a diminished cough and gag reflex, weaker respiratory muscles, and a reduced maximum breathing capacity. Because sedatives, cough suppressants, and narcotics suppress respiratory drive and the cough and gag reflexes, their use is commonly avoided in older adult patients.

- Assess respiratory status frequently, at least every 1 to 2 hours. Auscultate lungs for abnormal breath sounds, such as crackles, wheezes, and rhonchi. Encourage coughing and deep breathing.
- If respiratory status deteriorates, anticipate the need for ET intubation and mechanical ventilation.
- In severe pneumonia that requires ET intubation or a tracheostomy with or without mechanical ventilation, provide thorough respiratory care and suction as needed, using sterile technique, to remove secretions.
- Institute continuous cardiac monitoring as appropriate to detect the development of arrhythmias secondary to hypoxemia.
- Adhere to standard precautions and institute appropriate transmission based precautions depending on the causative organism.
- Obtain sputum specimens as needed. Use suction if the patient can't produce a specimen. Encourage incentive spirometry, coughing, and deep breathing. Periodically evaluate the patient's ability to perform bronchial hygiene. Anticipate the need for chest physiotherapy if the patient is having difficulty with coughing and deep breathing to mobilize and expectorate sputum.
- Administer pharmacotherapy, including antimicrobials, bronchodila-

tors, antipyretics, analgesics, I.V. fluids, and electrolyte replacement as ordered.
   – Evaluate the effectiveness of administered medications, and check the patient for adverse reactions.

ALERT *If the patient requires opiate analgesics for pleuritic pain, be alert for possible respiratory depression. Frequently monitor the patient's respiratory rate and depth and oxygen saturation closely for changes.*

■ Assess urine output hourly initially and then every 2 to 4 hours; notify the physician for a urine output of less than 0.5 ml/kg/hour; and monitor fluid intake and output closely; obtain daily weights.

■ Monitor vital signs at least every 1 to 2 hours initially, then less frequently as the patient's condition improves. Monitor hemodynamic status as indicated.

■ Provide a high-calorie, high-protein diet of soft foods. Supplement oral feedings with enteral or parenteral nutrition if needed.

■ If the patient is receiving nasogastric tube feedings, elevate the patient's head, check the tube position, and administer the feeding slowly to reduce the risk of aspiration. Don't give large volumes at one time because this could cause vomiting; if the patient has an ET tube, inflate the tube cuff before feeding. Keep his head elevated for at least 1 to 2 hours after feeding.

■ Organize all activities to provide maximum rest periods. Assess for signs of activity intolerance, such as increased shortness of breath, chest pain, changes in oxygen saturation, and tachycardia or tachypnea, and have patient stop activity. Provide a quiet, calm environment, with frequent rest periods.

■ Listen to the patient's fears and concerns, and remain with him during periods of severe stress and anxiety. Encourage him to identify actions and care measures that promote comfort and relaxation.

Patient teaching

■ Explain all procedures (especially intubation and suctioning) to the patient and his family, emphasizing the importance of adequate rest to promote full recovery and prevent a relapse.

■ Review the patient's medication. Stress the need to take the entire course of medication to prevent a relapse. Advise patients to avoid using antibiotics indiscriminately for minor infections. Doing so could result in upper airway colonization with antibiotic-resistant bacteria. If pneumonia develops, the organisms that produce the pneumonia may require treatment with more toxic antibiotics.

■ Teach the patient procedures and therapies for clearing lung secretions, such as deep-breathing and coughing exercises and chest physiotherapy; explain that postural drainage, percussion, and vibration help to mobilize and remove mucus from the patient's lungs.

■ Urge the patient to drink 2 to 3 qt (2 to 3 L) of fluid per day (unless contraindicated) to maintain adequate hydration and help with mucus expectoration.

■ Encourage the high-risk patient to ask his physician about an annual influenza vaccination and the pneumococcal pneumonia vaccination.

■ Discuss ways to avoid spreading the infection to others, such as good hand-

washing, use of tissues, and proper disposal of contaminated tissues.
■ Urge the patient to avoid irritants that stimulate secretions, such as cigarette smoke, dust, and significant environmental pollution. If necessary, refer him to community programs or agencies that can help him stop smoking.

Pneumothorax

Pneumothorax is an accumulation of air in the pleural cavity that leads to partial or complete lung collapse. When the air between the visceral and parietal pleurae collects and accumulates, increasing tension in the pleural cavity can cause the lung to progressively collapse. Air is trapped in the intrapleural space and determines the degree of lung collapse. Venous return to the heart may be impeded to cause a life-threatening condition called tension pneumothorax.

The most common types of pneumothorax are open, closed, and tension.

Common causes of open pneumothorax include:
■ penetrating chest injury (gunshot or stab wound)
■ insertion of a central venous catheter
■ chest surgery
■ transbronchial biopsy
■ thoracentesis or closed pleural biopsy.

Causes of closed pneumothorax include:
■ blunt chest trauma
■ air leakage from ruptured blebs

■ rupture resulting from barotrauma caused by high intrathoracic pressures during mechanical ventilation
■ tubercular or cancerous lesions that erode into the pleural space
■ interstitial lung disease, such as eosinophilic granuloma.

Tension pneumothorax may be caused by:
■ penetrating chest wound treated with an airtight dressing
■ fractured ribs
■ mechanical ventilation
■ high-level positive end-expiratory pressure that causes alveolar blebs to rupture
■ chest tube occlusion or malfunction.

Pathophysiology

A rupture in the visceral or parietal pleura and chest wall causes air to accumulate and separate the visceral and parietal pleurae. Negative pressure is destroyed and the elastic recoil forces are affected. The lung recoils by collapsing toward the hilus.

Open pneumothorax (also called sucking chest wound or communicating pneumothorax) results when atmospheric air (positive pressure) flows directly into the pleural cavity (negative pressure). As the air pressure in the pleural cavity becomes positive, the lung collapses on the affected side, resulting in decreased total lung capacity, vital capacity, and lung compliance. $\dot{V}/\dot{Q}$ imbalances lead to hypoxemia.

Closed pneumothorax occurs when air enters the pleural space from within the lung, causing increased pleural pressure, which prevents lung expansion during normal inspiration. Spontaneous pneumothorax is another type of closed pneumothorax.

Understanding tension pneumothorax

In tension pneumothorax, air accumulates intrapleurally and can't escape.

On inspiration, the mediastinum shifts toward the unaffected lung, impairing ventilation.

On expiration, the mediastinal shift distorts the vena cava and reduces venous return.

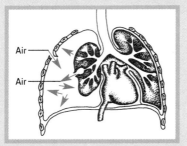

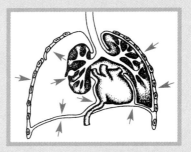

AGE ISSUE *Spontaneous pneumothorax is common in older patients with chronic pulmonary disease, but it may also occur in healthy, tall, young adults.*

Both types of closed pneumothorax can result in a collapsed lung with hypoxemia and decreased total lung capacity, vital capacity, and lung compliance. The range of lung collapse is between 5% and 95%.

Tension pneumothorax results when air in the pleural space is under higher pressure than air in the adjacent lung. The air enters the pleural space from the site of pleural rupture, which acts as a one-way valve. Air is allowed to enter into the pleural space on inspiration but can't escape as the rupture site closes on expiration. More air enters on inspiration and air pressure begins to exceed barometric pressure. Increasing air pressure pushes against the recoiled lung, causing compression atelectasis. Air also presses against the mediastinum, compressing and displacing the heart and great vessels. The air can't escape, and the accumulating pressure causes the lung to collapse. As air continues to accumulate and intrapleural pressures rise, the mediastinum shifts away from the affected side and decreases venous return. This forces the heart, trachea, esophagus, and great vessels to the unaffected side, compressing the heart and the contralateral lung. Without immediate treatment, this emergency can rapidly become fatal. (See *Understanding tension pneumothorax*.)

Comprehensive assessment

The patient history reveals sudden, sharp, pleuritic pain. The patient may report that chest movement, breathing, and coughing exacerbate the pain. He may also report shortness of breath.

Inspection typically reveals asymmetrical chest wall movement with overexpansion and rigidity on the affected side. The patient may appear cyanotic. Palpation may reveal crackling beneath the skin, indicating subcutaneous emphysema (air in tissues) and decreased vocal fremitus. Percussion may demonstrate hyperresonance on the affected side, and auscultation may disclose decreased or absent breath sounds over the collapsed lung. Spontaneous pneumothorax that releases only a small amount of air into the pleural space may cause no signs and symptoms.

Tension pneumothorax produces the most severe respiratory manifestations, including:

- decreased cardiac output (CO)
- hypotension due to decreased CO
- compensatory tachycardia
- tachypnea due to hypoxemia
- lung collapse due to air or blood in the intrapleural space
- mediastinal shift due to increasing tension
- tracheal deviation to the opposite side
- distended neck veins due to intrapleural pressure, mediastinal shift, and increased cardiovascular pressure
- pallor related to decreased CO
- anxiety related to hypoxemia
- weak and rapid pulse due to decreased CO.

Diagnosis

These tests help diagnose pneumothorax:

- Chest X-rays confirm the diagnosis by revealing air in the pleural space and, possibly, a mediastinal shift.
- Arterial blood gas (ABG) analysis may reveal hypoxemia, possibly with respiratory acidosis and hypercapnia. Partial pressure of arterial oxygen (PaO_2) levels may decrease at first, but

typically return to normal within 24 hours.

- Electrocardiogram may reveal decreased QRS amplitude, precordial T wave inversion, rightward shift of frontal QRS axis, and small precordial R voltage.

Collaborations

A multidisciplinary approach to care is needed, including medical, nursing, and respiratory therapy professionals, to ensure adequate oxygenation and pulmonary function. Surgery may be involved if the patient has experienced recurrent spontaneous pneumothoraces or if the pneumothorax hasn't resolved within a week. Physical therapy may be consulted to assist with energy conservation, range of motion, and strengthening if appropriate.

Treatment and care

Treatment depends on the type of pneumothorax.

Spontaneous pneumothorax with less than 30% of lung collapse, no signs of increased pleural pressure, and no dyspnea or indications of physiologic compromise, may be corrected with:

- bed rest to conserve energy and reduce oxygenation demands
- monitoring of blood pressure and pulse for early detection of physiologic compromise
- monitoring of respiratory rate to detect early signs of respiratory compromise
- oxygen administration to enhance oxygenation and improve hypoxemia
- aspiration of air with a large-bore needle attached to a syringe to restore negative pressure within the pleural space.

Correction of pneumothorax with more than 30% of lung collapse may include:

■ thoracostomy tube placed in the second or third intercostal space in the midclavicular line to try to reexpand the lung by restoring negative intrapleural pressure

■ connection of the thoracostomy tube to underwater seal or to low-pressure suction to reexpand the lung

■ if recurrent spontaneous pneumothorax, thoracotomy and pleurectomy may be performed, which causes the lung to adhere to the parietal pleura.

Open (traumatic) pneumothorax may be corrected with:

■ chest tube drainage to reexpand the lung

■ surgical repair of the lung.

Correction of tension pneumothorax typically involves:

■ immediate treatment with large-bore needle insertion into the pleural space through the second intercostal space to reexpand the lung

■ insertion of a thoracotomy tube if large amounts of air escape through the needle after insertion

■ analgesics to promote comfort and encourage deep breathing and coughing.

Complications

Possible complications of pneumothorax include:

■ decreased CO
■ hypoxemia
■ cardiac arrest.

Nursing considerations

■ Assess the patient's respiratory status frequently, including auscultation of bilateral breath sounds, at least every 1 to 2 hours. Monitor oxygen saturation levels closely for changes; obtain ABGs as ordered.

■ Monitor hemodynamic parameters frequently as appropriate and indicated; anticipate the need for continuous cardiac monitoring because hypoxemia can predispose the patient to arrhythmias.

■ Watch for complications, signaled by pallor, gasping respirations, and sudden chest pain. Carefully monitor vital signs at least every hour for indications of shock, increasing respiratory distress, or mediastinal shift. If patient's respiratory status deteriorates, anticipate the need for endotracheal intubation and mechanical ventilation and assist as necessary.

■ Assist with chest tube insertion and set up to suction. (See "Chest drainage," page 181.) Monitor patient for possible complications associated with chest tube insertion.

ALERT *Watch for signs of tension pneumothorax (especially if the patient has chest tubes inserted), including falling blood pressure and rising pulse and respiratory rates. This condition could be fatal without prompt treatment.*

■ Keep the patient as comfortable as possible, and administer analgesics as necessary. The patient with pneumothorax usually feels most comfortable sitting upright. Assess the effectiveness of administered analgesics, and monitor the patient for adverse reactions.

■ Change the patient's position every 2 hours to promote drainage and lung reexpansion.

■ Encourage the patient to perform deep-breathing exercises every hour when awake.

■ Listen to the patient's fears and concerns. Offer reassurance as appropri-

ate. Include the patient and his family in care-related decisions whenever possible. Provide opportunities for rest periods.
■ Prepare the patient for a thoracotomy as appropriate.

Patient teaching

■ Reassure the patient and provide explanations about the condition, causes, and treatment. If the patient is having surgery or chest tubes inserted, explain rationale for these procedures. Reassure him that the chest tubes will make him more comfortable.
■ Discuss the potential for recurrent spontaneous pneumothorax, and review its signs and symptoms, emphasizing the need for immediate medical intervention if these should occur.

Pulmonary embolism

An obstruction of the pulmonary arterial bed, pulmonary embolism (PE) occurs when a mass — such as a dislodged thrombus — lodges in a pulmonary artery branch, partially or completely obstructing it. This causes a ventilation-perfusion ($\dot{V}/\dot{Q}$) mismatch, resulting in hypoxemia as well as intrapulmonary shunting.

The prognosis varies. Although the pulmonary infarction that results from embolism may be so mild as to be asymptomatic, massive embolism (more than 50% obstruction of pulmonary arterial circulation) and infarction can cause rapid death.

Pathophysiology

In most patients, PE results from a dislodged thrombus that originates in the leg veins. More than half of such thrombi arise in the deep veins of the legs; usually, multiple thrombi arise. Other, less common sources of thrombi include the pelvic, renal, and hepatic veins; the right side of the heart; and the upper extremities.

Such thrombus formation results from vascular wall damage, venous stasis, or hypercoagulability of the blood. Trauma, clot dissolution, sudden muscle spasm, intravascular pressure changes, or a change in peripheral blood flow can cause the thrombus to loosen or fragment. The thrombus — now called an embolus — floats to the heart's right side and enters the lung through the pulmonary artery. There, the embolus may dissolve, continue to fragment, or grow.

By occluding the pulmonary artery, the embolus prevents alveoli from producing enough surfactant to maintain alveolar integrity. As a result, alveoli collapse and atelectasis develops. If the embolus enlarges, it may clog most or all pulmonary vessels and cause death.

Rarely, PE results from other types of emboli, including bone, air, fat, amniotic fluid, tumor cells, or a foreign object, such as a needle, catheter part, or talc (from drugs intended for oral administration that are injected I.V. by addicts).

The risk increases with long-term immobility, chronic pulmonary disease, heart failure or atrial fibrillation, thrombophlebitis, polycythemia vera, thrombocytosis, cardiac arrest, defibrillation, cardioversion, autoimmune hemolytic anemia, sickle cell disease, varicose veins, recent surgery, age over

Risk factors for pulmonary embolism

Many disorders and treatments heighten the risk of pulmonary embolism. At particular risk are surgical patients. For example, the anesthetic used during surgery can injure lung vessels, and surgery itself or prolonged bed rest can promote venous stasis, compounding the risk.

Predisposing disorders
● Lung disorders, especially chronic disorders
● Cardiac disorders
● Infection
● Diabetes mellitus
● History of thromboembolism, thrombophlebitis, or vascular insufficiency
● Sickle cell disease
● Autoimmune hemolytic anemia
● Polycythemia
● Osteomyelitis
● Long bone fracture
● Manipulation or disconnection of central lines

Venous stasis
● Prolonged bed rest or immobilization
● Obesity
● Age over 40 years
● Burns
● Recent childbirth
● Orthopedic casts

Venous injury
● Surgery, particularly of the legs, pelvis, abdomen, or thorax
● Leg or pelvic fractures or injuries
● I.V. drug abuse
● I.V. therapy

Increased blood coagulability
● Cancer
● Use of high-estrogen hormonal contraceptive agents

40, osteomyelitis, pregnancy, lower extremity fractures or surgery, burns, obesity, vascular injury, cancer, and oral contraceptive use. (See *Risk factors for pulmonary embolism.*)

Comprehensive assessment

The patient's history may reveal a predisposing condition. He may also complain of shortness of breath, often suddenly occurring for no apparent reason, as well as pleuritic or anginal pain. The patient's complaint of chest pain often is sudden and severe. The patient may also express a sense of impending doom. The severity of these symptoms depends on the extent of damage. The signs and symptoms produced by small or fragmented emboli depend on their size, number, and location. If the embolus totally occludes the main pulmonary artery, the patient will have severe signs and symptoms.

Initially, the patient is tachycardic. He may also have a low-grade fever. If circulatory collapse has occurred, he'll have a weak, rapid pulse rate and hypotension.

On inspection, a productive cough, possibly producing blood-tinged sputum may be noted. Less commonly, chest splinting, massive hemoptysis, leg edema and, with a large embolus, cyanosis, syncope, and distended neck veins may be observed.

Palpation may reveal a warm, tender area in the extremities, a possible area of thrombosis. On auscultation, a transient pleural friction rub and crackles at the embolus site may be heard. Additionally, an S_3 and S_4 gallop, with increased intensity of the pulmonic component of S_2 may also be noted.

In pleural infarction, the patient's history may include heart disease and left ventricular failure. He may complain of sudden, sharp pleuritic chest pain accompanied by progressive dyspnea. On inspection, you may note that the patient has a fever and is coughing up blood-tinged sputum. Auscultation may reveal a pleural friction rub.

Diagnosis

■ V/Q scan demonstrates a mismatching evidenced as decreased or absent perfusion in normally ventilated areas of the lung, highly suggestive of a PE.
■ Pulmonary angiography may show a pulmonary vessel filling defect or an abrupt vessel ending, both of which indicate PE. Although the most definitive test, it's only used if the diagnosis can't be confirmed any other way and anticoagulant therapy would put the patient at significant risk.
■ Twelve-lead electrocardiogram (ECG) helps distinguish PE from myocardial infarction. If the patient has an extensive embolism, the ECG shows right axis deviation; right bundle-branch block; tall, peaked P waves; depressed ST segments; T-wave inversions (a sign of right-sided heart failure); and supraventricular tachyarrhythmias.
■ Chest X-ray helps rule out other pulmonary diseases, although it's inconclusive in the 1 to 2 hours after embolism. It may also show areas of atelectasis, an elevated diaphragm, pleural effusion, a prominent pulmonary artery and, occasionally, the characteristic wedge-shaped infiltrate that suggests pulmonary infarction.
■ Arterial blood gas (ABG) analysis sometimes reveals decreased partial

pressure of arterial oxygen and partial pressure of arterial carbon dioxide levels from tachypnea.
■ Hemodynamic studies reveal an elevated pulmonary artery pressure (if due to a thrombotic emboli) and acutely elevated systolic, diastolic, and mean arterial pressure (if due to a venous air emboli).
■ Magnetic resonance imaging can identify blood flow changes that point to an embolus or identify the embolus itself.

Collaborations

A multidisciplinary approach to the patient's care is needed. Medical and nursing health care providers focus on maximizing oxygenation, maintaining cardiopulmonary function and hemodynamic status, and reducing oxygen demand with rest and limitation of activity. Surgical health care providers may be consulted for an embolectomy if other therapies have been ineffective and the patient is experiencing severe hemodynamic compromise. For the patient who has had recurrent emboli, surgical insertion of a vena caval filter may be necessary. Physical and occupational therapy may be necessary to help with activity limitations and energy conservation.

Treatment and care

The goal of treatment is to maintain adequate cardiovascular and pulmonary function until the obstruction resolves and to prevent any recurrence. (Most emboli resolve within 10 to 14 days.)

Treatment for an embolism caused by a thrombus generally consists of oxygen therapy, as needed, and anticoagulation with heparin to inhibit new thrombus formation. The patient on heparin therapy needs daily coagulation studies (partial thromboplastin time [PTT]). The patient may also receive warfarin for 3 to 6 months, depending on his risk factors. This patient's prothrombin time (PT) will be monitored daily and then biweekly.

If the patient has a massive PE and shock, he may need fibrinolytic therapy with urokinase, streptokinase, or alteplase. Initially, these thrombolytic agents dissolve clots within 12 to 24 hours. Seven days later, these drugs lyse clots to the same degree as heparin therapy alone.

If the embolus causes hypotension, the patient may need a vasopressor. A septic embolus requires antibiotic therapy, not anticoagulants, and evaluation for the infection's source (most likely endocarditis).

If the patient can't take anticoagulants or develops recurrent emboli during anticoagulant therapy, he'll need surgery consisting of vena cava ligation, plication, or insertion of a device (umbrella filter) to filter blood returning to the heart and lungs. If the patient has had a massive PE, a surgical embolectomy may be indicated. The procedure requires a thoracotomy and cardiopulmonary bypass. Angiographic demonstration of PE should take place before surgery.

To prevent postoperative venous thromboembolism, the patient may require a combination of heparin and dihydroergotamine, which is more effective than heparin alone.

If the patient has a fat embolus, he'll need oxygen therapy. He may also need mechanical ventilation, corticosteroids and, if pulmonary edema arises, diuretics.

Complications

If the embolus totally obstructs the arterial blood supply, pulmonary infarction (lung tissue death) occurs, a complication that affects about 10% of patients with PE. It's more likely to occur if the patient has chronic cardiac or pulmonary disease. Other complications include:

■ emboli extension, which blocks further vessels
■ hepatic congestion and necrosis
■ pulmonary abscess
■ shock and adult respiratory distress syndrome
■ massive atelectasis
■ venous overload
■ $\dot{V}/\dot{Q}$ mismatch
■ massive embolism, resulting in death.

Nursing considerations

■ Obtain the patient's vital signs and assess cardiopulmonary status closely, at least hourly. Auscultate for an S_4, crackles, and pleuritic rub.

ALERT *Keep in mind that many of the signs and symptoms of PE mimic those of myocardial infarction (MI). Obtain a 12-lead ECG to aid in ruling out MI.*

■ Institute continuous cardiac monitoring to detect arrhythmias that may occur secondary to hypoxemia.
■ Assess serial oxygen saturation levels and ABGs for hypoxemia. As ordered, give oxygen by nasal cannula or mask. Elevate the patient's head of the bed to maximize lung expansion and ease the work of breathing. If breathing is severely compromised, anticipate the need for endotracheal intubation and mechanical ventilation.
■ Monitor hemodynamic status closely. If one isn't already in place, antici-

pate the need for pulmonary artery or central venous catheter insertion.

■ Obtain coagulation studies to provide a baseline. Begin anticoagulant therapy, such as heparin, as ordered. Administer as an I.V. bolus or continuous infusion, titrating therapy based on coagulation studies. Effective heparin therapy raises PTT to about 2 to 2½ times normal. A therapeutic International Normalized Ratio ranges from 2.0 to 3.0. Alternatively, administer thrombolytic agents as ordered.

ALERT *Always be sure to have the antidotes for agents readily available. These include protamine sulfate for heparin, vitamin K for warfarin, and epsilon-aminocaproic acid for thrombolytics.*

■ During heparin therapy, assess the patient closely for epistaxis, petechiae, and other signs of abnormal bleeding. Check the patient's stools for occult blood. Watch for possible anticoagulant treatment complications, including gastric bleeding, stroke, and hemorrhage.

■ If the patient has pleuritic chest pain, administer the ordered analgesic.

■ Maintain bed rest in a comfortable position and organize activities to allow for periods of rest. Institute safety measures to prevent injury secondary to thrombolytic or anticoagulant therapy. Have the patient use a soft toothbrush or sponge applicator and an electric razor to minimize the risk of bleeding.

■ Apply pressure over any puncture sites for approximately 5 to 10 minutes for venous sites and 15 to 30 minutes for arterial sites, until bleeding stops.

ALERT *To reduce the risk of hematoma formation, avoid intramuscular injections.*

■ Expect to begin oral anticoagulant therapy while the patient is still receiving parenteral agents. Monitor PT.

ALERT *Avoid aspirin, aspirin-containing products, and nonsteroidal anti-inflammatory drugs while the patient is receiving anticoagulants. These products interfere with platelet aggregation and can increase the patient's risk for bleeding.*

■ Assist with gentle range-of-motion (ROM) exercises while the patient maintains bed rest.

After the patient's condition stabilizes, encourage him to move about and assist him with isometric and ROM exercises.

ALERT *Never vigorously massage the patient's legs; doing so could dislodge thrombi.*

■ Provide the patient with adequate nutrition and fluids to promote healing.

■ If needed, provide incentive spirometry to help the patient with deep breathing.

■ Offer the patient diversional activities to promote relaxation and relieve restlessness.

Patient teaching

■ Explain all procedures and treatments to the patient and his family including the rationale for anticoagulant therapy.

■ Instruct the patient and his family about anticoagulant therapy, danger signs and symptoms (bloody stools, blood in urine, large bruises), necessary safety precautions while receiving therapy (such as shaving with an electric razor and using a soft toothbrush), and measures to prevent a recurrence.

■ Make sure the patient understands the importance of taking his medication exactly as ordered. Tell him not to take any other medications, especially aspirin, without asking the physician. Instruct the patient taking warfarin not to significantly vary the amount of vitamin K he takes in daily. Doing so could interfere with anticoagulation stabilization.

■ Stress the importance of follow-up laboratory tests, such as PT, to monitor anticoagulant therapy.

■ Tell the patient that he must inform all of his health care providers — including dentists — that he's receiving anticoagulant therapy. He should also alert any specialists that he's taking anticoagulants before treatment.

■ To prevent PE in a high-risk patient, encourage him to walk and exercise his legs and to wear support or antiembolism stockings. Tell him not to cross or massage his legs.

Pulmonary hypertension

In both the rare primary form and the more common secondary form, pulmonary hypertension is indicated by a resting systolic pulmonary artery pressure (PAP) above 30 mm Hg and a mean PAP above 18 mm Hg.

Primary or idiopathic pulmonary hypertension is characterized by increased PAP and increased pulmonary vascular resistance, both without an obvious cause.

AGE ISSUE *Primary pulmonary hypertension is most com-*

mon in women between ages 20 and 40 and is usually fatal within 3 to 4 years; mortality is highest in pregnant women.

Secondary pulmonary hypertension results from existing cardiac or pulmonary disease or both. The prognosis in secondary pulmonary hypertension depends on the severity of the underlying disorder.

Although the cause of primary pulmonary hypertension remains unknown, the tendency for the disease to occur within families points to a hereditary defect. It also occurs more commonly in those with collagen disease and is thought to result from altered immune mechanisms. In primary pulmonary hypertension, the intimal lining of the pulmonary arteries thickens for no apparent reason. This narrows the artery and impairs distensibility, increasing vascular resistance.

Secondary pulmonary hypertension results from hypoxemia. (See *Causes of secondary pulmonary hypertension.*)

Pathophysiology
In primary pulmonary hypertension, the smooth muscle in the pulmonary artery wall hypertrophies for no reason, narrowing the small pulmonary artery (arterioles) or obliterating it completely. Fibrous lesions also form around the vessels, impairing distensibility and increasing vascular resistance. Pressures in the left ventricle, which receives blood from the lungs, remain normal. However, the increased pressures generated in the lungs are transmitted to the right ventricle, which supplies the pulmonary artery. Eventually, the right ventricle fails (cor pulmonale). Although oxygenation isn't severely affected initially,

hypoxemia and cyanosis eventually occur. Death results from cor pulmonale.

Alveolar hypoventilation can result from diseases caused by alveolar destruction or from disorders that prevent the chest wall from expanding sufficiently to allow air into the alveoli. The resulting decreased ventilation increases pulmonary vascular resistance. Hypoxemia resulting from this ventilation perfusion mismatch also causes vasoconstriction, further increasing vascular resistance and resulting in pulmonary hypertension.

Coronary artery disease or mitral valvular disease causing increased left ventricular filling pressures may cause secondary pulmonary hypertension. Ventricular septal defect and patent ductus arteriosus cause secondary pulmonary hypertension by increasing blood flow through the pulmonary circulation via left-to-right shunting. Pulmonary emboli and chronic destruction of alveolar walls, as in emphysema, cause secondary pulmonary hypertension by obliterating or obstructing the pulmonary vascular bed. Secondary pulmonary hypertension can also occur by vasoconstriction of the vascular bed, such as through hypoxemia, acidosis, or both. Conditions resulting in vascular obstruction can also cause pulmonary hypertension because blood isn't allowed to flow appropriately through the vessels.

Secondary pulmonary hypertension can be reversed if the disorder is resolved. If hypertension persists, hypertrophy occurs in the medial smooth muscle layer of the arterioles. The larger arteries stiffen and hypertension progresses. Pulmonary pressures begin to equal systemic blood pressure,

Causes of secondary pulmonary hypertension

Secondary pulmonary hypertension results from hypoxemia as the result of a variety of conditions.

Conditions causing alveolar hyperventilation:
- chronic obstructive pulmonary disease
- sarcoidosis
- diffuse interstitial pneumonia
- malignant metastases
- scleroderma
- obesity
- kyphoscoliosis.

Conditions causing vascular obstruction:
- pulmonary embolism
- vasculitis
- left atrial myxoma
- idiopathic veno-occlusive disease
- fibrosing mediastinitis
- mediastinal neoplasm.

Conditions causing primary cardiac disease:
- patent ductus arteriosus
- atrial septal defect
- ventricular septal defect.

Conditions causing acquired cardiac disease:
- rheumatic valvular disease
- mitral stenosis.

causing right ventricular hypertrophy and, eventually, cor pulmonale.

Primary cardiac diseases may be congenital or acquired. Congenital defects cause a left-to-right shunt, rerouting blood through the lungs twice and causing pulmonary hypertension. Acquired cardiac diseases, such as rheumatic valvular disease and mitral stenosis, result in left-sided heart failure that diminishes the flow of oxygenated blood from the lungs. This increases pulmonary vascular resistance and right ventricular pressure.

Comprehensive assessment

The patient with primary pulmonary hypertension may have no signs or symptoms until lung damage becomes severe. (In fact, the disorder may not be diagnosed until an autopsy.)

Usually, a patient with pulmonary hypertension complains of increasing dyspnea on exertion, weakness, syncope, and fatigue. He may also have difficulty breathing, feel short of breath, and report that breathing causes pain. Such signs may result from left ventricular failure.

Inspection may show signs of right-sided heart failure, including ascites and neck vein distention. The patient may appear restless and agitated and have a decreased level of consciousness (LOC). He may even be confused and have memory loss. Diaphragmatic excursion and respiration may be decreased, and the point of maximal impulse may be displaced beyond the midclavicular line.

On palpation, signs of right-sided heart failure such as peripheral edema may be noted. The patient typically has an easily palpable right ventricular lift and a reduced carotid pulse. He may also have a palpable and tender liver as well as tachycardia.

Auscultation findings are specific to the underlying disorder but may include a systolic ejection murmur, a widely split S_2, and S_3 and S_4. Decreased breath sounds and loud tubular sounds may be heard. The patient may have decreased blood pressure.

Diagnosis

These tests help to diagnose pulmonary hypertension:

■ Arterial blood gas analysis reveals hypoxemia.

■ Electrocardiography in right ventricular hypertrophy shows right axis deviation and tall or peaked P waves in inferior leads.

■ Cardiac catheterization reveals increased PAP, with systolic pressure above 30 mm Hg. It may also show an increased pulmonary capillary wedge pressure (PCWP) if the underlying cause is left atrial myxoma, mitral stenosis, or left-sided heart failure; otherwise, PCWP is normal.

■ Pulmonary angiography detects filling defects in pulmonary vasculature, such as those that develop with pulmonary emboli.

■ Pulmonary function studies may show decreased flow rates and increased residual volume in underlying obstructive disease; in underlying restrictive disease, they may show reduced total lung capacity.

■ Radionuclide imaging detects abnormalities in right and left ventricular functioning.

■ Open lung biopsy may determine the type of disorder.

■ Echocardiography allows the assessment of ventricular wall motion and possible valvular dysfunction. It can also demonstrate right ventricular enlargement, abnormal septal configuration consistent with right ventricular pressure overload, and reduction in left ventricular cavity size.

■ Perfusion lung scanning may produce normal or abnormal results, with multiple patchy and diffuse filling defects that don't suggest pulmonary embolism.

Collaborations

A multidisciplinary approach to the patient's care is needed. Medical and nursing health care providers focus on maintaining oxygenation, perfusion, cardiac output (CO), and hemodynamic stability with the administration of medications and reducing myocardial oxygen demand with rest and limitation of activity. If the patient's condition is severe, surgical health care providers may be contacted for possible consideration of heart-lung transplantation. Nutritional consultation may be necessary to help with dietary measures and fluid restriction. Physical and occupational therapy may be necessary to help with activity limitations and energy conservation.

Treatment and care

Managing this disorder typically involves:

■ oxygen therapy to correct hypoxemia and resulting increased pulmonary vascular resistance
■ fluid restriction in right-sided heart failure to decrease workload of the heart
■ digoxin to increase CO
■ diuretics to decrease intravascular volume and extravascular fluid accumulation
■ vasodilators to reduce myocardial workload and oxygen consumption
■ calcium channel blockers to reduce myocardial workload and oxygen consumption
■ bronchodilators to relax smooth muscles and increase airway patency
■ beta-adrenergic blockers to improve oxygenation
■ treatment of the underlying cause to correct pulmonary edema
■ heart-lung transplant in severe cases.

Nursing considerations

■ Administer pharmacologic agents as ordered to promote adequate heart and lung function.
■ Assess hemodynamic status, including PAP and PAWP as ordered, approximately every 2 hours or more frequently depending on the patient's condition; report any changes. Monitor the patient's vital signs, especially his blood pressure and heart rate. If hypotension or tachycardia develops, notify the physician.
■ Monitor intake and output closely and obtain daily weights; institute fluid restrictions as ordered.
■ Institute continuous cardiac monitoring to evaluate for arrhythmias and begin expected treatment should any occur.
■ Auscultate heart and lung sounds, being alert for S_3 heart sounds or murmurs, or crackles, rhonchi and wheezes indicative of heart failure; monitor vital signs for changes, especially a heart rate greater than 100 beats/minute, respiratory rate greater than 20 breaths/minute, and a systolic blood pressure less than 90 mm Hg and an elevated temperature, all of which suggest heart failure.
■ Assess patient for possible adverse effects of pharmacologic agents administered, such as postural hypotension with diuretics and beta-adrenergic blockers. Urge patient to change positions slowly.
■ Assist patient with activities of daily living to decrease oxygen demand. Assess patient's response to activity, such as complaints of shortness of breath, increases in heart rate or systolic blood pressure over resting rate, or changes in cardiac rhythm.

■ Administer supplemental oxygen as ordered; assess LOC for changes such as restlessness or decreased responsiveness indicating diminished cerebral perfusion. If patient has a pulmonary artery catheter in place, evaluate mixed venous oxygen saturation levels; if not, monitor oxygen saturation levels via pulse oximetry.

■ Organize care to promote periods of rest for the patient.

■ Listen to the patient's fears and concerns, and remain with him during periods of extreme stress and anxiety. Answer any questions he may have as best you can. Encourage him to identify care measures and activities that will make him comfortable and relaxed. Then try to perform these measures and encourage the patient to do so, too.

■ Include the patient in care decisions, and include the patient's family in all phases of his care.

Patient teaching

■ Teach the patient what signs and symptoms to report to his physician (increasing shortness of breath, swelling, increasing weight gain, increasing fatigue); review diet and fluid restrictions.

■ Fully explain the medication regimen, including dosage, action, possible adverse effects, and danger signs and symptoms to report to his physician. Teach the patient taking a potassium-wasting diuretic which foods are high in potassium.

■ If the patient needs special equipment for home use, such as oxygen equipment, refer him to the social service department.

Pulse oximetry

Performed intermittently or continuously, oximetry is a relatively simple procedure used to monitor arterial oxygen saturation noninvasively. Pulse oximeters usually denote arterial oxygen saturation values with the symbol SpO_2, whereas invasively measured arterial oxygen saturation values are denoted by the symbol SaO_2.

In this procedure, two diodes send red and infrared light through a pulsating arterial vascular bed, like the one in the fingertip. A photodetector slipped over the finger measures the transmitted light as it passes through the vascular bed, detects the relative amount of color absorbed by arterial blood, and calculates the exact mixed venous oxygen saturation without interference from surrounding venous blood, skin, connective tissue, or bone. Ear oximetry works by monitoring the transmission of light waves through the vascular bed of a patient's earlobe. Results will be inaccurate if the patient's earlobe is poorly perfused, as from a low cardiac output.

Equipment

Oximeter ■ finger or ear probe ■ alcohol pads ■ nail polish remover, if necessary

Essential steps

■ Review the manufacturer's instructions for assembly of the oximeter.

■ Explain the procedure to the patient.

■ For pulse oximetry select a finger for the test. Although the index finger is commonly used, a smaller finger may be selected if the patient's fingers are too large for the equipment.

AGE ISSUE *If you're testing a neonate or a small infant, wrap the probe around the foot so that light beams and detectors oppose each other. For a large infant, use a probe that fits on the great toe and secure it to the foot.*

– Make sure the patient isn't wearing false fingernails, and remove any nail polish from the test finger.

– Place the transducer (photodetector) probe over the patient's finger so that light beams and sensors oppose each other. If the patient has long fingernails, position the probe perpendicular to the finger, if possible, or clip the fingernail.

– Always position the patient's hand at heart level to eliminate venous pulsations and to promote accurate readings.

– Turn on the power switch. If the device is working properly, a beep will sound, a display will light momentarily, and the pulse searchlight will flash. The SpO_2 and pulse rate displays will show stationary zeros. After four to six heartbeats, the SpO_2 and pulse rate displays will supply information with each beat, and the pulse amplitude indicator will begin tracking the pulse.

■ For ear oximetry, use an alcohol pad to massage the patient's earlobe for 10 to 20 seconds. Mild erythema indicates adequate vascularization.

– Following the manufacturer's instructions, attach the ear probe to the patient's earlobe or pinna. Use the ear probe stabilizer for prolonged or exercise testing.

– Be sure to establish good contact on the ear; an unstable probe may set off the low-perfusion alarm. After the probe has been attached for a few seconds, a saturation reading and pulse waveform will appear on the oximeter's screen.

– Leave the ear probe in place for 3 or more minutes until readings stabilize at the highest point, or take three separate readings and average them. Make sure to revascularize the patient's earlobe each time.

■ After the procedure, remove the probe, turn off and unplug the unit, and clean the probe by gently rubbing it with an alcohol sponge.

Complications

Potential complications of pulse oximetry include:

■ skin irritation, which can develop from adhesives used to keep disposable probes in place and requires changing of the site

■ pulse oximeters, which sometimes fail to obtain a signal, indicating a poor connection or inadequate or intermittent blood flow problems to the site

■ equipment malfunctions.

Nursing considerations

■ If oximetry has been performed properly, know that readings are typically accurate. However, certain factors may interfere with accuracy. For example, an elevated bilirubin level may falsely lower SpO_2 readings, while elevated carboxyhemoglobin or methemoglobin levels, such as occur in heavy smokers and urban dwellers, can cause a falsely elevated SpO_2 reading.

■ Keep in mind that certain intravascular substances, such as lipid emulsions and dyes, can also prevent accurate readings. Other factors that may interfere with accurate results include hypothermia, hypotension, and vasoconstriction.

■ If light is a problem, cover the probes; if patient movement is a problem, move the probe or select a different probe; and if ear pigment is a problem, reposition the probe, revascularize the site, or use a finger probe.

■ If the patient has compromised circulation in his extremities, apply the photodetector across the bridge of his nose.

■ If SpO_2 is used to guide weaning the patient from forced inspiratory oxygen, obtain arterial blood gas analysis occasionally to correlate SpO_2 readings with SaO_2 levels.

■ If an automatic blood pressure cuff is used on the same extremity that is used for measuring SpO_2, the cuff will interfere with SpO_2 readings during inflation. Therefore evaluate levels when the cuff is deflated.

■ Be able to identify normal SpO_2 level. Normal SpO_2 levels for ear and pulse oximetry are 95% to 100% for adults.

■ **AGE ISSUE** *Normal SpO_2 values are 93.8% to 100% by 1 hour after birth for healthy, full-term neonates.*

Lower levels may indicate hypoxemia that warrants intervention. For such patients, follow the facility's policy or the physician's orders, which may include increasing oxygen therapy. If SaO_2 levels decrease suddenly, be prepared to initiate immediate resuscitative efforts. Notify the physician of any significant change in the patient's condition.

■ Document the procedure, including the date, time, procedure type, oximetric measurement, and any action taken. Record readings on appropriate flowcharts if indicated.

Status asthmaticus

Status asthmaticus is a life-threatening situation resulting from an acute asthmatic attack. Asthma is a chronic reactive airway disorder causing episodic airway obstruction that results from bronchospasms, increased mucus secretion, and mucosal edema. If left untreated or if the patient doesn't respond to treatment with pharmacotherapy after 24 hours, status asthmaticus is diagnosed. When the patient has an acute asthma attack, status asthmaticus may be heralded by progressive cyanosis, confusion, and lethargy. This complication begins with impaired gas exchange and may lead to respiratory failure and, eventually, death if rapid intervention isn't performed.

Asthma is a type of chronic obstructive pulmonary disease, a long-term pulmonary disease characterized by increased airflow resistance. Extrinsic, or atopic, asthma begins in childhood; typically, patients are sensitive to specific external allergens. Extrinsic allergens that can trigger an asthma attack include elements, such as pollen, animal dander, house dust or mold, kapok or feather pillows, food additives containing sulfites, and other sensitizing substances. Extrinsic asthma is commonly accompanied by other hereditary allergies, such as eczema and allergic rhinitis, in childhood populations. Intrinsic, or nonatopic, asthmatics react to internal, nonallergenic factors; external substances can't be implicated in patients with intrinsic asthma. Intrinsic allergens include irritants, emotional stress, fatigue, endocrine changes, temperature variations, humidity variations, exposure to noxious fumes, anxiety, coughing or laughing, and genetic factors. Most episodes occur after a severe respiratory tract infection, especially in adults. However, many asthmatics, especially children, have both intrinsic and extrinsic asthma.

A significant number of adults acquire an allergic form of asthma or exacerbation of existing asthma from exposure to agents in the workplace. Such irritants as chemicals in flour, acid anhydrides, toluene di-isocyanates, screw flies, river flies, and excreta of dust mites in carpet have been identified as agents that trigger asthma.

Pathophysiology

Two genetic influences are identified with asthma; namely, the ability of an individual to develop asthma (atopy) and the tendency to develop hyperresponsiveness of the airways independent of atopy. A locus of chromosome 11 associated with atopy contains an abnormal gene that encodes a part of the immunoglobulin (Ig) E receptor. Environmental factors interact with inherited factors to cause asthmatic reactions with associated bronchospasms.

Status asthmaticus begins with an asthma attack. In asthma, bronchial linings overreact to various stimuli, causing episodic smooth muscle spasms that severely constrict the airways. (See *Pathophysiology of asthma,* page 242.) IgE antibodies, attached to

histamine-containing mast cells and receptors on cell membranes, initiate intrinsic asthma attacks. When exposed to an antigen such as pollen, the IgE antibody combines with the antigen.

On subsequent exposure to the antigen, mast cells degranulate and release mediators. Mast cells in the lung interstitium are stimulated to release both histamine and the slow-reacting substance of anaphylaxis. Histamine attaches to receptor sites in the larger bronchi, where it causes swelling in smooth muscles. Mucous membranes become inflamed, irritated, and swollen. The patient may experience dyspnea, prolonged expiration, and an increased respiratory rate.

The leukotriene attaches to receptor sites in the smaller bronchi and causes local swelling of the smooth muscle. Leukotriene also causes prostaglandins to travel via the bloodstream to the lungs, where they enhance the effect of histamine. A wheeze may be audible during coughing; the higher the pitch, the narrower the bronchial lumen. Histamine stimulates the mucous membranes to secrete excessive mucus, further narrowing the bronchial lumen. Goblet cells secrete viscous mucus that's difficult to cough up, resulting in coughing, rhonchi, increased-pitch wheezing, and increased respiratory distress. Mucosal edema and thickened secretions further block the airways. (See *Looking at a bronchiole in asthma,* page 243.)

On inhalation, the narrowed bronchial lumen can still expand slightly, allowing air to reach the alveoli. On exhalation, increased intrathoracic pressure closes the bronchial lumen completely. Air enters but can't

Pathophysiology of asthma

In asthma, hyperresponsiveness of the airways and bronchospasms occur. The illustrations here show the progression of an asthma attack.

- Histamine (H) attaches to receptor sites in larger bronchi, causing swelling of the smooth muscles.

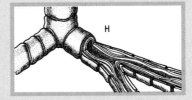

- Leukotrienes attach to receptor sites in the smaller bronchi and cause swelling of smooth muscle there. Leukotrienes also cause prostaglandins to travel via the bloodstream to the lungs, where they enhance histamine's effects.

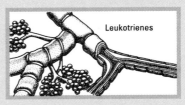

- Histamine stimulates the mucous membranes to secrete excessive mucus, further narrowing the bronchial lumen. On inhalation, the narrowed bronchial lumen can still expand slightly; however, on exhalation, the increased intrathoracic pressure closes the bronchial lumen completely.

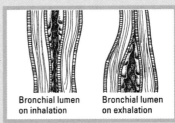

Bronchial lumen on inhalation   Bronchial lumen on exhalation

- Mucus fills lung bases, inhibiting alveolar ventilation. Blood is shunted to alveoli in other parts of the lungs, but it still can't compensate for diminished ventilation.

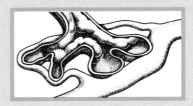

escape. The patient develops a barrel chest and hyperresonance to percussion.

Mucus fills the lung bases, inhibiting alveolar ventilation. Blood is shunted to alveoli in other lung parts, but still can't compensate for diminished ventilation.

Hyperventilation is triggered by lung receptors to increase lung volume because of trapped air and obstructions. Intrapleural and alveolar gas pressures rise, causing a decreased

Looking at a bronchiole in asthma

Asthma is characterized by broncho-spasms, increased mucus secretion, and mucosal edema, which contribute to airway narrowing and obstruction. Shown here is a normal bronchiole in cross section and an obstructed bronchiole, as it occurs in asthma.

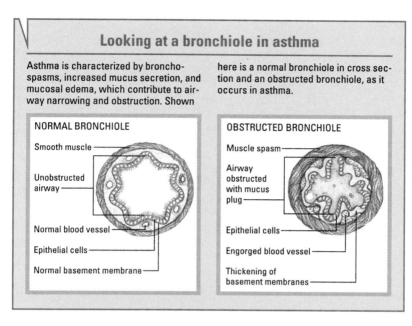

NORMAL BRONCHIOLE

- Smooth muscle
- Unobstructed airway
- Normal blood vessel
- Epithelial cells
- Normal basement membrane

OBSTRUCTED BRONCHIOLE

- Muscle spasm
- Airway obstructed with mucus plug
- Epithelial cells
- Engorged blood vessel
- Thickening of basement membranes

perfusion of alveoli. Increased alveolar gas pressure, decreased ventilation, and decreased perfusion result in uneven ventilation perfusion ($\dot{V}/\dot{Q}$) ratios and mismatching within different lung segments.

Hypoxemia triggers hyperventilation by stimulation of the respiratory center, which in turn decreases partial pressure of arterial carbon dioxide ($Paco_2$) and increases pH, resulting in a respiratory alkalosis. As the obstruction to the airways increases in severity, more alveoli are affected. $\dot{V}/\dot{Q}$ remains inadequate and CO_2 retention develops. Respiratory acidosis results and respiratory failure occurs.

When status asthmaticus occurs, hypoxemia worsens and expiratory flows and volumes decrease even further. Obstructed airways impede gas exchange and increase airway resistance. The patient labors to breathe. As

breathing and hypoxemia tire the patient, respiratory rate drops to normal, $Paco_2$ levels rise and the patient hypoventilates from exhaustion. Respiratory acidosis begins as partial pressure of arterial oxygen (Pao_2) levels drop and $Paco_2$ continues to rise. Acidosis develops as arterial CO_2 increases. The situation becomes life-threatening as no air becomes audible upon auscultation (a silent chest) and $Paco_2$ rises to over 70 mm Hg. Without treatment, the patient experiences acute respiratory failure.

Comprehensive assessment

An asthma attack may begin dramatically, with simultaneous onset of severe, multiple symptoms, or insidiously, with gradually increasing respiratory distress. Typically, the patient reports exposure to a particular allergen followed by a sudden onset of dyspnea, wheezing, and tightness in the chest accompanied by a cough that produces thick, clear or yellow sputum. The patient may complain of feeling suffocated and be visibly dyspneic, able to speak only a few words before pausing to catch his breath. He may use accessory muscles to breathe, sweat profusely, and exhibit an increased anteroposterior thoracic diameter.

Percussion may produce hyperresonance. Palpation may reveal vocal fremitus. Auscultation may disclose tachycardia, tachypnea, mild systolic hypertension, harsh respirations with inspiratory and expiratory wheezes, prolonged expiratory phase of respiration, and diminished breath sounds. Cyanosis, confusion, and lethargy commonly suggest status asthmaticus and respiratory failure.

Patients with asthma will vary in assessment, depending on the degree of the attack being experienced. Patients experiencing status asthmaticus typically have continuous signs and symptoms that include:

■ marked respiratory distress due to failure of compensatory mechanisms and decreased oxygenation levels

■ marked wheezing due to increased edema and increased mucus in the lower airways

ALERT *Be alert for the patient who was previously wheezing but then suddenly stops wheezing and continues to show signs of respiratory distress. In this case the absence of wheezing may be due to severe bronchial constriction that narrows the airways severely during inhalation and exhalation. As a result, so little air passes through the narrowed airways that no sound is made. This dangerous event signals the possibility of imminent respiratory collapse.*

■ absent breath sounds due to severe bronchoconstriction and edema

■ pulsus paradoxus greater than 10 mm Hg

■ chest wall contractions due to use of accessory muscles.

Diagnosis

These tests help diagnose status asthmaticus:

■ Pulmonary function studies reveal signs of airway obstructive disease, low-normal or decreased vital capacity, and increased total lung and residual capacities. (Pulmonary function may be normal between attacks). PaO_2 and $PaCO_2$ usually are decreased, except in severe asthma, when $PaCO_2$ may be normal or increased, indicating severe bronchial obstruction.

■ Peak end expiratory flow rate reveals a reading less than 60% of patient's baseline.

■ Pulse oximetry typically reveals an arterial oxygen saturation of less than 90%

■ Chest X-rays may show hyperinflation with areas of atelectasis and flat diaphragm due to increased intrathoracic volume, provide evidence to rule out other causes of respiratory failure, and can be used to diagnose or monitor the progress of asthma.

■ Arterial blood gas (ABG) analysis detects hypoxemia; initially PaO_2 is normal and then decreases with continued $\dot{V}/\dot{Q}$ mismatching; $PaCO_2$ is decreased early on because of hyperventilation but then increases as respiratory distress continues.

■ Electrocardiography shows sinus tachycardia during an attack; severe attack may show signs of cor pulmonale (right axis deviation, peaked P wave) that resolve after the attack.

- Serum IgE levels may increase from an allergic reaction.

- Sputum analysis may indicate increased viscosity, actual mucus plugs, presence of Curschmann's spirals (casts of airways), Charcot-Leyden crystals, and eosinophils; culture may identify causative organism if infection was the trigger.

- Complete blood count with differential reveals increased eosinophil count secondary to inflammation.

Collaborations

A multidisciplinary approach to care is essential. Most likely, emergency department personnel will be the first to see the patient. As a result of the patient's severe respiratory compromise, respiratory therapy will be closely involved. Most likely, an allergy and asthma specialist or pulmonologist will be consulted to assist with providing ongoing care as well as identifying causative factors and helping the patient alleviate or control them.

Treatment and care

In acute status asthmaticus, the patient is monitored closely for respiratory failure. Oxygen, bronchodilators, epinephrine, corticosteroids, and nebulizer therapies are administered as ordered. The patient may be intubated and placed on mechanical ventilation if his $PaCO_2$ rises or if respiratory arrest occurs.

Correcting asthma typically involves:

- prevention, by identifying and avoiding precipitating factors such as environmental allergens or irritants, which is the best treatment

- desensitization to specific antigens — helpful if the stimuli can't be removed entirely — which decreases the severity of attacks of asthma with future exposure

- bronchodilators (such as epinephrine, albuterol, metaproterenol, and terbutaline) to decrease bronchoconstriction, reduce bronchial airway edema, and increase pulmonary ventilation

- anticholinergics to increase the effects of bronchodilators

- corticosteroids (such as hydrocortisone and methylprednisolone) to decrease bronchoconstriction, reduce bronchial airway edema, and increase pulmonary ventilation

- subcutaneous epinephrine to counteract the effects of mediators of an asthma attack

- mast cell stabilizers (cromolyn sodium and nedocromil sodium), effective in patients with atopic asthma who have seasonal disease. When given prophylactically, they block the acute obstructive effects of antigen exposure by inhibiting the degranulation of mast cells, thereby preventing the release of chemical mediators responsible for anaphylaxis

- humidified oxygen, which may be needed to treat dyspnea, cyanosis, and hypoxemia to maintain oxygen saturation at greater than 90%

- mechanical ventilation — necessary if the patient doesn't respond to initial ventilatory support and drugs, or develops respiratory failure

- relaxation exercises to help increase circulation and to help a patient recover from an asthma attack.

Complications

Status asthmaticus may lead to these complications:

- arrhythmias
- metabolic acidosis
- barotrauma (if mechanical ventilation is required)
- respiratory failure.

Nursing considerations

- To reverse hypoxemia, administer oxygen as ordered at appropriate concentrations to maintain PaO_2 at a minimum pressure range of 50 to 60 mm Hg.
- Assess the patient's vital signs and respiratory status initially every 5 to 15 minutes and then less frequently as the patient's condition improves. Auscultate lungs for decreases in adventitious breath sounds. Observe for a positive response to oxygen therapy, such as improved breathing, color, and oximetry and ABG values.

ALERT *Remember that oxygen can be toxic and directly injure the lung if given too long or at excessive concentrations. Therefore, use the lowest fraction of inspired oxygen necessary to maintain adequate oxygenation for the shortest time possible.*

- Place the patient in a semi-Fowler's to high-Fowler's position to maximize lung expansion. Encourage slow deep breaths through pursed lips.

AGE ISSUE *If the patient is a child, the child and parents may find it more comforting for the child to sit on one of the parent's lap. The exception would be the child in impending respiratory failure.*

- Monitor oxygen saturation levels and ABG results for changes. Anticipate the need for endotracheal intubation and mechanical ventilation if PaO_2 continues to fall or $PaCO_2$ rises.
- If the patient requires mechanical ventilation, expect to use high inspiratory flow rates with minimal to no positive end-expiratory pressure. Monitor the patient closely for signs and symptoms of barotrauma.

ALERT *Due to expiratory airflow obstruction in status asthmaticus, gas is trapped and the alveoli become hyperinflated. Use of positive pressure ventilation can increase airway pressures, reducing alveolar emptying, thus increasing hyperinflation.*

- Administer beta-adrenergic agonist bronchodilators as ordered, I.V. or via intermittent (every 20 to 30 minutes) or continuous nebulization. Institute continuous cardiac monitoring to detect possible arrhythmias secondary to hypoxemia or bronchodilators.

AGE ISSUE *A child may be more compliant with oxygen and nebulizer therapy if his imagination can be spurred. For example, an oxygen mask with a bag reservoir resembles Santa's beard, or a space mask; if the child won't cooperate with these constrictive devices, flow-by oxygen can be implemented using the corrugated oxygen tubing inserted through a Styrofoam cup and held so that the child still receives the therapy.*

- Give corticosteroids I.V. as ordered to aid in reducing airway inflammation.
- Anticipate the need for an anticholinergic agent such as ipratropium given via nebulization, which may be ordered to supplement the action of the beta-adrenergic agonists and corticosteroids in patients not responding to these agents.

■ Administer I.V. fluids as ordered to liquefy secretions and replace insensible fluid lost via hyperventilation.

■ Monitor intake and output closely. Encourage intake of oral fluids when the patient is able to tolerate them.

■ Encourage the patient to cough at frequent intervals to help loosen secretions. After the acute phase is over, perform chest physiotherapy to help loosen secretions.

ALERT *During the acute phase of status asthmaticus, chest physiotherapy is contraindicated because of the patient's respiratory distress as well as the hyperreactiveness of his airways.*

■ Reassure the patient and stay with him. Assist him to relax as much as possible.

ALERT *Unless the patient is extremely agitated and is unable to cooperate with therapy, avoid the use of sedatives because these agents depress the central nervous system.*

■ Encourage the patient to express his fears and concerns about his illness. Answer his questions honestly. Encourage him to identify and comply with care measures and activities that promote relaxation.

Patient teaching

■ Instruct the patient in medications, including proper use of metered dose inhaler, daily peak flow monitoring, and measures to control asthma based on the peak flow readings.

■ Teach the patient and his family about diaphragmatic and pursed-lip breathing as appropriate. Advise him to perform relaxation exercises.

■ Teach the patient symptoms of cushingoid adverse effects from long-term corticosteroid therapy to report to his physician.

■ To prevent recurring attacks, instruct the patient about proper breathing techniques. Stress the need for fluid intake and a well-balanced diet. Advise him to avoid triggers, such as dust or pollen, to wear a mask if cold weather precipitates bronchospasm, to stay indoors when the outside air quality is poor, and to avoid contact with people who have respiratory infections.

Thoracic surgery

Thoracic surgery refers to the surgical opening of the chest. Thoracotomy, a surgical incision into the thoracic cavity, is done to perform a biopsy, to remove diseased lung tissue, or to locate and examine abnormalities, such as tumors, bleeding sites, or thoracic injuries. It's most commonly used to remove part or all of a lung to spare healthy lung tissue from disease. Other types of thoracic surgeries are performed for numerous reasons. Lung excision may involve pneumonectomy, lobectomy, segmental resection, or wedge resection.

A pneumonectomy is the excision of an entire lung. It's usually performed to treat bronchogenic cancer but may also be used to treat tuberculosis, bronchiectasis, or lung abscess. Pneumonectomy is used only when a less radical approach can't remove all diseased tissue. After pneumonectomy, chest cavity pressures stabilize and, over time, fluid fills the cavity where lung tissue was removed, preventing significant mediastinal shift.

Types of lung excision

Lung excision may be total (pneumonectomy), or partial (lobectomy, segmental resection, or wedge resection), depending on the patient's condition. The illustrations here show the extent of each of these surgeries for the right lung.

PNEUMONECTOMY

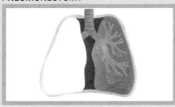

SEGMENTAL RESECTION

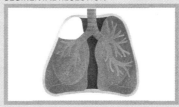

LOBECTOMY

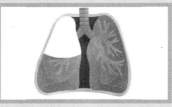

WEDGE RESECTION

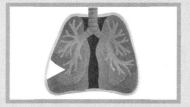

Lobectomy — the removal of one of the five lung lobes — is used to treat bronchogenic cancer, tuberculosis, lung abscess, emphysematous blebs, benign tumors, or localized fungal infections. After this surgery, the remaining lobes expand to fill the entire pleural cavity.

A segmental resection is the removal of one or more lung segments. This procedure preserves more functional tissue than lobectomy; it's commonly used to treat bronchiectasis.

The removal of a small portion of the lung without regard to segments, wedge resection preserves the most functional tissue of all the surgeries but can treat only a small, well-circumscribed lesion. Remaining lung tissue should be reexpanded. (See *Types of lung excision*.)

Other types of thoracic surgeries include:

■ *exploratory thoracotomy*, which is used to examine the chest and pleural space in evaluating chest trauma and tumors

■ *decortication*, which is used to help reexpand the lung in a patient with empyema (It involves removing or stripping the thick, fibrous membrane covering the visceral pleura.)

■ *thoracoplasty*, which is performed to remove part or all of one rib and to reduce the size of the chest cavity (It decreases the risk of mediastinal shift when tuberculosis has reduced lung volume.)

■ *bronchoplastic (sleeve) reduction,* which involves the excision of one lobar bronchus along with part of the right or left bronchus (The distal bronchus is then reanastomosed to the proximal bronchus or trachea.)

■ *lung reduction surgery,* which is used to treat emphysema. (Excision of giant bullae is performed, thereby reducing lung volume and allowing compressed alveoli to reexpand.)

Procedure

After the patient is anesthetized, the surgeon performs a thoracotomy using one of three approaches.

■ In a *posterolateral thoracotomy,* the incision starts in the submammary fold of the anterior chest, is drawn below the scapular tip and along the ribs, and then is curved posteriorly and up to the spine of the scapula. Any type of lung excision calls for a posterolateral incision through the fourth, fifth, sixth, or seventh intercostal space.

■ In an *anterolateral thoracotomy,* the incision begins below the breast and above the costal margins, extending from the anterior axillary line and then turning downward to avoid the axillary apex.

■ A *median sternotomy* involves a straight incision from the suprasternal notch to below the xiphoid process and requires the sternum to be transected with an electric or air-driven saw.

After the incision is made, the surgeon takes a biopsy, locates and ties off sources of bleeding, locates and repairs injuries within the thoracic cavity, or spreads the ribs and exposes the lung area for excision. For a pneumonectomy, the pulmonary arteries are ligated and severed. Next, the surgeon clamps the mainstem bronchus leading to the affected lung, divides it, and then closes it with nonabsorbable sutures or staples. He then removes the lung. To ensure airtight closure, he places a pleural flap over the bronchus and closes it. He then severs the phrenic nerve on the affected side, allowing it to reduce the size of the pleural cavity. After air pressure in the cavity stabilizes, he closes the chest.

In a lobectomy, the surgeon resects the affected lobe and ligates and severs the appropriate arteries, veins, and bronchial passages. He may insert one or two chest tubes for drainage and to aid lung reexpansion.

In a segmental resection, the surgeon removes the affected segment and ligates and severs the appropriate artery, vein, and bronchus. In a wedge resection, he clamps and excises the affected area and then sutures it. In both resections, he inserts two chest tubes to aid lung reexpansion.

After completing the procedure requiring the thoracotomy, the surgeon closes the chest cavity and applies a dressing.

Complications

Potential complications of thoracotomy include:

■ hemorrhage, infection, and tension pneumothorax

■ bronchopleural fistula and empyema.

A lung excision may also cause a persistent air space that the remaining lung tissue doesn't expand to fill. Removal of up to three ribs may be necessary to reduce chest cavity size and allow lung tissue to fit the space.

Nursing considerations

When caring for a patient undergoing a thoracotomy, your main responsibilities include patient teaching and postoperative care and monitoring.

Before thoracic surgery

■ Explain the procedure to the patient, and inform him that he'll receive a general anesthetic. Prepare him psychologically, according to his condition. A patient having a lung biopsy, for example, faces the fear of cancer as well as the fear of surgery and needs ongoing emotional support. In contrast, a patient with a chronic lung disorder, such as tuberculosis or a fungal infection, may view having a lung excision as a cure for his condition.

■ Inform the patient about postoperative events, such as chest tube insertion and oxygen therapy.

■ Teach him coughing and deep-breathing techniques, explaining that these will be used after surgery to facilitate lung reexpansion. Teach him how to use an incentive spirometer; record the volumes he achieves to provide a baseline.

■ Arrange for appropriate laboratory tests and ensure that the results are on the patient's medical record. For example, tests to assess cardiac function may include pulmonary function tests, electrocardiography, chest X-ray, arterial blood gas (ABG) analysis, bronchoscopy and, possibly, cardiac catheterization.

■ Ensure that the patient or a responsible family member has signed a consent form.

After thoracic surgery

■ Assess vital signs, cardiopulmonary status, and hemodynamic status frequently, at least every 15 minutes for the first hour and then every 30 minutes for the next hour, and then hourly as indicated. Auscultate heart and lung sounds for changes.

■ Monitor oxygen saturation levels and obtain ABGs as ordered. Administer oxygen as ordered based on results of pulse oximetry and ABGs.

■ Anticipate the need for continuous cardiac monitoring to detect possible arrhythmias.

■ Monitor chest tube insertion site and assess drainage amount and character frequently, at least every hour initially and then as ordered and indicated by the patient's condition. (See "Chest drainage," page 181.)

■ Ensure proper chest tube functioning.

ALERT *Monitor the patient for signs of tension pneumothorax, such as dyspnea, chest pain, an irritating cough, vertigo, syncope, or anxiety. If he develops any of these symptoms, palpate his neck, face, and chest wall for subcutaneous emphysema and palpate his trachea for deviation from midline. Auscultate his lungs for decreased or absent breath sounds on the affected side. Then percuss them for hyperresonance. If you suspect tension pneumothorax, notify the physician at once and help him to identify the cause.*

■ Inspect the surgical incision site dressing. Notify the physician if drainage on the dressing is bright red or increases in amount.

■ If the patient had a pneumonectomy, position him only on his operative side or his back until he's stabilized. This prevents fluid from draining into the unaffected lung if the sutured bronchus opens.

■ Administer analgesics as ordered for pain relief.

■ Have the patient begin coughing, deep-breathing exercises, and incentive spirometry as soon as he's stabilized. Auscultate his lungs, place him in semi-Fowler's position, and have him splint his incision to facilitate coughing and deep breathing. Have him cough every 2 to 4 hours until his breath sounds clear.

■ Perform passive range-of-motion (ROM) exercises the evening of surgery and two or three times daily thereafter. Progress to active ROM exercises. Assist with early ambulation.

■ Teach the patient to continue his coughing and deep-breathing exercises to prevent complications. Advise him to report any changes in sputum characteristics to his physician.

■ Instruct the patient to continue performing ROM exercises to maintain mobility of his shoulder and chest wall.

■ Provide the patient with instructions for wound care and dressing changes, and refer him to home health care as needed.

Tracheal cuff-pressure measurement

An endotracheal (ET) or tracheostomy cuff provides a closed system for mechanical ventilation, allowing a desired tidal volume to be delivered to the patient's lungs. To function properly, the cuff must exert enough pressure on the tracheal wall to seal the airway without compromising the blood supply to the tracheal mucosa.

The ideal pressure (known as *minimal occlusive volume*) is the lowest amount needed to seal the airway. Many authorities recommend maintaining a cuff pressure lower than venous perfusion pressure — usually 16 to 24 cm H_2O. (More than 24 cm H_2O may exceed venous perfusion pressure.) Actual cuff pressure will vary with each patient, however.

Equipment
10-ml syringe ■ three-way stopcock ■ cuff pressure manometer ■ stethoscope ■ suction equipment ■ gloves

Essential steps
■ Assemble all equipment at the patient's bedside. If measuring with a blood pressure manometer, attach the syringe to one stopcock port; then attach the tubing from the manometer to another port of the stopcock. Turn off the stopcock port where you'll be connecting the pilot balloon cuff so that air can't escape from the cuff. Use the syringe to instill air into the manometer tubing until the pressure reading reaches 10 mm Hg. This will prevent sudden cuff deflation when you open the stopcock to the cuff and the manometer.

■ Explain the procedure to the patient. Put on gloves and suction the ET or tracheostomy tube and the patient's oropharynx to remove accumulated secretions above the cuff. Then attach the cuff pressure manometer to the pilot balloon port.

■ Place the diaphragm of the stethoscope over the trachea and listen for an air leak.

ALERT *Slow deflation allows positive lung pressure to push secretions upward from the bronchi. Cuff deflation may also stimulate the patient's cough reflex, producing additional secretions.*

ALERT *Remember, a smooth, hollow sound indicates a sealed airway; a loud, gurgling sound indicates an air leak.*

■ If you don't hear an air leak, press the button under the dial of the cuff pressure manometer to slowly release air from the balloon on the tracheal tube and auscultate for an air leak.

■ As soon as you hear an air leak, release the button and gently squeeze the handle of the cuff pressure manometer to inflate the cuff. Continue to add air to the cuff until you no longer hear an air leak.

■ When the air leak ceases, read the dial on the cuff pressure manometer. This is the minimal pressure required to effectively occlude the trachea around the tracheal tube. In many cases, this pressure will fall within the green area (16 to 24 cm H_2O) on the manometer dial.

■ Disconnect the cuff pressure manometer from the pilot balloon port.

■ Document the pressure value.

ALERT *If pressure exceeds 25 mm Hg, notify the physician because you may need to change to a larger size tube, use higher inflation pressures, or permit a larger air leak. Recommended cuff pressure is about 18 mm Hg.*

Complications
Aspiration of upper airway secretions, underventilation, or coughing spasms

may occur if a leak is created during cuff pressure measurement.

Nursing considerations
■ Measure cuff pressure at least every 8 hours to avoid overinflation.

■ Keep in mind that some patients require less pressure, whereas others — for example, those with tracheal malacia (an abnormal softening of the tracheal tissue) — require more pressure. Maintaining the cuff pressure at the lowest possible level will minimize cuff-related problems.

■ When measuring cuff pressure, keep the connection between the measuring device and the pilot balloon port tight to avoid an air leak that could compromise cuff pressure. If you're using a stopcock, don't leave the manometer in the OFF position because air will leak from the cuff if the syringe accidentally comes off. Note the volume of air needed to inflate the cuff.

ALERT *Suspect a leak if injection of air fails to inflate the cuff or increase cuff pressure, if you're unable to inject the amount of air you withdrew, if the patient can speak, if ventilation fails to maintain adequate respiratory movement with pressures or volumes previously considered adequate, or if air escapes during the ventilator's inspiratory cycle.*

ALERT *A gradual increase in this volume indicates tracheal dilation or erosion. A sudden increase in volume indicates rupture of the cuff and requires immediate reintubation if the patient is being ventilated.*

■ Record the date and time of the measurement, total amount of air in cuff after the procedure, cuff pressure, any complications and actions taken, and patient's tolerance of the procedure.

Tracheal suction

Tracheal suction involves the removal of secretions from the trachea or bronchi by means of a catheter inserted through the mouth or nose, a tracheal stoma, a tracheostomy tube, or an endotracheal (ET) tube. In addition to removing secretions, tracheal suctioning also stimulates the cough reflex. This procedure helps maintain a patent airway to promote optimal exchange of oxygen and carbon dioxide and to prevent pneumonia that results from pooling of secretions. Performed as frequently as the patient's condition warrants, tracheal suction calls for strict aseptic technique.

Equipment
Oxygen source (wall or portable unit and handheld resuscitation bag with a mask, 15-mm adapter, or a positive end-expiratory pressure [PEEP] valve, if indicated) ■ wall or portable suction apparatus ■ collection container ■ connecting tube ■ suction catheter kit, or a sterile suction catheter, one sterile glove, one clean glove, and a disposable sterile solution container ■ 1-L bottle of sterile water or normal saline solution ■ sterile water-soluble lubricant (for nasal insertion) ■ syringe for deflating cuff of ET or tracheostomy tube ■ waterproof trash bag ■ optional: sterile towel

Essential steps
■ Before suctioning, determine whether your facility requires a physician's order and obtain one, if necessary.

■ Choose a suction catheter of appropriate size, one whose diameter is no larger than half the inside diameter of the tracheostomy or ET tube to minimize hypoxemia during suctioning. (A #12 or #14 French catheter may be used for an 8-mm or larger tube.) Place the suction apparatus on the patient's overbed table or bedside stand. Position the table or stand on your preferred side of the bed to facilitate suctioning.

■ Attach the collection container to the suction unit and the connecting tube to the collection container. Label and date the normal saline solution or sterile water. Open the waterproof trash bag.

■ Assess the patient's vital signs, breath sounds, and general appearance to establish a baseline for comparison after suctioning. Review the patient's arterial blood gas values and oxygen saturation levels and evaluate the patient's ability to cough and deep-breathe because this will help move secretions up the tracheobronchial tree.

◄ ALERT *If nasotracheal suctioning is ordered, check the patient's history for a deviated septum, nasal polyps, nasal obstruction, nasal trauma, epistaxis, or mucosal swelling to prevent injury during suctioning.*

■ Wash your hands. Explain the procedure to the patient even if he's unresponsive. Tell him that suctioning usually causes transient coughing or gagging but that coughing is helpful for removal of secretions. If the patient has been suctioned previously, summarize the reasons for suctioning. Continue to reassure the patient throughout the procedure to minimize anxiety, promote relaxation, and decrease oxygen demand.

■ Unless contraindicated, place the patient in semi-Fowler's or high Fowler's position to promote lung expansion and productive coughing.

■ Remove the top from the normal saline solution or water bottle.

■ Open the package containing the sterile solution container.

■ Using sterile technique, open the suction catheter kit and put on the gloves. If using individual supplies, open the suction catheter and the gloves, placing the nonsterile glove on your nondominant hand and then the sterile glove on your dominant hand.

■ Using your nondominant (nonsterile) hand, pour the normal saline solution or sterile water into the solution container.

■ Place a small amount of water-soluble lubricant on the sterile area. Lubricant may be used to facilitate passage of the catheter during nasotracheal suctioning.

■ Place a sterile towel over the patient's chest, if desired, to provide an additional sterile area.

■ Using your dominant (sterile) hand, remove the catheter from its wrapper. Keep it coiled so it can't touch a nonsterile object. Using your other hand to manipulate the connecting tubing, attach the catheter to the tubing.

■ Using your nondominant hand, set the suction pressure according to facility policy. Typically, pressure may be set between 80 and 100 mm Hg.

ALERT *Higher pressures don't enhance secretion removal and may cause traumatic injury.*

■ Occlude the suction port to assess suction pressure.

■ Dip the catheter tip in the saline solution to lubricate the outside of the catheter and reduce tissue trauma during insertion.

■ With the catheter tip in the sterile solution, occlude the control valve with the thumb of your nondominant hand. Suction a small amount of solution through the catheter to lubricate the inside of the catheter, thus facilitating passage of secretions through it.

■ For nasal insertion of the catheter, lubricate the tip of the catheter with the sterile, water-soluble lubricant to reduce tissue trauma during insertion.

■ Preoxygenate the patient.
  – If the patient isn't intubated or is intubated but isn't receiving supplemental oxygen or aerosol, instruct him to take three to six deep breaths to help minimize or prevent hypoxia during suctioning.
  – If the patient isn't intubated but is receiving oxygen, evaluate his need for preoxygenation. If indicated, instruct him to take three to six deep breaths while using his supplemental oxygen. (If needed, the patient may continue to receive supplemental oxygen during suctioning by leaving his nasal cannula in one nostril or by keeping the oxygen mask over his mouth.)
  – If the patient is being mechanically ventilated, preoxygenate him using either a handheld resuscitation bag or the sigh mode on the ventilator. To use the resuscitation bag, set the oxygen flow meter at 15 L/minute, disconnect the patient from the ventilator, and deliver three to six breaths with the resuscitation bag.

– If the patient is being maintained on PEEP, use a resuscitation bag with a PEEP valve.

– To pre-oxygenate using the ventilator, first adjust the fraction of inspired oxygen (FIO_2) and tidal volume according to facility policy and patient need. Then, either use the sigh mode or manually deliver three to six breaths. If you have an assistant for the procedure, the assistant can manage the patient's oxygen needs while you perform the suctioning.

■ If the patient isn't intubated and nasotracheal suctioning is ordered:
– Disconnect the oxygen from the patient, if applicable.
– Using your nondominant hand, raise the tip of the patient's nose to straighten the passageway and facilitate insertion of the catheter.
– Insert the catheter into the patient's nostril while gently rolling it between your fingers to help it advance through the turbinates.
– As the patient inhales, quickly advance the catheter as far as possible.

ALERT *To avoid oxygen loss and tissue trauma, don't apply suction during insertion.*

– If the patient coughs as the catheter passes through the larynx, briefly hold the catheter still and then resume advancement when the patient inhales.
■ If the patient is intubated:
– Using your nonsterile hand, disconnect the patient from the ventilator.
– Using your sterile hand, gently insert the suction catheter into the artificial airway, advancing the catheter, without applying suction,

until meeting resistance. If the patient coughs, pause briefly and then resume advancement.
– Alternatively, use a closed system. (See *Closed tracheal suctioning,* page 256.)
■ After inserting the catheter, apply suction intermittently by removing and replacing the thumb of your nondominant hand over the control valve. Simultaneously use your dominant hand to withdraw the catheter as you roll it between your thumb and forefinger. This rotating motion prevents the catheter from pulling tissue into the tube as it exits, thus avoiding tissue trauma.

ALERT *Never suction more than 10 seconds at a time to prevent hypoxemia.*

■ If the patient is intubated, use your nondominant hand to stabilize the tip of the ET tube as you withdraw the catheter to prevent mucous membrane irritation or accidental extubation.
■ If applicable, resume oxygen delivery by reconnecting the source of oxygen or ventilation and hyperoxygenating the patient's lungs before continuing to prevent or relieve hypoxemia.
■ Observe the patient and allow him to rest for a few minutes before the next suctioning. The timing of each suctioning and the length of each rest period depend on his tolerance of the procedure and the absence of complications. To enhance secretion removal, encourage the patient to cough between suctioning attempts.
■ After suctioning, hyperoxygenate the patient being maintained on a ventilator with the handheld resuscitation bag or by using the ventilator's sigh mode, as described earlier. Readjust the FIO_2 and, for ventilated patients,

Closed tracheal suctioning

The closed tracheal suction system can ease the removal of secretions and reduce patient complications. Consisting of a sterile suction catheter in a clear plastic sleeve, the system permits the patient to remain connected to the ventilator during suctioning.

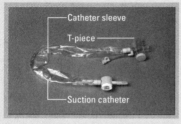

Catheter sleeve

T-piece

Suction catheter

As a result, the patient can maintain the tidal volume, oxygen concentration, and positive end-expiratory pressure delivered by the ventilator while being suctioned. In turn, this reduces the risk of suction-induced hypoxemia.

Another advantage of this system is a reduced risk of infection, even when the same catheter is used numerous times. The caregiver doesn't need to touch the catheter and the ventilator circuit remains closed.

To perform the closed tracheal suctioning, follow these steps:
● Gather a closed-suction control valve, a T-piece to connect the artificial airway to the ventilator breathing circuit, and a catheter sleeve that encloses the catheter and has connections at each end for the control valve and T-piece.
● Remove the closed-suction system from its wrapping and attach the control valve to the connecting tubing.
● Depress the thumb-suction control valve, keeping it depressed while setting the suction pressure to the desired level.
● Connect the T-piece to the ventilator breathing circuit, making sure that the irrigation port is closed, and then connect

the T-piece to the patient's endotracheal or tracheostomy tube, as shown.

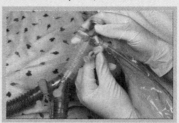

● With one hand keeping the T-piece parallel to the patient's chin, use the thumb and index finger of the other hand to advance the catheter through the tube and into the patient's tracheobronchial tree, as shown. It may be necessary to gently retract the catheter sleeve as the catheter is advanced.

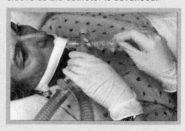

● While continuing to hold the T-piece and control valve, apply intermittent suction and withdraw the catheter until it reaches its fully extended length in the sleeve. Repeat as necessary.
● After suctioning is finished, flush the catheter by maintaining suction while slowly introducing normal saline or sterile water into the irrigation port.
● Place the thumb control valve in the OFF position.
● Dispose of and replace the suction equipment and supplies according to your facility's policy.
● Change the closed-suction system every 24 hours to minimize the risk of infection.

the tidal volume to the ordered settings.

■ After suctioning the lower airway, assess the patient's need for upper airway suctioning.

ALERT *If the cuff of the ET or tracheostomy tube is inflated, suction the upper airway before deflating the cuff with a syringe. Always change the catheter and sterile glove before suctioning the lower airway to avoid introducing microorganisms into the lower airway.*

■ Discard the gloves and catheter in the waterproof trash bag. Clear the connecting tubing by aspirating the remaining saline solution or water. Discard and replace suction equipment and supplies according to your facility's policy. Wash your hands.

Complications

Potential complications of tracheal suction include:

■ hypoxemia and dyspnea, which may occur due to oxygen being removed along with secretions

■ anxiety, which may alter the patient's respiratory patterns

■ cardiac arrhythmias, which can result from hypoxia and stimulation of the vagus nerve in the tracheobronchial tree

■ tracheal or bronchial trauma, which can result from traumatic or prolonged suctioning.

Nursing considerations

■ Auscultate the lungs bilaterally and take vital signs, if indicated, to assess the procedure's effectiveness.

■ During suctioning, observe the secretions. If they're thick, clear the catheter periodically by dipping the tip in the saline solution and applying

suction. Normally, sputum is watery and tends to be sticky. Tenacious or thick sputum usually indicates dehydration. Watch for color variations.

■ Keep in mind that white or translucent color is normal; yellow indicates pus; green indicates retained secretions or *Pseudomonas* infection; brown usually indicates old blood; red indicates fresh blood; and a "red currant jelly" appearance indicates *Klebsiella* infection.

■ When sputum contains blood, note whether it's streaked or well mixed. Indicate how often blood appeared.

■ If the patient's heart rate and rhythm are being monitored, observe for arrhythmias. If they occur, stop suctioning and ventilate the patient.

■ Raise the patient's nose into the sniffing position to help align the larynx and pharynx and facilitate passing the catheter during nasotracheal suctioning. If the patient's condition permits, have an assistant extend the patient's head and neck above his shoulders. The patient's lower jaw should be moved up and forward. If the patient is responsive, ask him to stick out his tongue so he won't be able to swallow the catheter during insertion.

■ During suctioning, advance the catheter typically as far as the mainstem bronchi. However, because of tracheobronchial anatomy, the catheter tends to enter the right mainstem bronchi instead of the left. Using an angled catheter (such as a coudé) may help you guide the catheter into the left mainstem bronchus. Rotating the patient's head to the right seems to have a limited effect.

■ Don't allow the collection container on the suction machine to become more than three-quarters full to keep from damaging the machine.

■ Use caution when suctioning patients who have increased intracranial pressure because suction may increase pressure further.

■ If the patient experiences laryngospasm or bronchospasm (rare) during suctioning, discuss with the patient's physician about the use of bronchodilators or lidocaine to reduce the risk.

■ Document the date and time of suctioning; the technique used; reason for suctioning; amount, color, consistency, and odor of secretions; any complications and actions to correct them; the patient's tolerance of procedure; and evidence of effectiveness of procedure.

Tracheostomy care

Whether a tracheotomy is performed in an emergency situation or after careful preparation, as a permanent measure or as temporary therapy, follow-up care has identical goals: to ensure airway patency by keeping the tube free from mucus buildup, to maintain mucous membrane and skin integrity, to prevent infection, and to provide psychological support.

The patient may have one of three types of tracheostomy tube — uncuffed, cuffed, or fenestrated. Tube selection depends on the patient's condition and the physician's preference.

An *uncuffed* tube, which may be plastic or metal, allows air to flow freely around the tracheostomy tube and through the larynx, reducing the risk of tracheal damage. A *cuffed* tube, made of plastic, is disposable. The cuff and the tube won't separate accidentally inside the trachea because the cuff is bonded to the tube. Also, it doesn't require periodic deflating to lower pressure because cuff pressure is low and evenly distributed against the tracheal wall. Although cuffed tubes may cost more than other tubes, they reduce the risk of tracheal damage. A plastic *fenestrated* tube permits speech through the upper airway when the external opening is capped and the cuff is deflated. It also allows easy removal of the inner cannula for cleaning. However, a fenestrated tube may become occluded.

Whichever tube is used, tracheostomy care should be performed using aseptic technique until the stoma has healed to prevent infection. As part of tracheostomy care you may be required to deflate and inflate a tracheostomy cuff. (See *Deflating and inflating a tracheostomy cuff.*)

For recently performed tracheotomies, use sterile gloves for all manipulations at the tracheostomy site. When the stoma has healed, clean gloves may be substituted for sterile ones.

Equipment

For aseptic stoma and outer-cannula care

Waterproof trash bag ■ two sterile solution containers ■ normal saline solution ■ hydrogen peroxide ■ sterile cotton-tipped applicators ■ sterile 4″ × 4″ gauze pads ■ sterile gloves ■ prepackaged sterile tracheostomy dressing (or 4″ × 4″ gauze pad) ■ equipment and supplies for suctioning and for mouth care ■ water-soluble lubricant or topical antibiotic cream ■ materials as

Deflating and inflating a tracheostomy cuff

As part of tracheostomy care, you may be required to deflate and inflate a tracheostomy cuff. If so, gather a 5-ml or 10-ml syringe, padded hemostat, and stethoscope and follow these steps:

1. Read the cuff manufacturer's instructions because cuff types and procedures vary.

2. Assess the patient's condition, explain the procedure to him, and reassure him. Wash your hands thoroughly.

3. Help the patient into semi-Fowler's position, if possible, or place him in a supine position so secretions above the cuff site will be pushed up into his mouth if he's receiving positive-pressure ventilation.

4. Suction the oropharyngeal cavity to prevent pooled secretions from descending into the trachea after cuff deflation.

5. Release the padded hemostat clamping the cuff inflation tubing, if a hemostat is present.

6. Insert a 5-ml or 10-ml syringe into the cuff pilot balloon and very slowly withdraw all air from the cuff. Leave the syringe attached to the tubing for later reinflation of the cuff.

7. Remove any ventilation device. Suction the lower airway through any existing tube to remove all secretions, and then reconnect the patient to the ventilation device.

8. Maintain cuff deflation for the prescribed time. Observe the patient for adequate ventilation, and suction as necessary. If the patient has difficulty breathing, reinflate the cuff immediately by depressing the syringe plunger very slowly. Use a stethoscope to listen over the trachea for the air leak, then inject the least amount of air needed to achieve an adequate tracheal seal.

9. When inflating the cuff, you may use the minimal-leak technique or the minimal occlusive-volume technique to help gauge the proper inflation point. (For more information, see "Endotracheal intubation," page 193.)

10. If you're inflating the cuff using cuff pressure measurement, be careful not to exceed 25 mm Hg.

11. After you've inflated the cuff, if the tubing doesn't have a one-way valve at the end, clamp the inflation line with a padded hemostat (to protect the tubing) and remove the syringe.

12. Check for a minimal-leak cuff seal. You shouldn't feel air coming from the patient's mouth, nose, or tracheostomy site, and a conscious patient shouldn't be able to speak. Be alert for air leaks from the cuff itself.

13. Note the exact amount of air used to inflate the cuff to detect tracheal malacia if more air is consistently needed.

14. Make sure the patient is comfortable and can easily reach the call button and communication aids.

15. Properly clean or dispose of all equipment, supplies, and trash according to your facility's policy. Replenish any used supplies and make sure all necessary emergency supplies are at the bedside.

needed for cuff procedures and for changing tracheostomy ties

For aseptic inner-cannula care
All of the preceding equipment plus a prepackaged commercial tracheostomy-care set, or sterile forceps ▪ sterile nylon brush ▪ sterile 6″ (15 cm) pipe cleaners ▪ clean gloves ▪ a third sterile solution container ▪ disposable temporary inner cannula (for a patient on a ventilator)

For changing tracheostomy ties
30″ (76-cm) length of tracheostomy twill tape ▪ bandage scissors ▪ sterile gloves ▪ hemostat

For emergency tracheostomy tube replacement
Sterile tracheal dilator or sterile hemostat ▪ sterile obturator that fits the tracheostomy tube in use ▪ extra sterile tracheostomy tube and obturator in appropriate size ▪ suction equipment and supplies (Keep these supplies in full view in the patient's room at all times for easy access in case of emergency. Consider taping an emergency sterile tracheostomy tube in a sterile wrapper to the head of the bed for easy access in an emergency.)

Essential steps
▪ Wash your hands and assemble all equipment and supplies in the patient's room.
— Check the expiration date on each sterile package and inspect the package for tears. Open the waterproof trash bag and place it next to you so that you can avoid reaching across the sterile field or the patient's stoma when discarding soiled items.
— Establish a sterile field near the patient's bed (usually on the overbed table) and place equipment and supplies on it. Pour normal saline solution, hydrogen peroxide, or a mixture of equal parts of both solutions into one of the sterile solution containers; then pour normal saline solution into the second sterile container for rinsing.
— For inner-cannula care, you may use a third sterile solution container to hold the gauze pads and cotton-

tipped applicators saturated with cleaning solution. If you'll be replacing the disposable inner cannula, open the package containing the new inner cannula while maintaining sterile technique.
— Obtain or prepare new tracheostomy ties, if indicated.
▪ Assess the patient's condition to determine his need for care. Prepare the patient.
— Explain the procedure to the patient even if he's unresponsive. Provide privacy.
— Place the patient in semi-Fowler's position (unless it's contraindicated) to decrease abdominal pressure on the diaphragm and promote lung expansion.
— Remove any humidification or ventilation device. Using sterile technique, suction the entire length of the tracheostomy tube to clear the airway of any secretions that may hinder oxygenation. (See "Tracheal suction," page 253.)
— Reconnect the patient to the humidifier or ventilator, if necessary.
▪ To clean the stoma and outer cannula:
— Put on sterile gloves if you aren't already wearing them.
— With your dominant hand, saturate a sterile gauze pad with the cleaning solution. Squeeze out the excess liquid to prevent accidental aspiration. Wipe the patient's neck under the tracheostomy tube flanges and twill tapes.
— Saturate a second pad and wipe until the skin around the tracheostomy is cleaned. Use more pads or cotton-tipped applicators to clean the stoma site and the tube's flanges.

ALERT *The stoma provides an open entry site for microorganisms. Wipe only once with each pad and then discard it to prevent contamination of a clean area with a soiled pad.*

– Rinse debris and peroxide (if used) with one or more sterile 4″ × 4″ gauze pads dampened in normal saline solution. Dry the area thoroughly with additional sterile gauze pads; then apply a new sterile tracheostomy dressing.

– Remove and discard your gloves.

■ To clean a nondisposable inner cannula:

– Put on sterile gloves.

– Using your nondominant hand, remove and discard the patient's tracheostomy dressing. Then, with the same hand, disconnect the ventilator or humidification device and unlock the tracheostomy tube's inner cannula by rotating it counterclockwise. Place the inner cannula in the container of hydrogen peroxide.

– Working quickly, use your dominant hand to scrub the cannula with the sterile nylon brush. If the brush doesn't slide easily into the cannula, use a sterile pipe cleaner.

– Immerse the cannula in the container of normal saline solution and agitate it for about 10 seconds to rinse it thoroughly.

– Inspect the cannula for cleanliness. Repeat the cleaning process if necessary. If it's clean, tap it gently against the inside edge of the sterile container to remove excess liquid and prevent aspiration. Don't dry the outer surface because a thin film of moisture acts as a lubricant during insertion.

– Reinsert the inner cannula into the patient's tracheostomy tube. Lock it in place and then gently pull on it to make sure it's positioned securely. Reconnect the mechanical ventilator. Apply a new sterile tracheostomy dressing.

– If the patient can't tolerate being disconnected from the ventilator for the time it takes to clean the inner cannula, replace the existing inner cannula with a clean one and reattach the mechanical ventilator. Then clean the cannula just removed from the patient and store it in a sterile container the next time.

■ To care for a disposable inner cannula:

– Put on clean gloves.

– Using your dominant hand, remove the patient's inner cannula. After evaluating the secretions in the cannula, discard it properly.

– Pick up the new inner cannula, touching only the outer locking portion. Insert the cannula into the tracheostomy and, following the manufacturer's instructions, lock it securely.

■ To change tracheostomy ties:

– Obtain assistance from another nurse or a respiratory therapist because of the risk of accidental tube expulsion during this procedure. Patient movement or coughing can dislodge the tube.

– Wash your hands thoroughly and put on sterile gloves.

– If you aren't using commercially packaged tracheostomy ties, prepare new ties from a 30″ (76-cm) length of twill tape by folding one end back 1″ (2.5 cm) on itself. Then, with the bandage scissors, cut

a ½″ (1.5-cm) slit down the center of the tape from the folded edge.
— Prepare the other end of the tape the same way.
— Hold both ends together and, using scissors, cut the resulting circle of tape so that one piece is approximately 10″ (25.5 cm) long and the other is about 20″ (51 cm) long.
— Help the patient into semi-Fowler's position if possible.
— After your assistant puts on gloves, instruct her to hold the tracheostomy tube in place to prevent its expulsion during replacement of the ties. If you must perform the procedure without assistance, fasten the clean ties in place before removing the old ties to prevent tube expulsion.
— With the assistant's gloved fingers holding the tracheostomy tube in place, cut the soiled tracheostomy ties with the bandage scissors or untie them and discard the ties. Be careful not to cut the tube of the pilot balloon.
— Thread the slit end of one new tie a short distance through the eye of one tracheostomy tube flange from the underside; use the hemostat, if needed, to pull the tie through. Then thread the other end of the tie completely through the slit end and pull it taut so it loops firmly through the flange. This avoids knots that can cause throat discomfort, tissue irritation, pressure, and necrosis at the patient's throat.
— Fasten the second tie to the opposite flange in the same manner.
— Instruct the patient to flex his neck while you bring the ties around to the side and tie them together with a square knot. Flexion produces the same neck circumference as coughing and helps prevent an overly tight tie. Instruct your assistant to place one finger under the tapes as you tie them to ensure that they're tight enough to avoid slippage but loose enough to prevent choking or jugular vein constriction. Placing the closure on the side allows easy access and prevents pressure necrosis at the back of the neck when the patient is recumbent.
— After securing the ties, cut off the excess tape with the scissors and instruct your assistant to release the tracheostomy tube.
— Make sure the patient is comfortable and can reach the call button easily.
— Check tracheostomy-tie tension frequently.

ALERT *Be alert that patients with traumatic injury, radical neck dissection, or cardiac failure may experience swelling in the neck area; check ties frequently to prevent constriction secondary to this swelling.*
— Check neonatal or restless patients frequently because ties can loosen and cause tube dislodgment.
■ To conclude tracheostomy care:
— Replace any humidification device.
— Provide mouth care as needed because the oral cavity can become dry and malodorous or develop sores from encrusted secretions.
— Observe soiled dressings and any suctioned secretions for amount, color, consistency, and odor.
— Properly clean or dispose of all equipment, supplies, solutions, and trash according to facility policy.

– Take off and discard your gloves.
– Make sure that the patient is comfortable and that he can easily reach the call button.

Complications

These complications can occur within the first 48 hours after tracheostomy tube insertion:
■ hemorrhage at the operative site, causing drowning
■ bleeding or edema in tracheal tissue, causing airway obstruction
■ aspiration of secretions
■ introduction of air into the pleural cavity, causing pneumothorax
■ hypoxemia or acidosis, triggering cardiac arrest
■ introduction of air into surrounding tissues, causing subcutaneous emphysema.

In addition, secretions collecting under dressings and twill tape can encourage skin excoriation and infection. Hardened mucus or a slipped cuff can occlude the cannula opening and obstruct the airway. Tube displacement can stimulate the cough reflex if the tip rests on the carina, or it can cause blood vessel erosion and hemorrhage. Just the presence of the tube or cuff pressure can produce tracheal erosion and necrosis.

Nursing considerations

■ Keep appropriate equipment at the patient's bedside for immediate use in an emergency.
■ Perform tracheostomy care at least once every 8 hours or as needed. Change the dressing as often as necessary regardless of whether you also perform the entire cleaning procedure, because a wet dressing with exudate or secretions predisposes the patient to skin excoriation, breakdown, and infection.

■ Consult the physician about first-aid measures to use should an emergency occur. Follow facility policy regarding procedure if a tracheostomy tube is expelled or if the outer cannula becomes blocked. If the patient's breathing is obstructed — for example, when the tube is blocked with mucus that can't be removed by suctioning or by withdrawing the inner cannula — call the appropriate code and provide manual resuscitation with a handheld resuscitation bag or reconnect the patient to the ventilator.

ALERT *Don't remove the tracheostomy tube entirely because this may allow the airway to close completely. Use extreme caution when attempting to reinsert an expelled tracheostomy tube because of the risk of tracheal trauma, perforation, compression, and asphyxiation.*

Reassure the patient until the physician arrives (usually a minute or less in this type of code or emergency).
■ Refrain from changing tracheostomy ties unnecessarily during the immediate postoperative period before the stoma track is well formed (usually 4 days) to avoid accidental dislodgment and expulsion of the tube. Unless secretions or drainage is a problem, ties can be changed once per day.
■ Refrain from changing a single-cannula tracheostomy tube or the outer cannula of a double-cannula tube. Because of the risk of tracheal complications, the physician usually changes the cannula, with the frequency of change depending on the patient's condition.
■ If the patient's neck or stoma is excoriated or infected, apply a water-

soluble lubricant or topical antibiotic cream as ordered. Remember not to use a powder or an oil-based substance on or around a stoma because aspiration can cause infection and abscess.

■ Replace all equipment, including solutions, regularly according to facility policy to reduce the risk of nosocomial infections.

■ Record the date and time of the procedure; type of procedure; the amount, consistency, color, and odor of secretions; stoma and skin condition; the patient's respiratory status; change of the tracheostomy tube; the duration of any cuff deflation; the amount of any cuff inflation; and cuff pressure readings and specific body position. Note any complications and action taken, any patient or family teaching and their comprehension and progress, and the patient's tolerance of the procedure.

■ If the patient is being discharged with a tracheostomy, start self-care teaching as soon as he's receptive. Teach the patient how to change and clean the tube. If he's being discharged with suction equipment (a few patients are), make sure he and his family feel knowledgeable and comfortable about using this equipment.

Tracheotomy

A tracheotomy involves the surgical creation of an external opening — called a *tracheostomy* — into the trachea and insertion of an indwelling tube to maintain the airway's patency. If all other attempts to establish an airway have failed, a physician may per-

form a tracheotomy at a patient's bedside. This procedure may be necessary when an airway obstruction results from laryngeal edema, foreign body obstruction, or a tumor. An emergency tracheotomy may also be performed when endotracheal (ET) intubation is contraindicated.

Use of a cuffed tracheostomy tube provides and maintains a patent airway, prevents the unconscious or paralyzed patient from aspirating food or secretions, allows removal of tracheobronchial secretions from the patient unable to cough, replaces an ET tube, and permits the use of positive-pressure ventilation.

Although tracheostomy tubes come in plastic and metal, plastic tubes are commonly used in emergencies because they have a universal adapter for respiratory support equipment, such as a mechanical ventilator, and a cuff to allow positive-pressure ventilation.

Equipment

Tracheostomy tube of the proper size (usually #13 to #38 French or #00 to #9 Jackson) with obturator ■ tracheostomy tape ■ sterile tracheal dilator ■ vein retractor ■ sutures and needles ■ 4″ × 4″ gauze pads ■ sterile drapes, gloves, mask, and gown ■ sterile bowls ■ stethoscope ■ sterile tracheostomy dressing ■ pillow ■ tracheostomy ties ■ suction apparatus ■ alcohol pad ■ povidone-iodine solution ■ sterile water ■ 5-ml syringe with 22G needle ■ local anesthetic such as lidocaine ■ oxygen therapy device ■ oxygen source ■ emergency equipment to be kept at bedside, including suctioning equipment, sterile obturator, sterile tracheostomy tube, sterile inner cannula, sterile tracheostomy tube and inner cannula one size smaller than tubes in use, sterile tracheal dilator or sterile hemostat (many hospitals use prepackaged sterile tracheotomy trays)

Essential steps

■ Have one person stay with the patient while another obtains the necessary equipment. Wash your hands; then, maintaining sterile technique, open the necessary supplies and equipment. Set up the suction equipment and make sure it works.

■ Explain the procedure to the patient even if he's unresponsive.

■ Assess his condition and provide privacy. Maintain ventilation until the tracheotomy is performed.

■ Place a pillow under the patient's shoulders and neck and hyperextend his neck.

■ Assist with the tracheotomy. (See *Assisting with a tracheotomy*, page 266.)

■ When the tube is in position, attach it to the appropriate oxygen therapy device, which is connected to an oxygen source.

■ Inject air into the distal cuff port to inflate the cuff.

■ Auscultate the patient's lungs using a stethoscope.

■ After the physician sutures the corners of the incision and secures the tracheostomy tube with tape, put on sterile gloves.

■ Apply the sterile tracheostomy dressing under the tracheostomy tube flange. Place the tracheostomy ties through the openings of the tube flanges and tie them on the side of the patient's neck. This allows easy access and prevents pressure necrosis at the back of the neck.

■ Clean or dispose of the used equipment according to facility policy. Replenish all supplies as needed.

■ Make sure that a chest X-ray is ordered to confirm tube placement.

Complications

Complications that may result from a tracheotomy include:

■ airway obstruction (from improper tube placement)
■ hemorrhage
■ edema
■ perforated esophagus
■ subcutaneous or mediastinal emphysema
■ aspiration of secretions
■ tracheal necrosis (from cuff pressure)
■ infection
■ lacerations of arteries, veins, or nerves.

Nursing considerations

■ Assess the patient's vital signs and respiratory status every 15 minutes for 1 hour, then every 30 minutes for 2 hours, and then every 2 hours until his condition is stable.

■ Monitor the patient carefully for signs of infection. Ideally, the tracheotomy should be performed using sterile technique as described. However, in an emergency, this may not be possible.

■ Make sure the following equipment is always at the patient's bedside:

– suctioning equipment, because the patient may need his airway cleared at any time
– the sterile obturator used to insert the tracheostomy tube in case the tube is expelled
– a sterile tracheostomy tube and obturator (the same size as the one

Assisting with a tracheotomy

When performing a tracheotomy, the physician:
• cleans the area from the chin to the nipples with an antiseptic solution
• places sterile drapes on the patient and determines the area for the incision, usually 1 to 2 cm below the cricoid cartilage
• administers a local anesthetic

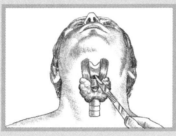

• makes either a horizontal or vertical incision (A vertical incision avoids arteries, veins, and nerves on the lateral borders of the trachea.)
• dissects the subcutaneous fat and muscle, moving the muscle aside to locate the tracheal rings
• makes an incision between the second and third tracheal rings and uses a hemostat to control bleeding
• injects a local anesthetic into the tracheal lumen to suppress the cough reflex
• creates a stoma in the trachea
• inserts the tracheostomy tube and obturator into the stoma

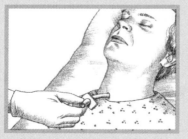

• removes the obturator.
During the process, the nurse:
• carefully applies suction while the physician creates the stoma in the trachea to remove any blood and secretions that could obstruct the airway or be aspirated into the lungs
• applies a sterile tracheostomy dressing after the obturator is removed and anchors the tube with tracheostomy ties

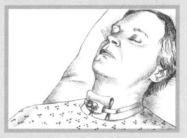

• checks for air movement through the tube and auscultate the lungs to ensure proper placement.

An alternative approach

The physician may insert the tracheostomy tube percutaneously at the bedside. Unlike the approach described previously, this method dilates rather than cuts the tissue structures. After preparing and anesthetizing the skin, the physician:
• makes a 1-cm midline incision
• creates a stoma for tube insertion using a series of dilators or a pair of forceps
• inserts the tracheostomy tube after the stoma reaches the desired size.
In this approach, the nurse:
• inflates the cuff after the tube is in place, secures the tube, and auscultates the patient's breath sounds
• arranges for a portable chest X-ray to verify proper placement.

used) in case the tube must be re-placed quickly
– a spare, sterile inner cannula that can be used if the cannula is expelled
– a sterile tracheostomy tube and obturator one size smaller than the one used, which may be needed if the tube is expelled and the trachea begins to close
– a sterile tracheal dilator or sterile hemostat to maintain an open airway before inserting a new tracheostomy tube.

■ Review emergency first-aid measures and always follow your facility's policy concerning an expelled or blocked tracheostomy tube. When a blocked tube can't be cleared by suctioning or withdrawing the inner cannula, policy may require you to stay with the patient while someone else calls the physician or the appropriate code. Continue trying to ventilate the patient with whatever method works; for example, a handheld resuscitation bag. Don't remove the tracheostomy tube entirely; doing so may close the airway completely.

■ Use extreme caution if you try to reinsert an expelled tracheostomy tube to avoid tracheal trauma, perforation, compression, and asphyxiation.

■ Record the reason for the procedure, the date and time it took place, and the patient's respiratory status before and after the procedure. Include any complications that occurred during the procedure, the amount of cuff pressure, and the respiratory therapy initiated after the procedure. Note the patient's response to respiratory therapy.

Weaning from mechanical ventilation

Weaning a patient from mechanical ventilation refers to the gradual removal of the patient's dependence on the ventilator for breathing. Weaning typically involves three aspects: weaning from the actual ventilator, weaning from the tube, and weaning from oxygen. The decision to wean a patient is based on the patient's physiologic status such as cardiopulmonary function, fluid and electrolyte balance, acid-base status, nutritional status, and comfort level. In addition, the patient's emotional status, such as anxiety level, coping abilities, and ability to cooperate, must be considered before and during the weaning process. Specific criteria must be met before weaning can occur. (See *Criteria for weaning,* page 268.)

There's no one best method for weaning a patient from a mechanical ventilator. Three methods are commonly used: intermittent mandatory ventilation (IMV); pressure support ventilation (PSV); and T-piece. (See *Methods of weaning,* page 269.)

Equipment
T-piece ■ ventilator ■ gloves (as necessary)

Essential steps
■ Assess the patient's pulmonary function status and ensure that the patient meets the necessary criteria for weaning; check the physician's order for specific instructions for the weaning process.

Criteria for weaning

Successful weaning depends on the patient's ability to breathe on his or her own. This means that the patient must have a spontaneous respiratory effort that can maintain ventilation, a stable cardiovascular system, and sufficient respiratory muscle strength and level of consciousness to sustain spontaneous breathing.

Pulmonary function criteria include:
- minute ventilation less than or equal to 10 L/minute, indicating that the patient is breathing at a stable rate with adequate tidal volume
- negative inspiratory force greater than or equal to –20 cm H_2O, indicating the patient's ability to initiate respirations independently
- maximum voluntary ventilation greater than or equal to twice the resting minute volume, indicating the patient's ability to sustain maximal respiratory effort
- tidal volume of 5 to 10 ml/kg, indicating the patient's ability to ventilate lungs adequately
- partial pressure of arterial oxygen (Pao_2) greater than or equal to 60 mm Hg (50 mm Hg or the ability to maintain baseline levels if the patient has chronic lung disease,)
- partial pressure of arterial carbon dioxide ($Paco_2$) less than or equal to 45 mm Hg (or normal for the patient)

- arterial pH ranging from 7.35 to 7.45 (or normal for the patient)
- fractional concentration of inspired oxygen less than or equal to 0.4.
  Other criteria include:
- adequate natural airway or functioning tracheostomy
- ability to cough and mobilize secretions
- successful withdrawal of any neuromuscular blocker such as pancuronium bromide
- clear or clearing chest X-ray
- absence of infection, acid-base or electrolyte imbalance, hyperglycemia, arrhythmia, renal failure, anemia, fever, or excessive fatigue.
  Ultimately, after being weaned, the patient should demonstrate:
- respiratory rate less than 24 breaths/minute
- heart rate and blood pressure within 15% of his or her baseline
- tidal volume of at least 3 to 5 ml/kg
- arterial pH greater than 7.35
- Pao_2 maintained at greater than 60 mm Hg
- $Paco_2$ maintained at less than 45 mm Hg
- oxygen saturation maintained at greater than 90%
- absence of cardiac arrhythmias
- absence of accessory muscle use.

- Explain the procedure to the patient, including expected patient activities during this time.
- Reassure the patient that someone will be with him at all times.
- Institute the appropriate and prescribed method for weaning.
- Assess the patient for signs and symptoms of hypoxemia including tachycardia, arrhythmias, restlessness, respiratory rate above 35 breaths per minute, accessory muscle use for breathing, and paradoxical chest movement.
- Obtain arterial blood gas (ABG) levels as ordered and compare with baseline levels.
- Expect to place the patient back on the ventilator if fatigue, exhaustion, or manifestations including ABG results suggest deterioration in the patient's status.
- After the patient is successfully weaned from the ventilator, prepare to

Methods of weaning

The three most commonly used methods of weaning are described here. In patients receiving long-term mechanical ventilation, intermittent mandatory ventilation with or without pressure support ventilation is used.

Intermittent mandatory ventilation

With intermittent mandatory ventilation (IMV), breaths produced by the ventilator are gradually decreased, allowing the patient to breath independently. Decreasing ventilator-produced breaths allows the patient to increase his respiratory muscle strength and endurance. As the number of ventilator breaths decrease, the patient increases the number of spontaneous breaths until he's breathing independently.

Pressure support ventilation

Pressure support ventilation (PSV) is often used as an adjunct to IMV in the weaning process. In this method, a set burst of pressure is applied during inspiration with the patient's normal breathing pattern. PSV helps to decrease the patient's work of breathing, thereby allowing him to build up respiratory muscle strength. As the patient's strength improves, PSV is gradually decreased.

T-piece

Weaning via a T-piece is commonly used for patients requiring short-term mechanical ventilation. The T-piece is attached to the end of the endotracheal tube. The patient is then disconnected from the ventilator and allowed to initiate spontaneous breaths. In the beginning, the amount of time the patient is off the ventilator is short, possibly 1 to 2 minutes. The time off the ventilator is gradually increased until the patient is breathing independently. During the weaning process, the patient receives supplemental oxygen therapy at or above the concentration that he was receiving while on the ventilator.

This method is sometimes used for patients receiving long-term mechanical ventilation. In these situations, the patient is weaned during the day and placed back on the ventilator when fatigue occurs, and during the night for rest.

---

wean the patient from the tracheostomy or endotracheal (ET) tube as ordered.

■ To remove the ET tube:
  – When authorized to remove the tube, obtain another nurse's assistance to prevent traumatic manipulation of the tube when it's untaped or unfastened.
  – Elevate the head of the patient's bed to approximately 90 degrees.
  – Suction the patient's oropharynx and nasopharynx to remove any accumulated secretions and to help prevent aspiration of secretions when the cuff is deflated.

  – Using a handheld resuscitation bag or the mechanical ventilator, give the patient several deep breaths through the ET tube to hyperinflate his lungs and increase his oxygen reserve.
  – Attach a 10-ml syringe to the pilot balloon port and aspirate air until you meet resistance and the pilot balloon deflates.

  ALERT *If you fail to detect an air leak around the deflated cuff, notify the physician immediately and don't proceed with extubation. Absence of an air leak may indicate marked tracheal edema, which can result in total* *airway obstruction if the ET tube is removed.*

   – If you detect the proper air leak, untape or unfasten the ET tube while an assistant stabilizes the tube.

   – Insert a sterile suction catheter through the ET tube. Then apply suction and ask the patient to take a deep breath and to open his mouth fully and pretend to cry out. This causes abduction of the vocal cords and reduces the risk of laryngeal trauma during withdrawal of the tube.

   – Simultaneously remove the ET tube and the suction catheter in one smooth, outward and downward motion, following the natural curve of the patient's mouth. Suctioning during extubation removes secretions retained at the end of the tube and prevents aspiration.

   – Give the patient supplemental oxygen. For maximum humidity, use a cool-mist, large-volume nebulizer to help decrease airway irritation, patient discomfort, and laryngeal edema.

   – Encourage the patient to cough and breathe deeply. Remind him that a sore throat and hoarseness are to be expected and will gradually subside.

   – Make sure the patient is comfortable and the airway is patent. Clean or dispose of equipment.

■ To wean the patient from a tracheostomy tube:

   – Have the patient perform a trial period of mouth or nose breathing.

   – Change to a smaller sized tube to increase air flow resistance and deflate the cuff at the same time.

   – Switch to a cuffless tracheostomy tube.

   – Change to a fenestrated tube which allows the patient to talk by permitting air to flow around and through the tube.

   – Change to a tracheostomy button.

   – Remove the tracheostomy tube entirely.

■ To wean the patient from oxygen, gradually reduce the flow rate or fraction of inspired oxygen until the patient's partial pressure of arterial oxygen ranges between 70 to 100 mm Hg while on room air.

Complications

Potential complications after weaning include:

■ respiratory failure

■ airway obstruction due to laryngospasm

■ marked tracheal edema secondary to extubation.

Nursing considerations

■ When weaning the patient, continue to assess the patient's status closely and frequently; observe for signs of hypoxemia and check tidal volume after the first 15 minutes of weaning and then as needed (ideally tidal volume should within 5 to 10 ml/kg). Assess ABGs and oxygen saturation levels as ordered. Notify the physician of any abnormalities.

■ Place the patient in a position that maximizes lung expansion and comfort, such as semi-Fowler's position.

■ Assess vital signs every 15 minutes for the 1st hour after weaning and then hourly as the patient's condition stabilizes.

■ Schedule weaning to fit comfortably and realistically with the patient's daily regimen. Avoid scheduling sessions after meals, baths, or lengthy therapeutic or diagnostic procedures. Have the patient help you set up the schedule to give him some sense of control over a frightening procedure.

■ As the patient's tolerance for weaning increases, help him sit up out of bed to improve his breathing and sense of well-being. Suggest diversionary activities to take his mind off breathing.

■ Assist the patient with measures to aid in relaxation during the weaning process to facilitate chest muscle relaxation; encourage the patient to take deep breaths if possible.

■ After extubation of a patient who has been intubated for an extended time, keep reintubation supplies readily available for at least 12 hours or until you're sure he can tolerate extubation.

ALERT *Never extubate a patient unless someone skilled at intubation is readily available.*

■ After extubation, auscultate the patient's lungs frequently and watch for signs of respiratory distress. Be especially alert for stridor or other evidence of upper airway obstruction. If ordered, draw a sample for ABG analysis.

■ During weaning, record the date and time of each session, the weaning method, and baseline and subsequent vital signs, oxygen saturation levels, and ABG values. Again, describe the patient's subjective and objective responses, including level of consciousness, respiratory effort, arrhythmia, skin color, and need for suctioning.

■ Record any complications and actions taken. If the patient was receiving PSV or using a T-piece or tracheostomy collar, note the duration of spontaneous breathing and the patient's ability to maintain the weaning schedule. If using IMV, with or without PSV, record the control breath rate, the time of each breath reduction, and the rate of spontaneous respirations.

■ Document the time and date of extubation or tracheostomy tube removal and cessation of oxygen. Record the patient's condition before removal and the patient's response after removal.

3 | *Neurologic system challenges*

Imagine a patient who presents with a severe headache. Does his pain signal a stress response, a sinus infection, or a neurologic problem, such as a rupture of a cerebral aneurysm or a hemorrhagic stroke? What would you do first? If the problem is a ruptured cerebral aneurysm, would you know how to grade it? If the problem is a stroke, would fibrinolytic therapy be indicated? If cerebral blood flow monitoring was indicated, would you know how to implement appropriate care and obtain readings? Additionally, once you've obtained the readings, could you identify abnormal values and reach a conclusion about the patient's status?

Suppose your patient has increased intracranial pressure (ICP) and requires ICP monitoring. Would you know which type of monitoring allows you to drain cerebrospinal fluid? Could you differentiate a normal ICP waveform from an abnormal one? What if the monitor displays A-waves? Is this an ominous sign, a problem with the equipment, or an insignificant finding? A patient who's receiving mechanical ventilation and being sedated requires bispectral index monitoring. Would you be able to apply the sensor correctly and interpret the bispectral index score to determine if the patient is adequately sedated? Imagine that

your patient is diagnosed with status epilepticus. How would you intervene, and what drugs would you expect to administer? What would you do for a patient with myasthenia gravis who experiences a myasthenic crisis? Answers to these questions are presented in this chapter, along with other essential information needed to address the major challenges involving the neurologic system that are commonly encountered in the critical care area.

 MULTISYSTEM DISORDER

Acute spinal cord injury

Usually the result of trauma to the head or neck, spinal cord injuries (SCI) — other than spinal cord damage — include fractures, contusions, and compressions of the vertebral column. Spinal cord injuries most commonly occur in the 12th thoracic, 1st lumbar, and 5th, 6th, and 7th cervical areas. The real danger from such injuries lies in associated damage to the spinal cord.

Most serious SCIs result from motor vehicle accidents, falls, diving into shallow water, and gunshot wounds; less serious injuries result from lifting heavy objects and minor falls. Approximately 10,000 persons per year suffer

SCIs, the majority of whom are males from age 18 to 25. Spinal dysfunction may also result from hyperparathyroidism and neoplastic lesions.

The prognosis for a patient following an SCI depends on the degree of injury. The majority of patients with SCIs eventually return home with some degree of independence. However, morbidity is high, most commonly the result of pulmonary or renal complications such as infection.

Pathophysiology

Spinal cord trauma results from acceleration, deceleration, or other deforming forces, usually applied from a distance. Mechanisms involved with spinal cord trauma include:

■ hyperextension from acceleration-deceleration forces and sudden reduction in the anteroposterior diameter of the spinal cord

■ hyperflexion from sudden and excessive force, propelling the neck forward or causing an exaggerated movement to one side

■ vertical compression from force applied from the top of the cranium along the vertical axis through the vertebra

■ rotational forces from twisting, which adds shearing forces.

Injury causes microscopic hemorrhages in the gray matter and pia-arachnoid. The hemorrhages gradually increase in size until all of the gray matter is filled with blood, which causes necrosis. From the gray matter, the blood enters the white matter, where it impedes the circulation within the spinal cord. Ensuing edema causes compression and decreases the blood supply; thus, the spinal cord loses perfusion and becomes ischemic.

The edema and hemorrhage are greatest approximately two segments above and below the injury. Edema temporarily adds to the patient's dysfunction by increasing pressure and compressing the nerves. If near the 3rd to 5th cervical vertebrae, edema may also interfere with phrenic nerve impulse transmission to the diaphragm, thereby inhibiting respiratory function.

In the white matter, circulation usually returns to normal in approximately 24 hours. However, in the gray matter, an inflammatory reaction prevents restoration of circulation. Phagocytes appear at the site within 36 to 48 hours after the injury, macrophages engulf degenerating axons, and collagen replaces the normal tissue. Scarring and meningeal thickening leaves the nerves in the area blocked or tangled.

Comprehensive assessment

The patient's history may reveal trauma, a neoplastic lesion, an infection that could produce a spinal abscess, or an endocrine disorder. The patient typically complains of muscle spasm and back or neck pain that worsens with movement. In cervical fractures, point tenderness may be present; in dorsal and lumbar fractures, pain may radiate to other body areas such as the legs.

Physical assessment (including a neurologic assessment) helps locate the level of injury and detect any cord damage. General observation of the patient reveals that he limits movements and activities that cause pain. Inspection may reveal surface wounds that occurred with the spinal injury.

Palpation can identify pain location and loss of sensation.

If the injury damaged the spinal cord, you'll note clinical effects that range from mild paresthesia to quadriplegia and shock. Specific signs and symptoms depend on injury type and degree. (See *Types of spinal cord injury,* pages 276 and 277.)

Diagnosis

Diagnosis is based on the following:
- Spinal X-rays — the most important diagnostic measure — detect the fracture.
- Myelography, magnetic resonance imaging, and computed tomography (CT) scans are used to locate the fracture and site of the compression. CT scans or magnetic resonance imaging also reveal spinal cord edema and may reveal a spinal mass.
- Thorough neurologic evaluation locates the level of injury and detects cord damage.
- Lumbar puncture may show increased cerebrospinal fluid (CSF) pressure from a lesion or trauma in spinal compression.

Collaborations

Acute SCI is a multisystem problem; therefore, a multidisciplinary approach to care is needed. Typically, emergency medical service personnel are involved outside the hospital, ensuring the patient's airway, breathing, and circulation and immediately immobilizing him to stabilize his spine and prevent cord damage. When he reaches the emergency department, one physician typically directs the team caring for the patient. The secondary airway, breathing, circulation, and defibrillation survey is reapplied, including vital signs,

level of consciousness (LOC), oxygen saturation, brief and targeted history, and continued immobilization to prevent further injury. The focus is on rapid but accurate diagnosis.

The amount and type of personnel involved depend on the level of injury. For example, respiratory therapy may be needed to assist with pulmonary hygiene and care of the ventilator-dependent patient. Surgery may be involved to relieve pressure or reduce a fracture. Physical therapy can assist with maintaining joint range of motion (ROM) and mobility training. Occupational therapy can assist with developing implements and retraining for activities of daily living. Speech therapy can help the patient learn to swallow more effectively, if necessary. Social services may also be contacted for assistance with rehabilitative services and care at home.

Treatment and care

The primary treatment after spinal injury is immediate immobilization to stabilize the spine and prevent cord damage; other treatment is supportive. Cervical injuries require immobilization, using sandbags on both sides of the patient's head, a hard cervical collar, skeletal traction with skull tongs, or a halo device. When a patient shows clinical evidence of a spinal cord injury, high doses of I.V. methylprednisolone (corticosteroids) are given to reduce inflammation.

Treatment of stable lumbar and dorsal fractures consists of bed rest on a firm surface (such as a bed board), analgesics, and muscle relaxants until the fracture stabilizes (usually in 10 to 12 weeks). Later treatment includes exercises to strengthen the back muscles and a back brace or corset to provide support while walking. An unstable dorsal or lumbar fracture requires a plaster cast, a turning frame and, in severe fracture, laminectomy and spinal fusion.

Neurosurgery may be required to relieve the pressure due to compression of the spinal column. If the cause of compression is a neoplastic lesion, chemotherapy and radiation may relieve the compression by shrinking the lesion. Surface wounds that accompany the spinal injury require wound care and tetanus prophylaxis unless the patient has recently been immunized.

Complications
The patient with acute SCI is at risk for complications affecting potentially every body system, including:
■ pulmonary, such as atelectasis and pneumonia
■ renal, such as urinary retention, urinary tract infection, pyelonephritis, renal calculi, and urosepsis
■ GI, such as gastric ulceration, constipation, fecal impaction, and paralytic ileus.

In addition, the patient is at risk for three other specific complications:
■ autonomic dysreflexia
■ spinal shock
■ neurogenic shock. (See *Complications of spinal cord injury,* page 278.)

Nursing considerations
■ Immediately stabilize the patient's spine.

ALERT *As in all spinal injuries, suspect cord damage until diagnosis is established.*

■ Perform a neurologic assessment to establish a baseline, including LOC

and motor and sensory function, to aid in determining the level of injury. Continually assess the patient's LOC for changes, such as increasing restlessness or anxiety.
■ Assist with obtaining spinal X-rays and other diagnostic tests to determine the level of injury.
■ Assess respiratory status closely — initially, at least every hour. Obtain baseline parameters for tidal volume, vital capacity, negative inspiratory forces, and minute volume. Monitor for signs of respiratory dysfunction, such as shallow, slow, or rapid respirations and decreases in vital capacity or tidal volume. Continue to monitor tidal volume at least every 8 hours.
■ Auscultate lung sounds for evidence of adventitious sounds, such as crackles or rhonchi, or absence of breath sounds, indicating ineffective airway clearance. Obtain chest X-rays as ordered.
■ Monitor oxygen saturation levels via pulse oximetry and arterial blood gas studies, as ordered.

ALERT *Partial pressure of arterial oxygen (PaO_2) less than 60 mm Hg and partial pressure of arterial carbon dioxide ($PaCO_2$) greater than 50 mm Hg accompanied by a decreasing pH suggest the need for mechanical ventilation secondary to atelectasis, pneumonia, or respiratory muscle fatigue. If the patient isn't intubated when admitted to the emergency department, hemorrhage and edema at the injury site can predispose him to increasing cord damage that ultimately leads to a higher level of dysfunction and altered respiratory function, necessitating mechanical ventilation.*

(Text continues on page 278.)

Types of spinal cord injury

Injury to the spinal cord can be classified as complete or incomplete. An incomplete spinal injury may be an anterior cord syndrome, central cord syndrome, or Brown-Séquard's syndrome, depending on the area of the cord affected. This chart highlights the characteristic signs and symptoms of each.

Type	Description	Signs and symptoms
Complete transsection 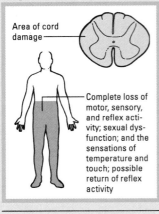 Area of cord damage — Complete loss of motor, sensory, and reflex activity; sexual dysfunction; and the sensations of temperature and touch; possible return of reflex activity	● All tracts of the spinal cord completely disrupted ● All functions involving the spinal cord below the level of transsection lost ● Complete and permanent loss	● Loss of motor function (quadriplegia) with cervical cord transsection; paraplegia with thoracic cord transsection ● Muscle flaccidity ● Loss of all reflexes and sensory function below the level of the injury ● Bladder and bowel atony ● Paralytic ileus ● Loss of vasomotor tone in lower body parts with low and unstable blood pressure ● Loss of perspiration below the level of the injury ● Dry, pale skin ● Respiratory impairment
Incomplete transsection: Central cord syndrome 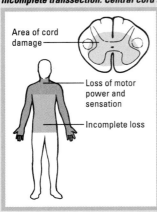 Area of cord damage — Loss of motor power and sensation — Incomplete loss	● Center portion of cord affected ● Typically from hyperextension injury	● Motor deficits greater in upper than lower extremities ● Variable degree of bladder dysfunction

Type	Description	Signs and symptoms
Incomplete transsection: Anterior cord syndrome		

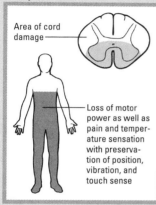

Area of cord damage

Loss of motor power as well as pain and temperature sensation with preservation of position, vibration, and touch sense

	Description	Signs and symptoms
	• Occlusion of anterior spinal artery • Occlusion from pressure of bone fragments	• Loss of motor function below the level of the injury • Loss of pain and temperature sensations below the level of the injury • Intact touch, pressure, position, and vibration senses

Incomplete transsection: Brown-Séquard's syndrome

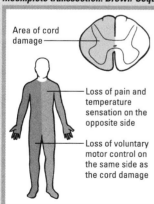

Area of cord damage

Loss of pain and temperature sensation on the opposite side

Loss of voluntary motor control on the same side as the cord damage

	Description	Signs and symptoms
	• Hemisection of cord affected • Most common in stabbing and gunshot wounds • Damage to cord on only one side	• Ipsilateral paralysis or paresis below the level of the injury • Ipsilateral loss of touch, pressure, vibration, and position sense below the level of the injury • Contralateral loss of pain and temperature sensations below the level of the injury

Complications of spinal cord injury

Of the following three sets of complications, only autonomic dysreflexia requires emergency attention.

Autonomic dysreflexia

Also known as autonomic hyperreflexia, autonomic dysreflexia is a serious medical condition that occurs after the resolution of spinal shock. Emergency recognition and management is a must.

Autonomic dysreflexia should be suspected in the patient with:

● spinal cord trauma at or above level T6
● bradycardia
● hypertension and a severe, pounding headache
● cold or goose-fleshed skin below the lesion.

Dysreflexia is caused by noxious stimuli, most commonly a distended bladder or skin lesion.

Treatment focuses on eliminating the stimulus; rapid identification and removal may eliminate the need for pharmacologic control of headache and hypertension.

Spinal shock

Spinal shock is the loss of autonomic, reflex, motor, and sensory activity below the level of the cord lesion. It occurs secondary to damage of the spinal cord.

Signs of spinal shock include:
● flaccid paralysis
● loss of deep tendon and perianal reflexes
● loss of motor and sensory function.

Until spinal shock has resolved (usually 1 to 6 weeks after injury), the extent of actual cord damage can't be assessed. The earliest indicator of resolution is the return of reflex activity.

Neurogenic shock

Neurogenic shock is an abnormal vasomotor response that occurs secondary to the disruption of sympathetic impulses from the brain stem to the thoracolumbar area. It's seen most frequently in patients with cervical cord injury. The temporary loss of autonomic function below the level of injury causes cardiovascular changes.

Signs of neurogenic shock include:
● orthostatic hypotension
● bradycardia
● loss of the ability to sweat below the level of the lesion.

Treatment is symptomatic. Symptoms resolve when spinal cord edema resolves.

■ Administer supplemental oxygen as indicated. Suction secretions as necessary, based on auscultation findings.

ALERT Always preoxygenate the patient before suctioning. Monitor his heart rate closely during tracheal suctioning because bradycardia can occur.

■ Anticipate the need for endotracheal intubation or tracheostomy and mechanical ventilation if the patient exhibits signs and symptoms of respiratory distress.

ALERT If a cervical spine injury hasn't been ruled out, don't hyperextend the patient's neck for intubation. Perform nasal intubation or orotracheal intubation with the cervical spine immobilized manually.

■ Assess cardiac status at least every hour initially; note cardiac rate and rhythm. Institute continuous cardiac monitoring to evaluate for possible arrhythmias due to hypoxemia. Monitor blood pressure and hemodynamic status frequently. Assist with insertion of a pulmonary artery catheter if indicated. Notify the physician of decreases in right atrial pressure, pulmonary artery pressure, pulmonary artery wedge pressure, and systemic vascular resistance, indicating neurogenic shock. If the patient becomes hypotensive, expect to administer vasopressors.

▰ **ALERT** *Hypotension occurs in the patient with SCI due to a loss of vascular motor control below the level of injury, causing vasodilation and a relative hypovolemia.*

▪ Administer methylprednisolone I.V., as ordered. (See *Administering methylprednisolone.*)

▪ Prepare the patient for surgical stabilization, if indicated.

▪ Assess GI status closely for indications of ulceration or bleeding. Anticipate nasogastric (NG) tube insertion attached to low intermittent suction for gastric decompression. Assess abdomen for possible distention; auscultate bowel sounds and report any decrease or absence of bowel sounds.

▰ **ALERT** *Paralytic ileus is a common problem for patients with SCI, usually occurring within the first 72 hours after the injury.*

▪ Check stools and NG drainage for blood every 8 hours. Administer histamine-2 receptor antagonists, as ordered.

▪ Anticipate the need for indwelling urinary catheter insertion and assess urine output hourly during the initial period; notify the physician if urine output is less than 0.5 ml/kg/hour for 2 consecutive hours. Monitor intake and output for discrepancies; maintain an intake of at least 2 to 3 L per day, unless contraindicated. Make sure that the urinary catheter drainage system is

Administering methylprednisolone

Methylprednisolone is a corticosteroid given to a patient with an acute spinal cord injury to improve his functional outcome by protecting the membranes of the nervous system from further destruction. The drug also has been shown to improve blood flow to the injured area, thereby facilitating tissue repair. Methylprednisolone is given to patients who arrive for treatment within 8 hours of the injury.

If methylprednisolone is ordered:
● Administer an initial loading dose of 30 mg/kg as a bolus I.V. injection over 15 minutes.
● After the bolus is completed, maintain the I.V. infusion with normal saline or other solution, as ordered, for 45 minutes.
● Next, administer a continuous infusion of the drug at a rate of 5.4 mg/kg/hour over the next 23 hours.
● Keep in mind that if the patient arrives for treatment within 3 hours of the injury, the infusion may be continued an additional 24 hours (for a total of 48 hours of treatment) because the additional time may provide further patient benefit.

Nursing implications
● Expect to administer histamine-2 receptor antagonists to reduce the risk of gastric ulceration resulting from the use of high-dose steroids in conjunction with the patient's increased production of gastric acid secondary to the injury.
● Monitor the I.V. infusion carefully.
● If for some reason the infusion is interrupted, recalculate the rate so that the entire dosage is infused by the end of the 23rd hour.
● Assess the patient's cardiac rate and rhythm closely for arrhythmias.
● Monitor serum electrolyte levels (especially sodium) for changes.

functioning and the tubing is without kinks or blockage. Palpate the bladder for distention.

ALERT Assess the patient frequently for signs and symptoms of autonomic dysreflexia. Be alert for throbbing headache, cutaneous vasodilation, and sweating above the level of the injury; sudden severe elevation in blood pressure; and piloerection, pallor, chills, and vasoconstriction below the level of injury. If any of these occur, immediately elevate the head of the bed, monitor blood pressure and heart rate every 3 to 5 minutes, and determine the underlying stimulus for the event, such as blocked catheter, fecal impaction, or urinary tract infection. Administer antihypertensive agents, as ordered.

■ Monitor laboratory and diagnostic test results, including blood urea nitrogen, creatinine, complete blood count, and urine culture, if indicated.

■ Institute measures to prevent skin breakdown from immobilization including turning (as appropriate), repositioning, padding, and care of any devices, such as a halo jacket (for example, pin-site care) or traction. Monitor insertion sites for signs of infection.

■ Institute bladder and bowel training program including intermittent catheterization and bowel retraining, as appropriate.

ALERT Autonomic dysreflexia can be precipitated by bowel distention or anal sphincter stimulation, such as from fecal impaction, enema administration, or rectal examination. Use an anesthetic lubricant to minimize the risk of stimulation when administering an enema or checking for fecal impaction.

■ Assist with measures to help the patient maintain body temperature because his ability to conserve (vasoconstrict) and lose (vasodilate) heat are lost.

■ Encourage mobility as appropriate within the restrictions of the patient's condition and injury.

ALERT Be alert for orthostatic hypotension, which may occur in patients with SCI to the cervical or high thoracic area. This sudden drop in blood pressure could lead to cerebral hypoxia and loss of consciousness. To prevent orthostatic hypotension, change the patient's position slowly and perform ROM exercises every 2 hours.

■ Monitor the patient for signs and symptoms of deep vein thrombosis and pulmonary embolism. Apply antiembolism stockings or intermittent sequential compression devices as ordered. Administer prophylactic heparin, as ordered.

■ Provide emotional support to the patient and his family; allow the patient to verbalize concerns.

■ Begin rehabilitation as soon as possible. Keep in mind that the patient with a spinal cord injury may need extensive rehabilitation depending on the level of, and prognosis for, the injury. If he requires ventilatory dependency, placement in an extended care facility may be necessary.

Patient teaching

■ Explain treatment methods to the patient and his family. For example, reassure them that a halo traction device or skull tongs don't penetrate the brain.

■ Explain the prescribed regimen for care, including rehabilitation, exercises to maintain physical mobility, medication therapy (including adverse effects), and the duration of treatment.

■ Instruct the patient about signs and symptoms of complications and the need to notify someone as soon as possible should any occur.

■ Teach the patient and his family how to perform necessary self-care activities, such as catheterization, tracheal suctioning, or fecal impaction removal.

Bispectral index monitoring

Bispectral index monitoring involves the use of an electronic device that converts EEG waves into a number. This number, statistically derived based on raw EEG data, indicates the depth or level of sedation in the patient and provides a direct measure of the effects of sedatives and anesthetics on the brain. Rather than relying on subjective assessments and vital signs, bispectral index monitoring provides clinicians with objective, reliable data on which to base care, thus minimizing the risks of over- or under-sedation.

Bispectral index consists of a monitor attached to a sensor applied to the patient's forehead. The sensor obtains information about the patient's electrical brain activity or EEG and then translates this information into a number from 0 (indicating no brain activity) to 100 (indicating a patient who is awake and alert). In the critical care unit, bispectral index monitoring is used to assess sedation when the patient is receiving mechanical ventilation or neuromuscular blockers or during barbiturate coma or bedside procedures.

Equipment

Bispectral index monitor and cable ■ bispectral index sensor ■ alcohol swabs ■ soap and water

Essential steps

■ Gather the necessary equipment, and explain the procedure and its purpose to the patient and his family. (See *Bispectral index monitoring,* page 282.)

■ Clean the patient's forehead with soap and water and allow it to dry. If necessary, wipe his forehead with an alcohol swab to ensure that the skin is oil-free. Allow the alcohol to dry.

■ Open the sensor package, and apply the sensor to the patient's forehead. Position the circle labeled as 1 midline approximately 1½″ (4 cm) above the bridge of the nose.

■ Position the circle labeled as 3 on the right or left temple area, at the level of the outer canthus of the eye, between the corner of the eye and the patient's hairline.

■ Make sure that the circle labeled as 4 and the line below it are parallel to the eye on the designated side.

■ Apply gentle, firm pressure around the edges of the sensor, including the areas in between the numbered circles, to ensure proper adhesion.

■ Press firmly on each of the numbered circles for approximately 5 seconds each to ensure that the electrodes are adhered to the skin.

■ Connect the sensor to the interface cable and monitor.

■ Turn on the monitor.

■ Watch the monitor for information related to impedance (electrical resistance) testing.

ALERT *Be aware that for the monitor to display a reading, impedance values must be below a speci-*

Bispectral index monitoring

Bispectral index monitoring consists of a monitor and cable connected to a sensor applied to the patient's forehead (as shown below).

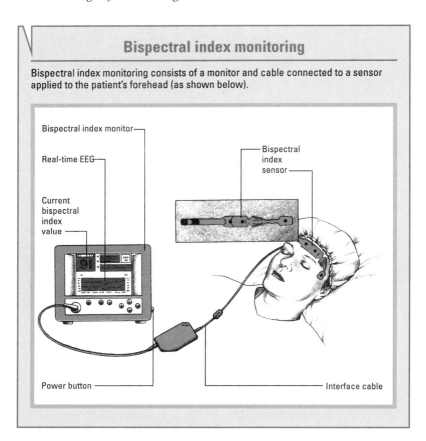

Bispectral index monitor

Real-time EEG

Current bispectral index value

Bispectral index sensor

Power button

Interface cable

---

fied threshold. If not, be prepared to troubleshoot sensor problems. (*See* Troubleshooting sensor problems.)

■ Select a smoothing rate (usually 15 or 30 seconds, during which data is analyzed for calculation of the bispectral index) using the advanced setup button, based on your facility's policy. Read and record the bispectral index value.

Complications

There are no complications associated with bispectral index monitoring.

Nursing considerations

■ Don't rely on the bispectral index value alone; always evaluate the bispectral index value in relation to other assessment findings. (*See Interpreting bispectral index values.*)

■ Keep in mind that movement may occur if bispectral index values are low. Be alert for possible artifacts that could falsely elevate bispectral index values.

ALERT *Bispectral index values may be elevated due to muscle shivering, tightening, or twitching or the use of mechanical devices, either*

Troubleshooting sensor problems

When initiating bispectral index monitoring, be aware that the monitor may display messages that indicate a problem. The chart below highlights these messages and offers possible solutions.

Message	Possible solutions
High impedance message	Check sensor adhesion; reapply firm pressure to each of the numbered circles on the sensor for 5 seconds each; if message continues, check the connection between the sensor and the monitor; if necessary, apply a new sensor
Noise message	Remove possible pressure on the sensor; investigate possible large stimulus such as electrocautery
Lead-off message	Check sensor for electrode displacement or lifting; reapply with firm pressure or, if necessary, apply a new sensor.

Interpreting bispectral index values

Use the following guidelines to interpret your patient's bispectral index value:

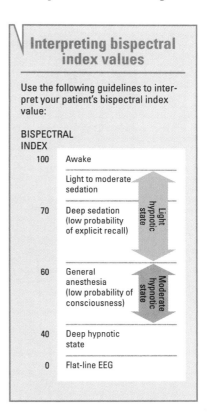

with the patient or in close proximity to the patient, bispectral index monitor, or sensor. Use caution when interpreting the bispectral index value in these situations.

■ Anticipate the need to adjust the dosage of sedation based on the patient's bispectral index value.

ALERT *Keep in mind that a decrease in stimulation, increased sedation, recent administration of a neuromuscular blocking agent or analgesia, or hypothermia may decrease the bispectral index and thus indicate the need for a decrease in sedative agents. Pain may cause an elevated bispectral*

index, indicating a need for an increase in sedation.

■ Check the sensor site according to your facility's policy. Change the sensor every 24 hours.

■ Document initiation of bispectral index monitoring, including baseline values and location of the sensor. Record assessment findings in conjunction with the bispectral index value to provide a clear overall picture of the patient's condition.

■ Record any increases or decreases in bispectral index values, along with actions instituted based on values and any changes in sedative agents administered.

Cerebral aneurysm and subarachnoid hemorrhage

In an intracranial, or cerebral, aneurysm, a weakness in the wall of a cerebral artery causes localized dilation. The majority of cerebral aneurysms are berry (saccular) aneurysms, a saclike outpouching in a cerebral artery. Cerebral aneurysms usually arise at an arterial junction in the circle of Willis, the circular anastomosis forming the major cerebral arteries at the base of the brain. (See *Common sites of cerebral aneurysm.*) Cerebral aneurysms commonly rupture, resulting in subarachnoid hemorrhage (SAH).

Cerebral aneurysms are much more common in adults than in children. Incidence is slightly higher in women than in men, especially those in their late 40s or early to mid-50s, but a cerebral aneurysm may occur at any age in either sex. Causes may include congenital defect, degenerative process, a combination of both, or trauma.

The prognosis is always guarded, but is affected by the patient's age and neurologic condition, the presence of other diseases, and the extent and location of the aneurysm. About one-half of all patients who suffer a subarachnoid hemorrhage die immediately. With new and better treatments being developed, the prognosis is improving.

Pathophysiology

Blood flow exerts pressure against a congenitally weak arterial wall, stretching it like an overblown balloon and causing a rupture. The rupture is followed by an SAH, in which blood spills into the space normally occupied by cerebrospinal fluid (CSF). Blood may also spill into brain tissue, where a clot can cause potentially fatal increased intracranial pressure (ICP) and brain tissue damage.

Most cerebral aneurysms occur at bifurcations of major arteries in the circle of Willis and its branches. An aneurysm can produce neurologic symptoms by exerting pressure on the surrounding structures such as the cranial nerves.

Comprehensive assessment

The patient may exhibit premonitory symptoms resulting from oozing of blood into the subarachnoid space. The symptoms, which may persist for several days, include:
- headache
- intermittent nausea
- nuchal rigidity
- stiff back and legs.

Usually, however, the rupture occurs abruptly and without warning, causing the following:
- sudden, severe headache caused by increased pressure from bleeding into a closed space
- nausea and projectile vomiting related to increased pressure
- altered level of consciousness (LOC), including deep coma, depending on the severity and location of bleeding, from increased pressure caused by increased cerebral blood volume
- meningeal irritation, resulting in nuchal rigidity, back and leg pain, fever, restlessness, irritability, occasional seizures, photophobia, and blurred

Common sites of cerebral aneurysm

Cerebral aneurysms usually arise at the arterial bifurcation in the circle of Willis and its branches. The illustration below shows the most common sites around this circle.

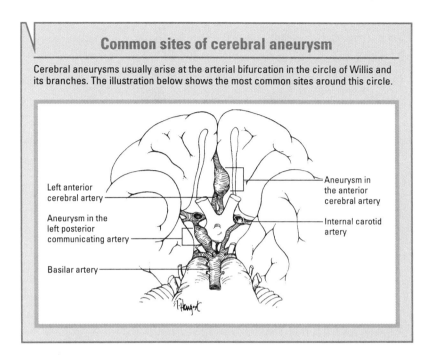

Left anterior cerebral artery

Aneurysm in the left posterior communicating artery

Basilar artery

Aneurysm in the anterior cerebral artery

Internal carotid artery

vision, secondary to bleeding into the meninges

■ hemiparesis, hemisensory defects, dysphagia, and visual defects from bleeding into the brain tissues

■ diplopia, ptosis, dilated pupil, and inability to rotate the eye from compression on the oculomotor nerve if the aneurysm is near the internal carotid artery.

Typically, the severity of a ruptured intracranial aneurysm is graded according to the patient's signs and symptoms. (See *Hunt-Hess classifications for subarachnoid hemorrhage,* page 286.)

Diagnosis

The following tests help diagnose cerebral aneurysm and SAH:

■ Cerebral angiography reveals altered cerebral blood flow, vessel lumen dilation, and differences in arterial filling.

■ Computed tomography (CT) scan identifies evidence of aneurysm and possible hemorrhage; it may also identify hydrocephalus, areas of infarction, and the extent of blood spillage within the cisterns around the brain.

■ Magnetic resonance imaging may help locate the aneurysm and the bleeding.

■ Positron emission tomography shows the chemical activity of the brain as well as the extent of tissue damage.

■ Electrocardiogram commonly shows flattened or depressed T waves.

■ Lumbar puncture (LP) and CSF analysis reveal blood in CSF; elevated

---

Hunt-Hess classifications for subarachnoid hemorrhage

The severity of symptoms accompanying subarachnoid hemorrhage (SAH) varies from patient to patient, depending on the site and the amount of bleeding. The Hunt-Hess classification identifies five grades that characterize an SAH from a ruptured cerebral aneurysm:

● *Grade I (minimal bleeding)*—The patient is alert and oriented without symptoms.
● *Grade II (mild bleeding)*—The patient is alert and oriented, with a mild to severe headache and nuchal rigidity.
● *Grade III (moderate bleeding)*—The patient is lethargic and confused or drowsy, with nuchal rigidity and, possibly, a mild focal deficit such as hemiparesis.
● *Grade IV (severe bleeding)*—The patient is stuporous, with nuchal rigidity and, possibly, moderate to severe focal deficits, hemiplegia, early decerebrate rigidity, and vegetative disturbances.
● *Grade V (moribund; often fatal)*—If the rupture is nonfatal, the patient is in a deep coma, with severe neurological deficits, such as decerebrate rigidity and moribund appearance.

CSF pressure, protein, and white blood cell count; and decreased glucose levels with SAH.

ALERT *Be aware that an LP, if performed in patients with SAH and increased ICP, increases the patient's risk for herniation and rebleeding. Therefore, it's performed only if the results of the CT scan are inconclusive.*

Collaborations

A multidisciplinary approach to care is essential. Care focuses on respiratory support, bed rest, ICP monitoring, fluid and electrolyte management, and pharmacologic therapy. In addition, a neurosurgeon may be involved to evaluate the need for surgery and help determine the best course of treatment. If the patient experiences neurologic deficits, he may require physical rehabilitation, nutritional therapy, occupational therapy, and respiratory therapy.

Treatment and care

Initial emergency treatment includes oxygenation and ventilation. To reduce the risk of rebleeding, the physician may then attempt to repair the aneurysm. Surgical repair is typically done by clipping, ligating, or wrapping the aneurysm neck with muscle. Newer surgical techniques include interventional radiology in conjunction with endovascular balloon therapy to occlude the aneurysm or the vessel, and cerebral angioplasty to treat arterial vasospasm. The timing of surgery is controversial; many patients with grade III or higher with anterior circulation aneurysms go to surgery within 1 to 3 days.

After surgical repair, the patient's condition depends on the extent of damage from the initial bleed and the degree of successful treatment of the resulting complications. Surgery can't improve the patient's neurologic condition unless it removes a hematoma or reduces the compression effect.

When surgical correction poses too much risk (in very elderly patients and those with heart, lung, or other serious diseases), when the aneurysm is in a particularly dangerous location, or when vasospasm necessitates a delay in surgery, the patient may receive conservative treatment. This includes:

■ bed rest in a quiet, darkened room with head of the bed flat or raised less than 30 degrees; if immediate surgery isn't possible, such bed rest may continue for 4 to 6 weeks

■ avoidance of coffee, other stimulants, and aspirin to reduce the risk of rupture and elevation of blood pressure, which increases the risk of rupture

■ codeine or another analgesics as needed to maintain rest and minimize the risk of pressure changes leading to rupture

■ hydralazine or another antihypertensive agent, if the patient is hypertensive, to reduce the risk of rupture

■ a vasoconstrictor to maintain blood pressure at the optimum level (20 to 40 mm Hg above normal), if necessary

■ corticosteroids to reduce cerebral edema and meningeal irritation

■ phenytoin or another anticonvulsant to prevent or treat seizures secondary to pressure and tissue irritation from bleeding

■ phenobarbital or another sedative to prevent agitation leading to hypertension and reduce the risk of rupture

■ aminocaproic acid, an inhibitor of fibrinolysis, to minimize the risk of rebleeding by delaying blood clot lysis (controversial).

Complications

If the patient develops increased ICP and brain herniation, rupture of a cerebral aneurysm could be fatal. Other major complications include:

■ vasospasm (most common cause of death after rupture, occurring in a large majority of patients after SAH,

usually between 4 to 14 days — peaking between 7 and 10 days — after SAH)

■ rebleeding (usually occurring within the first 24 to 48 hours after rupture, 7 to 10 days after the initial rupture, or anytime within the first 6 months)

■ hydrocephalus

■ hypothalamic dysfunction

■ hyponatremia. (See *Complications of cerebral aneurysm rupture,* page 288.)

Nursing considerations

■ Secure and maintain the patient's airway and anticipate the need for endotracheal intubation and mechanical ventilation, as necessary. Administer supplemental oxygen, as ordered. Monitor oxygen saturation levels via pulse oximetry and serial arterial blood gas studies, as ordered.

ALERT *Be sure to maintain adequate oxygenation because the development of cerebral hypoxia, along with hypoxemia and hypercapnia, can lead to increased cerebral vasodilation, subsequently increasing cerebral edema and ICP.*

■ Assess the patient's neurologic status frequently, at least every hour, or more frequently if indicated. Note the patient's LOC and ability to respond to stimuli, pupillary response, motor and sensory function, and reflexes. Observe for signs and symptoms of increased ICP and monitor ICP as ordered. (See "Intracranial pressure monitoring," page 312.)

ALERT *Watch for decreased LOC, unilaterally enlarged pupil, onset or worsening of hemiparesis or motor deficit, increased blood pressure, decreased heart rate, worsened or sudden headache, renewed or persistent*

Complications of cerebral aneurysm rupture

Complication	Pathophysiologic mechanism	Assessment findings
Vasospasm	Exact cause is unknown; it's believed that blood clots in the basal cisterns hemolyze, causing the release of substances that initiate spasms of the blood vessels	• Intense headaches • Decreased level of consciousness (LOC) • Aphasia • Partial paralysis
Rebleeding	Exact mechanism is unknown; it's believed that a dissolving blood clot and changes in arterial pressure lead to bleeding	• Sudden, severe headache • Nausea, vomiting • Decreased LOC • Neurologic deficits
Hydrocephalus	Blood in the subarachnoid space and ventricular system interferes with normal cerebrospinal (CSF) circulation and reabsorption, causing CSF pressure to rise	• Acute (occurring within 24 hours): loss of pupillary reflexes, sudden onset of coma • Subacute (occurring within 1 to 7 days): gradual changes in LOC, progressing from confusion, drowsiness, and lethargy to stupor • Delayed (occurring after 10 days): gradual change in LOC, incontinence, impaired balance, gait and mobility, slowing of intellectual function, diminished affect, and positive grasp and sucking reflexes (abnormal in adults)
Hypothalamic dysfunction	Dilated third ventricle exerts mechanical pressure on the hypothalamus, leading to dysfunction	• Vomiting • Glycosuria • Proteinuria • Flushing, diaphoresis • Pupillary dilation • Decreased gastric motility • Hyperglycemia • Fever • Hypertension • Tachycardia • Arrhythmias • Cardiac ischemia and infarction
Hyponatremia	Cerebral salt-wasting syndrome, syndrome of inappropriate antidiuretic hormone (SIADH), or other factors influence sodium and water metabolism, leading to increased sodium excretion	• Anxiety • Confusion • Agitation • Disorientation • Anorexia, nausea, vomiting • Abdominal pain • Cold clammy skin • Generalized weakness • Lower extremity muscle cramps • SIADH • Cerebral salt-wasting syndrome

vomiting, and renewed or worsened nuchal rigidity. These signs and symptoms may be indicative of an enlarging aneurysm, rebleeding, an intracranial clot, vasospasm, or another complication; report them to the patient's physician immediately.

■ Determine the patient's cerebral perfusion pressure (CPP). Institute cerebral blood flow monitoring as ordered to determine CPP. If not available, calculate CPP by subtracting the patient's ICP from mean arterial pressure — the systolic blood pressure plus twice the diastolic blood pressure divided by 3.

■ Assess vital signs, including heart rate, respiratory rate, and blood pressure, at least every 15 minutes until stabilized. Monitor temperature for increases.

ALERT *Be aware that if the aneurysm ruptures and blood accumulates in the subarachnoid space, it triggers an inflammatory response in the body that causes the patient's temperature to rise. Be ready to institute measures to reduce hyperthermia, such as cooling blankets and antipyretics.*

■ Assess hemodynamic status frequently, including central venous pressure (CVP) and pulmonary artery pressure (PAP). Give fluids as ordered and monitor I.V. infusions to avoid overhydration, which may increase ICP.

■ Administer antihypertensive agents such as hydralazine, propranolol, labetalol, or sodium nitroprusside as ordered to maintain blood pressure within the desired range. Anticipate the use of direct intra-arterial blood pressure monitoring.

■ If the patient develops vasospasm, as evidenced by increasing confusion, focal motor deficits, worsening head-

ache, and increasing blood pressure, anticipate the use of hypervolemic-hemodilution therapy, such as administration of normal saline, whole blood, packed red blood cells, albumin, plasma protein fraction (increase circulating volume to reverse or prevent ischemia secondary to vasospasm) and crystalloid solution (to decrease blood viscosity).

ALERT *Keep in mind that hypervolemic-hemodilution therapy is associated with numerous risks, including increased ICP with rerupture and rebleeding and cerebral edema and cerebral ischemia with additional neurologic deficits. When administering this therapy, monitor the patient's blood pressure and ICP continuously. Assess the patient closely for signs and symptoms of fluid overload; monitor urine output every hour, auscultate lungs for crackles, observe for jugular vein distention, and monitor CVP and PAP for increases.*

■ If the patient experiences a sudden increase in ICP, expect to administer mannitol I.V., as ordered; monitor renal function status, including urine output and electrolytes, before and during administration.

ALERT *Be alert for a rebound effect of mannitol and a subsequent rebound increase in ICP due to the increase in circulating volume, which may occur 8 to 12 hours after administration. Assess the patient closely. Anticipate the possible use of furosemide to reduce this effect.*

■ Position the patient to promote pulmonary drainage and prevent upper airway obstruction. Avoid placing the patient in the prone position or hyperextending his neck.

Aneurysm precautions

Aneurysm precautions are measures to help prevent increased intracranial pressure and reduce the risk of rebleeding by minimizing increases in blood pressure. Although the specific precautions may vary among facilities, the following general guidelines are helpful.

• Place the patient on immediate and complete bed rest in a dimly lit, quiet, nonstressful environment.

• Keep the head of the patient's bed flat or slightly elevated (15 to 30 degrees).

• Avoid hyperflexion, hyperextension, or hyperrotation of the neck (minimizes jugular venous compression).

• Have the patient avoid activities involving isometric muscle contraction, such as pulling or pushing on the side rails or against the foot of the bed. Provide passive range-of-motion exercises.

• Administer stool softeners to prevent straining. Advise the patient to avoid bearing down with bowel movements (Valsalva's maneuver); encourage the patient to exhale slowly when defecating or voiding.

• Avoid rectal temperature measurement, suppositories, enemas, or digital impaction removal.

• Urge the patient to avoid coughing; administer antitussives, if ordered.

• Administer antiemetics as ordered to prevent or manage vomiting.

• Eliminate coffee, tea, or other caffeinated beverages from the patient's intake.

• Assist with personal care and activities of daily living to prevent exertion.

• Eliminate exposure to external stimuli, such as television, radio, and books.

• Restrict visitors to family; encourage visitors to talk quietly with the patient, avoiding stressful topics as much as possible.

■ Following your facility's policy, suction secretions from the airway as necessary to prevent hypoxia and vasodilatation from carbon dioxide accumulation. Suction for less than 20 seconds to avoid increased ICP.

■ Institute aneurysm precautions to prevent increased ICP and minimize the risk for rebleeding. (See *Aneurysm precautions.*)

■ Administer analgesics for mild to moderate pain from headache and anticonvulsants to prevent seizures, as ordered.

■ Anticipate the use of aminocaproic acid by continuous infusion, approximately 1 to 2 weeks after rupture, if ordered to prevent lysis of the aneurysm's clot. Keep in mind that the use of this drug is controversial.

■ Turn the patient often. Apply antiembolism stockings or intermittent sequential compression devices to the patient's legs to reduce the risk of deep vein thrombosis.

■ Institute measures to prevent skin breakdown.

■ If the patient can eat, provide a high-fiber diet (bran, salads, and fruit) to prevent straining during defecation, which can increase ICP.

■ Administer a stool softener or mild laxative, as ordered. Implement a bowel elimination program based on previous habits. If the patient is receiving steroids to relieve cerebral edema, monitor for GI irritation and check the stool for blood.

■ Prepare the patient for surgery as appropriate. If the patient develops hydrocephalus, prepare him for ventriculostomy. (See "Ventriculostomy," page 348.)

■ Provide emotional support to the patient and his family. To minimize stress, encourage the patient to use relaxation techniques. Encourage him to express his concerns if he's able.

Patient teaching

■ Teach the patient, if possible, and his family about his condition. Encourage family members to adopt a realistic attitude but don't discourage hope. Answer questions honestly.

■ Explain all tests, neurologic examinations, treatments, and procedures to the patient, even if he's unconscious.

■ Warn the patient who will be treated conservatively to avoid all unnecessary physical activity.

■ If surgery will be performed, provide preoperative teaching if the patient's condition permits. Make sure that the patient, if possible, and his family understand the surgery and its possible complications. Reinforce the physician's explanations as necessary.

■ Teach family members to recognize and immediately report signs of rebleeding, such as headache, nausea, vomiting, and changes in LOC.

Cerebral blood flow monitoring

Traditionally, caregivers have estimated cerebral blood flow (CBF) in neurologically compromised patients by calculating cerebral perfusion pressure. However, modern technology permits continuous regional blood-flow monitoring at the bedside.

A sensor placed on the cerebral cortex calculates CBF in the capillary bed by thermal diffusion. Thermistors within the sensor detect the temperature differential between two metallic plates: one heated, one neutral. This differential is inversely proportional to CBF: As the differential decreases, CBF increases — and vice versa. This monitoring technique reveals important information about the effects of interventions on CBF. It also yields continuous real-time values for CBF, which are essential in conditions in which compromised blood flow may put the patient at risk for complications such as ischemia and infarction. The surgeon typically inserts the sensor in the operating room during or following a craniotomy. (Occasionally, he may insert it through a burr hole.) He implants the sensor far from major blood vessels and verifies that the metallic plates have good contact with the brain surface. (See *Inserting a cerebral blood flow sensor,* page 292.)

CBF monitoring is indicated whenever CBF alterations are anticipated. It's used most commonly in patients with subarachnoid hemorrhage (in which a vasospasm may restrict blood flow), trauma associated with high intracranial pressure, or vascular tumors.

Equipment

CBF monitoring requires a special sensor that attaches to a computer data system or to a small analog monitor that operates on a battery for patient transport. (See *Bedside cerebral blood flow monitor,* page 293.)

For care of site
Sterile 4″ × 4″ gauze pads ■ clean gloves ■ sterile gloves ■ povidone-

Inserting a cerebral blood flow sensor

The sensor used to monitor cerebral blood flow (CBF) does so by means of thermistors housed inside it. The thermistors consist of two metallic plates — one heated and one neutral. The sensor detects the temperature difference between the two plates, which is inversely proportional to CBF. As CBF increases, the temperature difference decreases, and vice versa.

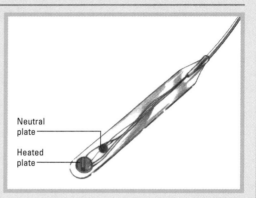

Neutral plate

Heated plate

Typically, the surgeon inserts a CBF sensor during a craniotomy. He tunnels the sensor toward the craniotomy site and then carefully inserts the metallic plates of the thermistor to ensure continuous contact with the surface of the cerebral cortex. After closing the dura and replacing the bone flap, he closes the scalp.

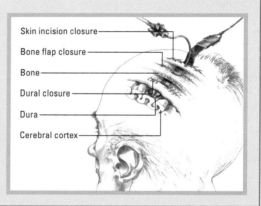

Skin incision closure

Bone flap closure

Bone

Dural closure

Dura

Cerebral cortex

iodine solution or ointment ▪ adhesive tape

For removing sensor
Sterile suture removal tray ▪ #19 adhesive tape ▪ sterile 4″ × 4″ gauze pads ▪ clean gloves ▪ sterile gloves ▪ suture material

Essential steps
▪ Make sure that the patient or a family member is fully informed about the procedures involved in CBF monitoring and obtain a signed consent form. If the patient will need CBF monitoring after surgery, advise him that a sensor will be in place for about 3 days. Tell the patient that the insertion site will be covered with a dry, sterile dressing. Mention that the sensor may be removed at the bedside.
▪ Set up the sensor monitor.
– Depending on the type of system you're using, ensure that a battery has been inserted in the monitor to

allow CBF monitoring during patient transport.

— Assemble the following equipment at the bedside: a monitor and sensor cable with an attached sensor. Attach the distal end of the sensor cable (from the patient's head) to the SENSOR CONNECT port on the monitor. When the sensor cable is securely in place, press the ON key to activate the monitor.

— Calibrate the system by pressing the CAL key. You should see the red light appear on the CAL button. Ideally, you'll begin by calibrating the sensor to 00.0 by pressing the directional arrows. Readouts of plus or minus 0.1 are also acceptable.

■ Press the RUN key to display the CBF reading. Observe the monitor's digital display and document the baseline value.

■ Record the CBF hourly. Be sure to watch for trends and correlate values with the patient's clinical status. Be aware that stimulation or activity may cause a 10% increase or decrease in CBF. If you detect a 20% increase or decrease, suspect poor contact between the sensor and the cerebral cortex.

■ Provide care for the insertion site.
— Wash your hands. Put on clean gloves, and remove the dressing from the sensor insertion site.
— Observe the site for cerebrospinal fluid (CSF) leakage, a potential complication; remove and discard your gloves.
— Put on sterile gloves. Using aseptic technique, clean the insertion site with a gauze pad soaked in antiseptic solution. Clean the site, starting at the center and working outward in a circular pattern.

Bedside cerebral blood flow monitor

Cerebral blood flow (CBF) monitoring at the patient's bedside often involves the use of a monitor attached to a sensor placed in the patient's cerebral cortex. This monitor measures CBF continuously. The monitor shown below has a digital display; some also display waveforms.

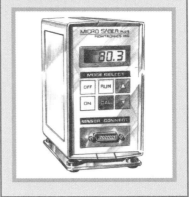

— Using a new gauze pad soaked with antiseptic solution, clean the exposed part of the sensor from the insertion site to the end of the sensor. Apply antiseptic ointment to the insertion site if your facility's policy permits.
— Place sterile 4″ × 4″ gauze pads over the insertion site to completely cover it. Tape all edges securely to create an occlusive dressing.

■ Assist with removing the sensor. (Keep in mind that in most cases, the CBF sensor remains in place for about 3 days when used for postoperative monitoring.)
— Explain the procedure to the patient. Wash your hands, and put on clean gloves. Remove the dressing,

and dispose of the gloves and dressing properly.
– Open the suture removal tray and the package of suture material. The surgeon will remove the anchoring sutures and then gently remove the sensor from the insertion site.
– After the surgeon closes the wound with stitches, put on sterile gloves, apply a folded gauze pad to the site, and tape it in place. Observe the condition of the site, including any leakage.

Complications
Possible complications associated with CBF monitoring include:
- infection
- CSF leakage
- equipment malfunction.

Nursing considerations
- Keep in mind that CBF fluctuates with the brain's metabolic demands, typically ranging from 60 to 90 ml/100 g/minute. However, the patient's neurologic condition dictates the acceptable range. For example, in a patient in a coma, the CBF may be one-half the normal value; in a patient in a barbiturate-induced coma with burst suppression on the EEG, CBF may be as low as 10 ml/100 g/minute.
- **ALERT** *Vasospasm secondary to subarachnoid hemorrhage may result in CBF below 40 ml/100 g/minute. In a patient who is awake, CBF above 90 ml/100 g/minute may indicate hyperemia.*
- If you suspect poor contact between the sensor and the cerebral cortex, turn the patient toward the side of the sensor or gently wiggle the catheter back and forth (using a sterile-gloved

hand). To determine whether these maneuvers have improved contact between the sensor and the cortex, observe the CBF value on the monitor as you perform them.
- If your patient has low CBF but no neurologic signs that indicate ischemia, suspect a fluid layer (a small hematoma) between the sensor and the cortex.
- Administer prophylactic antibiotics as ordered and maintain a sterile dressing around the insertion site to reduce the risk of infection; change the dressing at the insertion site daily.
- To prevent leakage, check to see if the surgeon placed an additional suture at the site.
- Record CBF values obtained at designated intervals along with patient assessment findings.
- Document cleaning of the site, appearance of the site, and dressing changes. After sensor removal, record any leakage from the site, including color, characteristics, and amount.

Craniotomy

Craniotomy involves creation of a surgical incision into the skull, thereby exposing the brain for treatment, such as ventricular shunting, excision of a tumor or abscess, hematoma aspiration, and aneurysm clipping.

Procedure
The surgical approach to a supratentorial craniotomy can be frontal, parietal, temporal, occipital, or a combination of these areas. If structures below the tentorium are involved, the surgical approach to an infratentorial cranioto-

my involves an incision slightly above the neck in the back of the skull. In the operating room just before surgery, the anesthetist will start a peripheral I.V. line, a central venous pressure (CVP) line, and an arterial line. The CVP line provides access to remove air should an air embolus occur—a particular risk when posterior fossa surgery is performed in the sitting position.

After the patient receives a general or local anesthetic, the surgeon marks an incision line and cuts through the scalp to the cranium, forming a scalp flap that he folds to one side. He then bores four or five holes through the skull in the corners of the cranial incision and cuts out a bone flap. After pulling aside or removing the bone flap, he incises and retracts the dura, exposing the brain. (See *Craniotomy: A window to the brain,* page 296.) The surgeon then proceeds with the surgery. Afterward, he reverses the incision procedure and covers the site with a sterile dressing.

Complications
Craniotomy has many potential complications, including:
■ infection
■ vasospasm
■ hemorrhage
■ air embolism
■ respiratory compromise
■ increased intracranial pressure (ICP)
■ diabetes insipidus
■ syndrome of inappropriate antidiuretic hormone (SIADH)
■ seizures
■ cranial nerve damage.

The degree of risk for these complications depends largely on the patient's condition and the surgery's complexity.

Nursing considerations
When preparing for, or managing a patient with, a craniotomy, expect to implement the following interventions.

Before craniotomy
■ Help the patient and his family cope with the surgery by clarifying the physician's explanation and encouraging them to ask questions. When answering their questions, be informative and honest. While you can't guarantee a complete and uncomplicated recovery, you can help instill a sense of confidence in the surgeon and a successful outcome.
■ Explain preoperative procedures, including hair washing and shaving and the use of steroids to reduce postoperative inflammation. Also explain about devices that may be inserted (such as a peripheral I.V. line, CVP line, and arterial line) and the possibility of endotracheal (ET) intubation and mechanical ventilation.
■ Inform the patient that antiembolism stockings or intermittent sequential compression devices may be applied to his legs to improve venous return and reduce the risk of thrombophlebitis. Explain that he may require an indwelling urinary catheter because craniotomy is a lengthy procedure.
■ Prepare the patient for postoperative recovery. Explain that he'll awaken from surgery with a large dressing on his head to protect the incision. He may also have a surgical drain implanted in his skull for at least 24

Craniotomy: A window to the brain

To perform a craniotomy, the surgeon incises the skin, clamps the aponeurotic layer, and retracts the skin flap. He then incises and retracts the muscle layer and scrapes periosteum off the skull.

Next, using an air-driven or electric drill, he drills a series of burr holes in the corners of the skull incision. During drilling, warm saline solution is dripped into the burr holes and the holes are suctioned to remove bone dust. When

drilling is complete, the surgeon uses a dural elevator to separate the dura from the bone around the margin of each burr hole. He then saws between the burr holes to create a bone flap. He either leaves this flap attached to the muscle and retracts it or detaches the flap completely and removes it. In either case, the flap is wrapped to keep it moist and protected. Finally, the surgeon incises and retracts the dura, exposing the brain.

INITIAL INCISION

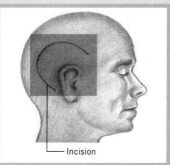

Incision

RETRACTION OF SKIN FLAP

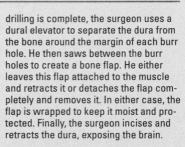

Skin flap

BURR HOLES DRILLED

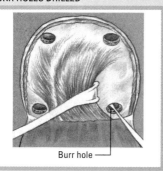

Burr hole

BRAIN EXPOSED

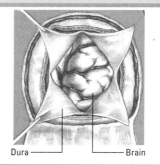

Dura ———— Brain

hours and will be receiving prophylactic antibiotics.

■ Warn him to expect a headache and facial swelling for 2 to 3 days after

surgery, and reassure him that he'll receive medication to reduce the pain.

■ Instruct him about the importance of postoperative leg exercises and deep breathing.

■ Before surgery, perform a complete neurologic assessment. Carefully record assessment data to use as a baseline for postoperative evaluation.

■ Arrange a preoperative visit to the critical care unit for the patient and his family, if not already there. Explain the equipment, and introduce them to the staff.

After craniotomy

■ After surgery, carefully monitor the patient's vital signs and neurologic status every 15 minutes for the first 4 hours, then once every 30 to 60 minutes for the next 24 to 48 hours.

■ Assess the patient's cardiopulmonary and hemodynamic status, as indicated. Administer supplemental oxygen as ordered, and monitor oxygen saturation via pulse oximetry and arterial blood gas analysis.

■ Closely observe the patient's respiratory status, noting rate and pattern. Immediately report abnormalities. Encourage him to deep-breathe and cough but warn him not to do this too strenuously. Suction gently, as ordered. If the patient's respiratory status is unstable or shows signs of deterioration, anticipate the need for ET intubation and mechanical ventilation.

■ Monitor ICP and CBF as ordered, and assess the monitoring insertion sites at least every 4 hours for signs and symptoms of infection and cerebrospinal fluid (CSF) leakage. Report any such symptoms to the physician. (See "Intracranial pressure monitoring," page 312, and "Cerebral blood flow monitoring," page 291.)

■ Position the patient on his side to help prevent increased ICP and protect his airway, if his level of consciousness is decreased. Elevate his head 15 to 30 degrees (if indicated) to increase venous return and help him breathe more easily. With another nurse's help, turn him carefully every 2 hours.

ALERT *Keep in mind that some cerebral edema is normal after a craniotomy, usually peaking at approximately 72 hours after surgery.*

■ Administer anticonvulsants as ordered, and maintain seizure precautions.

■ Provide other ordered medications, such as steroids to prevent or reduce cerebral edema, stool softeners to prevent increased ICP from straining during defecation, and analgesics to relieve pain.

■ Throughout the postoperative course, observe the patient closely for signs of increased ICP. Immediately notify the physician upon noting a worsening mental status, pupillary changes, or focal signs such as increasing weakness in an extremity.

ALERT *Be aware that neurologic deficits may occur or worsen after a craniotomy due to trauma response from surgical manipulation or cerebral edema. These deficits should improve over time as the edema and trauma response subside. Be sure to document these deficits and observe the patient for changes indicating improvement. Failure to resolve indicates permanent damage to the specific area of the brain.*

■ Carefully monitor the patient's fluid and electrolyte balance. Administer fluids as prescribed, to maintain normal fluid balance. Monitor and record intake and output, checking urine specific gravity every 2 hours and urine output every hour initially. Obtain daily weights.

■ Obtain serial serum electrolyte levels, and observe the patient for signs of imbalance.

ALERT *Diabetes insipidus and SIADH are two possible complications that can occur after a craniotomy. These two complications can cause severe fluid and electrolyte imbalances. Be alert for low potassium levels, which may cause confusion and stupor, and reduced sodium and chloride levels, which may produce weakness, lethargy, and even coma. Because fluid and electrolyte imbalance can precipitate seizures, report any of these signs immediately and prepare for I.V. replacement.*

■ Anticipate the need for continuous cardiac monitoring to detect arrhythmias secondary to cerebral hypoxia, ischemia, or electrolyte imbalances.

■ Assess the abdomen for distention and presence of bowel sounds. Decreased or absent bowel sounds may suggest paralytic ileus. If this occurs, prepare for nasogastric intubation and low intermittent suction. Anticipate the use of histamine-2 receptor antagonists to reduce the risk of GI bleeding secondary to cerebral trauma or use of corticosteroids.

■ Inspect the incision site at least every 4 hours, and provide good wound care. Make sure that the dressing stays dry and intact, without being too tight. A dressing that's too tight may cause soft-tissue swelling. If the patient has a closed drainage system, periodically check drain patency, and note and document the amount and characteristics of any discharge. Notify the physician of excessive bloody drainage, possibly indicating cerebral hemorrhage, or of clear or yellow drainage, which may indicate a CSF leak. Monitor the patient for signs of wound infection, such as fever and purulent drainage.

■ Provide supportive care. Ensure a quiet, calm environment to minimize anxiety and agitation and to help lower ICP.

■ Teach the patient proper wound care techniques, including keeping the suture line dry and clean. Instruct him to evaluate the incision regularly for redness, warmth, or tenderness and to report any of these findings to the physician.

■ Provide positive reinforcement about the patient's appearance, offering suggestions to aid in dealing with hair loss at the surgical site.

■ Remind the patient to continue taking prescribed anticonvulsant medications to minimize the risk of seizures. Depending on the type of surgery performed, he may need to continue anticonvulsant therapy for up to 12 months after surgery. Remind him to report any adverse drug effects, such as excessive drowsiness or confusion.

■ Instruct the patient to consult with the physician before consuming alcohol, driving, or participating in contact sports.

 MULTISYSTEM DISORDER

Guillain-Barré syndrome

Also known as infectious polyneuritis, Landry-Guillain-Barré syndrome, or acute idiopathic polyneuritis, Guillain-Barré syndrome is an acute, rapidly progressive, and potentially fatal form of polyneuritis that causes muscle weakness and mild distal sensory loss.

█ AGE ISSUE *Guillain-Barré syndrome can occur at any age but is most common between ages 30 and 50. It affects both sexes equally.*

Recovery is spontaneous and complete in about 95% of patients, although mild motor or reflex deficits may persist in the feet and legs. The prognosis is best when symptoms clear before 15 to 20 days after onset.

The precise cause of Guillain-Barré syndrome is unknown, but it may be a cell-mediated immune response to a virus. About 50% of patients with Guillain-Barré syndrome have a recent history of minor febrile illness, usually an upper respiratory tract infection or, less commonly, a GI infection such as gastroenteritis. When infection precedes the onset of Guillain-Barré syndrome, signs of infection subside before neurologic features appear.

Other possible precipitating factors include:
- surgery
- rabies or swine influenza vaccination
- Hodgkin's or other malignant disease
- systemic lupus erythematosus.

Pathophysiology

Guillain-Barré syndrome occurs in three phases:
- The *acute* phase begins with the onset of the first definitive symptom and ends 1 to 3 weeks later. Further deterioration doesn't occur after the acute phase.
- The *plateau* phase lasts several days to 2 weeks.
- The *recovery* phase is believed to coincide with remyelinization and re-

Understanding sensorimotor nerve degeneration

Guillain-Barré syndrome attacks the peripheral nerves so that they can't transmit messages to the brain correctly. The myelin sheath, which covers the nerve axons and conducts electrical impulses along the nerve pathways, degenerates. (The reason for this degeneration isn't known.) Degeneration brings inflammation, swelling, and patchy demyelination. As this disorder destroys myelin, the nodes of Ranvier (at the junction of the myelin sheaths) widen, delaying and impairing impulse transmission along both the dorsal and anterior nerve roots.

Because the dorsal nerve roots handle sensory function, the patient may experience tingling and numbness. Similarly, because the anterior nerve roots are responsible for motor function, impairment causes varying weakness, immobility, and paralysis.

growth of axonal processes. It extends over 4 to 6 months, but may last up to 2 to 3 years if the disease was severe.

The major pathologic manifestation is segmental demyelination of the peripheral nerves. This prevents normal transmission of electrical impulses along the sensorimotor nerve roots. Because this syndrome causes inflammation and degenerative changes in both the posterior (sensory) and the anterior (motor) nerve roots, signs of sensory and motor losses occur simultaneously. (See *Understanding sensorimotor nerve degeneration*.) Additionally, autonomic nerve transmission may be impaired.

Comprehensive assessment

Most patients seek treatment when Guillain-Barré syndrome is in the acute stage. The patient's history typically reveals that he has experienced a minor febrile illness (usually an upper respiratory tract infection or, less often, GI infection) 1 to 4 weeks before his current symptoms. The patient may report feelings of tingling and numbness (paresthesia) in the legs. If the syndrome has progressed further, he may report that the tingling and numbness began in the legs and progressed to the arms, trunk and, finally, the face. The paresthesia usually precedes muscle weakness but tends to vanish quickly; in some patients, it may never occur. Some patients may also report stiffness and pain in the calves (such as a severe charley horse) and back.

Neurologic examination uncovers muscle weakness (the major neurologic sign) and sensory loss, usually in the legs. If the syndrome has progressed, the weakness and sensory loss may also be present in the arms.

ALERT *Guillain-Barré syndrome progresses rapidly and symptoms may progress beyond the legs in 24 to 72 hours.*

If the cranial nerves are affected — as they often are — the patient may have difficulty talking, chewing, and swallowing. Subsequent cranial nerve testing may reveal paralysis of the ocular, facial, and oropharyngeal muscles.

ALERT *Muscle weakness sometimes develops in the arms first (descending type), rather than in the legs (ascending type) — or in the arms and legs simultaneously. Remember, too, that in milder forms of the syndrome, muscle weakness may affect* only the cranial nerves or may not occur at all.

Neurologic examination may reveal a loss of position sense and diminished or absent deep tendon reflexes. In addition, the following may be noted:

■ diplegia, possibly with ophthalmoplegia (ocular paralysis), from impaired motor nerve root transmission and involvement of cranial nerves III, IV, and VI
■ dysphagia or dysarthria and, less often, weakness of the muscles supplied by cranial nerve XI (spinal accessory nerve)
■ hypotonia and areflexia from interruption of the reflex arc.

Diagnosis

The following tests help diagnose Guillain-Barré syndrome:

■ Cerebrospinal fluid (CSF) analysis by lumbar puncture reveals elevated protein levels, peaking in 4 to 6 weeks, probably a result of widespread inflammation of the nerve roots; the CSF white blood cell count remains normal. However, in severe disease, CSF pressure may rise above normal.
■ Complete blood count shows leukocytosis with immature forms early in the illness, then quickly returns to normal.
■ Electromyography possibly shows repeated firing of the same motor unit, instead of widespread sectional stimulation.
■ Nerve conduction velocities show slowing soon after paralysis develops.
■ Serum immunoglobulin levels reveal elevated levels from inflammatory response.

Collaborations

The patient with Guillain-Barré syndrome will require a multidisciplinary approach to care; for example, a pulmonary specialist and respiratory specialist can help with clearing secretions and maintaining ventilation. The patient may also require a physical therapist to help maintain joint range-of-motion, an occupational therapist to assist with activities of daily living, and a registered dietitian to maintain nutrition. Social services may be involved to assist with continued care and follow-up and help with financial concerns and community support. A spiritual counselor or pastoral care associate can help the patient and his family during this highly stressful time.

Treatment and care

In Guillain-Barré syndrome, treatment is primarily supportive and may require endotracheal (ET) intubation or tracheotomy if the patient has difficulty clearing secretions or maintaining a patent airway. Mechanical ventilation is necessary if the patient has respiratory difficulties.

Continuous electrocardiogram (ECG) monitoring is necessary to identify cardiac arrhythmias. Pharmacologic therapy may include propranolol to treat tachycardia and hypotension and atropine to treat bradycardia. Marked hypotension may require volume replacement. A trial dose (7 days) of prednisone may be given to reduce inflammatory response if the disease is relentlessly progressive; if prednisone produces no noticeable improvement, the drug is discontinued.

Plasmapheresis involves the complete exchange of plasma whereby the abnormal circulating antibodies are re-

moved. As a result, a temporary reduction in circulating antibodies is produced in the hopes of attempting to lessen the severity and duration of the disease. This treatment is usually reserved for the most severely affected patients or those whose illness is progressing very rapidly. It's most effective if performed during the first few days of the illness.

Complications

Common complications of Guillain-Barré syndrome include:
- thrombophlebitis
- pressure ulcers
- muscle wasting
- sepsis
- joint contractures
- aspiration
- respiratory tract infections
- mechanical respiratory failure.
  Additionally, the patient may develop autonomic nervous system dysfunction, including:
- sinus tachycardia
- bradycardia
- hypotension or hypertension
- bowel and bladder retention and loss of sphincter control
- syndrome of inappropriate antidiuretic hormone
- cardiac arrhythmias.

Nursing considerations

- Continually assess the patient's respiratory function. Auscultate for breath sounds at least every 2 hours or more frequently if indicated. If respiratory muscles are weak, take serial vital capacity recordings. Use a respirometer with a mouthpiece or a face mask, for bedside testing.

ALERT *Vital capacity values less than 1 L suggest the potential need for mechanical ventilation.*

■ Obtain baseline and serial arterial blood gas studies as ordered and monitor pulse oximetry readings. Because neuromuscular disease results in primary hypoventilation with hypoxemia and hypercapnia, watch for partial pressure of arterial oxygen (PaO_2) below 70 mm Hg, which signals respiratory failure. Be alert for confusion and tachypnea — signs of rising partial pressure of carbon dioxide in arterial blood.

■ Administer supplemental oxygen, as ordered. Continue to monitor trends in the patient's respiratory status.

■ Turn and reposition the patient, and encourage coughing and deep breathing. Begin respiratory support at the first sign of dyspnea (in adults, this means a vital capacity less than 1 L or decreasing PaO_2).

■ If respiratory failure becomes imminent, establish an emergency airway with an ET tube. Be prepared to begin and maintain mechanical ventilation.

■ Institute continuous ECG monitoring; prepare to treat the development of arrhythmias as ordered. Monitor vital signs at least every 2 hours initially; if the patient develops hypertension or hypotension, administer antihypertensive agents or vasopressors as ordered.

■ Inspect the patient's skin regularly for evidence of skin breakdown. Give meticulous skin care to prevent skin breakdown and contractures. Establish a strict turning schedule and reposition the patient every 2 hours. Use alternating pressure pads at points of contact. Apply splints as appropriate to joint areas to reduce the risk of contractures. Remove splints approximately every 2 hours, keeping them off for 2 hours.

■ Assess deep tendon reflexes and monitor the patient's muscle function daily for pattern and degree of loss and later for return of muscle function. Perform passive range-of-motion (ROM) exercises within the patient's pain limits, possibly using a Hubbard tank. (Exercising little-used muscles will cause pain.)

ALERT *Remember that the proximal muscle group of the thighs, shoulders, and trunk will be the most tender and will cause the most pain on passive movement and turning.*

■ When the patient's condition stabilizes, change to gentle stretching and active assistance exercises.

■ Assess the abdomen for distention and presence of bowel sounds. If bowel sounds are absent, prepare to insert a nasogastric (NG) tube to intermittent suction. Administer parenteral nutrition until bowel sounds return. Assess gag reflex and elevate the head of the bed before giving the patient anything to eat. If the gag reflex is absent, give NG tube feedings until this reflex returns. Progress diet once the gag reflex returns and swallowing ability improves.

■ As the patient regains strength and can tolerate a vertical position, be alert for postural hypotension. Monitor blood pressure and pulse rate during tilting periods. As the patient regains strength and can tolerate a vertical position, apply toe-to-groin elastic bandages or an abdominal binder to prevent postural hypotension, if necessary.

■ Inspect the patient's legs regularly for signs and symptoms of thrombophlebitis (localized pain, tenderness, erythema, edema, and positive Homans' sign). To prevent thrombophlebitis, apply antiembolism stockings or intermittent sequential compression devices and give prophylactic anticoagulants as ordered.

■ If the patient has facial paralysis, give eye and mouth care every 4 hours. Protect the corneas with isotonic eye drops and conical eye shields.

■ Watch for urine retention. Measure and record intake and output every 8 hours or more frequently, as indicated by the patient's condition. Offer the bedpan every 3 to 4 hours unless an indwelling urinary catheter is in place. Encourage adequate fluid intake (2 qt/day [1.9 L/day]) unless contraindicated. If urine retention develops, begin intermittent catheterization as ordered. If the patient has an indwelling urinary catheter inserted, make sure that the catheter is patent and flowing freely without any kinks or obstructions. Palpate the bladder for distention.

ALERT *The patient with Guillain-Barré syndrome, like the patient with acute spinal cord injury, is at risk for autonomic system involvement when exposed to noxious stimuli. These stimuli may include a distended bladder, urinary tract infection, fecal impaction, use of enemas or suppositories, pressure on skin or bony prominences, or temperature changes. (See* "Acute spinal cord injury," *page 272.)*

■ To prevent or relieve constipation, offer prune juice and a high-fiber diet. If necessary, give daily or alternate-day suppositories (glycerin or bisacodyl) or enemas, as ordered.

■ If the patient can't communicate because of paralysis, tracheostomy, or intubation, try to establish some form of communication — for example, have the patient blink his eyes, once for yes and twice for no.

■ Provide emotional support to the patient and his family. Listen to their concerns. Stay with the patient during periods of severe stress.

Patient teaching

■ Explain the syndrome and its signs and symptoms, diagnostic tests that will be performed, and the treatments that are ordered, including the rationale for them. For example, if the patient loses his gag reflex, tell him that tube feedings are necessary to maintain nutritional status.

■ Advise the family to help the patient maintain mental alertness, fight boredom, and avoid depression. Suggest frequent visits, reading to the patient, using music or other activities enjoyed by the patient.

■ Assist with measures for rehabilitation including care at home and follow-up with physical therapy. Reinforce ROM exercises, position changes, and transfer techniques.

■ Instruct the family in adaptations, such as with eating and reducing the risk of skin breakdown.

■ Emphasize the importance of establishing a regular bowel and bladder elimination routine.

Head injury

Head injury refers to any traumatic insult to the brain that results in physical, intellectual, emotional, social, or vocational changes.

AGE ISSUE *Young children 6 months to age 2, people ages 15 to 24, and elderly people are at highest risk for head injury. The risk in men is double the risk in women.*

ALERT *Blacks and people of any ethnicity living in poor socioeconomic settings appear to be at greatest risk for head injury.*

Head injury is generally categorized as closed or open trauma. Closed trauma, or blunt trauma as it's sometimes called, is more common, typically occurring when the head strikes a hard surface or a rapidly moving object strikes the head. The dura is intact, and no brain tissue is exposed to the external environment. In open trauma, as the name suggests, an opening in the scalp, skull, meninges, or brain tissue, including the dura, exposes the cranial contents to the environment, and the risk of infection is high.

Head injury commonly results from the following:
- transportation or motor vehicle crashes (number one cause)
- falls
- sports-related accidents
- crime and assaults.

Mortality from head injury has declined with advances in preventive measures, such as seat belts and airbags, quicker response and transport times, and improved treatment, including the development of regional trauma centers. Advances in technology have increased the effectiveness of rehabilitative services, even for patients with severe head injuries.

Pathophysiology

The brain is shielded by the cranial vault — hair, skin, bone, meninges, and cerebrospinal fluid (CSF) — which intercepts the force of a physical blow. Below a certain level of force (the absorption capacity), the cranial vault prevents energy from affecting the brain. The degree of traumatic head injury usually is proportional to the amount of force reaching the cranial tissues. Furthermore, unless ruled out, neck injuries should be presumed present in patients with traumatic head injury.

Closed trauma is typically a sudden acceleration-deceleration or coup-contrecoup injury. In coup-contrecoup, the head hits a relatively stationary object, injuring cranial tissues near the point of impact (coup); then the remaining force pushes the brain against the opposite side of the skull, causing a second impact and injury (contrecoup). Contusions and lacerations may also occur during contrecoup as the brain's soft tissues slide over the rough bone of the cranial cavity. Also, the cerebrum may endure rotational shear, damaging the upper midbrain and areas of the frontal, temporal, and occipital lobes.

Open trauma may penetrate the scalp, skull, meninges, or brain. Open head injuries are usually associated with skull fractures, and bone fragments often cause hematomas and meningeal tears with consequent loss of CSF.

Comprehensive assessment

The patient's history (obtained from the patient, his family, eyewitnesses, or emergency personnel) reveals a traumatic injury to the head. A period of unconsciousness may follow the trauma. If unconscious, the patient may appear pale and motionless. If conscious, he may appear drowsy or easily disturbed by any form of stimulation, such as noise or light.

Assessment findings will vary, depending on the type and location of the head injury. Focus the examination on the patient's level of consciousness (LOC), pupillary responses, and strength of extremities. Vital signs aren't good indicators of neurologic status and don't correlate specifically with this type of injury unless the brain stem is involved. Types of head injury include concussion, contusion, epidural hematoma, subdural hematoma, intracerebral hematoma, and skull fractures. Each is associated with specific signs and symptoms. (See *Types of head injury,* pages 306 to 309.)

Diagnosis
Each type of head injury is associated with specific diagnostic findings. Possible diagnostic tests may include the following:

■ Skull X-rays will locate a fracture, if present, unless the fracture is of the cranial vault. (These fractures aren't visible or palpable.)

■ Cerebral angiography locates vascular disruptions from internal pressure or injuries that result from a cerebral contusion or skull fracture.

■ A computed tomography scan will disclose intracranial hemorrhage from ruptured blood vessels, ischemic or necrotic tissue, cerebral edema, areas of petechial hemorrhage, a shift in brain tissue, and subdural, epidural, and intracerebral hematomas that may have occurred from the head injury.

■ Magnetic resonance imaging and a radioisotope scan may also disclose intracranial hemorrhage from ruptured blood vessels in a patient with a skull fracture.

Collaborations
The patient with a head injury typically requires assistance from a multidisciplinary health care team. A neurosurgeon may coordinate care if the patient's head trauma is severe enough to require surgery or invasive intracranial pressure (ICP) monitoring. (See "Intracranial pressure monitoring," page 312.) Physical therapy, occupational therapy, and social services may be necessary if the patient has physical or cognitive deficits from the injury and requires assistance with activities of daily living. For children with head injuries, a child-life therapist may help facilitate normal growth and development through the use of play and self-expression therapy. In cases of an extremely severe injury, the family may require spiritual support as well as help in considering whether the patient may be a candidate for organ donation.

Treatment and care
Surgical treatment of head injury includes:

■ evacuation of the hematoma or a craniotomy to elevate or remove fragments that have been driven into the brain and to extract foreign bodies and necrotic tissue, thereby reducing the risk of infection and further brain damage from fractures.

Supportive treatment includes:

(Text continues on page 310.)

Types of head injury

Type	Description
Concussion (closed head injury)	• A blow to the head hard enough to make the brain hit the skull but not hard enough to cause a cerebral contusion causes temporary neural dysfunction. • Recovery is usually complete within 24 to 48 hours. • Repeated injuries exact a cumulative toll on the brain.
Contusion (bruising of brain tissue; more serious than concussion)	• Most common in people ages 20 to 40. • Most result from arterial bleeding. • Blood commonly accumulates between skull and dura. Injury to middle meningeal artery in parietotemporal area is most common and is frequently accompanied by linear skull fractures in temporal region over middle meningeal artery. • Less commonly arises from dural venous sinuses.
Epidural hematoma	• Acceleration-deceleration or coup-contrecoup injuries disrupt normal nerve functions in bruised area. • Injury is directly beneath the site of impact when the brain rebounds against the skull from the force of a blow (a beating with a blunt instrument, for example), when the force of the blow drives the brain against the opposite side of the skull, or when the head is hurled forward and stopped abruptly (as in an automobile accident when a driver's head strikes the windshield). • Brain continues moving and slaps against the skull (acceleration), then rebounds (deceleration). Brain may strike bony prominences inside the skull (especially the sphenoidal ridges), causing intracranial hemorrhage or hematoma that may result in tentorial herniation.

Signs and symptoms	Diagnostic test findings
• Short-term loss of consciousness secondary to disruption of reticular activating system (RAS), possibly due to abrupt pressure changes in the areas responsible for consciousness, changes in polarity of the neurons, ischemia, or structural distortion of neurons • Vomiting from localized injury and compression • Anterograde and retrograde amnesia (patient can't recall events immediately after the injury or events that led up to the traumatic incident) correlating with severity of injury; all related to disruption of RAS • Irritability or lethargy from localized injury and compression • Behavior out of character due to focal injury • Complaints of dizziness, nausea, or severe headache due to focal injury and compression	• Computed tomography (CT) scan reveals no sign of fracture, bleeding, or other nervous system lesion.
• Severe scalp wounds from direct injury • Labored respiration and loss of consciousness secondary to increased pressure from bruising • Drowsiness, confusion, disorientation, agitation, or violence from increased intracranial pressure (ICP) associated with trauma • Hemiparesis related to interrupted blood flow to the site of injury • Decorticate or decerebrate posturing from cortical damage or hemispheric dysfunction • Unequal pupillary response from brain stem involvement	• CT scan shows changes in tissue density, possible displacement of the surrounding structures, and evidence of ischemic tissue, hematomas, and fractures. • Lumbar puncture with cerebrospinal fluid (CSF) analysis reveals increased pressure and blood (not performed if hemorrhage is suspected). • EEG recordings directly over area of contusion reveal progressive abnormalities by appearance of high-amplitude theta and delta waves
• Brief period of unconsciousness after injury reflecting the concussive effects of head trauma, followed by a lucid interval varying from 10 to 15 minutes to hours or, rarely, days • Severe headache • Progressive loss of consciousness and deterioration in neurologic signs resulting from expanding lesion and extrusion of medial portion of temporal lobe through tentorial opening • Compression of brainstem by temporal lobe causing clinical manifestations of intracranial hypertension • Deterioration in level of consciousness resulting from compression of brainstem reticular formation as temporal lobe herniates on its upper portion • Respirations, initially deep and labored, becoming shallow and irregular as brainstem is impacted • Contralateral motor deficits reflecting compression of corticospinal tracts that pass through the brainstem	• CT scan or magnetic resonance imaging (MRI) identifies abnormal masses or structural shifts within the cranium.

(continued)

Types of head injury *(continued)*

Type	Description
Epidural hematoma *(continued)*	
Subdural hematoma	<ul><li>Meningeal hemorrhages, resulting from accumulation of blood in subdural space (between dura mater and arachnoid) are most common.</li><li>May be acute, subacute, and chronic: unilateral or bilateral.</li><li>Usually associated with torn connecting veins in cerebral cortex; rarely from arteries.</li><li>Acute hematomas are a surgical emergency.</li></ul>
Intracerebral hematoma	<ul><li>Subacute hematomas have better prognosis because venous bleeding tends to be slower.</li><li>Traumatic or spontaneous disruption of cerebral vessels in brain parenchyma cause neurologic deficits, depending on site and amount of bleeding.</li><li>Shear forces from brain movement frequently cause vessel laceration and hemorrhage into the parenchyma.</li><li>Frontal and temporal lobes are common sites. Trauma is associated with few intracerebral hematomas; most caused by result of hypertension.</li></ul>
Skull fracture	<ul><li>There are four types of skull fractures, including linear, comminuted, depressed, basilar.</li><li>Fractures of anterior and middle fossae are associated with severe head trauma and are more common than those of posterior fossa.</li><li>Blow to the head causes one or more of the types. May not be problematic unless brain is exposed or bone fragments are driven into neural tissue.</li></ul>

Signs and symptoms	Diagnostic test findings
• Ipsilateral (same-side) pupillary dilation due to compression of third cranial nerve • Seizures possible from high ICP • Continued bleeding leading to progressive neurologic degeneration, evidenced by bilateral pupillary dilation, bilateral decerebrate response, increased systemic blood pressure, decreased pulse, and profound coma with irregular respiratory patterns	
• Similar to epidural hematoma but significantly slower in onset because bleeding is typically of venous origin	• CT scan, X-rays, and arteriography reveal mass and altered blood flow in the area, confirming hematoma. • CT scan or MRI reveals evidence of masses and tissue shifting. • CSF is yellow and has relatively low protein (chronic subdural hematoma).
• Unresponsive immediately or experiencing a lucid period before lapsing into a coma from increasing ICP and mass effect of hemorrhage • Possible motor deficits and decorticate or decerebrate responses from compression of corticospinal tracts and brain stem	• CT scan or cerebral arteriography identifies bleeding site. CSF pressure elevated; fluid may appear bloody or xanthochromic (yellow or straw-colored) from hemoglobin breakdown.
• Possibly asymptomatic, depending on underlying brain trauma • Discontinuity and displacement of bone structure with severe fracture • Motor sensory and cranial nerve dysfunction with associated facial fractures • Persons with anterior fossa basilar skull fractures may have periorbital ecchymosis (raccoon eyes), anosmia (loss of smell due to first cranial nerve involvement) and pupil abnormalities (second and third cranial nerve involvement) • CSF rhinorrhea (leakage through nose), CSF otorrhea (leakage from the ear), hemotympanium (blood accumulation at the tympanic membrane), ecchymosis over the mastoid bone (Battle's sign), and facial paralysis (seventh cranial nerve injury) accompany middle fossa basilar skull fractures • Signs of medullary dysfunction, such as cardiovascular and respiratory failure, accompany posterior fossa basilar skull fracture	• CT scan and MRI reveal intracranial hemorrhage from ruptured blood vessels and swelling. • Skull X-ray may reveal fracture. • Lumbar puncture contraindicated by expanding lesions.

■ close observation to detect changes in neurologic status, suggesting further damage or expanding hematoma
■ cleaning and debridement of any wounds associated with skull fractures
■ diuretics (such as mannitol) and corticosteroids (such as dexamethasone) to reduce cerebral edema
■ analgesics (such as acetaminophen) to relieve complaints of headache
■ anticonvulsants (such as phenytoin) to prevent and treat seizures
■ respiratory support, including mechanical ventilation and endotracheal (ET) intubation as indicated for respiratory failure from brainstem involvement
■ prophylactic antibiotics to prevent the onset of meningitis from CSF leakage associated with skull fractures.

Complications

Overall, complications from a head injury may include:
■ increased ICP
■ infection (open trauma)
■ respiratory depression and failure
■ brain herniation.

In addition, different types of head injury are associated with specific complications. A concussion usually causes no significant anatomic brain injury. Seizures, persistent vomiting, or both may occur. Rarely, a concussion leads to intracranial hemorrhage (subdural, epidural, or parenchymal).

A cerebral contusion can cause intracranial hemorrhage or hematoma if the injury causes the brain to strike against bony prominences inside the skull (especially the sphenoidal ridges). Residual headaches and vertigo may complicate recovery. Secondary effects, such as brain swelling, may accompany serious contusions,

resulting in increased ICP and herniation.

Skull fractures can lead to infection, intracerebral hemorrhage and hematoma, brain abscess, and increased ICP from edema. Recovery from the injury can be further complicated by residual effects of the injury, such as seizure disorders, hydrocephalus, and organic mental syndrome.

Nursing considerations

■ Initially, monitor vital signs continuously and check for additional injuries.

ALERT *Abnormal respirations could indicate a breakdown in the brain's respiratory center and possibly an impending tentorial herniation — a neurologic emergency.*

■ Continue to check vital signs and neurologic status, including LOC and pupil size, every 15 minutes. If the patient's condition worsens or fluctuates, arrange for a neurosurgical consultation. Administer antipyretics and provide comfort measures for elevated temperature.
■ Maintain a patent airway. Monitor oxygenation saturation levels via pulse oximetry and serial arterial blood gas studies as ordered. Assist with ET intubation or tracheotomy, as necessary.
■ Assess hemodynamic parameters to aid in evaluating cerebral perfusion pressure (CPP).
■ Administer medications as ordered. If necessary, use continuous infusions of agents such as midazolam, fentanyl, morphine, or propofol to help reduce metabolic demand and reduce the risk of increased ICP.
■ Observe the patient closely for headache, dizziness, irritability, anxi-

ety, and changes in behavior, such as agitation, which may stem from hypoxia or increased ICP.

AGE ISSUE *Monitor the elderly patient especially closely. He may have brain atrophy and therefore more space for cerebral edema; ICP may increase, yet cause no signs.*

■ Assist with the insertion of the ICP monitoring system and continuously monitor ICP waveforms and pressure. Also, determine CPP either by calculation or via cerebral blood flow monitoring system. If ICP increases, administer mannitol and furosemide as ordered.

■ Carefully observe the patient for CSF leakage. Check the bed sheets for a blood-tinged spot surrounded by a lighter ring (halo sign). If the patient has CSF leakage or is unconscious, elevate the head of the bed up to 30 degrees. Such a patient is at risk for jugular compression, leading to increased ICP, when not positioned on his back. Be sure to keep his head properly aligned. Enforce strict bed rest.

■ Position the patient so that secretions drain properly. If you detect CSF leakage from the nose, place a gauze pad under the nostrils. If CSF leaks from the ear, position the patient so his ear drains naturally — don't pack the ear or nose. If the patient requires suctioning, suction him through the mouth, not the nose, to avoid introducing bacteria into the CSF.

■ If the patient is unconscious, insert a nasogastric tube to prevent aspiration — but only after a basilar skull fracture has been ruled out. Otherwise, the tube may be accidentally inserted into the cranial vault.

■ Monitor the patient's intake and output frequently to help maintain a normovolemic state. If necessary, insert an indwelling urinary catheter to monitor urine output more precisely and frequently. Obtain serum electrolyte levels and expect to replace fluids and electrolytes as necessary.

■ Institute seizure precautions, but don't restrain the patient. Administer anticonvulsants, such as phenytoin, as ordered to prevent seizure activity. Monitor serum phenytoin levels for therapeutic effectiveness. Institute safety precautions to minimize the risk of injury.

■ Cluster nursing activities to provide rest periods in between, thus reducing the metabolic demand and reducing the risk of sustained increases in ICP.

■ Prepare the patient for a craniotomy as indicated. (See "Craniotomy," page 294.)

■ After the patient is stabilized, clean and dress any superficial scalp wounds using strict aseptic technique. (If the skin has been broken, the patient may need tetanus prophylaxis.) Assist with suturing if needed. Carefully cover scalp wounds with a sterile dressing; control any bleeding as necessary. Monitor wounds for signs and symptoms of infection.

Patient teaching

■ Explain all treatment methods to the patient and his family.

■ Inform the patient and his family about the prescribed regimen for care, including monitoring, need for surgery, and other treatments.

■ Instruct the patient and his family in the signs and symptoms of complications and the need to notify someone as soon as possible should any occur.

- Teach the patient to recognize symptoms of postconcussion syndrome — headache, vertigo, anxiety, and fatigue. Tell him that the syndrome may persist for several weeks.
- Urge the patient with a cerebral contusion not to cough, sneeze, or blow his nose because these activities can increase ICP.
- Teach the patient and his family how to care for his scalp wound, if applicable, emphasizing the need for follow-up as appropriate.

Intracranial pressure monitoring

Intracranial pressure (ICP) monitoring measures the pressure exerted by the brain, blood, and cerebrospinal fluid (CSF) against the inside of the skull. Indications for monitoring ICP include head trauma with bleeding or edema, overproduction or insufficient absorption of CSF, cerebral hemorrhage, and space-occupying brain lesions. ICP monitoring can detect elevated ICP early, before clinical danger signs develop. Prompt intervention can then help avert or diminish neurologic damage caused by cerebral hypoxia and shifts of brain mass. (See *What happens when intracranial pressure rises.*)

The four basic ICP monitoring systems are intraventricular catheter, subarachnoid bolt, epidural sensor, and intraparenchymal pressure monitoring. (See *Types of intracranial pressure monitoring,* pages 314 and 315.) Regardless of which system is used, the procedure is typically performed by a neurosurgeon in the operating room, emergency department, or intensive care unit.

Insertion of an ICP monitoring device requires sterile technique to reduce the risk of central nervous system (CNS) infection. Setting up equipment for a monitoring system also requires strict asepsis.

Equipment
Monitoring unit and transducers as ordered ▪ 16 to 20 sterile 4″ × 4″ gauze pads ▪ linen-saver pads ▪ shave preparation tray or hair scissors ▪ sterile drapes ▪ sterile gown ▪ surgical mask ▪ sterile gloves ▪ head dressing supplies (including two rolls of 4″ elastic gauze dressing, one roll of 4″ roller gauze, and adhesive tape) ▪ optional: suction apparatus, I.V. pole, and yardstick

Essential steps
Monitoring units and setup protocols are varied and complex and differ among health care facilities. Check your facility's guidelines for your particular unit.

Various types of preassembled ICP monitoring units are also available, each with its own setup protocols. These units are designed to reduce the risk of infection by eliminating the need for multiple stopcocks, manometers, and transducer dome assemblies. Some facilities use units that have miniaturized transducers rather than transducer domes.

- Explain the procedure to the patient or his family. Make sure that the patient or a responsible family member has signed a consent form.
- Determine whether the patient is allergic to antiseptic skin preparations.

What happens when intracranial pressure rises

The pressure exerted within the intact skull by the intracranial volume — about 10% blood, 10% cerebrospinal fluid (CSF), and 80% brain tissue — is called intracranial pressure (ICP). The rigid skull has little space for expansion of these substances.

The brain compensates for increases in ICP by regulating the volume of the three substances in the following ways:
• limiting blood flow to the head

• displacing CSF into the spinal canal
• increasing absorption or decreasing production of CSF — withdrawing water from brain tissue and excreting it through the kidneys.

When compensatory mechanisms become overworked, small changes in volume lead to large changes in pressure. This flowchart will help you to understand the pathophysiology of increased ICP.

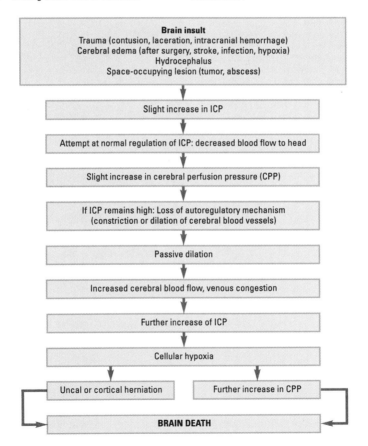

Types of intracranial pressure monitoring

Intracranial pressure (ICP) can be monitored by using one of four systems.

Intraventricular catheter monitoring

In intraventricular catheter monitoring, which monitors ICP directly, the physician inserts a small polyethylene or silicone catheter into the lateral ventricle through a burr hole.

This is the only type of ICP monitoring that allows evaluation of brain compliance and drainage of significant amounts of cerebrospinal fluid (CSF). Although this method measures ICP most accurately, it also carries the greatest risk of infection.

Contraindications usually include stenotic cerebral ventricles, cerebral aneurysms in the path of catheter placement, and suspected vascular lesions.

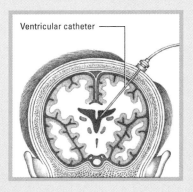

Ventricular catheter

Subarachnoid bolt monitoring

Subarachnoid bolt monitoring involves the insertion of a special bolt into the subarachnoid space through a twist-drill hole that's positioned in the front of the skull behind the hairline.

Placing the bolt is easier than placing an intraventricular catheter, especially if a computed tomography scan reveals that the cerebrum has shifted or the ventricles have collapsed. This type of ICP monitoring also carries less risk of infection and parenchymal damage because the bolt doesn't penetrate the cerebrum.

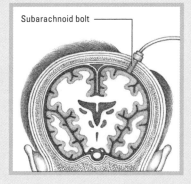

Subarachnoid bolt

■ Provide privacy if the procedure is being done in an open emergency department or intensive care unit. Wash your hands.

■ Obtain baseline routine and neurologic vital signs to aid in prompt detection of decompensation during the procedure.

■ Place the patient in the supine position and elevate the head of the bed 30 degrees (or as ordered). Document the number of bed crank rotations or hang a yardstick on an I.V. pole and mark the exact elevation.

■ Place linen-saver pads under the patient's head. Shave or clip his hair at the insertion site, as indicated by the physician, to decrease the risk of infection. Carefully fold and remove the linen-saver pads to avoid spilling loose

Epidural or subdural sensor monitoring

ICP can also be monitored from the epidural or subdural space. For epidural monitoring, a fiberoptic sensor is inserted into the epidural space through a burr hole. This system's main drawback is its questionable accuracy because ICP isn't being measured directly from a CSF-filled space.

For subdural monitoring, a fiber-optic transducer–tipped catheter is tunneled through a burr hole and its tip is placed on brain tissue under the dura mater. The main drawback to this method is its inability to drain CSF.

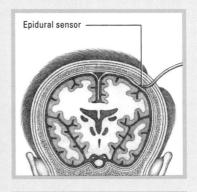

Epidural sensor

Intraparenchymal monitoring

In intraparenchymal monitoring, the physician inserts a catheter through a small subarachnoid bolt and, after puncturing the dura, advances the catheter a few centimeters into the brain's white matter. There's no need to balance or calibrate the equipment after insertion.

Although this method doesn't provide direct access to CSF, measurements are accurate because brain tissue pressure correlates well with ventricular pressures. Intraparenchymal monitoring may be used to obtain ICP measurements in patients with compressed or dislocated ventricles.

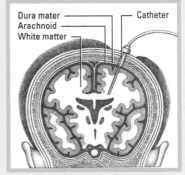

Dura mater
Arachnoid
White matter
Catheter

hair onto the bed. Drape the patient with sterile drapes. Then scrub the insertion site for 2 minutes with antiseptic skin solution.

■ Assist the physician with putting on a sterile gown, mask, and sterile gloves; opening the interior wrap of the sterile supply tray; and proceeding with insertion of the catheter or bolt.

■ To facilitate placement of the device, hold the patient's head in your hands or attach a long strip of 4″ roller gauze to one side rail and bring it across the patient's forehead to the opposite rail. Reassure the conscious patient to help ease his anxiety. Talk to him frequently to assess his level of consciousness (LOC) and detect signs of deterioration. Watch for cardiac ar-

Interpreting intracranial pressure waveforms

Three waveforms — A, B, and C — are used to monitor intracranial pressure (ICP). The illustrations below show these three types of waveforms, a normal waveform, and a waveform indicating an equipment problem.

Normal waveform

A normal ICP waveform typically shows a steep, upward systolic slope followed by a downward diastolic slope with a dicrotic notch. In most cases, this waveform occurs continuously and indicates an ICP between 0 and 15 mm Hg — normal pressure.

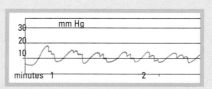

A waves

The most clinically significant ICP waveforms are A waves, which may reach elevations of 50 to 100 mm Hg, persist for 5 to 20 minutes, and then drop sharply — signaling exhaustion of the brain's compliance mechanisms. A waves may come and go, spiking from temporary rises in thoracic pressure or from any condition that increases ICP beyond the brain's compliance limits. Activities, such as sustained coughing or straining during defecation, can cause temporary elevations in thoracic pressure.

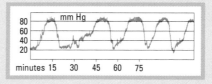

B waves

B waves appear sharp and rhythmic, with a sawtooth pattern; they occur every 1½ to 2 minutes and may reach elevations of 50 mm Hg. The clinical significance of B waves isn't clear, but the waves correlate with respiratory changes and may occur more frequently with decreasing compensation. Because B waves sometimes precede A waves, notify the physician if B waves occur frequently.

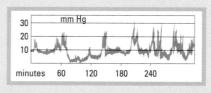

C waves

Like B waves, C waves are rapid and rhythmic, but they aren't as sharp. Clinically insignificant, they may fluctuate with respirations or systemic blood pressure changes.

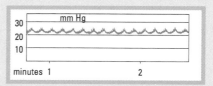

Interpreting intracranial pressure waveforms *(continued)*

Waveform showing equipment problem
A waveform such as the one shown signals a problem with the transducer or monitor. Check for line obstruction and determine whether the transducer needs rebalancing.

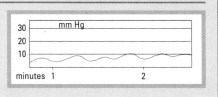

rhythmias and abnormal respiratory patterns.

■ After insertion, put on sterile gloves and apply antiseptic skin solution and a sterile dressing to the site. If not done by the physician, connect the catheter to the appropriate monitoring device, depending on the system used.

■ If the physician has set up a ventriculostomy drainage system, attach the drip chamber to the headboard or bedside I.V. pole, as ordered. (See "Ventriculostomy," page 348.)

ALERT *Positioning the drip chamber too high may raise ICP; positioning it too low may cause excessive CSF drainage.*

■ Inspect the insertion site at least every 24 hours (or according to your facility's policy) for redness, swelling, and drainage. Clean the site, reapply antiseptic solution, and apply a fresh sterile dressing.

Complications

CNS infection, the most common hazard of ICP monitoring, can result from contamination of the equipment setup or of the insertion site.

ALERT *Excessive loss of CSF can result from faulty stopcock placement or a drip chamber that's positioned too low. Such loss can rapidly decompress the cranial contents and*

damage bridging cortical veins, leading to hematoma formation. Decompression can also lead to rupture of existing hematomas or aneurysms, causing hemorrhage. Watch for signs of impending or overt decompensation: pupillary dilation (unilateral or bilateral); decreased pupillary response to light; decreasing LOC; rising systolic blood pressure and widening pulse pressure; bradycardia; slowed, irregular respirations; and, in late decompensation, decerebrate posturing.

Nursing considerations

■ Assess the patient's clinical status and take routine and neurologic vital signs every hour or as ordered. Make sure that you've obtained orders from the physician for the patient's waveforms and pressure parameters.

■ Calculate cerebral perfusion pressure (CPP) hourly or monitor cerebral blood flow if available; use the equation: CPP = MAP – ICP (MAP refers to mean arterial pressure).

■ Observe digital ICP readings and waves. Remember, the pattern of readings is more significant than any single reading. (See *Interpreting intracranial pressure waveforms.*) If you observe continually elevated ICP readings, note how long they're sustained. If they last several minutes, notify the physician immediately. Finally, record and describe any CSF drainage.

AGE ISSUE *In infants, ICP monitoring can be performed without penetrating the scalp. In this external method, a photoelectric transducer with a pressure-sensitive membrane is taped to the anterior fontanel. The transducer responds to pressure at the site and transmits readings to a bedside monitor and recording system. The external method is restricted to infants because pressure readings can be obtained only at fontanelles, the incompletely ossified areas of the skull.*

■ Administer (by I.V. infusion or bolus injection) osmotic diuretic agents, such as mannitol, to reduce cerebral edema by shrinking intracranial contents (mannitol draws water from tissues into plasma and doesn't cross the blood-brain barrier). Monitor serum electrolyte levels and osmolality readings closely because the patient may become dehydrated very quickly. Be aware that a rebound increase in ICP may occur. To avoid rebound increased ICP, administer 50 ml of albumin with the mannitol bolus. Note, however, that you'll see a residual rise in ICP before it decreases. If your patient has heart failure or severe renal dysfunction, monitor for problems in adapting to the increased intravascular volumes.

■ Restrict fluid intake, usually to 1,200 to 1,500 ml/day, to help prevent cerebral edema from developing or worsening.

■ Administer corticosteroids as ordered to lower elevated ICP by reducing sodium and water concentration in the brain. (Keep in mind that their use is controversial). If used, give with histamine-2 receptor antagonists to reduce the risk of GI irritation and bleeding. Observe for possible GI bleeding; check stools for occult blood. Monitor blood glucose levels because steroids may cause hyperglycemia.

■ Anticipate the use of a barbiturate-induced coma to depresses the reticular activating system and reduce the brain's metabolic demand. Reduced demand for oxygen and energy reduces cerebral blood flow, thereby lowering ICP. Anticipate using bispectral index monitoring to assess the patient's level of sedation.

■ Hyperventilate with oxygen from a handheld resuscitation bag or ventilator to help rid the patient of excess carbon dioxide, thereby constricting cerebral vessels and reducing cerebral blood volume and ICP. However, only normal brain tissues respond because blood vessels in damaged areas have reduced vasoconstrictive ability.

ALERT *Hyperventilation should be performed with care because it can cause ischemia.*

■ Before tracheal suctioning, hyperventilate the patient with 100% oxygen as ordered. Apply suction for a maximum of 15 seconds. Avoid inducing hypoxia because this condition greatly increases cerebral blood flow.

■ Because fever raises brain metabolism, which increases cerebral blood flow and subsequently ICP, reduce fever by administering acetaminophen as ordered, sponge baths, or a hypothermia blanket. However, rebound increases in ICP and brain edema may occur if rapid rewarming takes place after hypothermia or if cooling measures induce shivering.

■ Be aware that withdrawal of CSF through the drainage system reduces

CSF volume and thus reduces ICP. Although less commonly used, surgical removal of a skull-bone flap provides room for the swollen brain to expand. If this procedure is performed, keep the site clean and dry to prevent infection and maintain sterile technique when changing the dressing.

■ Record the time and date of the insertion procedure and the patient's response. Note the insertion site and the type of monitoring system used.

■ Record ICP digital readings and waveforms and CPP hourly. Document any factors that may affect ICP (for example, drug administration, stressful procedures, or sleep).

■ Record routine and neurologic vital signs hourly, and describe the patient's clinical status. Note the amount, character, and frequency of any CSF drainage (for example, "between 6 p.m. and 7 p.m., 15 ml of blood-tinged CSF"). Also record the ICP reading in response to drainage.

Lumbar drain insertion and care

Cerebrospinal fluid (CSF) is drained to reduce CSF pressure to the desired level and to maintain it at that level. Fluid can be withdrawn from the lumbar subarachnoid space (lumbar drain). Lumbar drainage is used to aid healing of the dura mater. External CSF drainage is used most commonly to manage increased intracranial pressure (ICP) and to facilitate spinal or cerebral dural healing after traumatic injury or surgery. In either case, CSF is drained by a catheter (see *Lumbar drainage of cerebrospinal fluid*) or a ven-

Lumbar drainage of cerebrospinal fluid

Cerebrospinal fluid (CSF) drainage aims to control intracranial pressure (ICP) during treatment for traumatic injury or other conditions that raise ICP. One method involves insertion of a lumbar drain.

In lumbar drainage of CSF, the physician inserts a catheter beneath the dura into the L3 to L4 interspace. The distal end of the catheter is connected to a sterile closed drainage system affixed securely to the bed or a bedside I.V. pole. The drip chamber is set at the level ordered by the physician.

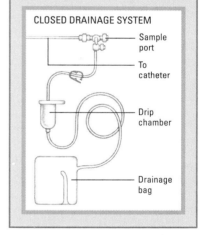

CLOSED DRAINAGE SYSTEM

- Sample port
- To catheter
- Drip chamber
- Drainage bag

triculostomy tube in a sterile, closed drainage collection system (see "Ventriculostomy," page 348).

Other therapeutic uses include direct instillation of medications, contrast media, or air for diagnostic radiology; and aspiration of CSF for laboratory analysis.

To place the lumbar subarachnoid drain, the physician may administer a local spinal anesthetic at bedside or in the operating room.

Equipment
Overbed table ▪ sterile gloves ▪ sterile cotton-tipped applicators ▪ antiseptic solution ▪ alcohol pads ▪ sterile fenestrated drape ▪ 3-ml syringe for local anesthetic ▪ 25G ¾″ needle for injecting anesthetic ▪ local anesthetic (usually 1% lidocaine) ▪ 18G or 20G sterile spinal needle or Tuohy needle ▪ #5 French whistle-tip catheter ▪ external drainage set (includes drainage tubing and sterile collection bag) ▪ suture material ▪ 4″ × 4″ dressings ▪ paper tape ▪ lamp or another light source ▪ bedside I.V. pole ▪ twist drill ▪ optional: pain medication and an anti-infective agent

Essential steps
▪ Gather the necessary equipment.
  – Open all equipment using sterile technique.
  – Check all packaging for breaks in seals and for expiration dates.
  – After the physician places the catheter, be prepared to connect it to the external drainage system tubing; secure connection points with tape or a connector; and place the collection system, including drip chamber and collection bag, on an I.V. pole.
▪ Explain the procedure to the patient and his family. Make sure that the patient or a responsible family member signs a consent form and document according to your facility's policy.
▪ Wash your hands thoroughly.
▪ Perform a baseline neurologic assessment, including vital signs, to help detect alterations or signs of deterioration.

▪ Assist with insertion of the lumbar subarachnoid drain.
  – Position the patient in a side-lying position with his chin tucked to his chest and knees drawn up to his abdomen, as for a lumbar puncture. Urge him to remain as still as possible during the procedure.
  – Observe as the physician inserts the drain by attaching a Tuohy needle (or spinal needle) to the whistle-tip catheter. After removing the needle, the physician connects the drainage system, sutures or tapes the catheter securely in place, and covers it with a sterile dressing.
▪ Monitor CSF drainage; maintain a continuous hourly output of CSF by raising or lowering the drainage system drip chamber.

ALERT *To maintain CSF outflow, the drip chamber should be slightly lower than or at the level of the lumbar drain insertion site. You may need to carefully raise or lower the drip chamber to increase or decrease CSF flow.*

▪ To drain CSF as ordered, put on gloves, and then turn the main stopcock on to drainage. This allows CSF to collect in the graduated flow chamber. Document the time and the amount of CSF obtained. Then turn the stopcock off to drainage.
▪ To drain the CSF from the graduated flow chamber into the drainage bag, release the clamp below the flow chamber.

ALERT *Never empty the drainage bag. Instead, replace it when full, using sterile technique.*

▪ Check the dressing frequently for drainage, which could indicate CSF leakage.

- Check the tubing for patency by watching the CSF drops in the drip chamber.
- Observe the CSF for color, clarity, amount, blood, and sediment. CSF specimens for laboratory analysis should be obtained from the collection port attached to the tubing, not from the collection bag.
- Change the collection bag when it's full or every 24 hours according to your facility's policy.

Complications

Signs and symptoms of excessive CSF drainage include:

- headache
- tachycardia
- diaphoresis
- nausea.

Acute overdrainage may result in collapsed ventricles, tonsillar herniation, and medullary compression.

ALERT *If drainage accumulates too rapidly, clamp the system and notify the physician immediately. This constitutes a potential neurosurgical emergency.*

Cessation of drainage may indicate clot formation. If you can't quickly identify the cause of the obstruction, notify the physician. If drainage is blocked, the patient may develop signs of increased ICP. Infection may cause meningitis. To prevent this, administer antibiotics, as ordered.

Nursing considerations

- Maintain a continual hourly output of CSF to prevent overdrainage or underdrainage. Underdrainage or lack of CSF may reflect kinked tubing, catheter displacement, or a drip chamber placed higher than the catheter insertion site. Overdrainage can occur if the drip chamber is placed too far below the catheter insertion site.
- Remember that raising or lowering the head of the bed can affect the CSF flow rate. When changing the patient's position, reposition the drip chamber.
- Assess patients for chronic headache during continuous CSF drainage. Reassure the patient that this isn't unusual; administer analgesics as appropriate.
- Record the date and time of the insertion procedure and the patient's response to it. Also record baseline and follow-up vital signs and neurologic assessment findings based on frequency of determination.
- Document the color, clarity, and amount of CSF drainage at least every 4 hours. Record hourly and 24 hour CSF output and describe the appearance and condition of the dressing.

Meningitis

In meningitis, the brain and the spinal cord meninges become inflamed. Such inflammation may involve all three meningeal membranes — the dura mater, the arachnoid membrane, and the pia mater.

For most patients, meningitis follows an onset of respiratory symptoms. In about 50% of patients, it develops over a period of 1 to 7 days; in just under 20% of patients, it occurs 1 to 3 weeks after respiratory symptoms appear. Unheralded by respiratory symptoms, meningitis has a sudden onset in about 25% of patients, who become seriously ill within 24 hours without respiratory symptoms.

Meningitis is almost always a complication of bacteremia, especially from the following:

- pneumonia
- empyema
- osteomyelitis
- endocarditis.

Other infections associated with the development of meningitis include:

- sinusitis
- otitis media
- encephalitis
- myelitis
- brain abscess, usually caused by *Neisseria meningitidis, Haemophilus influenzae, Streptococcus pneumoniae,* and *Escherichia coli.*

Meningitis may follow trauma or invasive procedures, including:

- skull fracture
- penetrating head wound
- lumbar puncture
- ventricular shunting.

Aseptic meningitis may result from a virus or other organism. Sometimes no causative organism can be found.

If the disease is recognized early and the infecting organism responds to treatment, the prognosis is good and complications are rare. However, mortality in untreated meningitis is 70% to 100%.

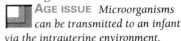 AGE ISSUE *Infants, children, and elderly people have the highest risk of developing meningitis, as do those living in close contact with large populations. The prognosis is poor for infants and elderly people.*

Pathophysiology

Meningitis often begins as an inflammation of the pia-arachnoid, which may progress to congestion of adjacent tissues and destroy some nerve cells.

The microorganism typically enters the central nervous system by one of four routes:

- the blood (most common)
- a direct opening between the cerebrospinal fluid (CSF) and the environment as a result of trauma
- along the cranial and peripheral nerves
- through the mouth or nose.

AGE ISSUE *Microorganisms can be transmitted to an infant via the intrauterine environment.*

The invading organism triggers an inflammatory response in the meninges. In an attempt to ward off the invasion, neutrophils gather in the area and produce an exudate in the subarachnoid space, causing the CSF to thicken. The thickened CSF flows less readily around the brain and spinal cord, and it can block the arachnoid villi, obstructing flow of CSF and causing hydrocephalus.

The exudate also:

- exacerbates the inflammatory response, increasing the pressure in the brain
- can extend to the cranial and peripheral nerves, triggering additional inflammation
- irritates the meninges, disrupting their cell membranes and causing edema.

The consequences are elevated intracranial pressure (ICP), engorged blood vessels, disrupted cerebral blood supply, possible thrombosis or rupture and, if ICP isn't reduced, cerebral infarction. Encephalitis may also ensue as a secondary infection of the brain tissue.

In aseptic meningitis, lymphocytes infiltrate the pia-arachnoid layers, but usually not as severely as in bacterial meningitis, and no exudate is formed. Thus, this type of meningitis is self-limiting.

Comprehensive assessment

Signs and symptoms of infection and increased ICP are the cardinal signs of meningitis. The patient's history may detail headache, stiff neck and back, malaise, photophobia, chills and, in some patients, vomiting, twitching, and seizures. The patient or a family member may also report altered level of consciousness (LOC), such as confusion and delirium. Vital signs may reveal fever.

In pneumococcal meningitis, the patient's history may uncover a recent lung, ear, or sinus infection or endocarditis. It may also reveal the presence of other conditions, such as alcoholism, sickle cell disease, basal skull fracture, recent splenectomy, or organ transplant.

In *H. influenzae* meningitis, patient history may reveal recent respiratory tract or ear infection. Physical findings vary, depending on the severity of the meningitis. The signs of meningitis typically include:

■ fever, chills, and malaise resulting from infection and inflammation
■ headache, vomiting and, rarely, papilledema (inflammation and edema of the optic nerve) from increased ICP.

Signs of meningeal irritation include:
■ nuchal rigidity
■ positive Brudzinski's and Kernig's signs (see *Assessing Brudzinski's and Kernig's signs,* page 324)
■ exaggerated and symmetrical deep tendon reflexes
■ opisthotonos (a spasm in which the back and extremities arch backward so that the body rests on the head and heels).

Other features of meningitis may include:
■ sinus arrhythmias from irritation of the nerves of the autonomic nervous system
■ irritability from increasing ICP
■ photophobia, diplopia, and other visual problems from cranial nerve irritation
■ delirium, deep stupor, and coma from increased ICP and cerebral edema.

AGE ISSUE *An infant may show signs of infection, but most are simply fretful and refuse to eat. In an infant, vomiting can lead to dehydration, which prevents formation of a bulging fontanel, an important sign of increased ICP. As the illness progresses, twitching, seizures (in 30% of infants), or coma may develop. Most older children have the same symptoms as adults. In subacute meningitis, onset may be insidious.*

Diagnosis

■ Lumbar puncture shows elevated CSF pressure (from obstructed CSF outflow at the arachnoid villi), cloudy or milky-white CSF, high protein level, positive Gram stain and culture (unless a virus is responsible), and decreased glucose concentration.
■ Positive Brudzinski's and Kernig's signs indicate meningeal irritation.
■ Cultures of blood, urine, and nose and throat secretions reveal the offending organism.
■ Chest X-ray may reveal pneumonitis or lung abscess, tubercular lesions, or granulomas secondary to a fungal infection.

Assessing Brudzinski's and Kernig's signs

When positive, Brudzinski's sign and Kernig's sign indicate meningeal irritation. Follow these guidelines to test for these two signs.

Brudzinski's sign
With the patient in the supine position, place your hand under his neck and flex it forward, chin to chest. This test is positive if he flexes his ankles, knees, and hips bilaterally. In addition, the patient typically complains of pain when the neck is flexed.

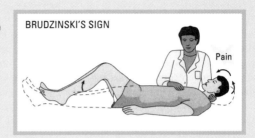

BRUDZINSKI'S SIGN

Pain

Kernig's sign
With the patient in the supine position, flex his hip and knee to form a 90-degree angle. Next, attempt to extend this leg. If he exhibits pain, resistance to extension, and spasm, the test is positive.

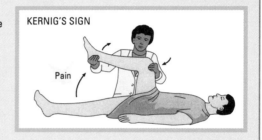

KERNIG'S SIGN

Pain

■ Sinus and skull X-rays may identify cranial osteomyelitis or paranasal sinusitis as the underlying infectious process, or skull fracture as the mechanism for entrance of microorganism.
■ White blood cell count reveals leukocytosis.
■ Computed tomography scan may reveal hydrocephalus or rule out cerebral hematoma, hemorrhage, or tumor as the underlying cause.

Collaborations

A multidisciplinary approach to care is necessary for the patient with meningitis. In addition to medical and nursing personnel, infection control personnel may be involved to assist with measures to prevent infection transmission. Nutritional therapy may be needed if the patient is unable to tolerate oral feedings. If the patient with meningitis exhibits neurologic defects after the acute phase has passed, consultation with appropriate health care team members, such as physical therapy, occupational therapy, and speech therapy may be indicated to assist with residual deficits that may have occurred. If the patient is a child, a pediatrician, speech therapist, physical therapist, and child-life therapist can help ensure that the patient receives appropriate therapies depending on the deficits incurred.

Treatment and care

Medical management of meningitis includes appropriate antibiotic therapy and vigorous supportive care. Usually, I.V. antibiotics are given for at least 2 weeks, followed by oral antibiotics selected by culture and sensitivity testing. Other drugs include a cardiac glycoside (such as digoxin) to control arrhythmias, corticosteroids to decrease cerebral inflammation and edema, an anticonvulsant (usually given I.V.) or a sedative to reduce restlessness and prevent or control seizure activity, and aspirin or acetaminophen to relieve headache and fever.

Supportive measures consist of bed rest to prevent increases in ICP, fever reduction to prevent hyperthermia and increased metabolic demands that may increase ICP, and fluid therapy to prevent dehydration (given cautiously if cerebral edema and increased ICP is present). Transmission based precautions also are indicated. For example, droplet precautions are implemented (in addition to standard precautions) for meningitis caused by *H. influenzae* and *N. meningitidis* until 24 hours after the start of effective therapy. Treatment also includes appropriate therapy for any coexisting conditions, such as endocarditis or pneumonia.

To prevent meningitis, prophylactic antibiotics are sometimes used after ventricular shunting procedures, skull fracture, or penetrating head wounds, but this use is controversial.

Complications

Complications of meningitis may include:
- increased ICP
- hydrocephalus
- cerebral infarction

- cranial nerve deficits including optic neuritis and deafness
- encephalitis
- paresis or paralysis
- endocarditis
- brain abscess
- syndrome of inappropriate antidiuretic hormone
- seizures
- coma.

AGE ISSUE *In children, complications of meningitis may include mental retardation, epilepsy, unilateral or bilateral sensory hearing loss, and subdural effusions.*

Nursing considerations

- Assess the patient's respiratory status, including the rate and depth of respirations, at least every 2 hours or more frequently if indicated. Monitor oxygen saturation via pulse oximetry and serial arterial blood gas studies as ordered. Administer supplemental oxygen as required to maintain partial pressure of oxygen at desired levels. If necessary, prepare for endotracheal intubation or tracheotomy and mechanical ventilation if the patient's respiratory status deteriorates. If these measures are initiated, provide appropriate care and suction as indicated.

- Continually assess the patient's clinical status, including neurologic function and vital signs. Monitor for changes in LOC and signs of increased ICP (plucking at the bedcovers, vomiting, seizures, and changes in motor function and vital signs) at least hourly. Watch for signs of cranial nerve involvement (ptosis, strabismus, and diplopia). Regularly observe the patient for signs of deterioration. (See *Meningitis care algorithm,* pages 326 and 327.)

Meningitis care algorithm

Use the algorithm shown below to help prioritize nursing care for the patient with meningitis.

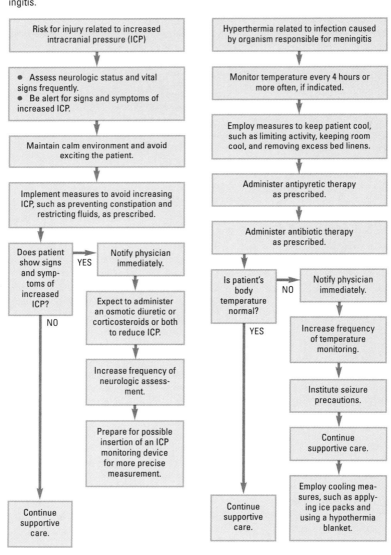

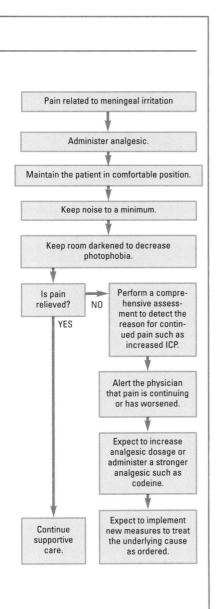

Pain related to meningeal irritation

↓

Administer analgesic.

↓

Maintain the patient in comfortable position.

↓

Keep noise to a minimum.

↓

Keep room darkened to decrease photophobia.

↓

Is pain relieved? → NO → Perform a comprehensive assessment to detect the reason for continued pain such as increased ICP.

↓ YES

↓

Alert the physician that pain is continuing or has worsened.

↓

Expect to increase analgesic dosage or administer a stronger analgesic such as codeine.

↓

Continue supportive care.

Expect to implement new measures to treat the underlying cause as ordered.

ALERT *Be especially alert for a temperature increase, deteriorating LOC, seizures, and altered respirations. All of these signs may herald an impending crisis.*

■ Institute continuous cardiac monitoring to assess for arrhythmias.

■ Assess the patient's fluid volume status including intake and output. Monitor hemodynamic parameters frequently, including central venous pressure and output. Maintain adequate fluid intake to avoid dehydration, but avoid fluid overload because of the danger of cerebral edema.

■ Assist with CSF analysis for culture. Administer I.V. fluid therapy and begin antimicrobial therapy, as ordered.

■ Administer anticonvulsants and other pharmacologic agents, such as antipyretics and corticosteroids, as ordered. Assess the patient for evidence of seizures.

ALERT *The goal is prevention of seizures because they increase metabolic rate, thereby increasing cerebral blood flow (CBF). This increased CBF is extremely dangerous in patients with meningitis who have cerebral edema.*

■ Position the patient carefully to prevent joint stiffness and neck pain. Turn him often, according to a planned positioning schedule. Make sure that the patient's environment is comfortable; dim the lights to alleviate photophobia. Provide for rest periods in between activities. Administer analgesics, as ordered.

■ Maintain adequate nutrition. Provide small, frequent meals. If the patient is unable to ingest orally, anticipate the need for supplemental enteral or parenteral feedings.

- To prevent constipation and minimize the risk of increased ICP from straining during defecation, give a mild laxative or stool softener as ordered.
- Provide reassurance and support. The patient may be frightened by his illness and frequent lumbar punctures. If he's delirious or confused, attempt to reorient him often. Reassure the patient's family that the delirium and behavior changes caused by meningitis usually disappear. However, if a severe neurologic deficit appears permanent, refer the patient to a rehabilitation program as soon as the acute phase of the illness has passed.

Patient teaching
- Inform the patient and his family of the contagion risks, and tell them to notify anyone who comes into close contact with the patient. Such people require antimicrobial prophylaxis and immediate medical attention if fever or other signs of meningitis develop.
- Explain all treatment methods to the patient and his family.
- Inform the patient and his family about the prescribed regimen for care, including monitoring, the need for surgery, and other treatments.
- Instruct the patient and his family in the signs and symptoms of complications and the need to notify the physician as soon as possible should any occur.

Myasthenia gravis

Myasthenia gravis causes sporadic but progressive weakness and abnormal fatigability of striated (skeletal) muscles; symptoms are exacerbated by exercise and repeated movement and relieved by anticholinesterase drugs. Usually, this disorder affects muscles innervated by the cranial nerves (face, lips, tongue, neck, and throat), but it can affect any muscle group.

Myasthenia gravis follows an unpredictable course of periodic exacerbations and remissions. There is no known cure. Drug treatment has improved the prognosis and allows patients to lead relatively normal lives, except during exacerbations. When the disease involves the respiratory system, it may be life threatening.

The exact cause of myasthenia gravis is unknown. However, it's believed to be the result of an autoimmune response, ineffective acetylcholine (ACh) release or, possibly, inadequate muscle fiber response to ACh.

AGE ISSUE *Myasthenia gravis affects 1 in 25,000 people. It can occur at any age, but incidence peaks between ages 20 and 40. It's three times more common in women than in men in this age group, but after age 40, the incidence is similar. About 20% of infants born to mothers with myasthenia gravis have transient (or occasionally persistent) myasthenia.*

This disease may coexist with immune and thyroid disorders; about 15% of myasthenic patients have thymomas. Remissions occur in about 25% of patients.

Pathophysiology
Myasthenia gravis causes a failure in the transmission of nerve impulses at the neuromuscular junction. The site of action is the postsynaptic mem-

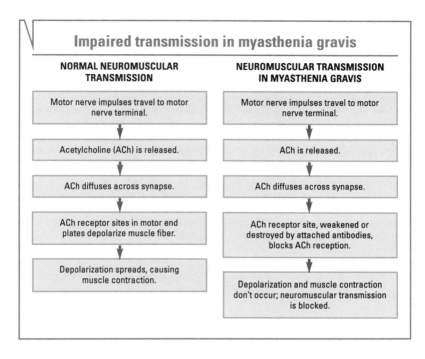

Impaired transmission in myasthenia gravis

NORMAL NEUROMUSCULAR TRANSMISSION	NEUROMUSCULAR TRANSMISSION IN MYASTHENIA GRAVIS
Motor nerve impulses travel to motor nerve terminal.	Motor nerve impulses travel to motor nerve terminal.
Acetylcholine (ACh) is released.	ACh is released.
ACh diffuses across synapse.	ACh diffuses across synapse.
ACh receptor sites in motor end plates depolarize muscle fiber.	ACh receptor site, weakened or destroyed by attached antibodies, blocks ACh reception.
Depolarization spreads, causing muscle contraction.	Depolarization and muscle contraction don't occur; neuromuscular transmission is blocked.

brane. Theoretically, antireceptor antibodies block, weaken, or reduce the number of ACh receptors available at each neuromuscular junction and thereby impair muscle depolarization necessary for movement. (See *Impaired transmission in myasthenia gravis.*)

Comprehensive assessment

Myasthenia gravis may occur gradually or suddenly. Depending on the muscles involved and the severity of the disease, assessment findings may vary. Muscle weakness is progressive, and eventually some muscles may lose function entirely. Expect the patient to complain of extreme muscle weakness and fatigue. The patient usually notes that symptoms are milder on awakening and worsen as the day progresses and that short rest periods temporarily restore muscle function. On questioning, she may report that symptoms become more intense during menses and after emotional stress, prolonged exposure to sunlight or cold, or infections.

Signs and symptoms typically include:

■ weak eye closure, ptosis, and diplopia from impaired neuromuscular transmission to the cranial nerves supplying the eye muscles

■ skeletal muscle weakness and fatigue, increasing through the day but decreasing with rest (In the early stages, easy fatigability of certain muscles may appear with no other findings. Later, it may be severe enough to cause paralysis.)

■ progressive muscle weakness and accompanying loss of function depending on muscle group affected

■ blank and expressionless facial appearance and nasal vocal tones secondary to impaired transmission of cranial nerves innervating the facial muscles

■ frequent nasal regurgitation of fluids, and difficulty chewing and swallowing from cranial nerve involvement

■ drooping eyelids from weakness of facial and extraocular muscles

■ weakened neck muscles with head tilting back to see (Neck muscles may become too weak to support the head without bobbing.)

■ weakened respiratory muscles and decreased tidal volume and vital capacity from impaired transmission to the diaphragm, making breathing difficult and predisposing the patient to pneumonia and other respiratory tract infections

■ respiratory muscle weakness (myasthenic crisis) possibly severe enough to require an emergency airway and mechanical ventilation.

Diagnosis

■ Tensilon test confirms diagnosis of myasthenia gravis, revealing temporarily improved muscle function within 30 to 60 seconds after I.V. injection of edrophonium or neostigmine and lasting up to 30 minutes.

■ Electromyography with repeated neural stimulation shows progressive decrease in muscle fiber contraction.

■ Serum anti-ACh antibody titer may be elevated.

■ Chest X-ray reveals thymoma (in approximately 15% of patients).

Collaborations

A multidisciplinary approach to care is essential. This disease can affect muscular functioning in any area, necessi-

tating the assistance from numerous health care providers. Respiratory therapy may be involved to assist with measure to improve respiratory muscle function and ventilation. Physical therapy may be consulted for assistance with exercises, muscle strengthening, and assistive devices for ambulation. Occupational therapy can help with adaptations needed for activities of daily living. Speech therapy may be necessary to assist the patient with swallowing. Because this disease involves remissions and exacerbations, social services may be necessary to assist the patient with referrals to community support groups, financial concerns, and home care issues and equipment.

Treatment and care

Treatment may include:

■ anticholinesterase drugs, such as neostigmine and pyridostigmine, to counteract fatigue and muscle weakness and allow about 80% of normal muscle function (drugs are less effective as disease worsens)

■ immunosuppressant therapy with corticosteroids, azathioprine, cyclosporine, and cyclophosphamide used in a progressive fashion (when the previous drug response is poor, the next one is used) to decrease the immune response toward ACh receptors at the neuromuscular junction

■ immunoglobulin G during acute relapses or plasmapheresis in severe exacerbations to suppress the immune system

■ thymectomy to remove thymomas and possibly induce remission in some cases of adult-onset myasthenia

■ tracheotomy, positive-pressure ventilation, and vigorous suctioning to re-

move secretions for treatment of acute exacerbations that cause severe respiratory distress
■ discontinuation of anticholinesterase drugs in myasthenic crisis, until respiratory function improves (Myasthenic crisis requires immediate hospitalization and vigorous respiratory support.)
■ plasmapheresis to remove abnormal circulating antibodies interfering with ACh receptors (typically used when medications have been ineffective).

Complications
Complications of myasthenia gravis may include:
■ respiratory distress
■ pneumonia
■ aspiration
■ myasthenic crisis.

Nursing considerations
■ Establish an accurate neurologic baseline, including level of consciousness, muscles affected, the severity of muscle weakness, and the location. Assess respiratory status to establish a baseline, including respiratory rate and rhythm, breath sounds, use of accessory muscles, and skin color. Obtain pulmonary function tests as ordered to establish ventilatory ability. Regularly monitor the patient's tidal volume, vital capacity, and inspiratory force.
■ Monitor oxygen saturation via pulse oximetry and arterial blood gas studies as ordered. Be alert for decreasing partial pressure of arterial oxygen values along with decreases in pulmonary function parameters. Anticipate the need for additional respiratory support, including supplemental oxygen administration, endotracheal (ET) in-

tubation, or tracheotomy and mechanical ventilation.
■ Position the patient with the head of bed elevated, in semi-Fowler's to high Fowler's position. Encourage coughing and deep breathing every 2 hours, or suction as necessary (hyperoxygenating before and after suctioning) to remove secretions; turn the patient every 2 hours to assist with lung expansion and decrease the risk of atelectasis and secretions.
■ If the patient has an ET or tracheostomy tube in place, keep the cuff inflated when suctioning the mouth and trachea to minimize the risk of aspiration.
■ Monitor for possible infection. Assess vital signs at least every 4 hours or more frequently if indicated. Watch for a temperature above 100° F (37.7° C). Obtain a white blood cell (WBC) count as ordered, and notify the physician if the WBC count is greater than 11,000/μl.
■ Assess for the presence of the gag reflex, swallowing reflex, and ability to chew. When swallowing is difficult, give soft, semisolid foods (applesauce, mashed potatoes) instead of liquids to lessen the risk of choking. Anticipate enteral or parenteral nutrition supplementation if swallowing is impaired. Consult with speech therapy to assist with swallowing.
■ Perform eye care as indicated, providing patches or lenses as necessary. Administer artificial tears in each eye at least every 4 to 6 hours or as ordered.
■ Administer medications on time and at evenly spaced intervals, as ordered, to prevent relapses. Be prepared to give atropine for anticholinesterase overdose or toxicity.

Myasthenic crisis and cholinergic crisis

Myasthenic crisis is an acute exacerbation of the muscular weakness that occurs in myasthenia gravis. It can be triggered by infection, surgery, emotional stress, drug interaction, alcohol ingestion, temperature extremes, or pregnancy. Insufficient anticholinesterase medication can also cause myasthenic crisis. Signs and symptoms of myasthenic crisis include:
● respiratory distress progressing to apnea
● extreme fatigue
● increased muscular weakness
● dysphagia
● dysarthria
● fever
● anxiety, restlessness, irritability
● inability to move jaw or raise one or both eyelids.

Cholinergic crisis results from an overdose of, or toxicity to, anticholinesterase agents that block the acetylcholine receptors, ultimately leading to a neuromuscular blockage. Typical signs and symptoms of cholinergic crisis include:
● increasing anxiety and apprehension
● anorexia, nausea, vomiting, abdominal cramps

● excessive salivation
● sweating
● fasciculation (twitching) around the eyes
● muscle cramps and spasms
● increasing muscle weakness
● dysarthria
● increasing dysphagia
● respiratory distress.

Both myasthenic and cholinergic crises are emergency situations that require immediate intervention.
● Notify the physician immediately.
● Maintain a patent airway; provide respiratory support as needed, including oxygen therapy or assisted ventilation.
● Assist with the administration of edrophonium (Tensilon) I.V.
● Provide supportive care, including parenteral fluids, antibiotics (if the crisis was due to infection), enteral feedings, or the insertion of an indwelling urinary catheter.
● Provide emotional support and be sure to explain all the events as they're happening to help allay some of the patient's fears and anxieties.

■ Plan exercise, meals, patient care, and activities to make the most of energy peaks. For example, administer the patient's medication 20 to 30 minutes before meals to facilitate chewing or swallowing.
■ Stay alert for signs of impending myasthenic or cholinergic crisis. (See *Myasthenic crisis and cholinergic crisis.*)

◤ ALERT *If the patient is experiencing a myasthenic crisis, edrophonium will cause his symptoms to improve. If he's experiencing a cholinergic crisis, the patient's symptoms will worsen. If this occurs, administer atropine to counteract the effects of edro-*

phonium and expect to withhold anticholinesterase agents.
■ If the patient is scheduled for plasmapheresis, assess the patient for possible complications including hypovolemia, clotting abnormalities, hypokalemia, hypocalcemia, myasthenic crisis, and cholinergic crisis.

Patient teaching
■ Teach the patient how to plan daily activities to coincide with energy peaks and stress the need for frequent rest periods throughout the day. Emphasize that periodic remissions, exacerba-

tions, and day-to-day fluctuations are common.

■ Instruct the patient about adverse effects of anticholinesterase drugs (headaches, weakness, sweating, abdominal cramps, nausea, vomiting, diarrhea, excessive salivation, and bronchospasm).

■ Warn the patient to avoid strenuous exercise, stress, infection, and needless exposure to the sun or cold weather. All of these things may worsen signs and symptoms. Wearing an eye patch or glasses with one frosted lens may help the patient with diplopia.

■ As appropriate, refer the patient to local support groups and the Myasthenia Gravis Foundation.

Status epilepticus

Status epilepticus is a continuous or recurrent seizure state lasting at least 20 to 30 minutes that can occur in all seizure types. The most life-threatening example is generalized tonic-clonic status epilepticus, a continuous generalized tonic-clonic seizure. With status epilepticus, the patient doesn't return to full consciousness before another seizure occurs.

Status epilepticus is accompanied by respiratory distress leading to hypoxia or anoxia. It can result from abrupt withdrawal of anticonvulsant medications, hypoxic encephalopathy, acute head trauma, metabolic encephalopathy, or septicemia secondary to encephalitis or meningitis. Most commonly, status epilepticus results from noncompliance with anticonvulsant medication therapy or decreased serum drug levels secondary to alcohol abuse or infection.

Epilepsy is believed to affect 1% to 2% of the population; approximately 2 million people have been diagnosed with epilepsy.

AGE ISSUE *The incidence of epilepsy is highest in childhood and old age.*

Pathophysiology

Some neurons in the brain may depolarize easily or be hyperexcitable. When stimulated, the neurons (called *epileptogenic focus*) fire more readily than normal, spreading electrical current to surrounding cells. These cells fire in turn and the impulse cascades to one side of the brain (a partial seizure), both sides of the brain (a generalized seizure), or cortical, subcortical, and brain stem areas.

The brain's metabolic demand for oxygen increases dramatically during a seizure. If this demand isn't met, hypoxia and brain damage ensue. Firing of inhibitory neurons causes the excitatory neurons to slow their firing and eventually stop. If this inhibitory action doesn't occur, the result is status epilepticus: one seizure occurring right after another and another; without treatment the anoxia is fatal.

Comprehensive assessment

Patient history reveals a history of epilepsy. Additional investigation may reveal inconsistent use of anticonvulsant medications, alcohol abuse, recent head injury, infection, or headaches.

Physical examination typically reveals ongoing seizure activity of either partial or generalized type. (See *Seizure types,* page 334.)

Seizure types

There are two major categories of seizures in status epilepticus — partial and generalized. Each has distinct signs and symptoms.

Partial seizures

Arising from a localized area of the brain, partial seizures cause focal symptoms. These seizures are classified by their effect on consciousness and whether they spread throughout the motor pathway, causing a generalized seizure.

- A *simple partial seizure* begins locally and usually doesn't cause an alteration in consciousness. It may cause sensory symptoms (lights, smells, and sounds that aren't actually present), autonomic symptoms (sweating, flushing, and pupil dilation), and psychic symptoms (dream states, anger, and fear). The seizure lasts for a few seconds and occurs without preceding or provoking events. Simple partial seizures can be motor or sensory.
- A *complex partial seizure* alters consciousness. Amnesia for events that occur during and immediately after the seizure is a differentiating characteristic. During the seizure, the patient may follow simple commands. A complex partial seizure generally lasts for 1 to 3 minutes.

Generalized seizures

As the term suggests, generalized seizures cause a generalized electrical abnormality within the brain. They can be convulsive or nonconvulsive, and include several types:

- *Absence seizures* occur most commonly in children, although they may also occur in adults. These seizures usually begin with a brief change in level of consciousness, indicated by blinking or rolling of the eyes, a blank stare, and slight mouth movements. The patient retains his posture and continues preseizure activity without difficulty. Typically, each seizure lasts from 1 to 10 seconds. If not properly treated, seizures can recur as often as 100 times a day. An absence seizure is a nonconvulsive seizure, but it may progress to a generalized tonic-clonic seizure.

- *Myoclonic seizures* (bilateral massive epileptic myoclonus) are brief, involuntary muscular jerks of the body or extremities that may be rhythmic. Consciousness isn't usually affected.

- *Generalized tonic-clonic seizures* typically begin with a loud cry, precipitated by air rushing from the lungs through the vocal cords. The patient then loses consciousness and falls to the ground. The body stiffens (tonic phase) and then alternates between episodes of muscle spasm and relaxation (clonic phase). Tongue biting, incontinence, labored breathing, apnea, and subsequent cyanosis may occur. The seizure stops in 2 to 5 minutes, when abnormal electrical conduction ceases. The patient is confused and may have difficulty talking when he regains consciousness. If he can talk, he may complain of drowsiness, fatigue, headache, muscle soreness, and arm or leg weakness. He may fall into a deep sleep after the seizure.

- *Atonic seizures* are characterized by a general loss of postural tone and a temporary loss of consciousness. They occur primarily in young children and are sometimes called "drop attacks" because they cause the child to fall.

Diagnosis

Typically, for the patient with a history of seizures, anticonvulsant drug levels often reveal a value below the therapeutic level. For those without a history of seizures, diagnostic tests are performed to rule out other possible underlying causes for the continuous seizure activity. These may include:

■ serum electrolyte and liver enzyme studies, glucose levels, complete blood count, and blood urea nitrogen, to rule out electrolyte and metabolic disturbances as the cause

■ arterial blood gas (ABG) analysis, to provide baseline levels for oxygenation status

■ EEG, to differentiate between absence and complete partial seizures

■ computed tomography scan, to rule out possible brain lesion or skull fracture.

Collaborations

A multidisciplinary approach to care is essential because the patient is at high risk for numerous complications. Numerous health care disciplines are involved to maintain the patient's vital functions. Respiratory therapy may be involved to assist with respiratory care measures, including mechanical ventilation. Anesthesiology may be necessary to provide general anesthesia or a barbiturate coma if the patient's condition fails to respond to usual drug therapy. Nutritional support may be necessary if the patient's underlying state is poor or if the patient experiences a prolonged duration of status epilepticus. Social services may be necessary to assist with ways to promote patient adherence to the medication regimen, as appropriate.

Treatment and care

Treatment focuses on maintaining ventilation and stopping the seizure activity:

■ airway maintenance (oral, endotracheal [ET] tube, or tracheotomy as appropriate), oxygen therapy, and mechanical ventilation as necessary

■ fast-acting anticonvulsants, such as diazepam or lorazepam I.V., and longer-acting anticonvulsants, such as phenytoin (or phenobarbital if the patient is allergic to phenytoin) or fosphenytoin (if phenytoin isn't used)

■ general anesthesia using pentobarbital coma, propofol, or midazolam if anticonvulsant therapy is ineffective

■ I.V. valproic acid, paraldehyde, lidocaine, or neuromuscular blockers to stop seizure activity.

Complications

Complications associated with status epilepticus include:

■ cardiac arrhythmias
■ hyperthermia
■ aspiration
■ hypertension or hypotension
■ hyperglycemia or hypoglycemia
■ dehydration
■ myoglobinuria
■ oral or musculoskeletal injuries
■ death.

Nursing considerations

■ Establish and maintain the patient's airway; assess respiratory status including rate, depth, and rhythm of respirations. Observe for accessory muscle use or labored respirations.

■ Assess neurologic status to establish a baseline and then frequently reassess the patient, at least every 5 to 10 minutes initially, until stabilized.

■ Use an oral airway to maintain patency; however, don't force it into the patient's mouth.

■ Assess oxygen saturation via pulse oximetry and ABG studies as ordered; report any indications of hypoxemia; administer supplemental oxygen as indicated; have ET intubation equipment and ventilatory assistance readily available at the bedside.

■ Monitor vital signs every 2 to 5 minutes; anticipate continuous direct intra-arterial blood pressure monitoring if appropriate.

■ Institute continuous cardiac monitoring to evaluate for arrhythmias.

■ Monitor blood glucose levels for hypoglycemia (a possible cause or effect of the patient's continued seizures) and administer glucose, as ordered.

■ If alcohol withdrawal is determined to be the underlying cause, administer thiamine I.V. to prevent Wernicke's encephalopathy.

■ Administer anticonvulsants agents I.V. as prescribed. Expect to administer fast-acting agents first, followed by long-acting agents.

ALERT *If phenobarbital is administered as the long-acting agent and it's given at the same time as the fast-acting agent, be alert for respiratory depression and hypotension. Have emergency intubation equipment readily available at the bedside if it isn't already being used.*

■ Maintain the I.V. infusion site.

■ Monitor the patient's response to anticonvulsant agents. If seizures continue, prepare for general anesthesia with pentobarbital, propofol, or midazolam. Keep in mind that these agents are tapered gradually to determine if seizure activity has abated.

ALERT *When anticonvulsant agents are given, expect to monitor cardiopulmonary status continuously. In addition, vasopressors are usually needed.*

■ Institute seizure precautions and ensure the patient's safety with raised, padded side rails, avoidance of restraints, and removal of dangerous objects.

Patient teaching

■ Answer any questions the patient and his family may have about the condition. Assure them that epilepsy is controllable for most patients who follow a prescribed regimen of medication and that most patients maintain a normal lifestyle.

■ Teach the patient about his medications and the need for compliance with dosage and schedule. Caution the patient to monitor the amount of medication remaining so that he doesn't run out of it.

■ Teach the patient about adverse effects and to report them immediately to the physician or health care provider.

■ Explain the importance of having anticonvulsant blood levels checked at regular intervals even if the seizures are under control.

■ Teach the patient measures to help him control and decrease the occurrence of seizures. These may include taking medication on time, eating balanced meals to avoid hypoglycemia, avoiding trigger factors (flashing lights, loud noises or music, video games, television), limiting alcohol intake or eliminating it altogether as advised, treating illnesses early, and decreasing stress.

■ Teach the patient's family how to care for the patient during a seizure to prevent him from being injured.

Stroke

A stroke, also known as a cerebrovascular accident or brain attack, is a sudden impairment of cerebral circulation in one or more blood vessels supplying the brain. A stroke interrupts or diminishes oxygen supply, and typically causes serious damage or necrosis in the brain tissues. The sooner the circulation returns to normal after the stroke, the better chances are for complete recovery. However, about one-half of the patients who survive a stroke remain permanently disabled and experience a recurrence within weeks, months, or years.

Stroke typically results from one of three causes:

■ thrombosis of the cerebral arteries supplying the brain or of the intracranial vessels occluding blood flow (see *Types of stroke,* page 338)

■ embolism from thrombus outside the brain, such as in the heart, aorta, or common carotid artery

■ hemorrhage from an intracranial artery or vein, such as from hypertension, ruptured aneurysm, arteriovenous malformation, trauma, hemorrhagic disorder, or septic embolism.

Risk factors that have been identified as predisposing a patient to stroke include:

■ hypertension

■ family history of stroke

■ history of transient ischemic attacks (TIAs) (see *Understanding transient ischemic attacks,* page 339)

■ cardiac disease, including arrhythmias, coronary artery disease, acute myocardial infarction, dilated cardiomyopathy, and valvular disease

■ diabetes

■ familial hyperlipidemia

■ cigarette smoking

■ increased alcohol intake

■ obesity, sedentary lifestyle

■ use of oral contraceptives.

AGE ISSUE *Although stroke may occur in younger persons, most patients experiencing stroke are over age 65. In fact, the risk of stroke doubles with each decade of life after age 55.*

The incidence of stroke is higher in Blacks than in Whites. In fact, Blacks have a 60% higher risk for stroke than Whites or Hispanics of the same age. This is believed to be the result of an increased prevalence of hypertension in Blacks. In addition, strokes in Blacks usually result from disease in the small cerebral vessels, while strokes in Whites are typically the result of disease in the large carotid arteries. Mortality rate for Blacks from stroke is twice that for Whites. Stroke is the third most common cause of death in the United States and the most common cause of neurologic disability. It strikes more than 500,000 persons per year and is fatal in approximately one-half of these persons.

Pathophysiology

Regardless of the cause of a stroke, the underlying event is deprivation of oxygen and nutrients. Normally, if the arteries become blocked, autoregulatory mechanisms help maintain cerebral circulation until collateral circulation develops to deliver blood to the affected area. If the compensatory mechanisms become overworked or if cerebral blood flow remains impaired for more than a few minutes, oxygen deprivation leads to infarction of brain tissue. The brain cells cease to func-

Types of stroke

Strokes are typically classified as ischemic or hemorrhagic depending on the underlying cause. The chart shown below describes the major types of strokes.

Type of stroke	Description
Ischemic: Thrombotic	• Most common cause of stroke • Frequently the result of atherosclerosis; also associated with hypertension, smoking, diabetes • Thrombus in extracranial or intracranial vessel blocks blood flow to the cerebral cortex • Carotid artery most commonly affected extracranial vessel • Common intracranial sites include bifurcation of carotid arteries, distal intracranial portion of vertebral arteries, and proximal basilar arteries • May occur during sleep or shortly after awakening, during surgery, or after a myocardial infarction
Ischemic: Embolic	• Second most common type of stroke • Embolus from heart or extracranial arteries floats into cerebral bloodstream and lodges in middle cerebral artery or branches • Embolus commonly originates during atrial fibrillation • Typically occurs during activity • Develops rapidly
Ischemic: Lacunar	• Subtype of thrombotic stroke • Hypertension creates cavities deep in white matter of the brain, affecting the internal capsule, basal ganglia, thalamus, and pons • Lipid-coated lining of the small penetrating arteries thickens and weakens wall, causing microaneurysms and dissections
Hemorrhagic	• Third most common type of stroke • Typically caused by hypertension or rupture of aneurysm • Diminished blood supply to area supplied by ruptured artery and compression by accumulated blood

tion because they can neither store glucose or glycogen for use, nor engage in anaerobic metabolism.

A thrombotic or embolic stroke causes ischemia. Some of the neurons served by the occluded vessel die from lack of oxygen and nutrients. This results in cerebral infarction, in which tissue injury triggers an inflammatory response that in turn increases intracranial pressure (ICP). Injury to surrounding cells disrupts metabolism and leads to changes in ionic transport, localized acidosis, and free radical formation. Calcium, sodium, and water accumulate in the injured cells, and excitatory neurotransmitters are released. Consequent continued cellular injury and swelling set up a vicious cycle of further damage.

When hemorrhage is the cause, impaired cerebral perfusion causes infarction, and the blood itself acts as a space-occupying mass, exerting pressure on the brain tissues. The brain's regulatory mechanisms attempt to maintain equilibrium by increasing blood pressure to maintain cerebral perfusion pressure. The increased ICP forces cerebrospinal fluid (CSF) out, thus restoring the balance. If the hemorrhage is small, this may be enough to keep the patient alive with only minimal neurologic deficits. But if the bleeding is heavy, ICP increases rapidly and perfusion stops. Even if the pressure returns to normal, many brain cells die.

Initially, the ruptured cerebral blood vessels may constrict to limit the blood loss. This vasospasm further compromises blood flow, leading to more ischemia and cellular damage. If a clot forms in the vessel, decreased blood flow also promotes ischemia. If the blood enters the subarachnoid space, meningeal irritation occurs. The blood cells that pass through the vessel wall into the surrounding tissue may also break down and block the arachnoid villi, causing hydrocephalus.

Comprehensive assessment

Clinical features of stroke vary with the artery affected (and, consequently, the portion of the brain it supplies), the severity of the damage, and the extent of collateral circulation that develops to help the brain compensate for decreased blood supply. (See *Assessment findings in stroke,* pages 340 and 341.)

When assessing a patient who may have experienced a stroke, remember this: If the stroke occurs in the left hemisphere, it produces signs and symptoms on the right side; if it occurs in the right hemisphere, signs and symptoms appear on the left side.

Understanding transient ischemic attacks

A transient ischemic attack (TIA) is an episode of neurologic deficit resulting from cerebral ischemia. The recurrent attacks may last from seconds to hours and clear within 12 to 24 hours. TIAs are commonly considered a warning sign for stroke and have been reported in more than one-half of the patients who later developed a stroke, usually within 2 to 5 years.

In a TIA, microemboli released from a thrombus may temporarily interrupt blood flow, especially in the small, distal branches of the brain's arterial tree. Small spasms in those arterioles may impair blood flow and also precede a TIA.

The most distinctive features of TIAs are transient focal deficits with complete return of function. The deficits usually involve some degree of motor or sensory dysfunction. They may progress to loss of consciousness and loss of motor or sensory function for a brief period. The patient typically experiences weakness in the lower part of the face and arms, hands, fingers, and legs on the side opposite the affected region. Other manifestations may include transient dysphagia, numbness or tingling of the face and lips, double vision, slurred speech, and vertigo.

However, a stroke that causes cranial nerve damage produces signs of cranial nerve dysfunction on the same side as the hemorrhage or infarct.

The patient's history, obtained from a family member or friend if necessary, may uncover one or more risk factors for stroke. The history may also reveal either a sudden onset of hemiparesis or hemiplegia or a gradual onset of

Assessment findings in stroke

A stroke can leave one patient with mild hand weakness and another with complete unilateral paralysis. In both patients, the functional loss reflects damage to the brain area normally perfused by the occluded or ruptured artery. In general, assessment findings associated with a stroke may include:

- unilateral limb weakness
- speech difficulties
- numbness on one side
- headache
- vision disturbances (diplopia, hemianopsia, ptosis)
- vertigo
- anxiety
- altered level of consciousness (LOC).

Typical assessment findings based on the artery affected are highlighted in the chart below.

Affected artery	Assessment findings
Middle cerebral artery	• Aphasia • Dysphasia • Visual field deficits • Hemiparesis of affected side (more severe in the face and arm than in the leg)
Carotid artery	• Weakness • Paralysis • Numbness • Sensory changes • Vision disturbances on the affected side • Altered LOC • Bruits • Headaches • Aphasia • Ptosis
Vertebrobasilary artery	• Weakness on the affected side • Numbness around lips and mouth • Visual field deficits • Diplopia • Poor coordination • Dysphagia • Slurred speech • Vertigo • Nystagmus • Amnesia • Ataxia
Anterior cerebral artery	• Confusion • Weakness • Numbness, especially in the leg on the affected side • Incontinence • Loss of coordination • Impaired motor and sensory functions • Personality changes

Assessment findings in stroke *(continued)*

Affected artery	Assessment findings
Posterior cerebral artery	• Visual field deficits (homonymous hemianopsia) • Sensory impairment • Dyslexia • Perseveration (abnormally persistent replies to questions) • Coma • Cortical blindness • Absence of paralysis (usually)

dizziness, mental disturbances, or seizures. The patient or a family member may also report that the patient lost consciousness or suddenly developed aphasia. Speaking with the patient during history-taking may reveal communication problems, such as dysarthria, dysphasia or aphasia, and apraxia.

Neurologic examination identifies most of the physical findings associated with stroke. These may include unconsciousness or changes in level of consciousness (LOC), such as a decreased attention span, difficulties with comprehension, forgetfulness, and a lack of motivation. If conscious, the patient may exhibit anxiety along with communication and mobility difficulties. Inspection may reveal related urinary incontinence.

Motor function and muscle strength tests commonly show a loss of voluntary muscle control and hemiparesis or hemiplegia on one side of the body. In the initial phase, flaccid paralysis with decreased deep tendon reflexes may occur. These reflexes return to normal after the initial phase, along with an increase in muscle tone and, in some cases, muscle spasticity on the affected side.

Vision testing commonly reveals hemianopsia on the affected side of the body and, in patients with left-sided hemiplegia, problems with visual-spatial relations.

Sensory assessment may reveal sensory losses, ranging from slight impairment of touch to the inability to perceive the position and motion of body parts. The patient may also have difficulty interpreting visual, tactile, and auditory stimuli.

Diagnosis

Diagnostic test findings may include the following:

■ Computed tomography (CT) scan identifies ischemic stroke within the first 72 hours of symptom onset; and evidence of hemorrhagic stroke (lesions larger than 1 cm) immediately.

■ Magnetic resonance imaging assists in identifying areas of ischemia or infarction and cerebral swelling.

■ Cerebral angiography reveals disruption or displacement of the cerebral circulation by occlusion, such as stenosis or acute thrombus, or hemorrhage.

■ Digital subtraction angiography shows evidence of occlusion of cerebral vessels, lesions, or vascular abnormalities.

■ Carotid duplex scan identifies stenosis greater than 60%.

■ Brain scan shows ischemic areas but may not be conclusive for up to 2 weeks after stroke.

■ Single photon-emission CT and positron emission tomography scans identify areas of altered metabolism surrounding lesions not yet able to be detected by other diagnostic tests.

■ Transesophageal echocardiogram reveals cardiac disorders, such as atrial thrombi, atrial septal defect, or patent foramen ovale, as causes of thrombotic stroke.

■ Lumbar puncture reveals bloody CSF when stroke is hemorrhagic.

■ Ophthalmoscopy may identify signs of hypertension and atherosclerotic changes in retinal arteries.

■ EEG helps identify damaged areas of the brain.

Collaborations

The patient with an acute stroke requires multidisciplinary care. Typically, outside of the hospital, emergency services (EMS) personnel are involved in confirming the signs and symptoms of an acute stroke, completing the primary survey, and then transporting the patient to the care facility. When the patient reaches the emergency department (ED), personnel are involved in completing the secondary survey, including vital signs, oxygen saturation and administration, brief and targeted history, I.V. access, and a decision regarding fibrinolytic therapy. The focus is on rapid, but accurate, diagnosis and prompt treatment.

After the acute phase has passed, the patient needs continued multidisciplinary care. The patient with a stroke needs specialized care from many health care professionals, including nursing, speech therapy, physical therapy, and occupational therapy. The nurse manages all aspects of the patient's care. In addition, the speech therapist assists the patient with deficits in swallowing as well as speaking while the physical therapist helps the patient regain mobility and maintain range of motion. An occupational therapist works with the patient to relearn basic activities of daily living, such as dressing, bathing, and cooking. The patient and his family may also benefit from pastoral or spiritual counsel and support groups. Social services plays an important role in ensuring continuity of care after discharge to home or to a rehabilitation facility and securing assistance with follow-up care and services and financial and emotional concerns.

Treatment and care

The essential steps to managing a patient with a stroke can be summarized as the seven D's: detection, dispatch, delivery, door, data, decision, and drug. *Detection* involves early identification of signs and symptoms by the patient or family members to ensure the best outcome. *Dispatch* involves EMS activation and *delivery* of the patient to the health care facility. *Door* involves the patient's arrival at the ED with rapid triage and assessment. *Data* refers to all of the information obtained to determine the course of therapy. *Decision* involves identifying the most appropriate treatment based on the patient's situation, assessment findings, and the type of injury. *Drug* refers to the initiation of appropriate pharmacologic treatment. Whenever a patient is suspected of having a stroke, the algorithm for treating a suspected stroke is initiated. (See *Suspected stroke treatment algorithm,* page 344.)

For ischemic strokes, the drug therapy of choice is fibrinolytics. This therapy is begun within 60 minutes of the patient's arrival in the ED. To be a candidate for fibrinolytic therapy, the patient must meet the following criteria:

■ acute ischemic stroke associated with significant neurologic deficit
■ onset of symptoms less than 3 hours before initiation of treatment.

Criteria that exclude a patient from receiving fibrinolytic therapy include:
■ evidence of intracranial hemorrhage during pretreatment evaluation
■ suspicion of subarachnoid hemorrhage during pretreatment
■ history of recent (within 3 months) intracranial or intraspinal surgery, serious head trauma, or previous stroke
■ history of intracranial bleeding
■ uncontrolled hypertension at time of treatment
■ seizure at stroke onset
■ active internal bleeding
■ intracranial neoplasm, arteriovenous malformation, or aneurysm
■ known bleeding diathesis, including but not limited to: current use of an anticoagulant such as warfarin, International Normalized Ratio greater than 1.7, or prothrombin time greater than 15 seconds; use of heparin within 48 hours before the onset of stroke with elevation of activated partial thromboplastin time; platelet count less than 100,000/μl.

Additional treatment measures may be used to minimize and prevent further cerebral damage. These include:

■ ICP management with monitoring, hyperventilation (to decrease partial pressure of arterial carbon dioxide, which lowers ICP), osmotic diuretics (mannitol, to reduce cerebral edema), and corticosteroids (dexamethasone, to reduce inflammation and cerebral edema)
■ stool softeners to prevent straining, which increases ICP
■ anticonvulsants to treat or prevent seizures
■ surgery for large cerebellar infarction to remove infarcted tissue and decompress remaining live tissue
■ aneurysm repair to prevent further hemorrhage
■ percutaneous transluminal angioplasty or stent insertion to open occluded vessels
■ anticoagulant therapy (heparin, warfarin) to maintain vessel patency and prevent further clot formation
■ antiplatelet agents (aspirin, ticlopidine) to reduce the risk of platelet aggregation and subsequent clot formation (for patients with TIAs)
■ carotid endarterectomy (for TIA) to open partially occluded carotid arteries
■ analgesics, such as acetaminophen, to relieve headache associated with hemorrhagic stroke.

Complications

Complications vary with the severity and type of stroke, but may include:
■ unstable blood pressure (from loss of vasomotor control)
■ cerebral edema
■ fluid imbalances
■ sensory impairment
■ infections such as pneumonia
■ altered LOC
■ aspiration
■ contractures

Suspected stroke treatment algorithm

This algorithm is used for suspected stroke. The patient's survival depends on prompt recognition of symptoms and treatment.

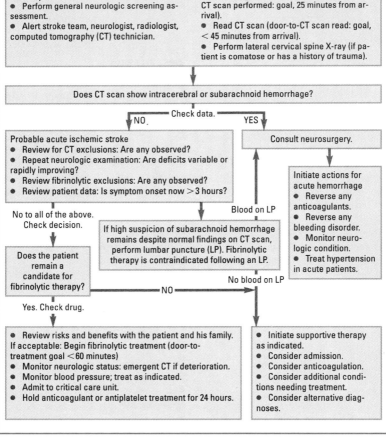

DETECTION, DISPATCH, DELIVERY TO DOOR

Immediate general assessment: first 10 minutes after arrival
- Assess ABCs and vital signs.
- Provide oxygen by nasal cannula.
- Obtain I.V. access; obtain blood samples (complete blood count, electrolyte levels, coagulation studies).
- Check blood glucose levels; treat if indicated.
- Obtain 12-lead electrocardiogram; check for arrhythmias.
- Perform general neurologic screening assessment.
- Alert stroke team, neurologist, radiologist, computed tomography (CT) technician.

Immediate neurologic assessment: first 25 minutes after arrival
- Review patient history.
- Establish onset (< 3 hours required for fibrinolytics).
- Perform physical examination.
- Perform neurologic examination: Determine level of consciousness (Glasgow Coma Scale) and level of stroke severity (NIH Stroke Scale or Hunt and Hess Scale).
- Order urgent noncontrast CT scan (door-to-CT scan performed: goal, 25 minutes from arrival).
- Read CT scan (door-to-CT scan read: goal, < 45 minutes from arrival).
- Perform lateral cervical spine X-ray (if patient is comatose or has a history of trauma).

Does CT scan show intracerebral or subarachnoid hemorrhage?

Check data.

NO. ⟶

YES ⟶

Probable acute ischemic stroke
- Review for CT exclusions: Are any observed?
- Repeat neurologic examination: Are deficits variable or rapidly improving?
- Review fibrinolytic exclusions: Are any observed?
- Review patient data: Is symptom onset now > 3 hours?

Consult neurosurgery.

Initiate actions for acute hemorrhage
- Reverse any anticoagulants.
- Reverse any bleeding disorder.
- Monitor neurologic condition.
- Treat hypertension in acute patients.

No to all of the above. Check decision.

Blood on LP

If high suspicion of subarachnoid hemorrhage remains despite normal findings on CT scan, perform lumbar puncture (LP). Fibrinolytic therapy is contraindicated following an LP.

Does the patient remain a candidate for fibrinolytic therapy?

No blood on LP

NO ⟶

Yes. Check drug.

- Review risks and benefits with the patient and his family. If acceptable: Begin fibrinolytic treatment (door-to-treatment goal <60 minutes)
- Monitor neurologic status: emergent CT if deterioration.
- Monitor blood pressure; treat as indicated.
- Admit to critical care unit.
- Hold anticoagulant or antiplatelet treatment for 24 hours.

- Initiate supportive therapy as indicated.
- Consider admission.
- Consider anticoagulation.
- Consider additional conditions needing treatment.
- Consider alternative diagnoses.

- pulmonary embolism
- death.

Nursing considerations

- Secure and maintain the patient's airway and anticipate the need for endotracheal intubation and mechanical ventilation as necessary. Monitor oxygen saturation levels via pulse oximetry and serial arterial blood gas studies as ordered. Administer supplemental oxygen as ordered to maintain oxygen saturation greater than 90%.
- Assess the patient's neurologic status frequently, at least every 15 to 30 minutes initially, then every hour as indicated. Note his LOC and ability to respond to stimuli, pupillary response, motor and sensory function, and reflexes. Observe for signs and symptoms of increased ICP and monitor ICP as ordered. (See "Intracranial pressure monitoring," page 312.) If the patient develops hydrocephalus, prepare him for a ventriculostomy. (See "Ventriculostomy," page 348.)
- If cerebral edema is suspected, maintain ICP sufficient for adequate cerebral perfusion but low enough to avoid brain herniation. Elevate the head of the bed 20 to 30 degrees; institute moderate fluid restriction; administer osmotic diuretics such as mannitol, as ordered. If necessary, anticipate the use of barbiturate coma to aid in lowering ICP.

ALERT *If barbiturate coma will be induced, mechanical ventilation and ICP monitoring are required because of the patient's subsequent respiratory suppression and inability to respond.*

Prepare to institute bispectral index monitoring, as appropriate, to monitor the patient's level of sedation. (See "Bispectral index monitoring," page 281.)

- Assess hemodynamic status frequently, including central venous pressure and pulmonary artery pressure. Assist with the insertion of a pulmonary artery catheter, if indicated, to monitor hemodynamic status. Give fluids as ordered and monitor I.V. infusions to avoid overhydration, which may increase ICP.
- Assess vital signs, including heart and respiratory rates, at least every 15 minutes until stabilized.
- Monitor blood pressure every 15 minutes. Anticipate the use of direct intra-arterial blood pressure monitoring.

ALERT *If the patient is receiving fibrinolytic therapy, maintain blood pressure below 185/110 mm Hg to minimize the risk of bleeding complications; if the patient isn't a candidate for fibrinolytic therapy, administer antihypertensive therapy only for markedly elevated blood pressures (diastolic pressure greater than 140 mm Hg, blood pressure greater than 220/120 mm Hg, or mean blood pressure about 130 mm Hg) because inducing lower perfusion pressures may increase ischemia and worsen the stroke.*

- If antihypertensive therapy is indicated, expect to administer labetalol 20 mg I.V. push over 1 to 2 minutes, then 40 to 80 mg every 10 minutes to a maximum dose of 300 mg; or sodium nitroprusside, 0.25 to 0.3 mg/kg/minute, titrating to maintain blood pressure within acceptable ranges without inducing hypotension.
- Monitor temperature for increases.

ALERT *Be aware that if the patient is experiencing a hemorrhagic stroke, blood can accumulate in* *the subarachnoid space. This blood triggers an inflammatory response in the body, causing the temperature to rise. Be ready to institute measures to reduce hyperthermia (such as cooling blankets) and antipyretics (such as acetaminophen).*

■ Institute continuous cardiac monitoring to detect arrhythmias.

■ For the patient receiving fibrinolytic therapy, assess the patient for signs and symptoms of bleeding every 15 to 30 minutes and institute bleeding precautions. Monitor results of coagulations studies. Ensure completion of type and cross match of patient's blood in case hemorrhage occurs and blood component replacement therapy is necessary.

■ Monitor the patient for seizures. Administer anticonvulsants, such as phenytoin, lorazepam, or diazepam, as ordered. Institute safety precautions to prevent injury.

■ Turn the patient often. Apply antiembolism stockings or intermittent sequential compression devices to the patient's legs to reduce the risk of deep vein thrombosis.

■ Institute measures to prevent skin breakdown.

■ Obtain an order for a stool softener or mild laxative and administer as ordered. Implement a bowel elimination problem based on previous habits. If the patient is receiving steroids to relieve cerebral edema, monitor for GI irritation and check the stool for blood; administer histamine-2 receptor antagonists as ordered to minimize the risk of GI bleeding.

■ If the patient experienced TIAs, expect to administer such antiplatelet agents as aspirin, ticlopidine, or clopidogrel as ordered, to reduce the risk of

stroke and decrease TIAs; administer anticoagulants, such as heparin, if the patient demonstrates signs of stroke progression, unstable signs and symptoms of stroke (such as TIAs), or evidence of embolic stroke. Monitor coagulation studies closely. Anticipate switching to an oral anticoagulant such as warfarin if long-term therapy is necessary.

■ Position the patient to promote pulmonary drainage and prevent upper airway obstruction. Encourage coughing and deep breathing and incentive spirometry (if not intubated) to prevent atelectasis. Avoid placing him in the prone position or hyperextending his neck.

■ Following your facility's policy, suction secretions from the airway as necessary to prevent hypoxia and vasodilatation from carbon dioxide accumulation. Suction for less than 20 seconds to avoid increasing ICP.

■ Monitor fluid intake and output and electrolyte balance. Assess urine output at least every 2 hours, or more frequently if indicated. Offer the urinal or bedpan every 2 hours. If necessary, insert an indwelling urinary catheter to allow for close monitoring. Administer I.V. fluids as ordered. If the patient can take liquids orally, offer them as often as fluid limitations permit.

■ Ensure adequate nutrition. If alert and awake, check for gag reflex before offering small oral feedings of semisolid foods. Place the food tray within the patient's visual field. Have the patient sit upright and tilt his head slightly forward when eating. If the patient has dysphagia or one-sided facial weakness, give him semisoft foods and tell him to chew on the unaffected side of his mouth. If oral feedings aren't possible or the patient can't swallow, administer enteral or parenteral nutrition, as ordered.

■ Manage GI problems. Prevent the patient from straining during defecation because this increases ICP. Modify his diet as appropriate, by increasing his fiber (bran, salads, fresh fruits) intake, administering stool softeners as ordered, and giving laxatives, if necessary. If the patient vomits (usually during the first few days), keep him positioned on his side to prevent aspiration and administer antiemetics as ordered because vomiting can increase ICP.

■ Provide careful mouth care. Clean and irrigate the patient's mouth to remove food particles. Care for his dentures as needed.

■ Provide meticulous eye care. Remove secretions with a cotton ball and normal saline solution. Instill eye drops as ordered. Patch the patient's affected eye if he can't close his eyelid.

■ Position the patient in correct body alignment. Use high-topped sneakers to prevent footdrop and contractures and specialized pressure reducing mattresses or overlays to minimize the risk of pressure ulcers. Elevate the affected hand to control dependent edema, and place it in a functional position.

■ Begin exercises as soon as possible. Perform passive range-of-motion exercises for both the affected and unaffected sides. Teach and encourage the patient to use his unaffected side to exercise his affected side.

■ Establish and maintain communication with the patient. If he's aphasic, set up a simple method of communicating basic needs. Use gestures if necessary to help him understand. Even the unresponsive patient can hear, so avoid saying anything in his presence that you wouldn't want him to hear and remember.

■ Provide psychological support and establish a rapport with the patient. Set realistic short-term goals. Spend time with him, involve his family in his care when possible, and explain his deficits and strengths.

ALERT *Remember that following a stroke a patient may experience emotional lability with mood fluctuations, which may result from brain damage or as a reaction to being dependent. Provide continued support and encouragement.*

■ Prepare the patient for surgery, such as carotid endarterectomy or craniotomy, as appropriate.

■ Provide emotional support to the patient and his family. Encourage them to express his concerns.

Patient teaching

■ Teach the patient, if possible, and his family about his condition. Encourage family members to adopt a realistic attitude, but don't discourage hope. Answer questions honestly.

■ Explain all tests, neurologic examinations, treatments (including medications), and procedures to the patient — even if he's unconscious — and his family.

■ Provide explanations about the use of fibrinolytic therapy; instruct in danger signs and symptoms and the need to report any such signs immediately.

■ If surgery will be performed, provide preoperative teaching if the patient's condition permits. Make sure that the patient, if possible, and his family understand the surgery and its possible complications. Reinforce the physician's explanations as necessary.

Ventriculostomy intracranial pressure monitoring

To set up a ventriculostomy intracranial pressure (ICP) monitoring system, use strict aseptic technique and follow these steps:

• Create a sterile field using a sterile towel, and place a 20-ml luer-lock syringe, 18-G needle, 250-ml I.V. bag filled with normal saline solution and disposable transducer on the field.

• Put on sterile gloves and gown, and fill the 20-ml syringe with normal saline solution from the I.V. bag.

• Remove the injection cap from the patient line and attach the syringe. Turn the system stopcock off to the short end of the patient line and flush through the drip chamber (as shown below). Allow a few drops to flow through the flow chamber (the manometer), the tubing, and the one-way valve into the drainage bag. (Fill the tubing and manometer slowly to minimize air bubbles. If air bubbles surface, make sure to force them from the system.)

• Attach the manometer to the I.V. pole at the head of the bed.

• Slide the drip chamber onto the manometer and align the chamber to the zero point (as shown below).

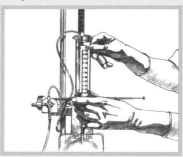

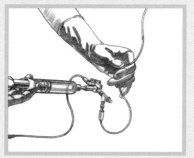

■ Provide information about rehabilitation and the need for continued follow-up and therapy.

Ventriculostomy

A ventriculostomy involves the placement of a catheter into one of the two lateral ventricles containing cerebrospinal fluid (CSF). This catheter then can be connected to a bedside monitor for intracranial pressure (ICP) monitoring and waveform evaluation. It can also be used to drain CSF to reduce pressure to the desired level and then to maintain it at that level. CSF is drained by a ventriculostomy tube in a sterile, closed drainage collection system.

Other therapeutic uses include direct instillation of medications, contrast media, or air for diagnostic radiology; and aspiration of CSF for laboratory analysis.

Ventriculostomy may be performed for patients with subacute and acute hydrocephalus, which developed, for

- Connect the transducer to the monitor.
- Put on a new pair of sterile gloves.
- Keeping one hand sterile, turn off the patient stopcock to the patient.
- Align the zero point with the center line of the patient's head, level with the middle of the ear (as shown below).

- Lower the flow chamber to zero, and turn off the stopcock to the dead-end cap. With a clean hand, balance the system according to the monitor's guidelines.
- Turn off the system stopcock to drainage, and raise the flow chamber to the ordered height (as shown below).

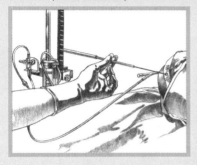

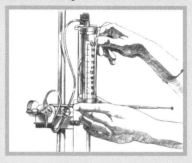

- Return the stopcock to the ordered position, and observe the monitor for the return of ICP patterns.

example, as a complication of cerebral aneurysm rupture.

Procedure

When a ventriculostomy is performed, the physician inserts a small flexible tube into one of the lateral ventricles. The ventriculostomy is then connected as a fluid filled system via a transducer to a monitor. If the ventriculostomy is done for placement of a ventricular drain, the physician inserts a ventricular catheter through a burr hole in the patient's skull. The catheter is then connected to a closed drainage collec-

tion system similar to that for a lumbar drain. (See "Lumbar drain insertion and care," page 319.) After completing the ventriculostomy, the physician will connect the drainage system and suture the catheter in place, covering the insertion site with a sterile dressing.

Complications

Complications of ventriculostomy may include:

- infection
- bleeding
- catheter malfunction.

Nursing considerations

Before ventriculostomy

■ Explain the procedure to the patient and his family.

■ Make sure that the patient or a responsible family member has signed a consent form, and document according to your facility's policy.

■ Perform a baseline neurologic assessment, including vital signs, to help detect alterations or signs of deterioration.

After ventriculostomy

■ Set up a ventriculostomy ICP monitoring system if ordered, and obtain pressures as indicated. (See *Ventriculostomy intracranial pressure monitoring,* pages 348 and 349, and "Intracranial pressure monitoring," page 312.)

■ Assess the patient's vital signs, respiratory status, and neurologic status at least every 15 minutes initially and then less frequently as the patient's condition stabilizes.

■ Maintain a continuous hourly output of CSF. Make sure that the flow chamber of the ICP monitoring setup remains positioned as ordered.

■ To drain CSF as ordered, put on gloves, and then turn on the main stopcock to drainage. This allows CSF to collect in the graduated flow chamber. Document the time and the amount of CSF obtained. Then turn off the stopcock to drainage. To drain the CSF from this chamber into the drainage bag, release the clamp below the flow chamber. Never empty the drainage bag. Instead, replace it when full using sterile technique.

■ Check the dressing for drainage (which could indicate CSF leakage) at least every hour initially and then less frequently as the patient's condition stabilizes.

■ Check the tubing for patency by watching the CSF drops in the drip chamber.

■ Observe the CSF for color, clarity, amount, blood, and sediment. CSF specimens for laboratory analysis should be obtained from the collection port attached to the tubing, not from the collection bag.

■ Change the collection bag when it's full or every 24 hours according to your facility's policy.

4 Gastrointestinal system challenges

Imagine you have a patient who presents with severe abdominal pain. Does this pain signal acute pancreatitis or peritonitis? What assessment information would be important to help determine the cause of the patient's pain? What laboratory test results would you evaluate to support a diagnosis of pancreatitis? Would nasogastric (NG) intubation be necessary? If so, what type of tube would you expect to be inserted? How would you prioritize the patient's care? Would these priorities be different if the patient was diagnosed with peritonitis?

Suppose your patient was to have a colonoscopy at the bedside. How would you prepare the patient for the procedure? Would your preparation be different if the patient had an NG tube inserted and wasn't being given anything orally (nothing by mouth)?

Another patient has hematemesis. What would you do first? Would your interventions be different if the patient had underlying hepatic disease and portal hypertension? Suppose the patient had bleeding esophageal varices and was scheduled for a transjugular intrahepatic portosystemic shunt procedure. Would you know how to prepare the patient, and how to care for him after the procedure? If liver transplantation was indicated, would you know how to care for the patient after the surgery?

What if another patient was receiving total parenteral nutrition? Could you administer the solutions correctly? What laboratory tests would you monitor? Would you know how to identify an occluded central venous catheter — and then clear it?

In this chapter, you'll find the answers to these questions, along with other information that will enable you to address the major challenges involving the GI system commonly encountered in the critical care area.

 MULTISYSTEM DISORDER

Acute GI bleeding

GI bleeding can occur anywhere in the GI tract. Upper GI bleeding occurs above the ligament of Treitz (where the duodenum meets the jejunum), and includes bleeding in the esophagus, stomach, and duodenum. Most commonly, upper GI bleeding results from peptic ulcer disease. Other common disorders associated with upper GI bleeding include:

- rupture of esophageal varices (see "Esophageal varices," page 376)
- esophagitis and esophageal ulcers
- Mallory-Weiss syndrome
- erosive gastritis
- angiodysplasias
- arteriovenous malformations.

Bleeding below the Treitz ligament is considered lower GI bleeding. The most common site of lower GI bleeding is the colon. Common causes include diverticulitis, inflammatory bowel disease, polyps, neoplasms, and arteriovenous malformations.

Although GI bleeding ceases spontaneously in most patients, acute GI bleeding accounts for significant morbidity and mortality. The incidence of upper GI bleeding is greater (100 patients per 100,000 adults) than that for lower GI bleeding (20 patients per 100,000 adults). On the average, just under one-fourth of the patients who develop upper GI bleeding are already hospitalized with another condition, whereas approximately 5% of those who develop lower GI bleeding are already hospitalized.

AGE ISSUE *In the older adult population, upper and lower GI bleeding are common. Incidence of upper GI bleeding increases 20% to 30% between ages 30 and 90. For lower GI bleeding, this increase is substantially more dramatic, increasing more than 200% during the same age span.*

Most patients requiring care in the critical care unit are experiencing upper GI bleeding. Additionally, the patient in the critical care unit commonly has underlying comorbidities that contribute to the risk of upper GI bleeding, such as:

■ coronary artery disease
■ history of myocardial infarction
■ renal failure
■ history of chronic liver damage secondary to alcohol abuse or hepatitis
■ history of radiation therapy
■ chronic pain condition (such as arthritis) requiring treatment with nonsteroidal anti-inflammatory drugs.

Pathophysiology

The patient experiences a loss of circulating blood volume regardless of the underlying cause of bleeding. The extensive arterial blood supply near the stomach and esophagus can lead to a rapid loss of large amounts of blood, subsequent hypovolemia, and shock.

Loss of circulating blood volume leads to a decrease in venous return. Subsequently, cardiac output (CO) and blood pressure decrease, resulting in inadequate tissue perfusion. In response, the body attempts to compensate by shifting interstitial fluids to the intravascular space. The sympathetic nervous system is stimulated, resulting in vasoconstriction and an increase in heart rate. Additionally, the renin-angiotensin-aldosterone system is activated, causing increased secretion of antidiuretic hormone, thereby leading to fluid retention.

These compensatory mechanisms together lead to an increase in blood pressure. However, if blood loss continues, these compensatory mechanisms ultimately fail; CO continues to decrease, leading to cellular hypoxia and a shift from aerobic to anaerobic metabolism with the subsequent buildup of lactic acid, causing metabolic acidosis. Eventually, all organs experience hypoperfusion and fail.

Comprehensive assessment

Because GI bleeding can occur anywhere along the GI tract, assessment of the patient with acute GI bleeding is crucial to determining the amount of bleeding and possible location. For example, bright red blood in nasogastric (NG) tube drainage or vomitus (hematemesis) typically indicates an upper GI source. However, if the blood has spent time in the stomach, where it was exposed to gastric acid, the drainage or vomitus looks like coffee grounds. Hematochezia, bright red blood from the rectum, typically indicates a lower GI source of bleeding. However, it may also suggest an upper GI source if the transit time through the bowel has been rapid. Melena — black, tarry, sticky stools — usually indicates an upper GI bleeding source. However, it can also result from bleeding in the small bowel or proximal colon.

In addition, the extent of blood loss, the rate of bleeding, and the patient's status before the bleeding influence the assessment findings. For example, a patient with underlying cardiac disease may develop angina following an acute GI bleeding episode. With severe GI bleeding, heart failure or diabetes may be aggravated. A patient with chronic GI bleeding may exhibit anemia or orthostatic blood pressure changes.

Typically, a patient exhibits signs and symptoms based on the amount and rate of bleeding. (See *Assessment findings related to blood loss*.) An acute GI bleeding episode is typically characterized by the loss of at least 25% to 30% of the person's blood volume (approximately 1500 ml). Usually, hematemesis is a primary clue. Additionally, with acute upper GI bleeding, the patient exhibits signs and symptoms of hypovolemic shock, including:

■ cool, clammy skin
■ pallor
■ restlessness, apprehension
■ tachycardia
■ diaphoresis
■ hypotension
■ syncope.

Assessment findings related to blood loss

Amount of blood lost (percentage of total blood volume)	Assessment findings
500 to 750 ml (10% to 15%)	● None; asymptomatic
750 to 1200 ml (15% to 25%)	● Anxiety, restlessness ● Tachycardia, hypotension ● Tachypnea ● Normal urine output
1200 to 1500 ml (25% to 35%)	● Anxiety, restlessness, agitation ● Tachycardia ● Tachypnea ● Orthostatic hypotension ● Reduction in urine output
1500 to 2000 ml (35% to 50%)	● Anxiety, agitation, confusion; continued deterioration with continued blood loss ● Tachycardia ● Tachypnea ● Hypotension with systolic blood pressure less than 60 mm Hg ● Oliguria ● Diaphoresis ● Cool, clammy skin ● Pallor

Diagnosis

■ Upper GI endoscopy reveals the source of the bleeding such as ulcer.
■ Complete blood count may reveal a decrease in hemoglobin level and

hematocrit (usually 6 to 8 hours after the initial symptoms), revealing the amount of blood lost (hematocrit may be normal initially, but then drops dramatically); increased reticulocyte and platelet levels; decreased red blood cell (RBC) count.

- Arterial blood gas (ABG) studies reveal low pH and bicarbonate levels, indicating lactic acidosis from massive hemorrhage and possible hypoxemia.
- A 12-lead electrocardiogram may reveal evidence of cardiac ischemia secondary to hypoperfusion.
- Abdominal X-ray may indicate air under the diaphragm, suggesting ulcer perforation.
- Angiography may aid in visualizing the site of bleeding, if it's from an artery or large vein.

Collaborations

Acute GI bleeding is a multisystem problem that requires a multidisciplinary approach to care. Medical and nursing care focus on maintaining all body functions. Respiratory therapy may be necessary to ensure a patent airway and improve respiratory functioning. Nutritional support is indicated to ensure that the patient gets adequate nutrients for maximum tissue healing. Enteral or parenteral nutritional therapy may be necessary. Physical therapy may be involved to help minimize the risks of bed rest. Surgical intervention may be necessary to repair the bleeding source. Social services may be involved to assist with emotional support for the patient and his family and follow-up care issues.

Treatment and care

Treatment focuses on halting the bleeding and providing fluid resuscita-

tion while maintaining the patient's vital functions.

Treatment may also include:
- fluid volume replacement with crystalloid solutions initially, followed by colloids and blood component therapy
- respiratory support as indicated, including supplemental oxygen and, possibly, mechanical ventilation for the patient who experiences respiratory failure
- gastric intubation with gastric lavage (unless the patient has esophageal varices) and gastric pH monitoring
- pharmacologic therapy, such as antacids, histamine-2 receptor antagonists, and other agents, such as sucralfate (Carafate), misoprostol (Cytotec), and omeprazole (Prilosec)
- endoscopic or surgical repair of bleeding sites.

Complications

Potential complications of acute GI bleeding include:
- rebleeding
- aspiration
- respiratory failure
- adult respiratory distress syndrome
- circulatory collapse
- death.

Nursing considerations

- Assess the patient for the extent of blood loss and begin fluid resuscitation as ordered. Obtain a type and crossmatch for blood component therapy.

ALERT *When massive bleeding occurs, lactated Ringer's solution is preferred for fluid volume replacement because its use minimizes the risk of electrolyte imbalances.*

- Ensure a patent airway and assess breathing and circulation. Monitor cardiac and respiratory status closely, at least every 15 minutes — or more frequently, depending on the patient's condition.

■ Administer supplemental oxygen as ordered. Monitor oxygen saturation via continuous pulse oximetry and serial ABG levels for evidence of hypoxemia, and anticipate the need for endotracheal intubation and mechanical ventilation should the patient's respiratory status deteriorate. Place the patient in semi-Fowler's position to maximize chest expansion. Keep the patient as quiet and comfortable as possible to minimize oxygen demands.

■ Monitor vital signs continuously for changes indicating hypovolemic shock. Observe skin color and check capillary refill. Notify the physician if capillary refill is greater than 2 seconds.

■ Assist with insertion of central venous or pulmonary artery catheter to evaluate hemodynamic status. Monitor hemodynamic parameters, including central venous pressure, pulmonary artery wedge pressure, CO, and cardiac index as often as every 15 minutes to evaluate the patient's status and response to treatment.

ALERT *Hemodynamic monitoring is essential in patients over age 50 and in patients with chronic heart, lung, liver, or kidney conditions. Rapid fluid volume replacement can quickly lead to fluid overload, resulting in heart failure and pulmonary edema in any patient, but especially in the older adult or one who has a chronic condition.*

■ Institute continuous cardiac monitoring to evaluate for possible arrhythmias, myocardial ischemia, or adverse effects of treatment.

■ When available, begin blood component therapy as ordered, being sure to warm the blood before transfusing to reduce the risk of hypothermia. Typically, packed RBCs and fresh frozen plasma are used for replacement.

ALERT *If the patient requires large volumes of blood, be alert for changes in calcium levels because calcium binds to the citrate in the stored blood, thereby decreasing the body's free calcium levels. Monitor serum calcium levels, and anticipate replacement if levels are low. Be alert for coagulation problems because transfusions of large amounts of blood can cause coagulopathy.*

■ Assess level of consciousness frequently — approximately every 30 minutes until the patient stabilizes, and then every 2 to 4 hours as indicated by the patient's status.

■ Obtain serial hemoglobin level and hematocrit; notify the physician of hematocrit below prescribed parameter. For every unit of packed RBCs given, the hematocrit typically rises 3%. Expect to administer albumin if the patient has hypoalbuminemia or if the hematocrit fails to stay above 28% even with packed RBC replacement therapy.

■ Monitor intake and output closely, including all losses from the GI tract. Insert an indwelling urinary catheter, and assess urine output hourly. Check stools and gastric drainage for occult blood.

■ Assist with or insert an NG tube, and perform lavage using room temperature saline to clear blood and clots from the stomach. Assess gastric pH every to 2 to 4 hours or continuously if indicated; maintain gastric pH between 4 and 5. Administer pharmacologic agents as prescribed to maintain pH.

ALERT *Gastric pH over 5 indicates excessive alkalinization, placing the patient at increased risk for aspiration pneumonia.*

■ Anticipate the use of parenteral nutrition if the patient is to remain nothing by mouth for several days or weeks. Assess abdomen for bowel sounds. Expect to resume enteral or oral feedings after the patient's bowel function has returned and there's no further evidence of bleeding.

■ As necessary, prepare the patient for endoscopic repair or surgery.

■ Provide emotional support and reassurance appropriately in the wake of massive GI bleeding, which is always a frightening experience.

Patient teaching

■ Review disease course with the patient and his family, including treatments and medications ordered and intended effects, dosage and adverse effects to report. Answer questions honestly and provide information as needed.

■ Teach the patient and his family about the signs and symptoms of actual or impending GI bleeding, such as blood in vomitus or stools, pallor, cool skin, and light-headedness; include instructions to notify the physician should any such signs occur.

■ Provide preoperative teaching as indicated.

 MULTISYSTEM DISORDER

Acute pancreatitis

Pancreatitis — inflammation of the pancreas — occurs in acute and chronic forms and may be due to edema, necrosis, or hemorrhage. In men, this disease is commonly associated with alcoholism, trauma, or peptic ulcer; in women, with biliary tract disease.

Causes of acute pancreatitis may include:
■ biliary tract disease
■ alcoholism
■ abnormal organ structure
■ metabolic or endocrine disorders, such as high cholesterol levels or overactive thyroid
■ pancreatic cysts or tumors
■ penetrating peptic ulcers
■ blunt trauma or surgical trauma
■ drugs, such as glucocorticoids, sulfonamides, thiazides, hormonal contraceptives, and nonsteroidal anti-inflammatory drugs
■ kidney failure or transplantation
■ endoscopic examination of the bile ducts and pancreas.

The prognosis is good in pancreatitis associated with biliary tract disease, but poor when associated with alcoholism. Mortality is as high as 60% when pancreatitis is associated with necrosis and hemorrhage. The severity of pancreatitis is predicted with Ranson's criteria. (See *Ranson's criteria.*) If the patient has fewer than three of these criteria, the mortality rate is less than 1%. When three or four of the criteria are present, the mortality rate increases to 15 to 20%. With five or six criteria, the mortality rate is 40%.

Pathophysiology

Acute pancreatitis occurs in two forms, edematous (interstitial) and necrotizing. Edematous pancreatitis causes fluid accumulation and swelling. Necrotizing pancreatitis causes cell death and tissue damage. The inflammation that occurs with both types is caused by premature activation of enzymes, which causes tissue damage.

Normally, the acini in the pancreas secrete enzymes in an inactive form. Two theories explain why enzymes become prematurely activated. According to one theory, a toxic agent, such as alcohol, alters the way the pancreas secretes enzymes. Alcohol probably increases pancreatic secretion, alters the metabolism of the acinar cells, and encourages duct obstruction by causing pancreatic secretory proteins to precipitate. Another theory is that a reflux of duodenal contents containing activated enzymes enters the pancreatic duct, activating other enzymes and setting up a cycle of more pancreatic damage.

If pancreatitis damages the islets of Langerhans, diabetes mellitus may result. Sudden, severe pancreatitis causes massive hemorrhage and total destruction of the pancreas, manifested as diabetic acidosis, shock, or coma.

Comprehensive assessment

Commonly, the patient describes intense epigastric pain centered close to the umbilicus and radiating to the back, between the 10th thoracic and 6th lumbar vertebrae. He typically reports that this pain is aggravated by eating fatty foods, consuming alcohol, or lying in a recumbent position. The pain is caused by the escape of inflammatory exudate and enzymes into the back of the peritoneum, edema and

Ranson's criteria

The severity of the patient's acute pancreatitis is determined by the existence of certain characteristics. The greater the number of criteria met by the patient, the more severe the episode of pancreatitis, and the greater the risk of mortality.

Admission criteria
- Age over 55
- White blood cell count greater than 16,000/mm^3
- Serum glucose greater than 200 mg/dl
- Lactate dehydrogenase greater than 350 IU/L
- Aspartate aminotransferase greater than 250 U/L

During initial 48 hours after admission
- 10% decrease in hematocrit
- Greater than 5 mg/dl increase in blood urea nitrogen
- Serum calcium less than 8 mg/dl
- Base deficit greater than 4 mEq/L
- Partial pressure of arterial oxygen less than 60 mm Hg
- Estimated fluid sequestration greater than 6 L

distention of the pancreatic capsule, and obstruction of the biliary tract. The patient may also complain of weight loss, with nausea and vomiting.

Investigation may uncover predisposing factors, such as alcoholism, biliary tract disease, or pancreatic disease. Other medical problems, such as peptic ulcer disease or hyperlipidemia, may also be discovered.

Upon physical examination, the following may be noted:
■ persistent vomiting (in a severe attack) from hypermotility or paralytic

ileus secondary to pancreatitis or peritonitis
■ abdominal distention (in a severe attack) from bowel hypermotility and the accumulation of fluids in the abdominal cavity
■ diminished bowel activity (in severe attack) suggesting altered motility secondary to peritonitis
■ crackles at lung bases (in a severe attack) secondary to heart failure
■ left pleural effusion (in a severe attack) from circulating pancreatic enzymes
■ mottled skin from hemorrhagic necrosis of the pancreas
■ tachycardia secondary to dehydration and possible hypovolemia
■ low-grade fever resulting from the inflammatory response
■ cold, sweaty extremities secondary to cardiovascular collapse
■ restlessness related to pain associated with acute pancreatitis
■ decreased pulmonary artery pressure and decreased cardiac output (CO) due to hemorrhage or dehydration
■ elevated CO and decreased systemic vascular resistance, in the presence of systemic inflammation or sepsis.

Diagnosis

■ Serum amylase levels are usually elevated approximately 3 to 5 times normal initially, and then decrease as healing advances.
■ Serum lipase levels, which are more specific for pancreatitis, are usually elevated 3 to 5 times the normal range for approximately 2 weeks; when viewed with serum amylase levels, these confirm the diagnosis.
■ Urine amylase level is increased for approximately 1 to 2 weeks.

■ Blood and urine glucose tests reveal transient glucose in urine and hyperglycemia (levels commonly greater than 200 mg/dl).
■ White blood cell count is elevated, ranging from 11,000 to 20,000 /mm^3, which reflects the inflammatory process; hemoglobin levels and hematocrit are decreased with hemorrhage and increased with dehydration.
■ Serum bilirubin levels are elevated.
■ Blood calcium levels may be decreased, possibly less than 8 mg/dl.
■ Coagulation studies reveal a decrease in platelets and fibrinogen.
■ Abdominal and chest X-rays detect pleural effusions and differentiate pancreatitis from diseases that cause similar symptoms; may detect pancreatic calculi; abdominal X-ray may reveal bowel dilation and ileus.
■ Computed tomography scan and ultrasonography show enlarged pancreas with fluid collections, cysts, abscesses, masses, and pseudocysts.
■ Endoscopic pancreatography identifies swelling, ductal system abnormalities, such as calcification or strictures, or evidence of stones or tumors; helps differentiate pancreatitis from other disorders such as pancreatic cancer.
■ Arterial blood gas (ABG) studies may reveal decreased partial pressure of arterial oxygen (Pao$_2$), mild respiratory alkalosis, and decreased oxygen saturation levels.
■ Electrocardiogram (ECG) may reveal S-T segment depression and T-wave inversion from coronary artery spasm (secondary to severe pain).

Collaborations

Multidisciplinary care is essential for the patient with acute pancreatitis. Medical and nursing care focus on maintaining circulation, relieving pain, and decreasing pancreatic secretions. Respiratory therapy may be included to help ensure a patent airway and improve respiratory functioning. Nutritional support is indicated to assist with tissue healing and maintain a positive nitrogen balance. A pain management team may be called upon to assist with pain management. Surgical intervention may be necessary if the patient has a biliary obstruction causing the acute pancreatitis or develops complications, such as an abscess or pseudocyst. Social services may be involved to assist with emotional support for the patient and his family and follow-up care issues.

Treatment and care

Treatment of acute pancreatitis may include:
■ I.V. replacement of fluids, protein, and electrolytes to treat shock
■ fluid volume replacement to help correct metabolic acidosis
■ blood transfusions to replace blood loss from hemorrhage
■ withholding of food and fluids to rest the pancreas and reduce pancreatic enzyme secretion
■ nasogastric (NG) tube suctioning to decrease stomach distention and suppress pancreatic secretions
■ meperidine or other analgesic to relieve abdominal pain
■ antacids to neutralize gastric secretions
■ histamine-2 (H_2) receptor antagonists to decrease hydrochloric acid production
■ antibiotics to fight bacterial infections

■ anticholinergics to reduce vagal stimulation, decrease GI motility, and inhibit pancreatic enzyme secretion
■ insulin to correct hyperglycemia
■ peritoneal lavage to remove toxins in peritoneal exudate
■ surgical drainage for a pancreatic abscess or a pseudocyst
■ laparotomy (if biliary tract obstruction causes acute pancreatitis) to remove obstruction.

Complications

Acute pancreatitis may lead to the following complications:
■ massive hemorrhage and hypovolemic shock
■ pancreatic fistula
■ pancreatic abscess
■ pancreatic pseudocyst
■ primary infections
■ secondary infections
■ pulmonary complications
■ disseminated intravascular coagulation. (See *Complications of acute pancreatitis,* page 360.)

Nursing considerations

■ Ensure a patent airway, and assess the patient's respiratory status at least every hour or more frequently as indicated by the patient's condition. Note respiratory rate, rhythm, and depth, reporting any dyspnea and accessory muscle use. Be alert for inspiratory retractions.
■ Auscultate lungs bilaterally for adventitious or diminished breath sounds.
■ Assess oxygen saturation continuously via pulse oximetry or mixed venous oxygen saturation via pulmonary artery (PA) catheter if in place. Monitor serial ABG levels; document and report changes in arterial oxygen satu-

Complications of acute pancreatitis

Complication	Pathophysiologic mechanism
Massive hemorrhage and hypovolemic shock	• Pancreatic tissue undergoes necrosis, which leads to rupture and hemorrhage. • Large amounts of fluid shift from the intravascular space to peritoneal and interstitial spaces. • Additional fluid loss may occur due to vomiting, diarrhea, hemorrhage, and nasogastric suction. • Third-space fluid shifting may occur due to hypoalbuminemia.
Pancreatic fistula	• Pancreatic enzymes disrupt a pancreatic duct exiting the pancreatic parenchyma, allowing pancreatic juice to pass and enter the peritoneal or retroperitoneal cavities, or remain within the pancreas.
Pancreatic abscess	• Pancreatic enzymes cause tissue necrosis with the collection of purulent material within the pancreas; this material can erode through the retroperitoneum into the bowel, pleural space, mediastinum, or pelvis, subsequently leading to sepsis.
Pancreatic pseudocyst	• Pancreatic enzymes cause the collection of pancreatic juices that become surrounded by a wall of fibrous granulation tissue; although these pseudocysts are usually sterile, they're treated as abscesses if infection occurs.
Primary infections	• Necrosed pancreatic tissue or the tissue surrounding the necrosed pancreas becomes infected.
Secondary infections	• Microorganisms—typically from other body areas, most commonly the colon—move to the necrosed pancreas.
Pulmonary complications	• Severe pain interferes with adequate lung expansion. • Pancreatic enzymes released into the circulation damage the pulmonary vessels, stimulate inflammation, and cause alveolocapillary leakage that results in intrapulmonary shunting and hypoxemia. • Movement of exudate across the diaphragm via the lymphatic system leads to subdiaphragmatic inflammation, which in turn leads to pleural effusions, atelectasis, and elevation of the diaphragm, further impairing ventilation.
Disseminated intravascular coagulation	• Pancreatic inflammation interferes with vitamin K absorption, leading to a vitamin K deficiency and impaired clotting mechanisms.

ration as well as changes in pH and Pao_2. If the patient's respiratory status deteriorates, assist with endotracheal intubation and mechanical ventilation. (See "Endotracheal intubation," in chapter 2, page 193, and "Mechanical ventilation," in chapter 2, page 213.)

■ Closely monitor the patient's heart rate and blood pressure at least every hour or more frequently as indicated by the patient's condition. Institute continuous cardiac monitoring and observe for arrhythmias that may result from fluid volume deficits, hypoxemia, acid-base disturbances, or electrolyte imbalance. Prepare to treat arrhythmias as ordered.

■ Assess hemodynamic status closely, at least every hour or more frequently, as indicated. Assist with insertion of PA catheter if one isn't in place. Monitor central venous pressure (CVP), pulmonary artery wedge pressure (PAWP), CO, and cardiac index for changes.

ALERT *Keep in mind that patients with acute pancreatitis commonly receive large amounts of fluid replacement therapy. In addition to assessing hemodynamic parameters for changes indicating continuing fluid losses, such as decreasing CVP, PAWP, CO, and a cardiac index less than 3 L/minute/m², be alert for changes suggesting fluid volume overload, such as elevations in CVP and PAWP.*

■ Place the patient in a comfortable position that maximizes air exchange such as semi-Fowler's to high Fowler's position. Use oxygen saturation levels as a guide to the effective position. Reposition the patient often.

■ Allow for periods of rest and activity to prevent fatigue and reduce oxygen demand.

■ If the patient develops adult respiratory distress syndrome, anticipate the need for additional therapies, such as extracorporeal membrane oxygenation or inhaled nitrous oxide, and prepare the patient and his family for these therapies. (See "Adult respiratory distress syndrome," in chapter 2, page 172, and "Extracorporeal membrane oxygenation," in chapter 2, page 205.)

■ Initiate I.V. fluid replacement therapy, including crystalloids and colloids, as ordered. Monitor serum electrolyte levels for changes, and administer replacement electrolytes as ordered.

ALERT *Be especially alert for signs and symptoms of hypokalemia (hypotension, muscle weakness, apathy, confusion, and cardiac arrhythmias), hypomagnesemia (hypotension, tachycardia, confusion, tremors, twitching, tetany, and hallucinations), hypocalcemia (positive Chvostek's and Trousseau's signs, seizures, and prolonged QT interval on ECG). Have emergency equipment readily available.*

■ Monitor intake and output closely. Assess urine output hourly, notifying the physician if the urine output is less than 0.5 ml/kg/hour. Obtain daily weights.

ALERT *When measuring output, be sure to include the drainage from all sources, including dressings that required changing because they became saturated. If necessary, weigh the dressing to determine the amount of fluid lost.*

■ Monitor the patient's level of consciousness (LOC), noting such changes as increasing confusion, lethargy, or mental sluggishness.

■ Maintain the patient in a normothermic state to reduce his body's demand for oxygen, monitor for fever, and inspect invasive access sites for signs and symptoms of infection. Use strict sterile technique when caring for these sites.

■ Assess the patient's level of pain and administer analgesics as a continuous infusion or intermittently as ordered.

ALERT *If the patient is alert and can participate in care, patient-controlled analgesia may be useful in controlling his pain. If his level of pain is severe and I.V. administered analgesics are ineffective, anticipate the insertion of an epidural catheter for analgesia.*

■ Institute nonpharmacologic pain methods as appropriate.

■ Provide emotional support to help alleviate the patient's, and his family's, anxiety.

■ Administer I.V. antibiotics as ordered; monitor serum peak and trough levels as appropriate.

ALERT *Aminoglycosides are commonly used to treat pancreatitis. Therefore, monitor the patient closely for signs and symptoms of ototoxicity and nephrotoxicity. Watch for complaints of tinnitus, dizziness, or vertigo, and monitor serum blood urea nitrogen and creatinine levels.*

■ Withhold oral fluids and food to prevent stimulation of pancreatic enzymes. Insert an NG tube (if not in place) as ordered, and connect to low intermittent suction. Check placement of the tube at least every 4 hours; irrigate the tube with normal saline as ordered to maintain patency.

■ Monitor any vomitus, stools, and drainage from the NG tube for frank bleeding, and test for occult blood at least every 4 hours until the patient's condition stabilizes, and then every 8 hours. Remember that the stools of a patient with pancreatitis are typically fatty and foul smelling due to pancreatic insufficiency and reduced release of lipase from the damaged pancreas.

■ Administer H_2-receptor antagonists, anticholinergic agents, and antacids as ordered; test gastric drainage for pH.

ALERT *Activity can stimulate gastric secretions, thereby increasing gastric pH. The goal is to maintain gastric pH above 5. Therefore, limit the patient's activity during the initial acute phase to minimize this risk. In addition, be prepared to adjust the medication regimen as ordered based on the patient's pH level.*

■ Assess the patient's abdomen for distention and evidence of bowel sounds, measure abdominal girth, and evaluate his present nutritional status and metabolic requirements.

■ Administer parenteral nutritional therapy as ordered during the acute phase of the disease. Monitor finger-stick blood glucose levels for hyperglycemia, and notify the physician about blood glucose levels greater than 200 mg/dl. Assess the patient for signs and symptoms of hyperglycemia, such as Kussmaul's respirations, fruity acetone breath, flushed, dry skin, and decreasing LOC. Administer insulin as ordered.

■ When bowel sounds become active, anticipate a switch to enteral or oral feedings as ordered. When beginning oral feedings, provide low-fat food choices.

■ Perform passive range-of-motion exercises to maintain joint mobility. If possible, help the patient perform active exercises. Monitor oxygen saturation levels throughout any activity for changes indicating deterioration in the patient's condition.

■ Provide meticulous skin care. To prevent skin breakdown, reposition the patient frequently.

■ Provide emotional support. Answer the patient's, and his family's, questions as fully as possible to allay their fears and concerns.

■ Prepare the patient for surgery as indicated.

Patient teaching

■ Explain the disorder to the patient and his family. Explain the signs and symptoms that may occur and review the treatments that may be required.

■ Orient the patient and his family to the unit and surroundings. Provide them with simple explanations and demonstrations of treatments and procedures. Involve the patient and his family in care as much as reasonably possible.

■ If the patient is receiving mechanical ventilation, explain why he can't speak. Suggest an alternative means of communication.

■ Inform the patient that recovery may take some time and that weakness may be present for a while. Urge him to share his concerns with the staff.

■ Teach the patient and his family about signs and symptoms to report immediately.

Endoscopy, lower GI

Endoscopy refers to the visualization of the mucosa via an endoscope. Three different types of endoscopy may be used to visualize the lower GI tract. These include a proctosigmoidoscopy, sigmoidoscopy, and colonoscopy. With these procedures, various sections of the lower portion of the colon can be viewed directly by using a rigid or flexible endoscope to evaluate bleeding, acute or chronic diarrhea, or changes in bowel habits. (See *Comparing flexible sigmoidoscopy and colonoscopy,* page 364.)

Currently, flexible fiber-optic scopes are used most often because they permit a larger area for examination — 16″ to 20″ (40.5 to 50.5 cm) from the anus — as compared to the rigid scopes which permit visualization of up to 10″ (25 cm) from the rectum.

Lower GI endoscopy is indicated for the following:

■ aid in diagnosis of inflammatory, infectious, and ulcerative bowel disease

■ diagnosis of malignant and benign neoplasms

■ detection of hemorrhoids, hypertrophic anal papilla, polyps, fissures, fistulas, and abscesses in the rectum and anal canal

■ location of the site of lower GI bleeding (colonoscopy)

■ evaluation of the colon postoperatively for recurrence of polyps or malignant lesions.

A proctosigmoidoscopic examination is a key cancer-prevention screening technique.

■ **AGE ISSUE** *Lower GI endoscopy is recommended routinely every 3 to 5 years for males and females over age 50.*

Procedure

For a proctosigmoidoscopy or sigmoidoscopy with a rigid scope, the patient is placed in the knee-chest position. If a flexible scope is used, the patient is placed in the left lateral position. The anus and rectum are examined digitally with a lubricated gloved finger. Upon withdrawing the gloved finger

Comparing flexible sigmoidoscopy and colonoscopy

The illustrations below depict the areas of the colon that are examined when a flexible sigmoidoscopy is performed and when a flexible colonoscopy is performed.

Flexible sigmoidoscopy
A flexible sigmoidoscopy allows visualization of the areas from the anus and rectum past the proximal sigmoid colon to the descending colon.

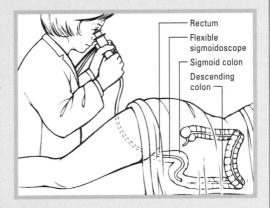

Rectum
Flexible sigmoidoscope
Sigmoid colon
Descending colon

Colonoscopy
A fiber-optic colonoscopy allows visualization of the entire large colon, from the anus and rectum through the sigmoid and into the descending, transverse, and ascending colon.

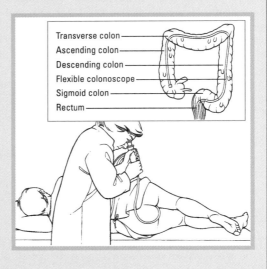

Transverse colon
Ascending colon
Descending colon
Flexible colonoscope
Sigmoid colon
Rectum

from the rectum, the physician examines the finger for mucus, blood, and fecal matter. Next, the physician inserts the proctoscope or sigmoidoscope into the anus and advances it to the rectum. Air may be instilled to open the bowel lumen and to aid visualization. As the scope is withdrawn, the mucosa is examined and specimens may be obtained for analysis.

For a colonoscopy, the patient typically receives conscious sedation and is placed in the left lateral or Sims' position with the knees drawn up close to the chest. The lubricated colonoscope is then inserted approximately 4¾" (12 cm) into the colon. Air may be introduced to help with visualization. The colonoscope is advanced through the colon with the patient being repositioned as necessary to aid in the passage of the scope and visualization. As the colonoscope is withdrawn, examination continues. Any specimens obtained are sent to the laboratory for immediate analysis.

Complications

Complications of lower GI endoscopy may include:
■ perforation
■ bleeding
■ cardiac arrhythmias (due to vagal stimulation)
■ hypotension (with colonoscopy secondary to overhydration or underhydration resulting from bowel preparation)
■ respiratory depression (with colonoscopy secondary to oversedation in conjunction with vagal stimulation from instrumentation).

Nursing considerations

Before lower GI endoscopy
■ Explain the purpose and procedure, including any sensations that the patient may experience.
■ Ensure that the patient or a family member has signed the consent form.
■ If possible, discontinue medications such as nonsteroidal anti-inflammatory drugs, aspirin, ticlopidine, and pentoxyfylline approximately 1 week before the test and for 2 weeks after the

procedure; discontinue iron therapy approximately 3 to 4 days before the test if possible.
■ Withhold food and fluids for approximately 6 to 8 hours before the test.
■ Administer bowel preparation as ordered. For example, Fleet enema the morning of a proctosigmoidoscopy; Fleet or tap water enemas 1 to 2 hours before sigmoidoscopy; and clear liquid diet and bowel cleansing with electrolyte lavage solution before a colonoscopy. If the patient can't swallow or is unconscious, administer electrolyte lavage solution via feeding or nasogastric (NG) tube.

ALERT *To minimize the risk of aspiration or regurgitation in patients receiving electrolyte lavage solution via NG tube, ensure proper tube placement and elevate the head of the bed or position the patient on his side and have suction equipment readily available.*

AGE ISSUE *Keep in mind that elderly patients may have difficulty ingesting the required amount of lavage solution because the solution can cause nausea, bloating, cramps, and abdominal fullness. In addition, these patients are at greater risk for fluid and electrolyte imbalances.*

■ Advise the patient that he may feel the urge to defecate when the scope is inserted; encourage slow, deep breathing through the mouth as appropriate.
■ Have necessary equipment readily available at the bedside if the procedure will be performed there.
■ Initiate an I.V. line if one isn't in place for the colonoscopy patient who'll be receiving conscious sedation.
■ Obtain baseline vital signs and oxygen saturation levels; have supplemen-

tal oxygen and emergency resuscitative equipment readily available.

■ Administer medications as ordered such as midazolam for sedation (for the patient undergoing a colonoscopy).

■ Be prepared to monitor the patient throughout the procedure, including vital signs, cardiac rate and rhythm, airway patency, abdominal distention, level of consciousness (LOC), pain tolerance, and skin color, temperature, and dryness.

After lower GI endoscopy

■ Assess the patient after a proctosigmoidoscopy or sigmoidoscopy for rectal bleeding and signs of possible perforation, such as fever, rectal drainage, abdominal distention and pain. If air was instilled, advise the patient that he may pass large amounts of flatus.

■ If the patient was placed in the knee-chest position, have the patient lie in a supine position for several minutes before sitting or standing up to reduce the risk of orthostatic hypotension.

■ Following a colonoscopy, assess vital signs and cardiopulmonary status including heart rate and rhythm, respiratory rate, breath sounds, oxygen saturation, and LOC every 15 minutes for the first hour then every 30 minutes for the next hour, then hourly until the patient stabilizes. Report hypotension or bradycardia.

■ Administer supplemental oxygen as ordered and as indicated by oxygen saturation levels.

■ Observe for adverse effects of sedation, such as respiratory depression, apnea, hypotension, excessive diaphoresis, bradycardia, and laryngospasm. Notify physician if such effects occur.

■ Assess stools for evidence of frank or occult bleeding.

■ Monitor for signs and symptoms of perforation, such as vomiting, severe abdominal pain, abdominal distention or rigidity, or fever. Immediately notify the physician if such signs occur.

Endoscopy, upper GI

The most common endoscopy used for visualizing the upper GI tract is the esophagogastroduodenoscopy (EGD). With this procedure, the lining of the esophagus, stomach, and upper duodenum are examined using a flexible fiber-optic or video endoscope. EGD is indicated for patients with GI bleeding, hematemesis, melena, substernal or epigastric pain, gastroesophageal reflux disease (GERD), dysphagia, anemia, strictures, or peptic ulcer disease. It may also be indicated for patients requiring foreign body retrieval and for postoperative patients with recurrent or new symptoms.

EGD eliminates the need for extensive exploratory surgery and can be used to detect small or surface lesions missed by radiography. Because the scope provides a channel for biopsy forceps or a cytology brush, it permits laboratory evaluation of abnormalities detected by radiography. Similarly, it allows removal of foreign bodies by suction (for small, soft objects) or by electrocautery snare of forceps (for large, hard objects).

Procedure

After receiving premedication, the patient's mouth and throat are sprayed with a local anesthetic, and he's placed in a left lateral position with head bent forward and mouth opened. The examiner guides the tip of the endoscope to the back of the patient's throat and downward. As the endoscope passes through the posterior pharynx and the cricopharyngeal sphincter, the patient's neck is slowly extended. When the endoscope is well into the esophagus (about 12″ [30 cm]), the patient's head is positioned with his chin toward the table so that saliva can drain out of his mouth.

After examination of the esophagus and the cardiac sphincter, the endoscope is advanced to allow examination of the stomach and duodenum. During the examination, air or water may be introduced through the endoscope to distend the area being examined. Suction may be applied to remove insufflated air and secretions. A measuring tube may be passed through the endoscope to determine a lesion's size. Biopsy forceps or a cytology brush may be passed through the scope to obtain specimens for histologic or cytologic study. A laser, a cauterizing device, or a sclerosing agent may be used to treat areas of bleeding or polyps.

The endoscope is slowly withdrawn, and suspicious-looking areas of the gastric and esophageal lining are reexamined. Specimens obtained are sent to the laboratory for immediate analysis.

Complications

Although rare, complications can occur with upper GI endoscopy. Observe the patient for possible perforation.

■ Perforation in the cervical area of the esophagus produces pain on swallowing and with neck movement.

■ Thoracic perforation causes substernal or epigastric pain that increases with breathing or movement of the trunk.

■ Diaphragmatic perforation produces shoulder pain and dyspnea.

■ Gastric perforation causes abdominal or back pain, cyanosis, fever, and pleural effusion.

Other complications of upper GI endoscopy may include:

■ bleeding or hemorrhage

■ local irritation (complaints of sore throat)

■ drug reactions, including possible adverse reactions to sedation

■ aspiration.

Nursing considerations

Before upper GI endoscopy

■ Explain the purpose and procedure, including sensations that the patient may experience.

■ Ensure that the patient or family member has signed an informed consent.

■ Withhold food and fluids for approximately 6 to 8 hours before the test.

ALERT *If the EGD is being done as an emergency, expect to insert a nasogastric tube to aspirate contents and minimize the risk of aspiration.*

■ Have necessary equipment readily available at the bedside if the procedure will be performed there.

■ Initiate an I.V. line if one isn't in place for conscious sedation.

■ Remove the patient's dentures and eyeglasses before the exam.
■ Obtain baseline vital signs and oxygen saturation levels; have supplemental oxygen and emergency resuscitative equipment readily available.
■ Administer medications as ordered, such as local anesthetic, sedation (for example, midazolam), and atropine (to reduce secretions).
■ Be prepared to monitor the patient throughout the procedure, including vital signs, cardiac rate and rhythm, airway patency, abdominal distention, level of consciousness (LOC), pain tolerance, and skin color, temperature, and dryness.

After upper GI endoscopy
■ Assess vital signs and cardiopulmonary status, including heart rate and rhythm, respiratory rate, breath sounds, oxygen saturation, and LOC every 15 minutes for the first hour, every 30 minutes for the next hour, and then hourly until the patient stabilizes.
■ Administer supplemental oxygen as ordered and as indicated by oxygen saturation levels.
■ Place the patient in the side-lying position with the head of the bed flat until sedation has worn off.
■ Check for gag reflex. Withhold food and fluids until gag reflex returns. When gag reflex returns, offer ice chips and sips of water, gradually increasing the patient's intake as tolerated and as allowed.
■ Observe for adverse effects of sedation, such as respiratory depression, apnea, hypotension, excessive diaphoresis, bradycardia, and laryngospasm. Notify the physician if such effects occur.

■ Monitor for signs and symptoms of perforation, such as unusual difficulty swallowing, pain, fever, or bleeding as evidenced by black stools or bloody vomitus.
■ Provide lozenges, saline gargles, or oral analgesics (if allowed) to help relieve complaints of sore throat after the gag reflex has returned.

Enteral nutrition

Enteral nutrition, also called tube feeding, involves delivery of a liquid feeding formula directly to the stomach (known as gastric gavage), duodenum, or jejunum. Gastric gavage is typically indicated for a patient who can't eat normally because of dysphagia or oral or esophageal obstruction or injury. Gastric feedings may also be given to a patient who's unconscious, intubated, or recovering from GI tract surgery and can't ingest food orally.

Duodenal or jejunal feedings decrease the risk of aspiration because the formula bypasses the pylorus. Jejunal feedings result in reduced pancreatic stimulation; thus, the patient may require an elemental diet.

Enteral nutrition can be administered on an intermittent schedule or as a continuous slow infusion. Liquid nutrient solutions come in various formulas for administration through a nasogastric (NG) tube, small-bore feeding tube, gastrostomy or jejunostomy tube, percutaneous endoscopic gastrostomy or jejunostomy tube, or gastrostomy feeding button. Tube feeding is contraindicated in patients who have no bowel sounds or a suspected intestinal obstruction.

Equipment

For gastric feedings

Feeding formula ▪ graduated container ▪ 120 ml of water ▪ gavage bag with tubing and flow regulator clamp ▪ towel or linen-saver pad ▪ 60-ml syringe ▪ stethoscope ▪ optional: infusion controller and tubing set (for continuous administration), adapter to connect gavage tubing to feeding tube

For duodenal or jejunal feedings

Feeding formula ▪ enteral administration set containing a gavage container, drip chamber, roller clamp or flow regulator, and tube connector ▪ I.V. pole ▪ 60-ml syringe with adapter hub ▪ water ▪ optional: pump administration set (for an enteral infusion pump), Y-connector

For nasal and oral care

Cotton-tipped applicators ▪ water-soluble lubricant ▪ sponge-tipped swabs ▪ petroleum jelly

Essential steps

▪ Obtain the necessary formula, checking the expiration date on the container.

▪ Allow the formula to warm to room temperature before administration.

ALERT *Never warm formula over direct heat or in a microwave because heat may curdle the formula or change its chemical composition. Hot formula may injure the patient. Never administer formula directly after removal from the refrigerator because cold formula can increase the chance of diarrhea.*

▪ Pour 60 ml of water into the graduated container.

▪ Close the flow clamp on the administration set, pour the appropriate

amount of formula into the gavage bag. Hang no more than a 6-hour supply at one time to prevent bacterial growth.

▪ Open the flow clamp on the administration set to remove air from the lines. This keeps air from entering the patient's stomach and causing distention and discomfort. If using an infusion pump or controller, thread the tubing from the formula through the controller or pump according to the manufacturer's directions, and purge the tubing of air.

▪ Provide privacy and wash your hands. Inform the patient that he'll receive nourishment through the tube, and explain the procedure to him. If possible, give him a schedule of subsequent feedings, or explain that the feedings will be continuous.

▪ If the patient has a nasal or oral tube, cover his chest with a towel or linen-saver pad to protect him and the bed linens from spills.

▪ Assess the patient's abdomen for bowel sounds and distention.

▪ When delivering a feeding, elevate the bed to semi-Fowler's or high Fowler's position to prevent aspiration by gastroesophageal reflux and to promote digestion.

▪ Check placement of the feeding tube to ensure it hasn't slipped out since the last feeding.

ALERT *Never give a tube feeding until you're sure the tube is properly positioned in the patient's stomach. Administering a feeding through a misplaced tube can lead to aspiration.*

▪ To check NG tube patency and position, remove the cap or plug from the feeding tube and use the syringe to aspirate gastric contents. Check the aspirate's pH, which should be less than 5. Additionally, inject 5 to 10 cc of air through the tube. At the same time, auscultate the patient's stomach with the stethoscope. Listen for a whooshing sound to confirm tube positioning in the stomach. Measure the length of a nasoduodenal tube to check for tube placement.

■ To assess gastric emptying, aspirate and measure residual gastric contents. Hold feedings if residual volume is greater then the predetermined amount specified in the physician's order (usually 50 to 100 ml). Reinstill any aspirate obtained. Remember that you may not get any residual when you aspirate a nasoduodenal tube.

■ Connect the formula tubing to the feeding tube, using an adapter if necessary. Substitute a bulb syringe or large catheter-tip syringe for a gavage bag after the patient demonstrates tolerance for a gravity drip infusion as appropriate. Use an infusion pump as necessary to ensure accurate delivery of the prescribed formula.

■ If using a bulb or catheter-tip syringe, remove the bulb or plunger and attach the syringe to the pinched-off feeding tube to prevent excess air from entering the patient's stomach, causing distention.

■ Open the regulator clamp on the formula tubing, and adjust the flow rate appropriately, or turn on the pump or controller if used. When using a bulb syringe, fill the syringe with formula, and release the feeding tube to allow formula to flow through it. The height at which you hold the syringe will determine the flow rate. When the syringe is three-quarters empty, pour more formula into it.

■ Always administer a tube feeding slowly — typically 200 to 350 ml over 15 to 30 minutes, depending on the patient's tolerance and the physician's order — to prevent sudden stomach distention, which can cause nausea, vomiting, cramps, or diarrhea. Most patients receive small amounts initially, with volumes increasing gradually after tolerance is established.

ALERT *To prevent air from entering the tube and the patient's stomach, never allow the syringe or formula bag to empty completely. If you're using an infusion pump or controller, set the flow rate according to the manufacturer's directions.*

■ After administering the appropriate amount of formula, flush the tubing by adding about 60 ml of water to the gavage bag or bulb syringe, or manually flush it using a barrel syringe. This maintains the tube's patency by removing excess formula, which could occlude the tube.

■ To discontinue an intermittent gastric feeding (depending on the equipment you're using), close the regulator clamp on the gavage bag tubing, disconnect the syringe from the feeding tube, or turn off the infusion controller.

■ Cover the end of the feeding tube with its plug or cap to prevent leakage and contamination of the tube.

■ Leave the patient in semi-Fowler's or high Fowler's position for at least 30 minutes.

■ Rinse all reusable equipment with warm water. Dry it and store it in a convenient place for the next feeding.

ALERT *Be sure to refrigerate formulas prepared in the dietary department or pharmacy. Refrigerate commercial formulas only after open-*

ing them. *When using powdered formula, always shake the container well to mix the solution thoroughly, and use the formula within 24 hours of mixing.*

Complications

Complications associated with enteral nutrition include:

■ erosion of esophageal, tracheal, nasal, and oropharyngeal mucosa if NG or nasoduodenal tubes are left in place for a long time
■ bloating, cramping, distention
■ dehydration
■ diarrhea and vomiting
■ metabolic and fluid and electrolyte imbalances
■ dumping syndrome
■ tube malfunction, such as occlusion or dislodgment
■ aspiration
■ tube exit site infection
■ vitamin and mineral deficiencies. (See *Troubleshooting tube-feeding problems,* page 372.)

Nursing considerations

■ Monitor the flow rate of a continuous feeding hourly to ensure correct infusion.
■ When administering a continuous feeding, flush the feeding tube every 4 hours to help prevent tube occlusion. Monitor gastric emptying every 4 hours. A needle catheter jejunostomy tube may require flushing every 2 hours to prevent formula buildup inside the tube. A Y-connector may be useful for frequent flushing. Attach the continuous feeding to the main port, and use the side port for flushes.
■ If a feeding tube becomes clogged, attempt to unclog the tube according to your facility's policy. Be aware that some facilities use carbonated cola or a

solution of meat tenderizer dissolved in water or a pancreatic enzyme solution (pancrelipase dissolved in water) to unclog a feeding tube. For example, after aspirating as much liquid as possible from the feeding tube, at least 5 ml of the appropriate solution is instilled into the tube, and then the tube is clamped. After waiting approximately 15 minutes, attempts to flush the tube with water or normal saline are made. If the tube remains clogged, the tube is removed and a new one is inserted.

■ Change equipment every 24 hours, or according to your facility's policy.
■ To prevent mucosal breakdown of the nose, esophagus, and oropharynx, use smaller-lumen tubes if possible. Check the facility's policy regarding the frequency of changing feeding tubes to prevent complications.
■ To reduce oropharyngeal discomfort from the tube, allow the patient to brush his teeth or care for his dentures regularly, and encourage frequent gargling. If the patient is unconscious, administer oral and nasal care at least every 4 hours. Be alert for dry mucous membranes, which may indicate dehydration.
■ If the feeding solution doesn't initially flow through a bulb syringe, attach the bulb and squeeze it gently to start the flow. Next, remove the bulb. Never use the bulb to force the formula through the tube.
■ During continuous feedings, assess the patient frequently for abdominal distention. Flush the tubing by adding about 50 ml of water to the gavage bag or bulb syringe. This maintains the tube's patency by removing excess formula, which could occlude the tube.

Troubleshooting tube-feeding problems

Problem	Interventions
Aspiration of gastric secretions	• Discontinue the feeding immediately. • Perform tracheal suctioning of aspirated contents if possible; anticipate the need for endotracheal intubation and mechanical ventilation if respiratory status deteriorates. • Notify the physician immediately. • Anticipate administration of prophylactic antibiotics as ordered. • Institute chest physiotherapy as ordered. • Always check tube placement before intermittent feeding, and periodically during continuous feedings, to prevent this problem. In addition, keep the head of the patient's bed elevated for at least 30 minutes after feeding is completed.
Hyperglycemia	• Monitor blood glucose levels frequently as indicated and compare to designated parameters. • Notify the physician of levels above designated parameters. • Administer insulin as ordered. • Anticipate changing to a feeding solution with a lower glucose content as ordered.
Tube obstruction	• Flush the tube with warm water, and follow your facility's policy for unclogging the tube. • If tube remains clogged after flushing, prepare to remove it and insert a new one. • Always flush tubing with at least 50 ml of water after intermittent feedings, and at least every 4 hours during continuous feedings, to prevent occlusion. • Ensure that medications given via the feeding tube are in liquid form; if mixed with water, make sure the medications are well dissolved. • Flush the feeding tube after medication administration.
Vomiting, bloating, diarrhea, or cramps	• Expect to reduce the flow rate of the feeding solution. • Administer GI motility agents as ordered to increase peristalsis. • Warm the feeding solution to room temperature before administering. • Maintain the patient on his right side with the head of the bed elevated approximately 30 degrees for at least 30 minutes after feeding is completed to promote gastric emptying. • Notify the physician for possible changes in orders, such as a decrease in the amount of feeding (for intermittent feedings) given at each interval or rate of flow for continuous feedings.

■ If the patient develops diarrhea, administer small, frequent, less concentrated feedings, or administer bolus feedings over a longer time. Make sure that the formula isn't cold and that proper storage and sanitation practices have been followed. The loose stools associated with tube feedings make extra perineal and skin care necessary. Anticipate the need for antidiarrheal agents or changing to a formula with more fiber.

■ If the patient becomes nauseated or vomits, stop the feeding immediately and assess his condition. The patient may vomit if the stomach becomes distended from overfeeding or delayed gastric emptying. Flush the feeding tube and attempt to restart the feeding in one hour. Be sure to check for gastric residuals and report if over specified parameters.

■ If the patient becomes constipated, the physician may increase the formula's fruit, vegetable, or sugar content. Assess the patient's hydration status because dehydration may produce constipation. Increase fluid intake as necessary. If the condition persists, administer an appropriate drug or enema as ordered.

■ Administer drugs as ordered through the feeding tube.

ALERT *Crush tablets or open and dilute capsules in water before administering them or use liquid forms. Be sure to flush the tubing afterward to ensure full instillation of medication. Never crush enteric-coated drugs, time-released, or sustained-release medications. Remember that some drugs may change the osmolarity of the feeding formula and cause diarrhea.*

■ Keep in mind that small-bore feeding tubes may kink, making instillation impossible. If you suspect this problem, try changing the patient's position, or withdraw the tube a few inches, and then restart.

ALERT *Never use a guidewire to reposition the feeding tube.*

■ Continuously monitor the flow rate of a blended or high-residue formula to determine if the formula is clogging the tubing as it settles. To prevent such clogging, squeeze the bag frequently to agitate the solution.

■ Monitor blood glucose levels to assess glucose tolerance. (A patient with a serum glucose level of less than 200 mg/dl is considered stable.) Monitor serum levels of electrolytes, blood urea nitrogen, and glucose as well as serum osmolality and other pertinent findings to determine the patient's response to therapy and to assess his hydration status.

■ Provide site care according to the type of tube — gastrostomy, jejunostomy, percutaneous endoscopic gastrostomy (PEG), or percutaneous endoscopic jejunostomy (PEJ). Gently remove the dressing by hand.

ALERT *Never cut away the dressing over the catheter because you might cut the tube or the sutures holding the tube in place.*

■ At least daily and as needed, clean the skin around the tube's exit site according to your facility's policy. When healed, wash the skin around the exit site daily with soap. Rinse the area with water and pat dry. Apply skin protectant if necessary.

■ Anchor a gastrostomy or jejunostomy tube to the skin with hypoallergenic tape to prevent peristaltic migration of the tube. This also prevents tension on the suture anchoring the tube in place. Coil the tube if necessary, and tape it to the abdomen to prevent pulling and contamination of the tube. PEG and PEJ tubes have toggle-bolt-like internal and external bumpers that make tape anchors un-

Caring for PEG and PEJ feeding-tube sites

The exit sites of percutaneous endo-scopic gastrostomy (PEG) or percuta-neous endoscopic jejunostomy (PEJ) feeding tubes require frequent observa-tion and care. Follow these guidelines:
● Change the dressing daily while the tube is in place.
● After removing the dressing, carefully slide the tube's outer bumper away from the skin (as shown below) about ½" (1.3 cm).

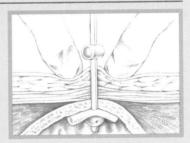

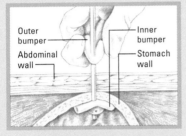

Outer bumper — Inner bumper
Abdominal wall — Stomach wall

● Inspect the skin around the tube, looking for redness and other signs of in-fection or erosion.
● Gently depress the skin surrounding the tube, and inspect for drainage (as shown top right). Expect minimal wound drainage initially after implantation; this should subside in approximately 1 week.

● Inspect the tube for wear and tear; expect replacement if signs are visible.
● Clean the site according to your facili-ty's policy.
● Rotate the outer bumper 90 degrees to avoid repeating the same tension on the same skin area, and slide the outer bumper back over the exit site.
● If leakage appears at the PEG site or if the patient risks dislodging the tube, apply a sterile gauze dressing over the site and secure with tape.
● Don't put a sterile gauze dressing un-der the outer bumper. This loosens the anchor and allows the feeding tube free play, possibly leading to wound abscess.
● Write the date and time of the dress-ing change on the tape.

necessary. (See *Caring for PEG and PEJ feeding-tube sites*.)
■ If the patient has a gastrostomy but-ton in place, flush it with 10 ml of wa-ter after the feeding. Clean the inside of the feeding catheter with a cotton-tipped applicator and water to pre-serve patency and to dislodge formula or food particles. Next, lower the sy-ringe or bag below stomach level to al-low burping. Remove the adapter and feeding catheter. The antireflux valve should prevent gastric reflux. Next, snap the safety plug into place to keep

the lumen clean and prevent leakage if the antireflux valve fails. If the patient feels nauseated or vomits after the feeding, vent the button with the adapter and feeding catheter to control emesis.
■ Be prepared to reinsert the gastros-tomy button if it pops out, for exam-ple, during feeding or with coughing. (See *Reinserting a gastrostomy feeding button*.) If this occurs during feeding, estimate the formula already delivered, reinsert the button and then resume feeding.

Reinserting a gastrostomy feeding button

If your patient's gastrostomy feeding button pops out, be prepared to reinsert it. Follow the guidelines provided here.
● Collect the feeding button, an obturator, and water-soluble lubricant. If the button will be reinserted, wash it with soap and water, and rinse it thoroughly.

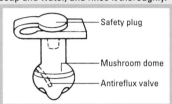

Safety plug

Mushroom dome

Antireflux valve

● Check the depth of the patient's stoma to ensure that the feeding button is the correct size. Then clean around the stoma.
● Lubricate the obturator with water-soluble lubricant, and distend the button several times to ensure patency of the antireflux valve within the button.
● Lubricate the mushroom dome and the stoma. Gently push the button through the stoma into the stomach.

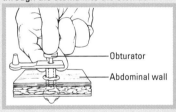

Obturator

Abdominal wall

● Remove the obturator by gently rotating it while withdrawing it. This keeps the antireflux valve from adhering to it. If the valve sticks, gently push the obturator back into the button until the valve closes.
● After removing the obturator, make sure the valve is closed. Then close the flexible safety plug, which should be relatively flat with the skin surface.

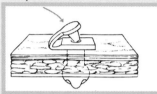

● If you need to administer a feeding right away, open the safety plug, and attach the feeding adapter and feeding tube. Deliver the feeding as ordered.

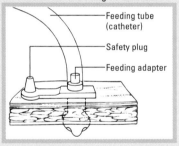

Feeding tube (catheter)

Safety plug

Feeding adapter

■ On the intake and output record, note the date, time, and amount of each feeding and the water volume instilled. Maintain total volumes for nutrients and water separately to allow calculation of nutrient intake.
■ In the patient's medical record, document the type of formula, the infusion method and rate, feeding time and duration, the patient's tolerance of the procedure and formula, and the amount of residual gastric contents. Record complications and abdominal assessment findings. Note patient-teaching topics covered and the patient's progress in self-care.
■ Record the appearance of the skin at the insertion or exit site and care of the site. For a gastrostomy button, document the stoma's appearance.

MULTISYSTEM DISORDER

Esophageal varices

Esophageal varices are dilated, tortuous veins in the submucosa of the lower esophagus resulting from portal hypertension. These varices can go undetected and result in sudden and massive bleeding. Care for the patient who has portal hypertension with esophageal varices focuses on careful monitoring for signs and symptoms of hemorrhage and subsequent hypotension, compromised oxygen supply, and altered level of consciousness (LOC).

Bleeding from esophageal varices accounts for approximately 10% of the cases of upper GI bleeding. If a patient experiences an episode of bleeding from esophageal varices, he has a 70% chance of experiencing further bleeding episodes. Moreover, of these rebleeding episodes, one-third typically end in death. In addition, comorbidities involving the renal, pulmonary, and cardiovascular systems further add to the mortality risk. If the patient experiences massive bleeding with a loss of approximately 40% of his blood volume, death can occur within 30 minutes.

Pathophysiology

Portal hypertension (elevated pressure in the portal vein) occurs when blood flow meets increased resistance. The disorder is a common result of cirrhosis, but may also stem from mechanical obstruction and occlusion of the hepatic veins (Budd-Chiari syndrome). As pressure in the portal vein rises, blood backs up into the spleen and flows through collateral channels to the venous system, bypassing the liver. Consequently, portal hypertension produces splenomegaly with thrombocytopenia and dilated collateral veins. (esophageal varices, hemorrhoids, or prominent abdominal veins), and ascites. (See *What happens in portal hypertension.*)

Comprehensive assessment

In many patients, bleeding from esophageal varices is the first sign of portal hypertension. The bleeding may be painless. The patient's history may reveal excessive use of alcohol or previously diagnosed cirrhosis. In addition, patient interview may reveal mechanical irritation, such as coarse or unchewed food, straining on defecation, or vigorous coughing preceding the bleeding episode. Bleeding esophageal varices commonly cause massive hematemesis, requiring emergency treatment to control hemorrhage and prevent hypovolemic shock. (See "Acute GI bleeding," page 351, and "Hypovolemic shock," in chapter 7, page 584.)

The patient's LOC varies, depending on the degree of bleeding. Melena, with or without hematemesis, may be noted. If the patient presents in hypovolemic shock, he may be tachycardic, tachypneic, and hypotensive with weak peripheral pulses. He may be pale, with circumoral pallor and pale, dry mucous membranes. Skin turgor is poor and urine output diminished. Jaundice is typically noted. Palpation commonly reveals splenomegaly.

Diagnosis

The following aid in diagnosing bleeding esophageal varices:

What happens in portal hypertension

Portal hypertension (elevated pressure in the portal vein) occurs when blood flow meets increased resistance, which can occur at any level. Normally, pressure in the portal vein is between 5 mm Hg and 10 mm Hg. When portal venous pressure exceeds 10 mm Hg, veins proximal to the site of the blockage distend, increasing capillary pressure in the organs that are drained by the obstructed veins. Resistance at any level between the right side of the heart and the splanchnic vessels occurs because the portal venous system lacks valves. Thus, blood flows in a retrograde pattern at increased pressure.

In many patients, the first sign of portal hypertension is bleeding esophageal varices (dilated tortuous veins in the submucosa of the lower esophagus). Esophageal varices commonly cause massive hematemesis, requiring emergency care to control hemorrhage and prevent hypovolemic shock.

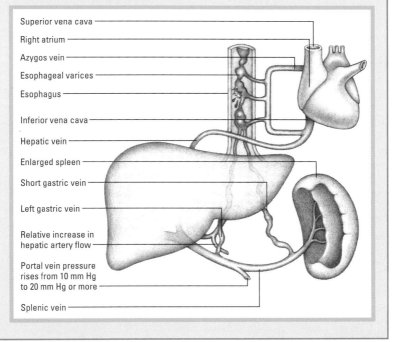

Superior vena cava
Right atrium
Azygos vein
Esophageal varices
Esophagus
Inferior vena cava
Hepatic vein
Enlarged spleen
Short gastric vein
Left gastric vein
Relative increase in hepatic artery flow
Portal vein pressure rises from 10 mm Hg to 20 mm Hg or more
Splenic vein

■ Endoscopy identifies the ruptured varix as the bleeding site and excludes other potential sources in the upper GI tract.
■ Complete blood count reveals decreased hemoglobin levels, hematocrit, and red blood cell (RBC) count; decreased white blood cell and platelet counts initially due to splenomegaly.
■ Coagulation studies reveal prolonged prothrombin time secondary to hepatocellular disease.
■ Serum chemistry tests may reveal elevated blood urea nitrogen, sodium,

total bilirubin and ammonia levels, and decreased serum albumin due to liver damage as well as elevated liver enzyme levels.

■ Angiography helps to identify patency of the portal vein and development of collateral vessels.

Collaborations

Multidisciplinary care is essential for the patient experiencing bleeding esophageal varices because of the high risk of massive blood loss. Management focuses on stabilizing the bleeding varices and replacing and maintaining fluid volume. Respiratory therapy may be involved to manage the patient's oxygenation, including the need for intubation and mechanical ventilation. A GI specialist may collaborate with a pulmonary specialist for ventilatory management, especially if the patient requires endotracheal intubation and mechanical ventilation. Nutritional therapy may be needed after the patient's condition stabilizes to ensure adequate caloric intake in conjunction with any restrictions such as protein or sodium as indicated. If appropriate, social services may be consulted for assistance with rehabilitation programs if the patient has a substance abuse problem, support of the patient and his family, and for referrals to community support groups.

Treatment and care

Treatment of portal hypertension with esophageal varices includes:

■ fluid volume replacement therapy with dextrose 5% and water, normal saline or lactated Ringer's solution initially

■ blood component therapy including packed RBCs, platelets (if indicat-

ed), and albumin for hypoalbuminemia or if the patient continues to be hypovolemic despite fluid and blood component therapy

■ I.V. vasopressin therapy (infused into the superior mesenteric artery) to stop bleeding temporarily

■ beta-adrenergic blockers such as propranolol to decrease portal venous pressure

■ somastatin therapy to decrease splanchic blood flow

■ nasogastric (NG) intubation with gastric lavage using room temperature water or saline

■ sclerotherapy via endoscopy to cause fibrosis and obliteration of the varices

■ endoscopic banding to ligate the varices which then leads to strangulation, sloughing and, eventually, fibrosis of the varices and subsequent obliteration

■ balloon tamponade, for example a Minnesota or Sengstaken-Blakemore tube, to help control hemorrhage by applying pressure on the bleeding site

■ portal systemic shunts when bleeding can't be controlled by endoscopic or pharmacologic methods or balloon tamponade

■ percutaneous transhepatic embolization to block the collateral vessels of the stomach that supply blood to the varices

■ transjugular intrahepatic portosystemic shunts to decrease portal hypertension, allowing blood to bypass the liver when returning to the heart. (see "Transjugular intrahepatic portosystemic shunt," page 414)

■ lactulose therapy to promote elimination of old blood from the GI tract, which combats excessive production and accumulation of ammonia.

Complications

If bleeding from esophageal varices isn't controlled, hypovolemic shock and, subsequently, death can occur. In addition, the underlying problem, such as cirrhosis or liver damage can lead to hepatic failure. (See "Hepatic failure," page 392.) Plus, the various treatments used to control esophageal bleeding can lead to complications. For example, vasopressin is a potent vasoconstrictor. It's associated with cardiotoxic effects, including reduced cardiac output, impaired cardiac contractility myocardial ischemia and infarction, and fatal arrhythmias. In addition, bowel ischemia, mesenteric artery infarction, and necrosis can result from its systemic vasoconstrictive effects.

If NG intubation is used, additional bleeding may occur because of the potential irritation of the mucosa by the tube.

Sclerotherapy is associated with the following complications:
- stricture formation
- perforation
- aspiration, pleural effusion
- bronchoesophageal fistula
- gastric wall necrosis
- pneumothorax or subcutaneous emphysema.

With balloon tamponade, the following may occur:
- esophageal necrosis
- esophageal rupture
- tissue necrosis.

Nursing considerations

- Assess the patient for the extent of blood loss. (See "Acute GI bleeding," page 351.)
- Ensure a patent airway and assess breathing and circulation. Monitor cardiac and respiratory status closely, at least every 15 minutes or more frequently, depending on the patient's condition.
- Administer supplemental oxygen as ordered. Monitor oxygen saturation via continuous pulse oximetry and serial arterial blood gas levels for evidence of hypoxemia, and anticipate the need for endotracheal intubation and mechanical ventilation should the patient's respiratory status deteriorate. Place the patient in semi-Fowler's position to maximize chest expansion.
- Monitor vital signs continuously for changes indicating hypovolemic shock. Observe skin color and check capillary refill. Notify the physician if capillary refill is greater than 2 seconds.
- Administer fluid replacement and blood component therapy as ordered. If necessary, assist with central venous line or pulmonary artery catheter insertion.

ALERT *Because the patient retains sodium, avoid excessive infusions of I.V. solutions containing sodium. Additionally, because the patient most likely had underlying liver damage, his ability to convert lactate (a component of lactated Ringer's solution) to bicarbonate is impaired. Therefore, avoid infusing lactated Ringer's solution.*

- Obtain serial hemoglobin level and hematocrit; notify the physician of hematocrit below 28%. Expect to administer albumin if the patient has hypoalbuminemia or if the hematocrit fails to stay above 28% even with packed RBC replacement therapy.
- Monitor intake and output closely, including all losses from the GI tract. Insert an indwelling urinary catheter,

Administering vasopressin

When your patient with bleeding esophageal varices requires vasopressin, be sure to do the following:

• Administer vasopressin I.V. at a rate of 0.1 to 0.4 U/minute; expect to continue this therapy for at least 12 hours after the bleeding is controlled.

• Monitor the patient's electrocardiogram continuously; be alert for bradycardia, myocardial ischemia, ventricular arrhythmias, or ST-segment changes; notify the physician if the patient complains of chest pain.

• Expect to administer nitroglycerin I.V. in conjunction with vasopressin to minimize the risks of cardiotoxic effects.

• Assess the patient's urine output carefully. Expect the urine output to drop after the first dose of vasopressin and diuresis to occur when vasopressin is discontinued.

• Monitor hemodynamic parameters closely; be alert for signs and symptoms of fluid overload and water intoxication.

• Monitor results of serum electrolyte levels, especially sodium. Hyponatremia can occur.

• Assess abdomen for distention and auscultate abdomen for presence of bowel sounds. Note any increase in distention or hyperactive or hypoactive bowel sounds, which may suggest bowel ischemia.

ALERT *Increases in central venous pressure, pulmonary artery pressure, and pulmonary artery wedge pressure indicate fluid overload.*

■ Institute continuous cardiac monitoring to evaluate for possible arrhythmias or adverse effects of treatment.

■ Assess LOC approximately every 15 to 30 minutes until the patient's condition stabilizes, and then every 4 hours as indicated.

ALERT *Be sure to establish a baseline for the patient's LOC. If he has underlying hepatic disease, his LOC may be altered due to hepatic encephalopathy, making it difficult to determine whether changes are due to hypovolemia alone. Correlate changes in LOC with additional findings, such as prolonged capillary refill, decreased distal pulses, cool, pale extremities, and hemodynamic parameters to evaluate for continued hypovolemia.*

■ Institute safety measures to protect patient from self-harm.

■ Administer pharmacologic agents as ordered. (See *Administering vasopressin*.) Assist with sclerotherapy as necessary, monitoring the patient's respiratory status closely for complications.

■ If the patient requires balloon tamponade, assist with insertion. Maintain balloon pressure as ordered, usually between 20 and 45 mm Hg and deflating the balloon at ordered intervals.

ALERT *After an esophageal balloon has been inserted, be alert for respiratory complications because the inflated balloon can partially or totally obstruct the airway. Suction any oral secretions from above the inflated balloon using a proximal tube or additional lumen of the tube, and ensure that this tube or lumen is labeled for suction purposes only. Assess breath sounds at least every hour, and keep*

and assess urine output hourly. Check urine osmolality and specific gravity as ordered.

■ Assess for signs and symptoms of fluid overload; auscultate lungs for crackles and observe for neck vein distention.

■ Monitor hemodynamic parameters as often as every 15 minutes to evaluate the patient's status and response to treatment.

scissors at the bedside (to cut all lumens) should total airway occlusion occur. Ensure that the tube and all connections are secure and taped, with firm traction applied to the tube. Check traction and balloon pressure at least every 2 hours.

■ As necessary, prepare the patient for shunting procedure or surgery.

■ Provide emotional support and reassurance appropriately in the wake of massive GI bleeding, which is always a frightening experience.

■ Keep the patient as quiet and comfortable as possible to minimize oxygen demands, but remember that tolerance for sedatives and tranquilizers may be decreased because of liver damage.

■ Clean the patient's mouth, which may be dry and flecked with dried blood.

Patient teaching

■ Review disease course with the patient and his family, including treatments and medications ordered and intended effects, dosage, and adverse effects to report. Answer questions honestly and provide information as needed.

■ Prepare the patient for surgery as indicated.

■ Provide information for spiritual counseling and support groups as indicated.

GI intubation, nasoenteric

A nasoenteric-decompression tube is inserted nasally and advanced beyond the stomach into the intestinal tract. It's used to aspirate intestinal contents for analysis and to treat intestinal obstruction. The tube may also help to prevent abdominal distention after GI surgery. A physician usually inserts or removes a nasoenteric-decompression tube; however, a nurse may occasionally remove it.

A balloon or rubber bag at one end of the tube holds mercury (or air or water) to stimulate peristalsis and facilitate the tube's passage through the pylorus and into the intestinal tract. (See *Common types of nasoenteric-decompression tubes,* page 382).

Equipment

Sterile 10-ml syringe ■ 21G needle ■ nasoenteric-decompression tube ■ container of water ■ 5 to 10 ml of mercury or water as ordered ■ suction-decompression equipment ■ gloves ■ towel or linen-saver pad ■ water-soluble lubricant ■ 4″ × 4″ gauze pad ■ 1″ hypoallergenic tape ■ bulb syringe or 60-ml catheter-tip syringe ■ rubber band ■ safety pin ■ clamp ■ specimen container ■ basin of ice or warm water ■ penlight ■ waterproof marking pen ■ glass of water with straw ■ optional: ice chips and local anesthetic

Essential steps

■ Prepare the necessary equipment for insertion.

  – Stiffen a flaccid tube by chilling it in a basin of ice to facilitate insertion. To make a stiff tube flexible, dip it into warm water.

  – Check the tube's balloon for leaks. If using a Cantor or Harris tube, inject 10 cc of air into the balloon with a 10-ml syringe and 21G needle. If you're using a Miller-Abbott or Dennis tube, attach a 10-ml syringe to the distal balloon port. Immerse the balloon in a con-

Common types of nasoenteric-decompression tubes

The type of nasoenteric-decompression tube chosen depends on the size of the patient and his nostrils, the estimated duration of intubation, and the reason for the procedure. Whichever tube is used, provide good mouth care, and check the patient's nares frequently for signs of irritation. If any are noted, retape the tube so that it doesn't cause tension and then lubricate the nostril. Alternatively, the tube may be inserted through the other nostril.

Most tubes are impregnated with a radiopaque mark so that placement can easily be confirmed by X-ray or other imaging technique. The most commonly used nasoenteric tubes are described here.

Cantor tube
The Cantor tube is a 10′ (3 m)-long, single-lumen tube with a balloon that can hold mercury at its distal tip. The tube may be used to relieve bowel obstructions and to aspirate intestinal contents.

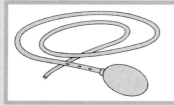

Harris tube
Measuring only 6′ (1.8 m) long, the Harris tube is a single-lumen tube that also ends with a balloon that holds mercury. Used primarily for treating a bowel obstruction, the tube allows lavage of the intestinal tract, usually with a Y-tube attached.

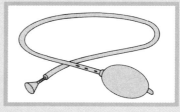

Miller-Abbott tube
The Miller-Abbott tube is a 10′-long tube with two lumens: one for inflating the distal balloon with air and one for instilling mercury or water. Also used for bowel obstruction, the tube allows aspiration of intestinal contents.

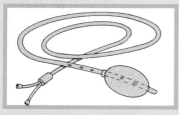

Dennis tube
The Dennis tube is a 10′-long, three-lumen sump tube used to decompress the intestinal tract before or after GI surgery. Each lumen is marked to denote its use: irrigation, drainage, or balloon inflation.

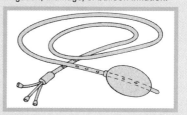

tainer of water, and watch for air bubbles. Bubble-free water means that the balloon is free from leaks. Next, remove the balloon from the water. Mercury, air, or water is added to the balloon either before or after insertion of the tube, depending on the type of tube used.

Follow the manufacturer's recommendations.

– Set up suction-decompression equipment, if ordered, and make sure it works properly.

■ Explain the procedure to the patient, forewarning him that he may experience some discomfort. Provide privacy and adequate lighting. Wash your hands and put on gloves.

■ Position the patient properly, usually in semi-Fowler's or high Fowler's position. You may also need to help the patient hold his neck in a hyperextended position. Protect the patient's chest with a linen-saver pad or towel.

■ Determine with the patient a signal that can be used to stop the insertion briefly if necessary.

■ Apply a local anesthetic, if ordered, to the nostril or the back of the throat to dull sensations and the gag reflex for intubation. Letting the patient gargle with a liquid anesthetic or hold ice chips in his mouth for a few minutes serves the same purpose.

■ Assist with insertion (or insert the tube if properly trained):

– After determining which nostril will be used for insertion, measure the length of tube to be inserted by holding the tube's distal end at the tip of the patient's nose and then extending the tube to the earlobe and down to the xiphoid process; mark this measurement on the tube with a waterproof marking pen or hold it at this point.

– Apply water-soluble lubricant to the first few inches of the tube to reduce friction and tissue trauma and to facilitate insertion.

– If the balloon already contains mercury or water, hold it so the fluid runs to the bottom. Next, pinch the balloon closed to retain the fluid as the insertion begins.

– Tell the patient to breathe through his mouth or to pant as the balloon enters his nostril. After the balloon begins its descent, release grip on it, allowing the weight of the fluid to pull the tube into the nasopharynx. When the tube reaches the nasopharynx, instruct the patient to lower his chin and to swallow. In some cases, the patient may sip water through a straw to facilitate swallowing as the tube advances, but not after the tube reaches the trachea. This prevents injury from aspiration. Continue to advance the tube slowly to prevent it from curling or kinking in the stomach.

– To confirm the tube's passage into the stomach, aspirate stomach contents with a bulb syringe. (If using a Miller-Abbott tube, after verifying passage, inject the appropriate amount of mercury [commonly between 2 and 5 ml] into the balloon lumen.)

– To keep the tube out of the patient's eyes and to help avoid undue skin irritation, fold a 4″ × 4″ gauze pad in half and tape it to the patient's forehead with the fold directed toward the patient's nose. Next, slide the tube through this sling, leaving enough slack for the tube to advance.

– Position the patient as directed to help advance the tube. He'll typically lie on his right side until the tube clears the pylorus (about 2 hours). Anticipate confirming passage by X-ray.

– After the tube clears the pylorus, expect to advance it 2″ to 3″ (5 to

7.5 cm) every hour and to reposition the patient until the premeasured mark reaches the patient's nostril. Gravity and peristalsis will help advance the tube. (Notify the physician if you can't advance the tube.)

– Keep the remaining premeasured length of tube well lubricated to ease passage and prevent irritation. Don't tape the tube while it advances to the premeasured mark unless ordered to do so.

– After the tube progresses the necessary distance, obtain an X-ray as ordered to confirm tube positioning. When the tube is in place, secure the external tubing with tape to help prevent further progression.

– Loop a rubber band around the tube, and pin the rubber band to the patient's gown with a safety pin.

– If ordered, attach the tube to intermittent suction.

■ Remove the tube when indicated or as ordered.

– Assist the patient into semi-Fowler's or high Fowler's position. Drape a linen-saver pad or towel across the patient's chest.

– Wash your hands and put on gloves.

– Clamp the tube and disconnect it from the suction. This prevents the patient from aspirating any gastric contents that leak from the tube during withdrawal.

– If your patient has a double-lumen Miller-Abbott tube or a triple-lumen Dennis tube, attach a 10-ml syringe to the balloon port and withdraw the mercury. Place the mercury in a specimen container and follow your facility's protocol for safe disposal. (If working with a single-lumen Cantor or Harris tube, withdraw the mercury after removing the tube.)

– Slowly withdraw between 6″ to 8″ (15 and 20.5 cm) of the tube. Wait 10 minutes and withdraw another 6″ to 8″. Wait another 10 minutes. Continue this procedure until the tube reaches the patient's esophagus (with about 18″ [45.5 cm] of the tube remaining inside the patient). At this point, gently withdraw the tube completely with the mercury in the balloon.

– Alternatively, for a single-lumen tube, withdraw it gently into the pharynx. Ask the patient to open his mouth. Next, grasp the tube and mercury balloon and gently pull them outside of the patient's mouth. Remove mercury from the bag with a needle and syringe, and pull the tube and empty balloon through the patient's nose.

Complications
Potential complications of nasoenteric-decompression tubes may include:
■ reflux esophagitis
■ nasal or oral inflammation and nasal, laryngeal, or esophageal ulceration
■ fluid volume deficit
■ electrolyte imbalance
■ pneumonia.

In addition, mercury poisoning (from a ruptured mercury-filled balloon) and intussusception of the bowel (from the weight of the mercury in the balloon) can occur.

Nursing considerations
■ For a double- or triple-lumen tube, note which lumen accommodates bal-

loon inflation and which accommodates drainage.

■ Never forcibly remove a tube if you meet resistance. Notify the physician immediately.

■ Properly dispose of mercury. It can be disposed of only by a licensed hazardous-waste disposal company. Put the container of mercury into a plastic bag, and send it to the appropriate department for disposal, according to the facility's policy.

■ Maintain slack in the tubing so the patient can move comfortably and safely in bed. Show him how far he can move without dislodging the tube.

■ Check the suction machine at least every 2 hours to confirm proper functioning and to ensure tube patency and bowel decompression.

ALERT *Excessive negative pressure may draw the mucosa into the tube openings, impair the suction's effectiveness, and injure the mucosa. To check functioning in an intermittent suction unit, look for drainage in the connecting tube and dripping into the collecting container. Empty the container at least every 8 hours, and measure the contents.*

■ Auscultate for presence of bowel sounds. Watch for peristalsis to resume, signaled by bowel sounds, passage of flatus, decreased abdominal distention and, possibly, a spontaneous bowel movement. These signs may require tube removal. After decompression and before extubation, as ordered, provide a clear-to-full liquid diet to assess bowel function.

ALERT *If the tip of the balloon falls below the ileocecal valve (confirmed by X-ray), the tube can't be removed nasally — it must be advanced and removed through the anus. If the*

balloon at the end of the tube protrudes from the anus, notify the physician. Most likely, the tube can be disconnected from suction, the proximal end severed, and the remaining tube removed gradually through the anus either manually or by peristalsis.

■ Record intake and output accurately to monitor fluid balance. If the tube is to be irrigated, its length may prohibit aspiration of the irrigant, so record the amount of instilled irrigant as "intake." Typically, normal saline solution supersedes water as the preferred irrigant because water, which is hypotonic, may increase electrolyte loss through osmotic action, especially if the tube is irrigated often.

■ If the tube becomes obstructed, attempt to clear it. (See *Clearing an obstructed nasoenteric-decompression tube,* page 386.)

■ Observe the patient for signs and symptoms of disorders related to suctioning and intubation including dehydration, a fluid volume deficit, or a fluid-electrolyte imbalance.

■ Assess respiratory status, noting any signs and symptoms of pneumonia related to the patient's inability to clear his pharynx or cough effectively with a tube in place. Be alert for fever, chest pain, tachypnea or labored breathing, and diminished breath sounds over the affected area.

■ Observe drainage characteristics: color, amount, consistency, odor, and any unusual changes.

■ Provide mouth care at least every 4 hours to increase the patient's comfort and promote a healthy oral cavity. If possible, encourage the patient to brush his teeth or rinse his mouth with the mouthwash and water mixture, and lubricate the patient's lips

Clearing an obstructed nasoenteric-decompression tube

If the patient's nasoenteric-decompression tube appears obstructed, notify the physician, and expect the following steps to be ordered to restore patency quickly and efficiently.

● Disconnect the tube from the suction source, and irrigate with normal saline solution. Use gravity flow to help clear the obstruction unless ordered otherwise.

● If irrigation doesn't reestablish patency, suspect that the tube may be obstructed by its position against the mucosa. Tug slightly and gently on the tube to move it away from the mucosa.

● If gentle tugging doesn't restore patency, suspect that the tube is kinked. However, before proceeding, take the following precautions:

– Never reposition or irrigate a nasoenteric-decompression tube without a physician's order in a patient who has had GI surgery.

– Avoid manipulating a tube in a patient who has had the tube inserted during surgery; to do so may disturb new sutures.

– Don't try to reposition a tube in a patient who was difficult to intubate, for example, because of an esophageal stricture.

and label it DO NOT TOUCH. Label the other lumen SUCTION. Marking the tube may prevent accidentally instilling irrigant into the wrong lumen.

■ If the suction machine works improperly, replace it immediately. If the machine works properly but no drainage accumulates in the collection container, suspect an obstruction in the tube.

■ If the tubing irritates the patient's throat or makes him hoarse, offer relief with mouthwash, gargles, viscous lidocaine, throat lozenges, an ice collar, sour hard candy, or gum as appropriate.

■ Record the date and time the nasoenteric-decompression tube was inserted and by whom. Note the patient's tolerance of the procedure, the type of tube used, the suction type and amount, and the color, amount, and consistency of drainage. Record the frequency and type of mouth and nose care provided.

■ Record the amount of drainage on the intake and output sheet. Always document the amount of irrigant or other fluid introduced through the tube or taken orally by the patient.

■ If the suction machine malfunctions, note the length of time it wasn't functioning and the actions taken. Describe the amount and character of any vomitus.

■ Document the date, time, and name of the person removing the tube and the patient's tolerance of the removal procedure.

with either wet sponge-tipped swabs or petroleum jelly applied with a cotton-tipped applicator.

■ At least every 4 hours, gently clean and lubricate the patient's external nostrils with either petroleum jelly or water-soluble lubricant on a cotton-tipped applicator to prevent skin breakdown.

■ For a Miller-Abbott tube, clamp the lumen leading to the mercury balloon

GI intubation, nasogastric

Usually inserted to decompress the stomach, a nasogastric (NG) tube can prevent vomiting after major surgery. An NG tube is typically in place for 48 to 72 hours after surgery, by which time peristalsis usually resumes. The tube may remain in place for shorter or longer periods, however, depending on its use.

The NG tube has other diagnostic and therapeutic applications, especially in assessing and treating upper GI bleeding, collecting gastric contents for analysis, performing gastric lavage, aspirating gastric secretions, and administering medications and nutrients.

Inserting an NG tube requires close observation of the patient and verification of proper placement. Removing the tube requires careful handling to prevent injury or aspiration. The tube must be inserted with extra care in pregnant patients and in those with an increased risk of complications. For example, the physician will order an NG tube for a patient with aortic aneurysm, myocardial infarction, gastric hemorrhage, or esophageal varices only if he believes that the benefits outweigh the risks of intubation.

Most NG tubes have a radiopaque marker or strip at the distal end so that the tube's position can be verified by X-ray. If the position can't be confirmed, the physician may order fluoroscopy to verify placement.

The most common NG tubes are the Levin tube, which has one lumen, and the Salem sump tube, which has two lumens, one for suction and drainage and a smaller one for ventilation. Air flows through the vent lumen continuously. This protects the delicate gastric mucosa by preventing a vacuum from forming should the tube adhere to the stomach lining. The Moss tube, which has a triple lumen, is usually inserted during surgery. (See *Types of nasogastric tubes,* page 388.)

Equipment
For inserting an NG tube
Tube (usually #12, #14, #16, or #18 French for a normal adult) ▪ towel or linen-saver pad ▪ facial tissues ▪ emesis basin ▪ penlight ▪ 19 or 29 hypoallergenic tape ▪ gloves ▪ water-soluble lubricant ▪ cup or glass of water with straw (if appropriate) ▪ stethoscope ▪ tongue blade ▪ catheter-tip or bulb syringe or irrigation set ▪ safety pin ▪ ordered suction equipment ▪ optional: metal clamp, ice, alcohol pad, warm water, large basin or plastic container, and rubber band

For removing an NG tube
Stethoscope ▪ gloves ▪ catheter-tip syringe ▪ normal saline solution ▪ towel or linen-saver pad ▪ adhesive remover ▪ optional: clamp

Essential steps
▪ Prepare the equipment.
  – Inspect the NG tube for defects, such as rough edges or partially closed lumens. Next, check the tube's patency by flushing it with water.
  – To ease insertion, increase a stiff tube's flexibility by coiling it around your gloved fingers for a few seconds or by dipping it into warm water. Stiffen a limp rubber tube by briefly chilling it in ice.

Types of nasogastric tubes

The Levin and Salem sump tubes are commonly used nasogastric tubes.

Levin tube
The Levin tube is a rubber or plastic tube with a single lumen, a length of 42" to 50" (106.5 to 127 cm), and holes at the tip and along the side.

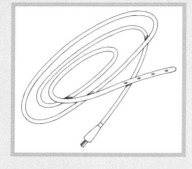

The Salem sump tube
The Salem sump tube is a double-lumen tube made of clear plastic. It has a colored sump port (pigtail) that allows atmospheric air to enter the patient's stomach; therefore, the tube floats freely and doesn't adhere to or damage gastric mucosa. The larger port of this 48" (122 cm) tube serves as the main suction conduit. The tube has openings at 45, 55, 65, and 75 cm as well as a radiopaque line to verify placement.

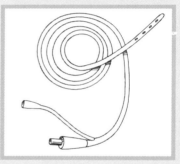

■ Provide privacy, wash your hands, and put on gloves before inserting the tube. Check the physician's order to determine the type of tube that should be inserted.
■ Insert the NG tube.
  – Explain the procedure to the patient, including the possibility of nasal discomfort, gagging, and eye tearing, to ease anxiety and promote cooperation. Emphasize that swallowing will ease the tube's advancement.
  – Agree on a signal that the patient can use if he wants you to stop briefly during the procedure.

—Help the patient into high Fowler's position unless contraindicated.
– Stand at the patient's right side if right-handed or at his left side if left-handed to ease insertion.
– Drape the towel or linen-saver pad over the patient's chest to protect gown and bed linens from spills. Have the patient gently blow his nose to clear the nostrils. Place the facial tissues and emesis basin well within the patient's reach.
– Help the patient face forward with his neck in a neutral position.

– Determine the length of tube for insertion. (See *Measuring nasogastric tube length*.)

– Mark this distance on the tubing with the tape. (Average measurements for an adult range from 22″ to 26″ [56 to 66 cm].) It may be necessary to add 2″ (5 cm) to this measurement in tall individuals to ensure entry into the stomach.

– Determine which nostril will allow easier access by using a penlight and inspecting for a deviated septum or other abnormalities. Ask the patient if he ever had nasal surgery or a nasal injury. Assess airflow in both nostrils by occluding one nostril at a time while the patient breathes through his nose. Choose the nostril with the better airflow.

– Lubricate the first 3″ (7.6 cm) of the tube with a water-soluble gel to minimize injury to the nasal passages.

◤ **ALERT** *Using a water-soluble lubricant prevents lipoid pneumonia, which may result from aspiration of an oil-based lubricant or from accidental slippage of the tube into the trachea.*

– Instruct the patient to hold his head straight and upright.

– Grasp the tube with the end pointing downward, curve it if necessary, and carefully insert it into the more patent nostril aiming the tube downward and toward the ear closer to the chosen nostril. Advance it slowly to avoid pressure on the turbinates and resultant pain and bleeding.

– When the tube reaches the nasopharynx, expect to feel resistance. Instruct the patient to lower his

Measuring nasogastric tube length

To determine how long the nasogastric tube must be to reach the stomach, hold the end of the tube at the tip of the patient's nose. Extend the tube to the patient's earlobe and then down to the xiphoid process.

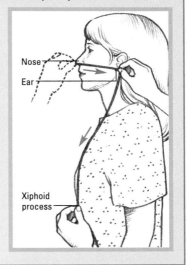

head slightly to close the trachea and open the esophagus. Next, rotate the tube 180 degrees toward the opposite nostril to redirect it so that the tube won't enter the patient's mouth.

– Unless contraindicated, offer the patient a cup or glass of water with a straw. Direct him to sip and swallow as you slowly advance the tube. This helps the tube pass to the esophagus. (If you aren't using water, ask the patient to swallow.) Keep an emesis basin and facial tissues readily available for the patient.

– Use a tongue blade and penlight to examine the patient's mouth and throat for signs of a coiled section of tubing (especially in an unconscious patient). Coiling indicates an obstruction.

– As you carefully advance the tube and the patient swallows, watch for respiratory distress signs, which may mean the tube is in the bronchus and must be removed immediately.

– Stop advancing the tube when the tape mark reaches the patient's nostril.

– Attach a catheter-tip or bulb syringe to the tube, and try to aspirate stomach contents. If you don't obtain stomach contents, position the patient on his left side to move the contents into the stomach's greater curvature, and aspirate again.

ALERT *When confirming tube placement, never place the tube's end in a container of water. If the tube should be mispositioned in the trachea, the patient may aspirate water. Water without bubbles doesn't confirm proper placement. Instead, the tube may be coiled in the trachea or the esophagus.*

—If you still can't aspirate stomach contents, advance the tube 1″ to 2″ (2.5 to 5 cm). Next, inject 10 cc of air into the tube. At the same time, auscultate for air sounds with your stethoscope placed over the epigastric region. You should hear a whooshing sound if the tube is patent and properly positioned in the stomach.

– Further confirm tube placement with X-ray verification.

– Secure the NG tube to the patient's nose with hypoallergenic tape, designated tube holder, or commercial device that secures and cushions it at the nose.

– Attach the tube to suction equipment if ordered, and set the designated suction pressure.

■ Remove the NG tube when ordered or indicated.

– Explain the procedure to the patient, including the possibility of nasal discomfort and sneezing or gagging.

– Assess bowel function by auscultating for peristalsis or flatus.

– Help the patient into semi-Fowler's position. Next, drape a towel or linen-saver pad across the chest to protect the gown and bed linens from spills.

– Wash your hands and put on gloves.

– Using a catheter-tip syringe, flush the tube with 10 ml of normal saline solution to ensure that the tube doesn't contain stomach contents that could irritate tissues during tube removal.

– Untape the tube from the patient's nose, and then unpin it from his gown.

– Clamp the tube by folding it in your hand.

– Ask the patient to hold his breath to close the epiglottis. Next, withdraw the tube gently and steadily. (When the distal end of the tube reaches the nasopharynx, you can pull it quickly.)

– When possible, immediately cover and remove the tube because its sight and odor may nauseate the patient.

– Assist the patient with thorough mouth care, and clean the tape residue from the patient's skin.

– For the next 48 hours, monitor the patient for signs of GI dysfunction, including nausea, vomiting, abdominal distention, and food intolerance. GI dysfunction may necessitate reinsertion of the tube.

Complications

Potential complications of prolonged intubation with an NG tube may include:

■ skin erosion at the nostril
■ sinusitis
■ esophagitis
■ esophagotracheal fistula
■ gastric ulceration
■ pulmonary and oral infection.

Additional complications that may result from suction include electrolyte imbalances and dehydration.

Nursing considerations

■ To reduce discomfort from the weight of the tube, tie a slipknot around the tube with a rubber band, and then secure the rubber band to the patient's gown with a safety pin, or wrap another piece of tape around the end of the tube and leave a tab. Next, fasten the tape tab to the patient's gown.

■ If necessary, use a helpful device such as Ross-Hanson tape for calculating the correct tube length. Place the narrow end of this measuring tape at the tip of the patient's nose. Extend the tape to the patient's earlobe and down to the tip of the xiphoid process. Mark this distance on the edge of the tape labeled "nose to ear to xiphoid." The corresponding measurement on the opposite edge of the tape is the proper insertion length.

■ Provide frequent nose and mouth care while the tube is in place.

■ If the patient has a deviated septum or other nasal condition that prevents nasal insertion, pass the tube orally after removing any dentures if necessary. Sliding the tube over the tongue, proceed as you would for nasal insertion. When using the oral route, remember to coil the end of the tube around your hand. This helps curve and direct the tube downward at the pharynx.

■ If the patient is unconscious or unresponsive, tilt his chin toward the chest to close the trachea. Next, advance the tube between respirations to ensure that it doesn't enter the trachea. While advancing the tube in an unconscious patient (or in a patient who can't swallow), stroke his neck to encourage the swallowing reflex and facilitate passage down the esophagus.

■ While advancing the tube, observe for signs that it has entered the trachea, such as choking or breathing difficulties in a conscious patient, and cyanosis in an unconscious patient or a patient without a cough reflex. If these signs occur, remove the tube immediately. Allow the patient time to rest, and then try to reinsert the tube.

■ After tube placement, vomiting suggests tubal obstruction or incorrect position. Assess immediately to determine the cause.

■ Irrigate the tube with the specified amount of solution as ordered, usually every 2 to 4 hours. Always check for proper placement before instilling any solution into the NG tube.

■ Slowly instill the irrigant into the NG tube. (When irrigating the Salem sump tube, you may instill small amounts of solution into the vent lumen without interrupting suction; however, you should instill greater amounts into the larger, primary lumen.) Gently aspirate the solution with the bulb syringe or 60-ml catheter-tip syringe or connect the tube to the suction equipment as ordered. Gentle aspiration prevents excessive pressure on a suture line and on delicate gastric mucosa. Report any bleeding. Reconnect the tube to suction after completing irrigation.

■ Assess bowel sounds regularly (every 4 to 8 hours) to verify GI function.

■ Inspect gastric drainage and note its color, consistency, odor, and amount. Normal gastric secretions have no color or appear yellow-green from bile and have a mucoid consistency. Immediately report any drainage with a coffee color because this may suggest GI bleeding. Check drainage for occult blood according to your facility's policy.

■ When administering medications through an NG tube, irrigate the tube with 30 ml of irrigant before and after instilling medication. Wait for about 30 minutes, or as ordered, after instillation, before reconnecting the suction equipment to allow sufficient time for the medication to be absorbed.

⚡ **ALERT** *If an NG tube malfunctions, usually due to a clog or an incorrect position, attempt to irrigate the tube, reposition the patient, or rotate and reposition the tube. However, if the tube was inserted during surgery, avoid this maneuver to ensure that the movement doesn't interfere with gastric or esophageal sutures. Instead, notify the physician.*

■ If the patient has a Salem sump tube, watch for gastric reflux in the vent lumen when pressure in the stomach exceeds atmospheric pressure. This problem may result from a clogged primary lumen or from a suction system that's set up improperly. Assess the suction equipment for proper functioning. Next, irrigate the NG tube, and instill 30 cc of air into the vent tube to maintain patency. Don't attempt to stop reflux by clamping the vent tube. Unless contraindicated, elevate the patient's torso more than 30 degrees, and keep the vent tube above his midline to prevent a siphoning effect.

■ Record the type and size of the NG tube and the date, time, and route of insertion and removal. Note the type and amount of suction, if used, and describe the drainage, including the amount, color, character, consistency, and odor. Note the patient's tolerance of the procedure.

■ Note any signs and symptoms of complications and actions taken while the tube is in place and after removal.

■ Document any irrigation procedures and continuing problems after irrigation.

⭐ **MULTISYSTEM DISORDER**

Hepatic failure

Hepatic (liver) failure can be the end result of any liver disease. The liver performs more than 100 separate functions in the body. When it fails, a complex syndrome involving the impairment of many different organs and body functions ensues. Failure may be caused by viral hepatitis, nonviral hepatitis, cirrhosis, or liver cancer. (See *Viral hepatitis — from A to E, plus G,* pages 394 and 395.) Hepatic encephalopathy and hepatorenal syndrome are two conditions occurring in liver failure.

Prognosis is generally poor. The only cure for liver failure is a liver transplant.

Pathophysiology

Manifestations of liver failure include hepatic encephalopathy and hepatorenal syndrome. Hepatic encephalopathy, a set of central nervous system disorders, results when the liver can no longer detoxify the blood. Liver dysfunction and collateral vessels that shunt blood around the liver to the systemic circulation permit toxins absorbed from the GI tract to circulate freely to the brain. Ammonia is one of the main toxins causing hepatic encephalopathy. Ammonia is a byproduct of protein metabolism. The normal liver transforms ammonia to urea, which the kidneys excrete. When the liver fails and can no longer transform ammonia to urea, ammonia blood levels rise and the ammonia is delivered to the brain. Short-chain fatty acids, serotonin, tryptophan, and false neurotransmitters may also accumulate in the blood and contribute to hepatic encephalopathy.

Hepatorenal syndrome is renal failure concurrent with liver disease; the kidneys appear normal but abruptly cease functioning. It causes expanded blood volume, accumulation of hydrogen ions, and electrolyte disturbances. It's most common in patients with alcoholic cirrhosis or fulminating hepatitis. The cause may be the accumulation of vasoactive substances that cause inappropriate constriction of renal arterioles, leading to decreased glomerular filtration and oliguria. The vasoconstriction may also be a compensatory response to portal hypertension and the pooling of blood in the splenic circulation.

Comprehensive assessment

Clinical features of hepatic encephalopathy vary depending on the severity of neurologic involvement. The disorder usually progresses through four stages or grades, but the patient's symptoms can fluctuate from one stage to another.

In the *prodromal stage* or grade I, early symptoms are typically overlooked because they're so subtle. The patient's history may reveal slight personality changes, such as agitation, belligerence, disorientation, or forgetfulness. The patient may also have trouble concentrating or thinking clearly. He may report feeling fatigued or drowsy, or may have slurred or slowed speech. On inspection, you may observe a slight tremor.

In the *impending stage* or grade II, the patient undergoes continuing mental changes. He may be confused and disoriented as to time, place, and person. Inspection continues to reveal tremor that has progressed to asterixis (liver flap, flapping tremor). The hallmark of hepatic encephalopathy, asterixis is quick, irregular extensions and flexions of the wrists and fingers when the wrists are held out straight and the hands flexed upward. On inspection, you may observe lethargy and aberrant behavior. Some patients demonstrate apraxia. When asked, the patient can't reproduce a simple design such as a star.

In the *stuporous stage* or grade III, the patient shows marked mental confusion. On inspection, he appears drowsy and stuporous. Yet he can still be aroused and is commonly noisy and

Viral hepatitis — from A to E, plus G

The chart shown below compares the features of each type of viral hepatitis characterized to date. Other types are emerging.

Feature	Hepatitis A	Hepatitis B	Hepatitis C
Incubation	15 to 45 days	30 to 180 days	15 to 160 days
Onset	Acute	Insidious	Insidious
Age-group most affected	Children, young adults	Any age	More common in adults
Transmission	Fecal-oral, sexual (especially oral-anal contact), nonpercutaneous (sexual, maternal-neonatal), percutaneous (rare)	Blood-borne; parenteral route, sexual, maternal-neonatal; virus is shed in all body fluids	Blood-borne; parenteral route
Severity	Mild	Commonly severe	Moderate
Prognosis	Generally good	Worsens with age and debility	Moderate
Progression to chronicity	None	Occasional	10% to 50% of cases

abusive when aroused. Hyperventilation, muscle twitching, and asterixis are also evident.

In the *comatose stage* or grade IV, the patient can't be aroused and is obtunded with no asterixis. Seizures, though uncommon, may occur. Palpation may reveal hyperactive reflexes and demonstrate a positive Babinski's reflex. The patient typically has fetor hepaticus (musty odor of the breath and urine). Fetor hepaticus may occur in other stages also. Eventually this stage progresses to coma, and is usually fatal.

In addition, other clinical findings may be noted, depending upon the degree of hepatic failure. They may include:

■ jaundice from the liver's failure to conjugate bilirubin
■ abdominal pain or tenderness from liver inflammation
■ nausea and anorexia from systemic effects of inflammation
■ fatigue and weight loss from failure of hepatic metabolism

Hepatitis D	Hepatitis E	Hepatitis G
14 to 64 days	14 to 60 days	2 to 6 weeks
Acute and chronic	Acute	Presumed insidious
Any age	Ages 20 to 40	Any age, primarily adults
Parenteral route; most people infected with hepatitis D are also infected with hepatitis B	Primarily fecal-oral	Blood-borne; similar to Hepatitis B and C
Can be severe and lead to fulminant hepatitis	Highly virulent with common progression to fulminant hepatitis and hepatic failure, especially in pregnant patients	Moderate
Fair, worsens in chronic cases; can lead to chronic hepatitis D and chronic liver disease	Good unless pregnant	Generally good; no current treatment recommendations
Occasional	None	Not known; no association with chronic liver disease

- pruritus due to the accumulation of bilirubin in the skin
- oliguria from intrarenal vasoconstriction
- splenomegaly secondary to portal hypertension
- ascites due to portal hypertension and decreased plasma proteins
- peripheral edema from accumulation of fluid retained because of decreased plasma protein production and loss of albumin with ascites
- varices of the esophagus, rectum, and abdominal wall secondary to portal hypertension
- bleeding tendencies from thrombocytopenia (secondary to blood accumulation in the spleen) and prolonged prothrombin time (PT) (from the impaired production of coagulation factors)
- petechiae resulting from thrombocytopenia
- amenorrhea secondary to altered steroid hormone production and metabolism

■ gynecomastia in males, from estrogen buildup due to failure of hepatic biotransformation functions.

Diagnosis

■ Liver function tests reveal elevated levels of aspartate aminotransferase, alanine aminotransferase, alkaline phosphatase, and bilirubin.
■ Blood studies reveal anemia, impaired red blood cell production, elevated bleeding and clotting times, low platelet levels, low blood glucose levels, low albumin, decreased blood urea nitrogen (BUN), and increased serum ammonia levels.
■ Serum electrolyte studies commonly reveal hyponatremia and hypokalemia in patients with ascites.
■ Urinalysis reveals increased urobilinogen, bilirubin, and osmolarity.
■ Electroencephalogram is typically abnormal with hepatic encephalopathy, but the changes are nonspecific.

Collaborations

Hepatic failure is a multisystem disorder that requires multidisciplinary care involving numerous members of the health care team. Respiratory therapy is consulted for airway and ventilation maintenance, especially if the patient is experiencing problems such as impaired gag reflex, aspiration, or difficulty with respirations due to ascites. Nutritional therapy is crucial in providing a high-calorie, protein-restricted, and possibly moderately sodium-restricted diet. Enteral or parenteral nutritional therapy may be necessary. Physical therapy may be involved to assist with measures to maintain joint function while the patient is maintained on strict bed rest. Various specialists, including neurolo-

gists and nephrologists, may be consulted for assistance depending on the involvement of the patient's organs and prognosis. The patient and his family may benefit from supportive counseling and a referral for social services.

Treatment and care

Treatment for hepatic failure may include:
■ liver transplantation
■ low-protein, high-carbohydrate diet to correct nutritional deficiencies and prevent overtaxing liver
■ lactulose to reduce ammonia blood levels and help alleviate some symptoms of hepatic encephalopathy
■ neomycin therapy (as short-term therapy) to destroy intestinal bacteria that breaks down protein into ammonia.

For ascites, treatment includes:
■ salt restriction and potassium-sparing diuretics to increase water excretion
■ potassium supplements to reverse the effects of high aldosterone
■ paracentesis to remove ascitic fluid and alleviate abdominal discomfort
■ shunt placement to aid in removal of ascitic fluid and alleviate abdominal discomfort.

For portal hypertension, treatment includes:
■ shunt placement between the portal vein and another systemic vein to divert blood flow and relieve pressure.

For variceal bleeding, treatment includes:
■ vasoconstrictor drugs to decrease blood flow
■ balloon tamponade to control bleeding by exerting pressure on the varices with the use of a balloon catheter

- surgery to tie off bleeding collaterals sprouting from the portal vein. (See "Esophageal varices," page 376.)

Complications

Potential complications of hepatic failure may include:
- GI hemorrhage
- encephalopathy
- coma
- death.

Nursing considerations

- Assess the patient's airway and respiratory status every 1 to 2 hours or more frequently if indicated. Maintain a patent airway, and institute measures to promote adequate ventilation and oxygenation such as elevating the head of the bed.
- Monitor oxygen saturation levels via pulse oximetry and arterial blood gas studies as ordered. Administer supplemental oxygen to prevent hypoxemia. If the patient's respiratory status deteriorates, expect endotracheal intubation and mechanical ventilation.
- Assess neurologic status, including level of consciousness, to establish a baseline. Reassess and reorient the patient frequently. As appropriate, evaluate the patient's ability to write his name at least every 8 hours to track progression (if any) of encephalopathy. Report any changes to the physician immediately.
- Monitor cardiovascular system and vital signs at least every hour. If the patient's vital signs aren't stable, monitor blood pressure every 15 minutes.
- Assess hemodynamic parameters at least every hour. Anticipate insertion of a central venous catheter or pulmonary artery catheter for monitoring. Monitor changes in central venous

pressure, pulmonary artery wedge pressure, cardiac output, and cardiac index, and report significant increases or decreases.

ALERT *The patient with hepatic failure may have a fluid volume deficit or excess. A deficit may exist because of restrictions prescribed as well as related to decreased intake. In addition, hypoalbuminemia, fluid shifting and sequestration, diuretic therapy, diarrheal effects of lactulose and, possibly, bleeding from varices also contribute to this deficit. A fluid volume excess may develop from malfunctioning regulatory mechanisms or as a response to treatment of the deficit. Therefore, establish a baseline for the patient's hemodynamic parameters, and then monitor them closely, looking for trends to indicate what exactly is occurring.*

- Institute continuous cardiac monitoring to evaluate electrocardiogram for changes indicative of electrolyte imbalances and hypoxemia.
- Assess urine output every hour. Expect to insert an indwelling urinary catheter, especially if the patient's neurologic status is compromised. Notify the physician of any output less than 0.5 ml/kg/hour.

ALERT *Assess the patient's neurologic and renal status carefully if he requires diuretic therapy. Rapid diuresis and changes in electrolyte levels secondary to diuretic therapy may further compound the patient's encephalopathy or renal dysfunction.*

- Monitor intake and output, comparing 24-hour totals. Measure abdominal girth daily for changes. Obtain daily weights and compare to previous day's weight to estimate degree of fluid loss. Keep in mind that daily weight loss should be less than 1 lb (0.5 kg). Otherwise, the patient is at risk for intravascular volume depletion and further impairment in renal function.

■ If fluids are restricted, offer ice chips (if appropriate and gag reflex is present) and provide frequent mouth care.

■ Assess for signs and symptoms of fluid excess including severity and location of peripheral edema, jugular vein distention, tachypnea, crackles that don't clear with coughing, labored breathing, and a third heart sound.

■ Obtain laboratory studies as ordered, including renal function studies, hepatic enzyme levels, serum albumin, total protein, and serum electrolyte levels. Notify the physician of abnormalities.

■ Monitor the patient's nutritional intake and maintain calorie count. Evaluate meals and food for adherence to restrictions such as protein and sodium restrictions. Administer enteral or parenteral nutrition as ordered.

ALERT *Be careful when inserting a nasogastric (NG) feeding tube for enteral feedings because esophageal varices are common in patients with hepatic failure. Insertion of the NG tube increases the risk of variceal rupture, which could result in massive hemorrhage.*

■ Check fingerstick blood glucose levels every 4 hours or as ordered, and assess for signs and symptoms of hyperglycemia and hypoglycemia.

ALERT *Don't confuse signs of hypoglycemia with those of hepatic encephalopathy. Always confirm suspicions and validate assessment with blood glucose levels. Administer*

insulin as ordered for blood glucose level greater than 160 mg/dl.

■ Institute bleeding precautions and monitor the patient for signs and symptoms of bleeding. Avoid I.M. injections and minimize trauma to skin. Obtain daily coagulation studies and platelet levels as ordered. Notify the physician of increased PT or decrease in platelet count.

■ Administer prescribed medications. Check with the physician to adjust dose of lactulose to allow for 2 to 3 semi-formed stools per day. Give neomycin as ordered to decrease intestinal bacteria. Watch for signs and symptoms of ototoxicity and renal toxicity. If the patient is receiving neomycin, monitor BUN and creatinine levels every 6 hours.

■ Assist with paracentesis as indicated. Be sure to record the amount of fluid obtained from paracentesis.

■ Begin emergency treatment to control bleeding if variceal rupture occurs. (See "Esophageal varices," page 376.)

■ Prepare the patient for surgery or shunting procedure.

■ Provide supportive care to the patient. Promote comfort measures, and prevent skin breakdown and contractures by turning and repositioning, padding bony prominences, and using specialty beds and pillows.

Patient teaching

■ Review disease course and proposed plan of treatment with the patient and his family, including medications and surgery as appropriate. Answer questions honestly and provide information as needed.

■ Inform the patient and his family about dietary restrictions, including protein restrictions as ordered.

■ Teach the patient and his family about signs and symptoms of complications or worsening symptoms with instructions to notify the physician immediately.

■ Provide information for spiritual counseling and support groups as indicated.

 MULTISYSTEM DISORDER

Liver transplantation

Liver transplantation involves removal of a patient's diseased liver and replacing it with a healthy liver from a donor. Liver transplantation is most commonly performed for patients with end-stage liver disease secondary to conditions such as hepatitis B and C, alcoholic cirrhosis, primary sclerosing cholangitis, primary biliary cirrhosis, and metabolic disorders. Additional indications for liver transplantation include:

■ acute fulminant hepatic failure related to drug toxicity

■ hepatitis A

■ autoimmune disorders

■ mushroom poisoning.

 The following are absolute contraindications to liver transplantation:

■ human immunodeficiency virus

■ spontaneous bacterial peritonitis (as confirmed by presence of more than 200 polymorphonuclear leukocytes, the identification of bacteria in the fluid by light microscopy, or subsequent positive bacterial culture results) or other active infection

■ severely advanced cardiopulmonary disease

■ extrahepatic malignancy that doesn't meet cure criteria

■ currently active alcohol or substance abuse problem

■ demonstrated inability to comply with immunosuppression protocols because of psychosocial situations.

 All of these conditions are indicators of a poor prognosis and increased mortality rates.

 According to statistics, hepatitis C and alcoholic cirrhosis account for almost one-half of the liver transplants in the United States. The prognosis after liver transplantation is good. According to the United Network for Organ Sharing, overall patient survival rates at 1 year are approximately 85.6%. At 3 years, the survival rate is 75.9%. Unfortunately, with longer survival rates and improved quality of life when compared to pretransplant status, concerns are arising involving the long-term effects of immunosuppressant therapy on the cardiovascular system, infection risks and rates, and increased risk of malignancy.

Procedure

Four techniques for liver transplantation exist. One major technique, called orthotopic transplantation, consists of removing the patient's diseased liver and surgically implanting a donor liver in its place. In an orthotopic liver transplant, the donor liver is removed and transported to the recipient's location. The surgeon makes bilateral subcostal incisions and extends the midline incision to the xiphoid process. After the vessels, ligaments, and other attachments are properly severed, the patient is placed on venovenous bypass, and the diseased liver is removed. To attach the donor liver, the suprahepatic vena cava is typically anastomosed, and then the recipient

Alternative liver transplant techniques

In addition to orthotopic liver transplant, three other techniques may be used. Each of these techniques was developed because of the shortage of donor organs available for the number of candidates requiring a liver transplant.

Reduced-size liver transplant
A donor liver from a cadaver is resected to create a right lobe, left lobe, or left lateral segment, which is then anastomosed to the recipient. The remainder of the liver tissue is discarded. This is usually done for pediatric patients because the availability of donors for this population is small.

Split-liver transplant
With a split-liver transplant, an entire adult donor liver is transected or split into two pieces to provide grafts for two recipients. The liver can be split through the falciform ligament, creating a small (left lateral segment) graft for a child and a larger (extended right lobe) graft for an adult. The liver may also be split through the main portal fissure and gall bladder bed to create right and left lobe grafts.

Living-donor transplant
With a living-donor transplant, a portion of the liver from a living donor is removed and transplanted to the recipient. At one time, this technique was used only with children. However, because of its success with children, it's now used for adults as well. For transplantation in children, left lateral segments or left lobes are typically used; for adults, right lobe grafts are commonly used.

ter which the hepatic artery is anastomosed in an end-to-end fashion. Next, the surgeon reconstructs the biliary duct by connecting the bile duct of the donor to that of the recipient (with or without T-tube stent brought out to the exterior of the abdomen through a stab wound) or by using a Roux-en-Y anastomosis to the recipient's jejunum (usually if the recipient's biliary duct is diseased or too small). Several drains are placed around the liver and brought out to the exterior abdominal wall to allow for drainage of ascitic fluid and assess for bleeding.

In other cases, a reduced-sized liver transplant, split liver transplant, or living donor liver transplant may be done. (See *Alternative liver transplant techniques*.)

AGE ISSUE *Children requiring liver transplants typically receive either living-donor transplants or reduced-sized liver transplants.*

AGE ISSUE *To ensure the best possible outcome for the recipient, donors for a split-liver transplant typically meet the following criteria: age over 50 with normal liver function, hospitalized for fewer than 3 days, with required minimal support with vasopressors and no evidence of fatty degeneration of the liver.*

Complications
Potential complications of liver transplantation may include:
- rejection, acute or chronic
- primary graft failure
- biliary malfunction
- hepatic artery thrombosis
- infection
- posttransplant lymphoproliferative disorder
- posttransplant malignancies

portal vein is cleared and anastomosed to the donor portal vein. Blood flow through these vessels is evaluated, af-

■ recurrent, metabolic, or autoimmune liver disease.

Nursing considerations

When caring for the patient undergoing a liver transplant, nursing care focuses on preparing the patient and his family physically and emotionally for the procedure, including instructing the patient about the procedure and events after surgery as well as instituting measures to prevent postoperative complications.

ALERT *Be ready to act rapidly when a donor liver becomes available.*

Before liver transplantation

■ Instruct the patient and his family about the transplant and necessary diagnostic tests such as antigen typing.

■ Reinforce the surgeon's explanation of the surgery, equipment, and procedures used in the critical care unit or postanesthesia care unit. If one hasn't been inserted already, inform the patient that he'll most likely awaken from surgery with an endotracheal tube in place and be connected to a mechanical ventilator. Review other equipment such as continuous cardiac monitoring, nasogastric (NG) tube, an indwelling urinary catheter, arterial lines and, possibly, a pulmonary artery catheter. Tell him that discomfort will be minimal and the equipment will be removed as soon as possible.

■ Administer medications, including immunosuppressant agents, as ordered.

■ Review techniques of incentive spirometry and range of motion with the patient.

■ Ensure that the patient or a responsible family member has signed a consent form.

■ Instruct family members in measures used to control infection and minimize rejection after transplant.

■ Provide emotional support to the patient and his family, especially because the waiting for a donor liver may seem endless.

After liver transplantation

■ Assess cardiopulmonary and hemodynamic status closely at least every 15 minutes for at least the first 2 hours in the postoperative period, and then hourly or more frequently as indicated by the patient's condition. Institute continuous cardiac monitoring if not in place, evaluating waveforms frequently. Monitor hemodynamic parameters for changes indicating changes in fluid volume status.

■ In the immediate postoperative period, monitor laboratory test results closely, especially liver enzyme and bilirubin levels.

ALERT *Expect liver enzyme levels to be elevated in the immediate postoperative period. Usually, these elevations reflect the effects of the donor liver undergoing cold preservation while being transported to the recipient's location. Enzyme levels, along with bilirubin levels, typically return to normal within 1 week; however, a marked rise in these levels after they begin to decrease suggests possible acute rejection.*

■ Other important laboratory tests may include complete blood count, hemoglobin level, hematocrit, platelet count, serum electrolyte studies, blood urea nitrogen and creatinine levels, and arterial blood gas and coagulation studies.

🔺 **ALERT** *Following liver transplantation, the patient is at high risk for bleeding. Monitor laboratory studies, such as hemoglobin levels, hematocrit, prothrombin time, partial thromboplastin time, International Normalized Ratio, and platelet count frequently. Be sure to evaluate the results in light of any blood component therapy such as fresh frozen plasma that the patient has received. Platelet count usually decreases during the first week after transplantation, but then begins to return to normal during the second week.*

■ Assess insertion sites, such as I.V. lines and drains, for indications of bleeding. Assess incision site closely for oozing or active bleeding. If the patient has an NG tube, assess color and character of drainage at least every 2 hours.

■ Institute strict infection control precautions; perform meticulous hand washing.

■ Administer prophylactic antimicrobial agents as ordered. The postoperative liver transplant patient is continuously trying to balance the risk of infection with the risk of rejection. Cytomegalovirus is one of the most common viral infections seen in postoperative liver transplant patients.

■ Monitor temperature at least every hour initially and then every 2 to 4 hours. If the patient exhibits a fever and an infection is suspected, expect to obtain cultures of all body fluids, X-rays of the chest and abdomen, and a Doppler ultrasound of the hepatic vessels.

🔺 **ALERT** *Sudden onset of high fever and a rise in liver enzyme levels suggests hepatic artery thrombosis. Prepare the patient for a Doppler ultrasound to determine vessel patency.*

■ Assist with extubating as soon as possible (usually within 4 to 6 hours), and administer supplemental oxygen as needed, based on mixed venous oxygen saturation or pulse oximetry levels. Encourage coughing and deep breathing and use of incentive spirometry after extubation, splinting and premedicating for pain as necessary.

■ Monitor intake and output at least hourly and notify the physician if output is less than 30 ml/hour. Maintain fluids at 2000 to 3000 ml/day or as ordered to prevent fluid overload.

■ Administer postoperative drugs, such as corticosteroids (Solu-Medrol, prednisone) (used to suppress T-cell and B-cell function, reduce or prevent edema, promote normal capillary permeability, and prevent vasodilation), cyclosporine (immunosuppressant), azathioprine (immunosuppressant), OKT3 (immunosuppressant used in place of cyclosporine), and tacrolimus (highly potent immunosuppressant used in place of cyclosporine when multiple rejections occur while on cyclosporine).

■ Maintain nothing-by-mouth status with NG decompression to low intermittent suction until bowel sounds return. Administer histamine blockers to suppress gastric acid secretion. Begin clear liquids after the patient is extubated and bowel sounds are active.

■ Change the patient's position at least every 2 hours, getting him out of bed to the chair within 24 hours if his condition is stable. Gradually increase the patient's activity as tolerated.

■ Continually assess the patient for signs and symptoms of acute rejection such as malaise, fever, graft enlarge-ment, and diminished graft function (typically occurs 7 to 14 days after the transplant).

 ALERT *Be alert for a rise in bilirubin and transaminase levels in conjunction with a change in T-tube biliary drainage, which may become thin and lighter in color. Note any abdominal pain or tenderness, jaundice, dark yellow or orange urine, and clay-colored stools. Notify the physician and prepare the patient for a graft biopsy.*

■ To ease emotional stress, plan care to allow frequent rest periods and provide as much privacy as possible. Allow family members to visit and comfort the patient as much as possible.

■ Allow the family to express their anger, anxiety, and fear.

■ Teach the patient and his family about danger signs and symptoms and the need to report immediately. Stress the need for continued follow-up.

MULTISYSTEM DISORDER

Peritonitis

An acute or chronic disorder, peritonitis is an inflammation of the peritoneum, the membrane that lines the abdominal cavity and covers the visceral organs. Such inflammation may extend throughout the peritoneum or be localized as an abscess. Peritonitis commonly decreases intestinal motility and causes intestinal distention with gas. Mortality is about 10%, with bowel obstruction as the usual cause of death.

Pathophysiology

Although the GI tract normally contains bacteria, the peritoneum is ster-ile. In peritonitis, bacteria invade the peritoneum. Generally, such an infection results from inflammation and perforation of the GI tract, usually as a result of appendicitis, diverticulitis, peptic ulcer, ulcerative colitis, volvulus, strangulated obstruction, abdominal neoplasm, or abdominal trauma. These conditions expose the peritoneum to bacterial invasion. Peritonitis can also result from chemical inflammation after rupture of a fallopian tube, ovarian cyst, or the bladder, perforation of a gastric ulcer, or released pancreatic enzymes.

In both bacterial and chemical inflammation, fluid containing protein and electrolytes accumulates in the peritoneal cavity and makes the transparent peritoneum opaque, red, inflamed, and edematous. Because the peritoneal cavity is so resistant to contamination, such an infection is commonly localized as an abscess instead of disseminated as a generalized infection.

In some cases, however, such as when the peritoneum becomes weakened or injured, the area of inflammation and infection spreads throughout the peritoneal cavity. Peristaltic action decreases, leading to obstruction. Large amounts of fluid from the intravascular space move into the peritoneal cavity, causing hypovolemia and hemoconcentration. Subsequently, shock, oliguria, and possibly renal failure can result.

Comprehensive assessment

The patient's symptoms depend on whether the disorder is assessed early or late in its course. In the early phase, the patient may report vague, generalized abdominal pain. If peritonitis is localized, he may describe pain over a specific area (usually over the site of inflammation); if it's generalized, he may complain of diffuse pain over the abdomen.

As the disorder progresses, the patient typically reports increasingly severe and unremitting abdominal pain. Pain usually increases with movement and respirations. Occasionally, pain may be referred to the shoulder or the thoracic area. Other signs and symptoms include abdominal distention, anorexia, nausea, vomiting, and an inability to pass feces and flatus.

Assessment of vital signs may reveal fever, tachycardia (a response to the fever), and hypotension. On inspection, the patient usually appears acutely distressed. He may lie very still in bed, typically with his knees flexed to try to alleviate abdominal pain. He tends to breathe shallowly and move as little as possible to minimize pain. If he loses excessive fluid, electrolytes, and proteins into the abdominal cavity, excessive sweating, cool, clammy skin, pallor, abdominal distention, and such signs of dehydration as dry mucous membranes may be noted.

Early in peritonitis, auscultation usually discloses bowel sounds; as the inflammation progresses, these sounds tend to disappear. Abdominal rigidity is usually felt on palpation. If peritonitis spreads throughout the abdomen, palpation may disclose general tenderness; if peritonitis stays in a specific area, you may detect local tenderness. Rebound tenderness may also be present.

Diagnosis

■ White blood cell count shows leukocytosis (commonly more than 20,000/mm^3).
■ Serum electrolyte levels may be abnormal; albumin levels may be decreased, suggesting bacterial peritonitis.
■ Abdominal X-rays demonstrate edematous and gaseous distention of the small and large bowel. With perforation of a visceral organ, the X-ray shows air in the abdominal cavity.
■ Chest X-ray may reveal elevation of the diaphragm.
■ Abdominal ultrasound may reveal fluid collections.
■ Paracentesis discloses the nature of the exudate and permits bacterial culture so appropriate antibiotic therapy can be instituted.

Collaborations

Because peritonitis can ultimately affect multiple systems, a multidisciplinary approach to care is needed. Moreover, peritonitis is usually a complication of another condition or underlying disorder. Thus, numerous health care professionals may be involved. For example, a GI specialist can help manage the patient's disorder. An infectious disease specialist can help identify and treat the specific agent responsible for peritonitis. As the patient's systems are affected, respiratory, renal, and cardiology specialists may be called in to help manage the patient. Additionally, social services may be necessary to assist with discharge plans and follow-up care such as home care referrals.

Treatment and care

To prevent peritonitis, early treatment of GI inflammatory conditions and preoperative and postoperative antibiotic therapy are important. After peritonitis develops, emergency treatment must maintain hemodynamic stability, combat infection, restore intestinal motility, and replace fluids and electrolytes.

■ The type of antibiotic therapy depends on the infecting organism, but usually includes administration of third-generation cephalosporin in conjunction with an aminoglycoside, or penicillin G and clindamycin with an aminoglycoside.

■ Nothing-by-mouth (NPO) status decreases peristalsis and prevents perforation; the patient will be given supplemental parenteral fluids and electrolytes.

■ Analgesics are used for pain management.

■ Nasogastric (NG) intubation is used to decompress the bowel, and a rectal tube may be used to facilitate the passage of flatus.

In addition, surgery is usually performed as soon as the patient's condition is stable enough to tolerate it to control the source of the peritonitis. The source of infection is eliminated by evaluating the spilled contents and inserting drains. The surgical procedure varies with the cause of peritonitis. For example, an appendectomy may be performed for a ruptured appendix or a colon resection for a ruptured colon. Occasionally, abdominocentesis may be necessary to remove accumulated fluid. Irrigation of the abdominal cavity with antibiotic solutions during surgery may be appropriate.

Complications

Potential complications of peritonitis include:

■ abscess formation
■ septicemia
■ respiratory compromise
■ bowel obstruction
■ shock
■ death.

Nursing considerations

■ Ensure a patent airway and assess the patient's respiratory status at least every hour, or more frequently as indicated by the patient's condition. Note respiratory rate, rhythm, and depth, reporting any dyspnea and accessory muscle use. Be alert for inspiratory retractions.

■ Auscultate lungs bilaterally for adventitious or diminished breath sounds.

■ Assess oxygen saturation continuously via pulse oximetry or mixed venous oxygen saturation via pulmonary artery (PA) catheter if in place. Monitor serial arterial blood gas levels; document and report changes in arterial oxygen saturation as well as changes in pH and partial pressure of arterial oxygen. If the patient's respiratory status deteriorates, assist with endotracheal intubation and mechanical ventilation. (See "Endotracheal intubation," in chapter 2, page 193, and "Mechanical ventilation," in chapter 2, page 213.)

■ Place the patient in a comfortable position that maximizes air exchange, such as semi-Fowler's to high Fowler's position. Use oxygen saturation levels as a guide to the most effective position. Reposition the patient often.

■ Closely monitor the patient's heart rate and blood pressure at least every hour or more frequently as indicated by the patient's condition. Institute continuous cardiac monitoring and observe for arrhythmias that may result from fluid volume deficits, hypoxemia, acid-base disturbances, or electrolyte imbalance. Prepare to treat arrhythmias as ordered.

▨ **ALERT** *If the patient develops hypovolemia, monitor his electrocardiogram for sinus tachycardia; if hypokalemia is present, be alert for ventricular ectopy, a prominent U wave, and ST-segment depression.*

■ Monitor the patient's temperature every 1 to 2 hours. Administer antipyretics as ordered; institute measures to aid in reducing the patient's temperature, such as a hypothermia blanket and tepid sponge baths.

■ Assess hemodynamic status closely, at least every hour or more frequently, as indicated. Assist with insertion of a PA catheter if one isn't in place. Monitor central venous pressure, pulmonary artery wedge pressure, cardiac output and cardiac index for changes.

■ Insert or assist with GI intubation with NG or nasoenteric tube, if not in place. (See "GI intubation, nasoenteric," page 381, and "GI intubation, nasogastric," page 387.) Monitor tube drainage every 1 to 2 hours for color, amount, and characteristics. Notify the physician if drainage appears bright red or looks like coffee grounds.

■ Assess abdomen for evidence of bowel sounds and distention. If distention occurs, measure abdominal girth for changes. Maintain NPO status until bowel function returns. Expect to administer histamine-2 receptor antagonists to reduce the risk of gastric ulcer formation.

■ Administer I.V. fluid and electrolyte replacement as ordered. If the patient

exhibits signs and symptoms of hemorrhage, prepare to administer blood component therapy such as packed red blood cells.

■ Give I.V. antimicrobial agents as ordered. If the patient is receiving aminoglycosides, assess for ototoxicity and nephrotoxicity; also monitor serum peak and trough levels for therapeutic effectiveness.

■ Monitor intake and output closely. Assess urine output hourly, notifying the physician if urine output is less than 0.5 ml/kg/hour. Obtain daily weights.

▨ **ALERT** *When measuring output, be sure to include the drainage from all sources, including any tubes, catheters, drains, and dressings that required changing because they became saturated. If necessary, weigh the dressing to determine the amount of fluid lost.*

■ Monitor the patient's level of consciousness, noting such changes as increasing confusion, lethargy, or mental sluggishness, which suggest hypovolemia.

■ Assess patient's complaints of pain.

▨ **ALERT** *Be alert for changes in how the patient describes or rates the pain, including its location and severity. A sudden increase in the severity of the pain may indicate imminent rupture of an organ. Conversely, be alert for a sudden change in the patient's pain level, for example, previously severe, but now significantly decreased, which may also signal that a rupture has occurred.*

■ Administer analgesics as ordered based on patient's degree of pain.

▨ **ALERT** *The abdominal pain associated with peritonitis can be severe and can interfere with the pa-*

tient's ability to breathe deeply and fully, placing him at risk for respiratory dysfunction. Moreover, opioid analgesics can depress respirations. Therefore, carefully assess the patient's level of pain, and administer opioid analgesics carefully, being sure to evaluate his respiratory function frequently.

■ Prepare the patient for surgery as indicated. Provide preoperative teaching, and monitor the patient for surgical complications as appropriate.

■ Provide emotional support and offer encouragement as indicated.

Patient teaching

■ Teach the patient about peritonitis, the possible causes, and necessary treatments.

■ Instruct the patient in signs and symptoms to report immediately, such as changes in pain characteristics, difficulty breathing, nausea or vomiting, or light-headedness.

■ Provide preoperative teaching. Review postoperative care procedures.

■ Discuss the proper use of prescribed medications, reviewing their correct administration, desired effects, and possible adverse effects.

Total parenteral nutrition

When a patient can't meet his nutritional needs by oral or enteral feedings, he may require I.V. nutritional support, or parenteral nutrition. The patient's diagnosis, history, and prognosis determine the need for parenteral nutrition. Generally, this treatment is prescribed for any patient who can't absorb nutrients through the GI tract

for more than 10 days. More specific indications include:

■ debilitating illness lasting longer than 2 weeks

■ loss of 10% or more of pre-illness weight

■ serum albumin level below 3.5 g/dl

■ excessive nitrogen loss from wound infection, fistulas, or abscesses

■ renal or hepatic failure

■ nonfunctioning GI tract for 5 to 7 days in a severely catabolic patient.

Parenteral nutrition may be given through a peripheral or central venous (CV) line. Depending on the solution, it may be used to boost the patient's caloric intake, to supply full caloric needs, or to surpass the patient's caloric requirements.

The type of parenteral solution prescribed depends on the patient's condition and metabolic needs and on the administration route. The solution usually contains protein, carbohydrates, electrolytes, vitamins, and trace minerals. A lipid emulsion provides the necessary fat. (See *Types of parenteral nutrition,* pages 408 and 409.)

Total parenteral nutrition (TPN) refers to any nutrient solution, including lipids, given through a CV line. Peripheral parenteral nutrition (PPN), which is given through a peripheral line, supplies full caloric needs while avoiding the risks that accompany a CV line. To keep from sclerosing the vein through which it's administered, the dextrose in PPN solution must be limited to 10% or less. Therefore, the success of PPN depends on the patient's tolerance for the large volume of fluid necessary to supply his nutritional needs.

Typically, you'll need to increase the glucose content beyond the level a pe-

Types of parenteral nutrition

Type	Solution components/liter	Special considerations
Standard I.V. therapy	• Dextrose, water, electrolytes in varying amounts, for example: -- dextrose 5% in water (D_5W) = 170 calories/L -- $D_{10}W$ = 340 calories/L -- normal saline = 0 calories • Vitamins as ordered	• Nutritionally incomplete; doesn't provide sufficient calories to maintain adequate nutritional status
Total parenteral nutrition (TPN) by way of central venous (CV) line	• $D_{15}W$ to $D_{25}W$ (1 L dextrose 25% = 850 non-protein calories) • Crystalline amino acids 2.5% to 8.5% • Electrolytes, vitamins, trace elements, and insulin as ordered • Lipid emulsion 10% to 20% (usually infused as a separate solution)	*Basic solution* • Nutritionally complete • Requires minor surgical procedure for CV line insertion (can be done at bedside by the doctor) • Highly hypertonic solution • May cause metabolic complications (glucose intolerance, electrolyte imbalance, essential fatty acid deficiency) *I.V. lipid emulsion* • May not be used effectively in severely stressed patients (especially burn patients) • May interfere with immune mechanisms; in patients suffering respiratory compromise, reduces carbon dioxide buildup • Given by way of CV line; irritates peripheral vein in long-term use
Protein-sparing therapy	• Crystalline amino acids in same amounts as TPN • Electrolytes, vitamins, minerals, and trace elements as ordered	• Nutritionally complete • Requires little mixing • May be started or stopped any time during the hospital stay • Other I.V. fluids, medications, and blood by-products may be administered through the same I.V. line • Not as likely to cause phlebitis as peripheral parenteral nutrition • Adds a major expense; has limited benefits
Total nutrient admixture	• One day's nutrients are contained in a single, 3-L bag (also called 3:1 solution)	• See TPN (above) • Reduces need to handle bag, cutting risk of contamination

Type	Solution components/liter	Special considerations
Total nutrient admixture *(continued)*	● Combines lipid emulsion with other parenteral solution components	● Decreases nursing time and reduces need for infusion sets and electronic devices, lowering facility costs, increasing patient mobility, and allowing easier adjustment to home care ● Has limited use because not all types and amounts of components are compatible ● Precludes use of certain infusion pumps because they can't accurately deliver large volumes of solution; precludes use of standard I.V. tubing filters because a 0.22-micron filter blocks lipid and albumin molecules
Peripheral parenteral nutrition (PPN)	● D_5W to $D_{10}W$ ● Crystalline amino acids 2.5% to 5% ● Electrolytes, minerals, vitamins, and trace elements as ordered ● Lipid emulsion 10% or 20% (1 L of dextrose 10% and amino acids 3.5% infused at the same time as 1 L of lipid emulsion = 1,440 nonprotein calories) ● Heparin or hydrocortisone as ordered	*Basic solution* ● Nutritionally complete for a short time ● Can't be used in nutritionally depleted patients ● Can't be used in volume-restricted patients because PPN requires large fluid volume ● Doesn't cause weight gain ● Avoids insertion and care of CV line but requires adequate venous access; site must be changed every 72 hours ● Delivers less hypertonic solutions than CV line TPN ● May cause phlebitis and increases risk of metabolic complications ● Less chance of metabolic complications than with CV line TPN *I.V. lipid emulsion* ● As effective as dextrose for caloric source ● Diminishes phlebitis if infused at the same time as basic nutrient solution ● Irritates vein in long-term use ● Reduces carbon dioxide buildup when pulmonary compromise is present

ripheral vein can handle. For example, most TPN solutions are six times more concentrated than blood. As a result, they must be delivered into a vein with a high rate of blood flow to dilute the solution.

The most common delivery route for TPN is through a central venous catheter (CVC) into the superior vena cava. The catheter may also be placed via the infraclavicular approach or, less commonly, via the supraclavicular, internal jugular, or antecubital fossa approach. (See *Central venous catheter pathways*.)

Equipment

Bag or bottle of prescribed parenteral nutrition solution ▪ sterile I.V. tubing with attached extension tubing ▪ 0.22-micron filter (or 1.2-micron filter if solution contains lipids or albumin) ▪ reflux valve ▪ time tape ▪ alcohol pads ▪ electronic infusion pump ▪ portable glucose monitor ▪ scale ▪ intake and output record ▪ sterile gloves ▪ optional: mask

Essential steps

▪ Prepare the necessary equipment.
  – Remove the solution from the refrigerator at least 1 hour before use to avoid pain, hypothermia, venous spasm, and venous constriction, which can result from delivery of a chilled solution.
  – Check the solution against the physician's order for correct patient name, expiration date, and formula components. Observe the container for cracks and the solution for cloudiness, turbidity, and particles. If any of these is present, return the solution to the pharmacy.
  – If administering a total nutrient admixture solution, look for a brown layer on the solution, which indicates that the lipid emulsion has "cracked," or separated from the solution. If present, return the solution to the pharmacy.
  – Assist with insertion of CVC as necessary. Ensure follow-up chest X-ray to confirm catheter placement

▪ Explain the procedure to the patient. Check the name on the solution container against the name on the patient's wristband. Next, put on gloves and, if specified by facility policy, a mask. Throughout the procedure, use strict sterile technique.

▪ In sequence, connect the pump tubing, the micron filter with attached extension tubing (if the tubing doesn't contain an in-line filter), and the reflux valve. Insert the filter as close to the catheter site as possible. If the tubing doesn't have luer-lock connections, tape all connections to prevent accidental separation, which could lead to air embolism, exsanguination, or sepsis. Next, squeeze the I.V. drip chamber and, holding it upright, insert the tubing spike into the I.V. bag or bottle. Next, release the drip chamber. Squeeze the drip chamber before spiking an I.V. bottle to prevent accidental dripping of the parenteral nutrition solution. An I.V. bag, however, shouldn't drip.

▪ Next, prime the tubing. Invert the filter at the distal end of the tubing and open the roller clamp. Let the solution fill the tubing and the filter. Gently tap it to dislodge air bubbles trapped in the Y-ports. Record the date and time you hung the fluid, and initial the parenteral nutrition solution container.

▪ Attach the setup to the infusion pump, and prepare it according to the manufacturer's instructions. Remove and discard gloves.

▪ With the patient in the supine position, flush the catheter with normal saline solution, according to the facility's policy. Next, put on gloves, and clean the catheter injection cap with an alcohol pad.

Central venous catheter pathways

A central venous catheter (CVC) is a sterile catheter made of polyurethane, polyvinyl chloride, or silicone rubber. It's inserted through a large vein such as the subclavian vein or, less commonly, the jugular vein. By providing access to the central veins, central venous (CV) therapy offers several benefits, such as allowing:
- CV pressure monitoring, which indicates blood volume or pump efficiency and permits aspiration of blood samples for diagnostic tests
- administration of I.V. fluids (in large amounts if necessary) in emergencies or when decreased peripheral circulation makes peripheral vein access difficult; when prolonged I.V. therapy reduces the number of accessible peripheral veins; when solutions must be diluted (for large fluid volumes or for irritating or hypertonic fluids such as total parenteral nu-

trition solutions); and when a patient requires long-term venous access
- multiple blood sampling without repeated venipuncture, thus helping to decrease the patient's anxiety and preserve or restore peripheral veins.

Peripheral CV therapy, a variation of CV therapy, involves the insertion of a catheter into a peripheral vein instead of a central vein, but with the catheter tip still lying in the CV circulation. A peripherally inserted central catheter usually enters at the basilic vein and terminates in the superior vena cava.

The illustrations below show several common pathways for CVC insertion. A CVC is typically inserted into the subclavian veins or in the internal jugular vein. The catheter usually terminates in the superior vena cava. If long-term placement is needed, the CVC is tunneled.

Insertion: subclavian vein
Termination: superior vena cava

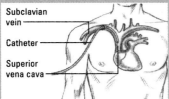

Insertion: internal jugular vein
Termination: superior vena cava

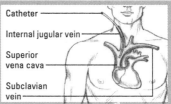

Insertion: basilic vein (peripheral)
Termination: superior vena cava

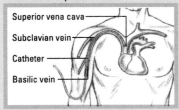

Insertion: through a subcutaneous tunnel to the subclavian vein (Dacron cuff holds catheter in place)
Termination: superior vena cava

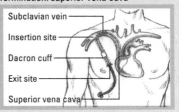

- If attaching the container of parenteral nutrition solution to a CV line, clamp the CV line before disconnecting it to prevent air from entering the catheter.

ALERT *If a clamp isn't available, ask the patient to perform Valsalva's maneuver just as you change the tubing if possible. If the patient is being mechanically ventilated, change the I.V. tubing immediately after the machine delivers a breath at peak inspiration. Both of these measures increase intrathoracic pressure and prevent air embolism, manifested as sudden onset of pallor, cyanosis, dyspnea, coughing, and tachycardia, progressing to syncope and shock. If any of these signs occur, place the patient on his left side in Trendelenburg's position, and notify the physician.*

- Using sterile technique, attach the tubing to the designated luer-locking port. After connecting the tubing, remove the clamp if applicable.
- Make sure the catheter junction is secure. Set the infusion pump at the ordered flow rate, and start the infusion.
- Label the tubing with the date and time of change.
- Because parenteral nutrition solution usually contains a large amount of glucose, start the infusion slowly to allow the patient's pancreatic beta cells time to increase their output of insulin. Depending on the patient's tolerance, parenteral nutrition is usually initiated at a rate of 40 to 50 ml/hour and then advanced by 25 ml/hour every 6 hours (as tolerated) until the desired infusion rate is achieved. Allow the solution to hang for no more than 24 hours.
- Change the solution as appropriate.

- Flush the catheter according to your facility's policy to maintain patency. Most facilities use a heparin flush solution available in premixed 10-ml multidose vials. Recommended concentrations vary from 10 to 100 units of heparin per milliliter. Use normal saline solution instead of heparin to maintain patency in two-way valved devices, such as the Groshong type of catheter, because research suggests that heparin isn't always needed to keep the line open.

ALERT *Before flushing a CVC, always aspirate to confirm the patency of the CVC, then inject the recommended type and amount of flush solution. After flushing the catheter, maintain positive pressure by keeping the thumb on the plunger of the syringe while withdrawing the needle. This prevents blood backflow and clotting in the line. If flushing a valved catheter, close the clamp just before the last of the flush solution leaves the syringe.*

Complications

Complications can occur at any time during infusion therapy. Traumatic complications, such as pneumothorax, typically occur on catheter insertion but may not be noticed until after the procedure is completed. Systemic complications, such as sepsis, typically occur later during infusion therapy. Other complications may include:

- phlebitis (especially in peripheral CV therapy)
- thrombus formation
- air embolism.

Catheter-related sepsis is the most serious complication of parenteral nutrition. Although rare, a malpositioned subclavian or jugular vein catheter may lead to thrombosis or sepsis. An air embolism, a potentially fatal complication, can occur during I.V. tubing changes if the tubing is inadvertently disconnected. It may also result from undetected hairline cracks in the tubing. Extravasation of parenteral nutrition solution can cause necrosis and then sloughing of the epidermis and dermis.

Nursing considerations

■ If you can't aspirate to check CVC patency before flushing, meet resistance when trying to flush the CVC, or the TPN solution doesn't flow right, suspect blockage. Follow the facility's policy for clearing a blocked CVC. (See *Clearing a blocked CVC,* page 414.)

■ Always infuse parenteral nutrition solution at a constant rate, without interruption, to avoid blood glucose fluctuations. If the infusion slows, consult the physician before changing the infusion rate.

■ Monitor the patient's vital signs every 2 to 4 hours or more often if indicated. Watch for an increased temperature, an early sign of catheter-related sepsis.

■ Check the patient's blood glucose level every 6 hours. Some patients may require supplementary insulin, which the pharmacist may add directly to the solution. The patient may require additional subcutaneous doses.

■ Record daily intake and output accurately. Specify the volume and type of each fluid, and calculate the daily caloric intake.

■ Monitor the results of routine laboratory tests, and report abnormal findings to the physician to allow for appropriate changes in the parenteral nutrition solution. Such tests typically include measurement of serum electrolyte levels, cal-

cium, blood urea nitrogen (BUN) levels, and creatinine levels at least three times weekly; serum magnesium and phosphorus levels twice weekly; liver function studies, complete blood count and differential, and serum albumin and transferrin levels weekly; and urine nitrogen balance and creatinine-height index studies weekly. A serum zinc level is obtained at the start of parenteral nutrition therapy. The physician may also order serum prealbumin levels, total lymphocyte count, amino acid levels, fatty acid-phospholipid fraction, skin testing, and expired gas analysis.

■ Monitor kidney function by monitoring BUN and creatinine levels; increases can indicate excess amino acid intake. Assess nitrogen balance with 24-hour urine collection.

■ Assess liver function by periodically monitoring liver enzyme, bilirubin, triglyceride, and cholesterol levels. Abnormal values may indicate an intolerance or excess of lipid emulsions or a problem with metabolizing the protein or glucose in the TPN formula.

■ Physically assess the patient daily. If ordered, measure arm circumference and skin-fold thickness over the triceps. Weigh him at the same time each morning after voiding, in similar clothing, and on the same scale. Suspect fluid imbalance if he gains more than 1 lb (0.5 kg) daily.

■ Change the dressing over the catheter according to your facility's policy or whenever the dressing becomes wet, soiled, or nonocclusive. Always use strict sterile technique. When performing dressing changes, watch for signs of phlebitis and catheter retraction from the vein. Measure the catheter length from the insertion site to the hub for verification.

Clearing a blocked CVC

Maintaining a free-flowing central venous catheter (CVC) is essential. Usually, this is accomplished by adhering to a specified policy for flushing the catheter. Unfortunately, even with the most meticulous care, occlusion or blockage of a CVC can occur. Many types of infusion pumps sound an alarm to signify an occlusion. It most commonly results from one of the following:

• formation of fibrin sheath (due to an inflammatory-like response by the body sensing the catheter as a foreign object and attempting to wall it off by producing fibrin)

• development of a clot within the catheter

• deposition of drugs, minerals, or lipids inside the catheter.

If you encounter difficulty flushing the catheter, check for mechanical problems before attempting to flush it. Look for kinks in the tubing anywhere along it, such as in the extension tubing or the catheter itself. Check to make sure that all of the clamps are opened, that there is solution in the I.V. container leading to the tubing, and that the infusion pump is working properly. If you determine that there's no mechanical problem, attempt to clear the catheter following your facility's policy.

At one time, urokinase was the drug of choice to clear an occluded catheter; however, it's no longer used for this purpose. Recently, a new drug has been approved for use in clearing occluded CVCs, alteplase (Activase), a tissue plasminogen activator. This drug is indicated for restoring the function of a CVC that's occluded due to fibrin sheath or thrombus. It isn't indicated for clearing occlusions due to deposits of lipids, minerals, or drug precipitates.

If your facility's policy allows the use of alteplase, follow these guidelines to clear the catheter:

• Reconstitute the alteplase according to the manufacturer's instructions, yielding a concentration of 1 mg/1 ml; be sure to reconstitute the drug just before use.

• For patients weighing 66 lb (30 kg) or more, prepare 2 mg of the drug (2 ml) in a syringe.

• Aspirate the contents of the CVC.

• Instill the dose into the CVC and allow the drug to remain (dwell) in the catheter for 30 minutes. If appropriate, follow the drug with 1 ml of normal saline to allow the alteplase to flow out of the catheter to the fibrin sheath.

• After 30 minutes, attempt to aspirate the catheter.

• If successful (as demonstrated by a blood return), aspirate 4 to 5 ml of blood from the catheter to ensure that the drug and any residual clots are removed; irrigate the CVC with normal saline.

• If unsuccessful, allow the drug to remain in the catheter for 120 minutes, and then attempt to aspirate. If successful, follow the method described above; if the catheter still isn't clear, instill a second dose of the drug, and allow it to dwell for 30 minutes. If this second dose doesn't clear the catheter, prepare the patient for contrast X-rays involving the veins and catheter.

■ Change the tubing and filters every 24 hours or according to your facility's policy.

■ Closely monitor the catheter site for swelling, which may indicate infiltration. Extravasation of parenteral nutrition solution can lead to tissue necrosis.

ALERT *Use caution when using the parenteral nutrition line for other functions. Don't use a single-lumen CVC to infuse blood or blood products, to give a bolus injection, to administer simultaneous I.V. solutions, to measure CV pressure, or to draw blood for laboratory tests.*

■ Provide regular mouth care. Provide emotional support. Keep in mind that patients commonly associate eating with positive feelings and become disturbed when they can't eat.

■ When discontinuing TPN, decrease the infusion rate slowly, depending on the patient's current glucose intake, to minimize the risk of hyperinsulinemia and resulting hypoglycemia. Weaning usually takes place over 24 to 48 hours but can be completed in 4 to 6 hours if the patient receives sufficient oral or I.V. carbohydrates.

■ Teach the patient the potential adverse effects and complications of parenteral nutrition. Encourage the patient to inspect his mouth regularly for signs of parotitis, glossitis, and oral lesions. Tell him that he may have fewer bowel movements while receiving parenteral nutrition therapy. Encourage him to remain physically active to help his body use the nutrients more fully.

■ Document the times of the dressing, filter, and solution changes; the condition of the catheter insertion site; your observations of the patient's condition; and any complications and interventions.

■ Document results of serial laboratory test monitoring on the appropriate flowchart to determine the patient's progress and response. Note any abnormal, adverse, or altered responses. While weaning from TPN, document his dietary intake.

Transjugular intrahepatic portosystemic shunt

Transjugular intrahepatic portosystemic shunt (TIPS) is a procedure performed to relieve portal hypertension in patients with hepatic disease. It's indicated for patients who have active variceal bleeding even after emergency endoscopic or pharmacologic treatment and those with recurrent variceal bleeding despite adequate endoscopic treatment. It may be used for patients with isolated bleeding from the gastric fundus and continued ascites unresponsive to other therapies. TIPS may also be used to control portal hypertension until a suitable donor for a liver transplant can be found.

Insertion of the shunt allows blood to flow from the portal vein to the hepatic vein and subsequently into the vena cava. As a result, blood returning to the heart from the spleen and intestine bypasses the liver, thereby reducing portal hypertension.

Procedure

TIPS is performed by an interventional radiologist using general anesthesia or conscious sedation. A catheter is placed into the right jugular vein and threaded through the superior and inferior vena cava to the hepatic vein using fluoroscopy and ultrasonography to guide the catheter placement. A guide wire with an attached needle located inside the catheter is passed through the wall of the hepatic vein, across a small gap, and then into the portal vein. Dye is injected through the catheter to ensure that the portal vein has been accessed.

A balloon is used to dilate the tract, and one to three stents are placed in the area connecting the veins and overlapping the liver. The stents are opened to their maximum diameter with a balloon. Dye is injected to ensure that the stents are positioned and secured properly and that blood flows from the portal vein through the stents into the hepatic vein, and then into the vena cava. (See *Transjugular intrahepatic portosystemic shunt insertion*.)

Complications

Complications can occur due to the technique used to insert the shunt as well as from the effects of shunting of the blood. Complications from the technique may include:

- hematoma of the neck or liver area
- cardiac arrhythmias
- liver capsule rupture
- fistula.

Complications associated with the effects of shunting may include:

- hepatic encephalopathy
- bacteremia
- hepatic failure.

Additionally, infection of the stent may occur.

Nursing considerations

When caring for the patient undergoing a TIPS procedure, nursing care focuses on ensuring that the patient is at the optimal level of functioning based on his liver disease and on preparing the patient and his family physically and emotionally for the procedure, including instructing the patient about the procedure and events after it as well as instituting measures to prevent postprocedural complications.

Before TIPS insertion

- Instruct the patient and his family about the transplant and necessary diagnostic tests such as antigen typing.
- Reinforce the physician's explanation of the procedure, anesthesia and sedation, equipment, and techniques used.
- Keep the patient nothing by mouth (NPO), if he isn't already, for approximately 6 hours before the procedure.
- Administer medications such as sedatives as ordered.

ALERT *Administer sedatives cautiously in a patient with underlying liver disease. Be sure to establish a baseline for the patient's level of consciousness (LOC) before administering the medication to ensure valid assessments of the patient's LOC after the medication has been given.*

- Review techniques of incentive spirometry and range of motion with the patient.
- Ensure that he or a responsible family member has signed a consent form.
- Provide emotional support to the patient and his family, especially when the patient has experienced variceal bleeding without effective treatment.

After TIPS insertion

- Assess vital signs at least every 15 minutes for the first hour, then every 30 minutes for the next hour, and then every hour until stable.
- Monitor the patient's LOC, including observations for increasing level of alertness; reorient patient as necessary. Continue to monitor LOC frequently for changes that may indicate adverse effects of the procedure or possible bleeding.
- Inspect catheter insertion site closely for signs and symptoms of bleeding

Transjugular intrahepatic portosystemic shunt insertion

A transjugular intrahepatic portosystemic shunt (TIPS) can be used to relieve portal hypertension in patients with variceal bleeding, or in patients with portal hypertension who are waiting for a liver transplant. The illustration below shows the placement of the shunt.

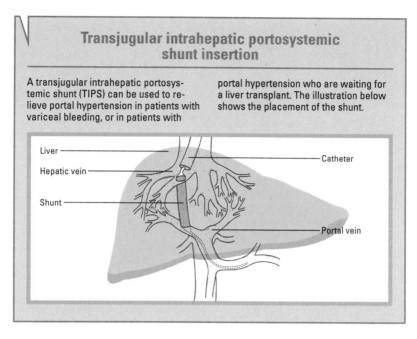

Liver
Hepatic vein
Shunt
Catheter
Portal vein

and infection. Change dressing as ordered.

🔆 **ALERT** *Keep in mind that because of the patient's underlying liver disease, coagulation may be altered. Monitor the dressing at least every 30 minutes initially, and then every 1 to 2 hours. Immediately report any bright red drainage on the dressing.*

■ Assess cardiopulmonary status at least every hour, noting changes in heart or breath sounds. Institute continuous cardiac monitoring to evaluate for possible arrhythmias secondary to the TIPS procedure or to possible variceal bleeding. Monitor hemodynamic parameters as ordered to evaluate the patient's fluid-volume status.

■ Assess abdomen for bowel sounds and distention. Measure abdominal girth. When bowel sounds return, expect to begin oral feedings.

🔆 **ALERT** *Insertion should cause the patient's abdominal girth to gradually decrease. However, because of the underlying liver disease, bleeding can occur at the site of the catheter insertion into the hepatic and portal veins. Be alert to increases in abdominal girth, and notify the physician immediately. This increase may indicate bleeding, or it could suggest that the stent isn't functioning.*

■ Assess for complaints of abdominal cramping (an expected finding after the procedure), and administer medication as ordered.

■ Check gag reflex, and maintain NPO status until gag reflex returns.

5

Renal system challenges

Imagine that a patient demonstrates a dramatic decrease in urine output. Does this indicate an infection of the urinary tract or a more serious condition such as acute renal failure? How would you go about assessing this patient? If the patient informed you that he had type 1 diabetes, would the information influence your assessment? If acute renal failure were diagnosed, would you be able to classify it as prerenal, intrarenal, or postrenal? While caring for this patient, you notice tall, peaked T waves. What electrolyte imbalance might be occurring? What measures would you expect to institute to correct this imbalance?

A patient is scheduled for peritoneal dialysis. How would you prepare the patient? What if the patient has a column disk peritoneal catheter inserted? Would you expect the patient to be more or less comfortable during dialysis? Another patient is to undergo hemodialysis with arteriovenous (AV) fistula. What key assessments do you need to make? How does hemodialysis with an AV fistula differ from that with a AV shunt?

Suppose a patient required continuous renal replacement therapy, specifically continuous venovenous hemofiltration? Would you know how to perform this procedure? For which complications would you be alert?

What if the arterial pressure alarm sounds? What would you do first? Another patient is scheduled for a renal transplant using a living donor organ. Would you expect the patient's diseased kidney to be removed? How would you prepare the patient for the surgery? Suppose the patient develops a high fever, oliguria, hypertension, and elevated white blood cell count approximately 2 weeks after the transplant. Is the patient experiencing an infection or rejection? And if a rejection, what type of rejection is occurring? In this chapter, you'll find answers to these questions and additional information that will allow you to address the major challenges involving the renal system commonly encountered by critical care nurses.

 MULTISYSTEM DISORDER

Acute renal failure

Acute renal failure refers to the sudden interruption of renal function resulting from obstruction, reduced circulation, or renal parenchymal disease. About 5% of all hospitalized patients develop acute renal failure. Renal failure is typically classified as prerenal, intrarenal, or postrenal, and each classification has a different cause. (See *Causes of acute renal failure*.)

Causes of acute renal failure

Acute renal failure may be prerenal, intrarenal, or postrenal. All conditions that lead to prerenal failure involve impaired renal perfusion, resulting in a decreased glomerular filtration rate and increased proximal tubular reabsorption of sodium and water. Intrarenal failure results from damage to the kidneys themselves, whereas postrenal failure results from obstruction of urine flow.

Causes of prerenal failure
- Antihypertensive drugs
- Arrhythmias
- Arterial embolism
- Arterial or venous thrombosis
- Burns
- Cardiac tamponade
- Cardiogenic shock
- Dehydration
- Disseminated intravascular coagulation
- Diuretic overuse
- Eclampsia
- Heart failure
- Hemorrhage
- Hypovolemic shock
- Malignant hypertension
- Myocardial infarction
- Sepsis
- Severe vasoconstriction
- Trauma
- Tumor
- Vasculitis

Causes of intrarenal failure
- Acute glomerulonephritis
- Acute interstitial nephritis
- Acute pyelonephritis
- Bilateral renal vein thrombosis
- Crush injuries
- Malignant nephrosclerosis
- Myopathy
- Nephrotoxins
- Obstetric complications
- Papillary necrosis
- Polyarteritis nodosa
- Poorly treated prerenal failure
- Renal myeloma
- Sickle cell disease
- Systemic lupus erythematosus
- Transfusion reaction
- Vasculitis

Causes of postrenal failure
- Bladder obstruction
- Ureteral obstruction
- Urethral obstruction

Renal failure is usually reversible with treatment. However, it can take as long as 6 months to 1 year for the patient's kidney function to return to his baseline level. If not treated, it may progress to end-stage renal disease, uremia, and death.

Pathophysiology

Each classification of acute renal failure — prerenal, intrarenal, and postrenal — has its own pathophysiology. Prerenal failure occurs when a condition that diminishes blood flow to the kidneys leads to hypoperfusion. Examples include hypovolemia, hypotension, vasoconstriction, and inadequate cardiac output. When renal blood flow is interrupted, so is oxygen delivery. The ensuing hypoxemia and ischemia can rapidly and irreversibly damage the kidney. The tubules are most susceptible to the effects of hypoxemia: Between 40% and 80% of all cases of acute renal failure are caused by prerenal azotemia, a consequence of renal hypoperfusion. The impaired blood flow results in decreased glomerular filtration rate (GFR) and increased tubular reabsorption of sodium and water. A decrease in GFR causes electrolyte imbalances and metabolic acidosis. Usually, restoring renal blood flow and glomerular filtration reverses azotemia.

Intrarenal failure, also called intrinsic or parenchymal renal failure, results from damage to the kidneys themselves, usually from acute tubular necrosis. Causes of intrarenal failure are classified as nephrotoxic, inflammatory, or ischemic. When the damage is caused by nephrotoxicity or inflammation, the delicate layer under the epithelium (the basement membrane) becomes irreparably damaged, commonly leading to chronic renal failure. Severe or prolonged lack of blood flow by ischemia may lead to renal damage (ischemic parenchymal injury) and excess nitrogen in the blood (intrinsic renal azotemia). Acute tubular necrosis, the precursor to intrarenal failure, can result from ischemic damage to renal parenchyma during unrecognized or poorly treated prerenal failure, or from obstetric complications, such as eclampsia, postpartum renal failure, septic abortion, or uterine hemorrhage. The fluid loss causes hypotension, which leads to ischemia. The ischemic tissue generates toxic oxygen-free radicals, which cause swelling, injury, and necrosis.

Another cause of intrarenal failure is the use of nephrotoxins, including analgesics, anesthetics, heavy metals, radiographic contrast media, organic solvents, and antimicrobials, particularly aminoglycoside antibiotics. These drugs accumulate in the renal cortex, causing renal failure that manifests well after treatment or other toxin exposure. The necrosis caused by nephrotoxins tends to be uniform and limited to the proximal tubules, whereas ischemia

necrosis tends to be patchy and distributed along various parts of the nephron.

Postrenal failure results from bilateral obstruction of urine outflow. The cause may be in the bladder, ureter, or urethra. Bladder obstruction can result from anticholinergic drugs, autonomic nerve dysfunction, infection, or tumors. Ureteral obstructions, which restrict blood flow from the kidneys to the bladder, can result from blood clots, calculi, edema or inflammation, necrotic renal papillae, retroperitoneal fibrosis or hemorrhage, surgery (accidental ligation) and tumor, or uric acid crystals. Urethral obstruction can be the result of prostatic hyperplasia, tumor, or strictures.

Regardless of the classification of acute renal failure (prerenal, intrarenal, or postrenal), the patient usually passes through three distinct phases: oliguric, diuretic, and recovery. During the oliguric phase, oliguria may be the result of one factor or several factors. Necrosis of the tubules can cause sloughing of cells, cast formations, and ischemic edema. The resulting tubular obstruction causes a retrograde increase in pressure and a decrease in GFR. Renal failure can occur within 24 hours from this effect. Glomerular filtration may remain normal in some cases of renal failure, but tubular reabsorption of filtrate may be accelerated. In this instance, ischemia may increase tubular permeability and cause backleak. Another concept is that intrarenal release of angiotensin II or redistribution of blood flow from the cortex to the medulla may constrict the afferent arterioles, increasing glomerular permeability and decreasing GFR.

Urine output may remain at less than 30 ml/hour or 400 ml/day for a few days to weeks. Before damage occurs, the kidneys respond to decreased blood flow by conserving sodium and water. Damage impairs the kidney's ability to conserve sodium. Fluid (water) volume excess, azotemia (elevated serum levels of urea, creatinine, and uric acid), and electrolyte imbalance occur. Ischemic or toxic injury leads to the release of mediators and intrarenal vasoconstriction. Medullary hypoxia results in the swelling of tubular and endothelial cells, adherence of neutrophils to capillaries and venules, and inappropriate platelet activation. Increasing ischemia and vasoconstriction further limit perfusion. Injured cells lose polarity, and the ensuing disruption of tight junctions between the cells promotes back-leak of filtrate. Ischemia impairs the function of energy-dependent membrane pumps, and calcium accumulates in the cells, further stimulating vasoconstriction and activating proteases and other enzymes. Untreated prerenal oliguria may lead to acute tubular necrosis.

As the kidneys become unable to conserve sodium and water, the diuretic phase, marked by increased urine secretion of more than 400 ml/24 hours, ensues. GFR may be normal or increased, but tubular support mechanisms are abnormal. Excretion of dilute urine causes dehydration and electrolyte imbalances. High blood urea nitrogen (BUN) levels produce osmotic diuresis and consequent deficits of potassium, sodium, and water. The diuretic phase may last days or weeks. The recovery phase is a gradual return to normal or near-normal renal function over 3 to 12 months. If the cause of the diuresis is corrected, azotemia gradually disappears and the patient recovers.

AGE ISSUE *Even with treatment, an elderly patient is particularly susceptible to volume overload, precipitating acute pulmonary edema, hypertensive crisis, hyperkalemia, and infection.*

Comprehensive assessment

The patient's history may include a disorder that can cause renal failure, and he may have a recent history of fever, chills, central nervous system (CNS) problems such as headache, and GI problems, such as anorexia, nausea, vomiting, diarrhea, and constipation. He may appear irritable, drowsy, and confused or demonstrate other alterations in his level of consciousness caused by altered cerebral perfusion. In advanced stages, seizures and coma may occur. Depending on the stage of renal failure, his urine output may be oliguric (less than 400 ml/24 hours) or anuric (less than 100 ml/24 hours).

Inspection may uncover evidence of bleeding abnormalities, such as petechiae and ecchymosis from bleeding abnormalities. Hematemesis may occur. The skin may be dry and pruritic (due to buildup of toxins) and, rarely, you may note urea frost. Mucous membranes may be dry (because of stimulation of the sympathetic nervous system), and the patient's breath may have a uremic odor. If the patient has hyperkalemia, muscle weakness may occur.

Auscultation may detect tachycardia and, possibly, an irregular rhythm. Bibasilar crackles may be heard if the patient has heart failure. Palpation and percussion may reveal abdominal pain, if pancreatitis or peritonitis occurs, and peripheral edema, if the patient has heart failure.

Diagnosis

Diagnosis of acute renal failure is based on the following:

■ Blood test results indicating acute intrarenal failure include elevated BUN, serum creatinine, and potassium levels as well as low hematocrit and hemoglobin levels.

■ Urine studies reveal casts, cellular debris, and decreased specific gravity; in glomerular diseases, proteinuria and urine osmolality close to serum osmolality. The urine sodium level is under 20 mEq/L if oliguria results from decreased perfusion and above 40 mEq/L if it results from an intrarenal problem.

■ Creatinine clearance test (which measures the GFR) provides an estimate of the number of remaining functioning nephrons.

■ Serum electrolyte levels reveal evidence of electrolyte imbalances

■ Arterial blood gas (ABG) values reveal decreased pH and bicarbonate levels indicating metabolic acidosis

■ Electrocardiogram (ECG) shows tall, peaked T waves; a widening QRS complex; and disappearing P waves if hyperkalemia is present.

■ Other studies, such as kidney ultrasonography, plain films of the abdomen, kidney-ureter-bladder radiography, excretory urography, renal scan, retrograde pyelography, computed tomography scans, and nephrotomography, help determine the cause of renal failure.

Collaborations

Because acute renal failure affects many of the body processes, a multidisciplinary approach to care is needed. Numerous professionals may be required to work in conjunction with medical and nursing personnel. A renal specialist or nephrologist can help evaluate, treat, and manage the patient's kidney function. Respiratory and cardiology specialists may be consulted, depending on the patient's history and complications he may develop. Nutritional therapy may be involved to help institute necessary restrictions or supplementations. Physical and occupational therapy may be necessary to help with energy conservation and rehabilitation depending on the patient's condition and length of stay. If a prolonged hospital stay is expected and the patient requires long-term care or home care, social services may be consulted early on in the patient's care. The patient may also benefit from psychological or spiritual counseling if he's acutely ill or will require continued care even on discharge.

Treatment and care

Supportive measures include a diet high in calories and low in protein, sodium, and potassium, with supplemental vitamins and restricted fluids. Meticulous electrolyte monitoring is essential to detect hyperkalemia. If hyperkalemia occurs, acute therapy may include hypertonic glucose-and-insulin infusions and sodium bicarbonate administered I.V. as well as sodium polystyrene sulfonate, by mouth or enema, to remove potassium from the body.

If the initial treatment fails to control uremic symptoms, the patient may require hemodialysis, peritoneal dialysis, or continuous renal replacement therapy. Early initiation of diuretic

Drugs and acute renal failure

Many drugs are eliminated by the kidneys. Therefore, when your patient has acute renal failure, drug dosages may need to be adjusted to avoid overburdening the patient's already compromised kidney function. Highlighted below are some commonly used drugs that require a reduction in dosage and some examples of drugs that should be avoided for the patient with acute renal failure.

Drugs requiring reduced dosage may include:
- ACE inhibitors
- cefazolin
- ciprofloxacin
- digoxin
- histamine-2 receptor antagonists, such as cimetidine, famotidine, nizatidine, and ranitidine
- magnesium-containing antacids and laxatives
- meperidine
- penicillins
- phenobarbital
- sulfonamides.

The following drugs should be avoided in patients with acute renal failure:
- amikacin and other aminoglycosides, such as gentamicin, kanamycin, neomycin (oral form), netilmicin, tobramycin (parenteral form), because of the increased risk of nephrotoxicity
- amiloride and other potassium-sparing diuretics, such as spironolactone, because of the increased risk of potassium retention, which compounds and increases the patient's risk of life-threatening hyperkalemia
- cisplatin, because of the increased risk of nephrotoxicity
- lithium carbonate, because of the increased risk of nephrotoxicity as well as drug toxicity. (Renal dysfunction increases the plasma half life of the drug, predisposing the patient to possible toxic drug levels.)

therapy during the oliguric phase may benefit the patient. Because there are no specific therapies for the treatment of acute renal failure due to ischemia or nephrotoxicity, identifying high-risk groups and taking preventive measures are important. After major surgery or trauma, aggressive restoration of fluid volume can help reduce acute renal failure. Aggressive fluid restoration is also important in cases of burns or of infection such as cholera. Careful and prudent administration of drug dosages can help prevent nephrotoxicity (See *Drugs and acute renal failure*.)

Monitoring blood levels and adjusting medication dosages accordingly is helpful in limiting injury. Allopurinol and forced diuresis may be helpful in individuals at high risk such as those undergoing cancer chemotherapy.

Complications
Complications of acute renal failure may include:
- chronic renal failure
- ischemic parenchymal injury
- intrinsic renal azotemia
- electrolyte imbalance
- metabolic acidosis
- pulmonary edema
- hypertensive crisis
- infection.

Nursing considerations
- Monitor level of consciousness at least every 2 to 4 hours and vital signs every hour, or more frequently if indi-

cated. Notify the physician of any changes.

![ALERT icon] **ALERT** *Keep in mind that fever increases the breakdown of protein, which causes potassium to be released from the cells, increasing the patient's risk of hyperkalemia. Moreover, patients with acute renal failure commonly exhibit mild hypothermia. Be alert for rises in temperature of 1° or 2°, which could be significant.*

■ Assess fluid balance status, including skin turgor, evidence of peripheral, sacral, or periorbital edema (and degree of pitting if any), and intake and output, including wound drainage, nasogastric tube output, and diarrhea. Monitor urine output every hour; insert an indwelling urinary catheter if indicated. Assess daily weight for trends.

■ Anticipate insertion of central venous or pulmonary artery catheter to assess patient's hemodynamic status. Monitor parameters as ordered.

■ Maintain fluid restrictions as ordered. Expect fluid to be replaced in the exact amount to that of the fluid lost. Provide the patient with ice chips, chewing gum, or hard candy to alleviate thirst.

![ALERT icon] **ALERT** *Be sure to include the amount of ice chips consumed by the patient as part of the patient's intake and fluid allotment. When determining the amount of intake as ice, consider the fluid intake to be half the amount of the ice chips. For example, 2 oz ice chips is equivalent to 1 oz fluid intake.*

■ Check urine specific gravity and osmolality as ordered.

![ALERT icon] **ALERT** *Be aware that with prerenal failure, urine specific gravity is usually greater than 1.020 and urine osmolality is increased up to 500 mOsm; with intrarenal failure, specific gravity usually is less than 1.010 and osmolality is approximately 350 mOsm.*

■ Assess cardiopulmonary status frequently, including heart and breath sounds. Report any shortness of breath, basilar crackles, gallops, pericardial friction rub, or the presence of an S_3 or S_4 since these may be signs of fluid overload.

■ Obtain laboratory and diagnostic tests as ordered. Monitor results of serum BUN and creatinine levels, ABGs, and serum electrolyte levels closely; be prepared to intervene based on the imbalance that occurs. (See *Electrolyte and acid-base imbalances associated with acute renal failure*, pages 426 to 429.)

■ Institute continuous cardiac monitoring, and monitor for arrhythmias secondary to electrolyte imbalances; continuously assess the patient for signs and symptoms of electrolyte imbalances. Have emergency resuscitative equipment readily available.

■ Administer diuretic agents as ordered.

![ALERT icon] **ALERT** *Diuretics promote water excretion, which may predispose the patient to a fluid volume deficit. In addition, diuretics affect electrolyte reabsorption and excretion, further compounding the risk of electrolyte imbalances. Moreover, treatment for one imbalance can ultimately lead to the opposite imbalance. Monitor the patient closely.*

■ Assess the patient frequently, especially during emergency treatment to lower potassium levels. If he's hyperkalemic, avoid any potassium-containing medications. Administer sodium polystyrene sulfonate, orally or rectally as ordered. If given rectally, encourage the patient to retain the enema for approximately 30 to 60 minutes to ensure maximum effectiveness. If he receives hypertonic glucose-and-insulin infusions, monitor potassium and glucose levels.

■ Administer phosphate binders, such as aluminum hydroxide antacids, to bind phosphorus and treat hyperphosphatemia. Monitor the patient for constipation, a possible adverse effect of phosphate binders. Expect to administer bulk laxatives and stool softeners as ordered.

■ Assess the patient for signs and symptoms of GI bleeding. Test all drainage for occult blood. Monitor hemoglobin level and hematocrit for decreases.

ALERT *A patient with acute renal failure already has a low hemoglobin level and hematocrit because of the anemia associated with decreased erythropoietin production, minor ulcerative bleeding, repeated blood specimens, and shortened life of the red blood cells (RBCs). In addition, platelet function is altered, causing them to be less adhesive, resulting in an increased risk of bleeding. Be alert for continued decreases in hemoglobin level and hematocrit, along with a rise in BUN but without a corresponding rise in serum creatinine. These findings suggest GI bleeding that requires immediate intervention. Administer erythropoietin and packed RBCs as ordered.*

■ Institute bleeding precautions to minimize the patient's risk of bleeding.

■ Prepare the patient for hemodialysis, peritoneal dialysis, or continuous renal replacement therapy, as indicated. (See "Continuous renal replacement therapy," page 430, "Hemodialysis," page 435, and "Peritoneal dialysis," page 445.) Administer prescribed medications after treatment is completed, because many medications are removed from the blood during treatment.

■ Institute infection control measures during care, because the patient with acute renal failure is highly susceptible to infection. Don't allow staff members or visitors with upper respiratory tract infections to come in contact with the patient. Use standard precautions when handling blood and body fluids.

■ Evaluate and maintain nutritional status. Provide a diet high in calories and low in protein, sodium, and potassium, with vitamin supplements. Give the anorectic patient small, frequent meals.

■ Prevent complications of immobility by encouraging frequent coughing and deep breathing and by performing passive range-of-motion exercises. Help the patient walk as soon as possible. Add lubricating lotion to his bath water to combat skin dryness.

■ Provide mouth care frequently to lubricate dry mucous membranes. If stomatitis occurs, use an antibiotic solution, if ordered, and have the patient swish it around in his mouth before swallowing.

■ Provide meticulous perineal care to reduce the risk of ascending urinary tract infection in women and to protect skin integrity caused by frequent loose, irritating stools, particularly when sodium polystyrene sulfonate is used.

■ Use appropriate safety measures, such as side rails and restraints, be-

(Text continues on page 430.)

Electrolyte and acid-base imbalances associated with acute renal failure

Imbalance	Cause
Hypernatremia (serum level greater than 145 mEq/L)	Inability of kidneys to excrete sodium; decreased intake of water or increased water losses; overuse of sodium-containing parenteral solutions
Hyponatremia (serum level less than 135 mEq/L)	Sodium loss via vomiting, diarrhea, excessive sweating, use of potent diuretics; use of sodium-free I.V. solutions
Hyperkalemia (serum level greater than 5 mEq/L)	Inability of kidneys to excrete potassium; catabolism leading to release of potassium from cells
Hypokalemia (serum level less than 3.5 mEq/L)	Inadequate intake over a prolonged period of time; use of potassium-reducing diuretics without replacement; excessive losses due to diarrhea, vomiting, or GI suctioning

Assessment findings	Treatment
• Severe thirst • Fatigue • Restlessness • Agitation • Low-grade fever • Flushed skin • Increased serum osmolality • Increased urine specific gravity	• Water replacement orally or I.V. • Diuretics • Seizure precautions
• Abdominal cramps • Diarrhea • Postural hypotension • Cool, clammy skin • Irritability • Apprehension • Headache • Seizures • Coma • Decreased serum osmolality • Decreased urine sodium	• Sodium and water replacements (water restriction if extracellular fluid volume is increased) • Administration of other, corresponding electrolytes, if low • Hypertonic sodium chloride I.V., if serum level severely decreased • Seizure precautions • Safety precautions
• Tall peaked T waves, loss of P waves, prolonged PR interval, widening of QRS complex • Irritability • Abdominal cramps and distention • Paresthesia • Irregular pulse • Cardiac standstill if level greater than 8.5 mEq/L	• I.V. calcium gluconate to reverse neuromuscular and cardiac effects of potassium • I.V. glucose and insulin to move potassium back into the cells (temporarily lowers serum potassium level) • I.V. sodium bicarbonate to move potassium back into the cells (temporarily lowers serum potassium level) • Administration of cation exchange resins such as Kayexalate orally or as a retention enema • Avoidance of high-potassium foods • Protein-restricted intake with adequate intake of carbohydrates to spare protein • Serum potassium level monitoring
• Prolonged PR interval, flattened or inverted T wave, depressed ST segment, presence of U wave • Ventricular arrhythmias • Muscle weakness, paresthesia • Decreased bowel sounds • Weak, irregular pulse • Decreased reflexes	• Potassium replacement orally or as I.V. infusion (never administered I.V. push) • Dietary intake of foods high in potassium • Potassium-sparing diuretics

(continued)

Electrolyte and acid-base imbalances associated with acute renal failure (continued)

Imbalance	Cause
Hypocalcemia (serum level less than 8.5 mg/dl)	Inadequate calcium absorption in diet; elevated phosphorus levels causing calcium to precipitate out of tissues; lack of conversion of vitamin D leading to inadequate absorption and utilization of calcium
Hyperphosphatemia (serum level greater than 2.4 mEq/L)	Inability of kidneys to excrete excessive phosphorous
Hypermagnesemia (serum level greater than 2.5 mEq/L)	Use of magnesium-containing medications
Retention of magnesium as a result of decreased glomerular filtration rate and destruction of the tubules
Metabolic acidosis	Inability of the kidneys to remove excess acid (hydrogen ions) produced normally by metabolic activities; reduction in nephron function leading to decreased production and absorption of bicarbonate in the tubules and to inhibition of ammonia and hydrochloric acid conversion for excretion; formation of lactic acid from hypoxemia

Assessment findings	Treatment
• Circumoral numbness and tingling • Muscle twitching and spasms • Altered mental status • Positive Chvostek's and Trousseau's signs • Prolonged QT interval secondary to elongated ST segment • Hyperactive reflexes • Tetany	• Calcium replacement orally or I.V. • I.V. calcium gluconate, if tetany is present • Magnesium replacement, if indicated • Administration of vitamin D to promote calcium absorption from GI tract • Use of phosphorus-binder antacids, if elevated before administering calcium
• Anorexia • Nausea, vomiting • Muscle weakness • Hyperreflexia • Tetany • Tachycardia • Electrocardiogram changes similar to that for hypocalcemia	• Administration of phosphorus-binding antacids (calcium acetate and calcium carbonate preferred) • Dialysis, if severe • Dietary restrictions of phosphorus-containing foods and products
• Diaphoresis • Flushing • Hypotension • Drowsiness • Weak to absent deep tendon reflexes • Bradycardia • Lethargy • Respiratory compromise • Prolonged PR, QRS, and QT intervals (if level greater than 5 mEq/L); heart block and cardiac arrest (if level greater than 15 mEq/L)	• Discontinuation of causative agent • Avoidance of foods high in magnesium • Diuretic therapy along with I.V. infusion of 0.45% sodium chloride solution • I.V. administration of calcium gluconate to counteract the neuromuscular effects of magnesium • Dialysis with magnesium-free dialysate (for severely elevated levels and diminished renal function)
• pH less than 7.35; bicarbonate level less than 24 mEq/L • Hyperkalemia (possible) • Weakness • Altered mental status • Fatigue • Shortness of breath and Kussmaul's respirations • Tachycardia (unless pH less than 7 then bradycardia) • Anorexia • Headache • Arrhythmias such as ventricular fibrillation • Seizures • Coma	• Seizure precautions • Treatment of underlying disorder such as hemodialysis or peritoneal dialysis in acute renal failure • I.V. fluid administration; I.V. infusion of bicarbonate (or I.V. push in emergencies) • Mechanical ventilation

cause the patient with CNS involvement may become dizzy or confused.

■ Assess the patient's ability to resume normal activities of daily living, and plan for the gradual resumption of activity; arrange for consultations with physical and occupational therapy as ordered.

■ Provide emotional support to the patient and his family.

Patient teaching

■ Reassure the patient and his family by clearly explaining diagnostic tests, treatments, and procedures.

■ Explain to the patient about prescribed medications and avoidance of over-the-counter medications unless allowed by the physician. Stress the importance of complying with the regimen, including following the prescribed diet, fluid allowance, and laboratory testing.

■ Instruct the patient about monitoring daily weight and how to recognize edema along with the need to report changes of 3 lb (1.4 kg) or more in weight or evidence of edema immediately.

■ Advise the patient against overexertion. Advise him to report any dyspnea or shortness of breath during normal activity.

Continuous renal replacement therapy

Continuous renal replacement therapy (CRRT) is used to treat patients who suffer from acute renal failure. Unlike the more traditional intermittent hemodialysis (IHD), CRRT is administered around the clock, providing patients with continuous therapy and sparing them the destabilizing hemodynamic and electrolytic changes characteristic of IHD. CRRT is used for patients who are unable to tolerate traditional hemodialysis, for example, those with hypotension. For such patients, CRRT is commonly the only choice of treatment. (Of course, CRRT can also be used on many patients who can tolerate IHD.) Patients who have had abdominal surgery and can't receive peritoneal dialysis because of the overwhelming risk of infection are also candidates for CRRT.

CRRT methods vary in complexity. The techniques include the following:

■ Slow continuous ultrafiltration (SCUF) uses arteriovenous access and the patient's blood pressure to circulate blood through a hemofilter. Since the goal with this therapy is the removal of fluids, the patient doesn't receive any replacement fluids.

■ Continuous arteriovenous hemofiltration (CAVH) uses the patient's blood pressure and arteriovenous access to circulate blood through a flow resistance hemofilter. However, in order to maintain the patency of the filter and the systemic blood pressure, the patient receives replacement fluids.

■ Continuous arteriovenous hemodialysis (CAVH-D) is a similar procedure, combining hemodialysis with hemofiltration. In this technique, the infusion pump moves dialysate solution concurrent to blood flow, adding the ability to continuously remove solute while removing fluid. Like CAVH, it can also be performed in patients with hypotension and fluid overload.

■ Continuous venovenous hemofiltration (CVVH) fuses SCUF and CAVH. A double-lumen catheter is used to provide access to a vein, and a pump moves blood through the hemofilter.

■ Continuous venovenous hemodialysis (CVVH-D) is similar to CAVH-D, except that a vein provides the access while a pump is used to move dialysate solution concurrent with blood flow. (See *CAVH and CVVH setup*, pages 432 and 433.)

🔆**ALERT** *Continuous venovenous hemofiltration (CVVH or CVVH-D) is being used instead of CAVH or CAVH-D in many facilities to treat critically ill patients. CVVH has several advantages over CAVH: it doesn't require arterial access, it can be performed in patients with low mean arterial pressures, and it has a better solute clearance.*

Equipment
CRRT equipment ■ heparin flush solution ■ occlusive dressings for catheter insertion sites ■ sterile gloves ■ sterile mask ■ povidone-iodine solution ■ sterile 4″ × 4″ gauze pads ■ tape ■ filter replacement fluid (FRF) as ordered ■ infusion pump

Essential steps
■ Prime the hemofilter and tubing according to the manufacturer's instructions.

■ Wash your hands. Assemble the equipment at the patient's bedside, and explain the procedure.

■ If necessary, assist with catheter insertion, using strict sterile technique.

– If ordered, flush both catheters with the heparin flush solution to prevent clotting.

– Apply occlusive dressings to the insertion sites, and mark the dressings with the date and time. Secure the tubing and connections with tape.

■ Weigh the patient, take baseline vital signs, and make sure that all necessary laboratory studies have been done (usually, electrolyte levels, coagulation factors, complete blood count, blood urea nitrogen, and creatinine studies). Monitor the patient's weight and vital signs hourly.

■ Put on the sterile gloves and mask. Prepare the connection sites by cleaning them with gauze pads soaked in povidone-iodine solution; then connect them to the exit port of each catheter.

■ Using sterile technique, connect the catheters to the hemofilter.

■ Turn on the hemofilter, and monitor the blood flow rate through the circuit.

■ Assess all pulses in the affected leg every hour for the first 4 hours, then every 2 hours afterward.

🔆**ALERT** *When using CVVH, begin with a slow flow rate of approximately 50 ml/minute for the first several minutes and then gradually increase the flow rate at a rate of approximately 25 ml/minute every minute until the prescribed flow rate is achieved. Throughout this initial period, monitor the patient's blood pressure continuously; if the blood pressure drops, reduce the flow rate and notify the physician immediately.*

■ Inspect the ultrafiltrate during the procedure. It should remain clear yellow, with no gross blood.

🔆**ALERT** *Pink-tinged or bloody ultrafiltrate may signal a membrane leak in the hemofilter, which per-*

(Text continues on page 434.)

CAVH and CVVH setup

Continuous arteriovenous hemofiltration

In continuous arteriovenous hemofiltration (CAVH), as shown below, the physician inserts two large-bore, single-lumen catheters. One catheter is inserted into an artery—most commonly, the femoral artery. The other catheter is inserted into a vein, usually the femoral, subclavian, or internal jugular vein. During CAVH, the patient's arterial blood pressure serves as a natural pump, driving blood through the arterial line. A hemofilter removes water and toxic solutes (ultrafiltrate) from the blood. Replacement fluid is infused into a port on the arterial side. This same port can be used to infuse heparin. The venous line carries the replacement fluid and purified blood to the patient.

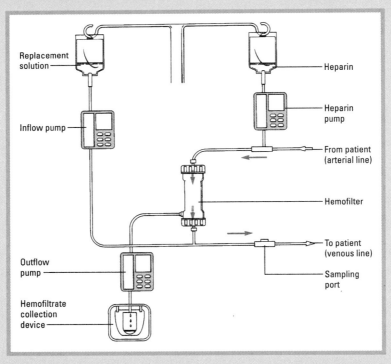

Continuous venovenous hemofiltration

With continuous venovenous hemofiltration (CVVH), as shown below, the physician inserts a special double-lumen catheter into a large vein, commonly the subclavian, femoral, or internal jugular vein. Because the catheter is in a vein, an external pump is used to move blood through the system. The patient's venous blood moves through the "arterial" lumen to the pump, which then pushes the blood through the catheter to the hemofilter. Here, water and toxic solutes (ultrafiltrate) are removed from the patient's blood and drain into a collection device. Blood cells aren't removed because they are too large to pass through the filter. As the blood exits the hemofilter, it is then pumped through the "venous" lumen back to the patient. Several components of the pump provide safety mechanisms. Pressure monitors on the pump maintain the flow of blood through the circuit at a constant rate. An air detector traps air bubbles before the blood returns to the patient. A venous trap collects any blood clots that may be in the blood. A blood-leak detector signals when blood is found in the ultrafiltrate; a venous clamp operates if air is detected in the circuit or if there is any disconnection in the blood line.

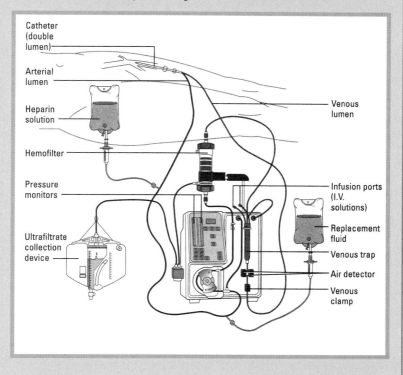

Catheter (double lumen)

Arterial lumen

Heparin solution

Hemofilter

Pressure monitors

Ultrafiltrate collection device

Venous lumen

Infusion ports (I.V. solutions)

Replacement fluid

Venous trap

Air detector

Venous clamp

mits bacterial contamination. With a CVVH system, look for the blood-leak detector to signal this. If a leak occurs, notify the physician so he can have the hemofilter replaced.

■ Assess the affected leg for signs of obstructed blood flow, such as coolness, pallor, and weak pulse. Check the groin area on the affected side for signs of hematoma. Ask the patient whether he has pain at the insertion sites.

■ Calculate the amount of FRF every hour, or as ordered, according to facility policy. Infuse the prescribed amount and type of FRF through the infusion pump into the arterial side of the circuit.

Complications

In addition to fluid imbalance, other possible complications of CRRT include:
■ bleeding
■ hemorrhage
■ hemofilter occlusion
■ infection
■ thrombosis.

Nursing considerations

■ Assess hemodynamic parameters, including pulmonary artery pressure (PAP), central venous pressure (CVP) and pulmonary artery wedge pressure (PAWP), and blood pressure hourly, or more frequently if indicated. Be alert for indications of hypovolemia (such as dropping blood pressure and decrease in PAP, CVP, and PAWP) from too-rapid removal of ultrafiltrate, or hypervolemia due to excessive fluid replacement with a decrease in ultrafiltrate.

■ Institute continuous cardiac monitoring for arrhythmias indicative of electrolyte imbalances.

■ Calculate the amount of replacement fluid needed every hour.

ALERT *When calculating the amount of replacement fluid, total the amount of fluid in the collection device from the previous hour with any other fluid losses the patient may have, for example, blood loss, emesis, or nasogastric drainage. From this total, subtract the patient's fluid intake for the past hour and the net fluid loss prescribed by the physician.*

■ Remember that because blood flows through an extracorporeal circuit during CAVH and CVVH, the blood in the hemofilter most likely requires anticoagulation. To do this, infuse heparin in low doses (usually starting at 500 U/hour) into an infusion port on the arterial side of the setup.

■ Measure thrombin clotting time or the activated clotting time (ACT). This ensures that the circuit, not the patient, is anticoagulated. A normal ACT is 100 seconds; during CRRT, keep it between 100 and 300 seconds, depending on the patient's clotting times. If the ACT is too high or too low, the physician will adjust the heparin dose accordingly.

■ Make sure the patient doesn't bend the affected leg more than 30 degrees at the hip to prevent catheter kinking.

■ Use another line to infuse medications or blood products.

■ Obtain serum electrolyte levels every 4 to 6 hours or as ordered; anticipate adjustments in replacement fluid or dialysate based on the results.

■ If the patient is receiving CVVH and the pressure alarm sounds, check the catheter for kinks, disconnections, or other problems. Determine which alarm sounded — the arterial, or venous, pressure alarm. If the arterial pressure alarm sounds, check the arterial lumen; if the venous pressure alarm sounds, check the venous lumen. A sudden rise in pressure indicates some blockage in the catheter or tubing. A dramatic and significant drop in pressure suggests a disconnection or opening of a port.

■ Inspect the site dressing every 4 to 8 hours for infection and bleeding. To prevent infection, perform skin care at the catheter insertion sites every 48 hours, using sterile technique. Cover the sites with an occlusive dressing.

■ If the ultrafiltrate flow rate decreases, raise the bed to increase the distance between the collection device and the hemofilter. Lower the bed to decrease the flow rate.

ALERT *Clamping the ultrafiltrate line is contraindicated with some types of hemofilters because pressure may build up in the filter, clotting it and collapsing the blood compartment.*

■ Record the time the treatment began and ended, fluid balance, vital signs, information, times of dressing changes, complications, medications given, and the patient's tolerance.

Hemodialysis

Hemodialysis is performed to remove toxic wastes from the blood of patients in renal failure. This potentially life-saving procedure removes blood from the body, circulates it through a purifying dialyzer, and then returns the blood to the body. Various access sites can be used for this procedure. (See *Hemodialysis access sites*, page 436.) The most common access device for long-term treatment is an arteriovenous (AV) fistula.

The underlying mechanism in hemodialysis is differential diffusion across a semipermeable membrane, which extracts by-products of protein metabolism, such as urea and uric acid as well as creatinine and excess body water. This process restores or maintains the balance of the body's buffer system and electrolyte level. Hemodialysis thus promotes a rapid return to normal serum values and helps prevent complications associated with uremia. (See *How hemodialysis works*, pages 438 and 439.)

Hemodialysis provides temporary support for patients with acute reversible renal failure. It's also used for regular long-term treatment of patients with chronic end-stage renal disease. A less common indication for hemodialysis is acute poisoning, such as a barbiturate or analgesic overdose. The patient's condition (including rate of creatinine accumulation and weight gain) determines the number and duration of hemodialysis treatments.

Specially trained personnel usually perform this procedure in a hemodialysis unit. However, if the patient is acutely ill and unstable, hemodialysis can be done at bedside in the critical care unit. Special hemodialysis units are available for use at home.

Equipment
For preparing the hemodialysis machine

Hemodialysis machine with appropriate dialyzer ■ I.V. solution, administration sets, lines, and related equipment

Hemodialysis access sites

Hemodialysis requires vascular access. The site and type of access may vary, depending on the expected duration of dialysis, the surgeon's preference, and the patient's condition.

Subclavian vein catheterization
Using the Seldinger technique, the physician or surgeon inserts an introducer needle into the subclavian vein. He then inserts a guidewire through the introducer needle and removes the needle. Using the guidewire, he then threads a 5″ to 12″ (12.5 to 30.5 cm) plastic or Teflon catheter with a Y-hub into the patient's vein.

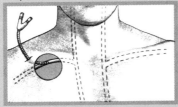

Femoral vein catheterization
Using the Seldinger technique, the physician or surgeon inserts an introducer needle into the right or left femoral vein. He then inserts a guidewire through the introducer needle and removes the needle. Using the guidewire, he then threads a 5″ to 12″ (12.5 to 30.5 cm) plastic or Teflon catheter with a Y-hub or two catheters, one for inflow and another, placed about ½″ (1.5 cm) distal to the first, for outflow.

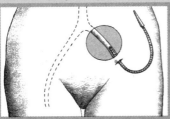

Arteriovenous fistula
To create a fistula, the surgeon makes an incision in the patient's wrist or lower forearm, then a small incision in the side of an artery and another in a side of a vein. He then sutures the edges of the incisions together to make a common opening approximately 1″ to 3″ (2.5 to 7.5 cm) long.

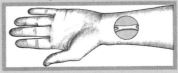

Arteriovenous shunt
To create a shunt, the surgeon makes an incision in the patient's wrist, lower forearm, or (rarely) ankle. He then inserts a 6″ to 10″ (15 to 25.5 cm) transparent Silastic cannula into an artery and another into a vein. Finally, he tunnels the cannulas out through incisions and joins them with a piece of Teflon tubing.

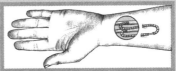

Arteriovenous graft
To create a graft, the surgeon makes an incision in the patient's forearm, upper arm, or thigh. He then tunnels a natural or synthetic graft under the skin and sutures the distal end to an artery and the proximal end to a vein.

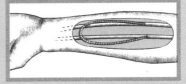

■ dialysate ■ optional: heparin, 3-ml syringe with needle, medication label, and hemostat

For hemodialysis with an AV fistula

Two winged fistula needles (each attached to a 10-ml syringe filled with heparin flush solution) ■ linen-saver pad ■ povidone-iodine pads or other skin antiseptic ■ sterile 4″ × 4″ gauze pads ■ tourniquet ■ gloves ■ adhesive tape

For discontinuing hemodialysis with an AV fistula

Gloves ■ sterile 4″ × 4″ gauze pads ■ two adhesive bandages ■ two hemostats ■ optional: sterile absorbable gelatin sponges (Gelfoam)

Essential steps

■ Prepare the hemodialysis equipment following the manufacturer's instructions and your facility's protocol. Maintain strict sterile technique to prevent introducing pathogens into the patient's bloodstream during dialysis. Make sure to test the dialyzer and dialysis machine for residual disinfectant after rinsing, and test all the alarms.

■ Weigh the patient. To determine ultrafiltration requirements, compare present weight to weight after the last dialysis and target weight.

■ Record baseline vital signs, taking blood pressure while sitting and standing. Auscultate heart for rate, rhythm, and abnormalities. Observe respiratory rate, rhythm, and quality. Assess for edema. Check mental status and the condition and patency of the access site. Check for problems since the last dialysis, and evaluate previous laboratory data.

■ Help the patient into a comfortable position (such as supine or sitting in recliner chair with feet elevated). Make sure the access site is well supported and resting on a clean drape.

■ If the patient is undergoing hemodialysis for the first time, explain the procedure in detail.

■ Adhere to standard precautions in all cases to prevent transmission of infection. Wash hands before beginning the procedure.

■ Begin hemodialysis with an AV fistula. (See *Hemodialysis with a double-lumen catheter or an AV shunt*, pages 440 to 442.)

– Flush the fistula needles, using attached syringes containing heparin flush solution, and set them aside.

– Place a linen-saver pad under the patient's arm.

– Using sterile technique, clean a 3″ × 10″ (7.5 × 25.5 cm) area of skin over the fistula with povidone-iodine or other antiseptic pads. Discard each pad after one wipe. (If the patient is sensitive to iodine, use chlorhexidine [Hibiclens] or alcohol instead.)

– Apply a tourniquet above the fistula to distend the veins and facilitate venipuncture. Be sure to avoid occluding the fistula.

– Put on gloves. Perform the venipuncture with a fistula needle. Remove the needle guard and squeeze the wing tips firmly together. Insert the arterial needle at least 1″ (2.5 cm) above the anastomosis, being careful not to puncture the fistula.

– Release the tourniquet, and flush the needle with heparin flush solution to prevent clotting. Clamp the arterial needle tubing with a hemostat, and secure the wing tips of the

How hemodialysis works

In hemodialysis, blood flows from the patient to an external dialyzer (or artificial kidney) through an arterial access site. Inside the dialyzer, blood and dialysate flow countercurrently, divided by a semipermeable membrane. The composition of the dialysate resembles normal extracellular fluid. The blood contains an excess of specific solutes (such as metabolic waste products and electrolytes), and the dialysate contains electrolytes that may be at abnormal levels in the patient's bloodstream. The dialysate's electrolyte composition can be modified to raise or lower electrolyte levels, depending on need.

Excretory function and electrolyte homeostasis are achieved by diffusion — the movement of a molecule across the dialyzer's semipermeable membrane — from an area of higher solute concentration to an area of lower concentration. Water (solvent) crosses the membrane from the blood into the dialysate by ultrafiltration. This process removes excess water, waste products, and other metabolites through osmotic pressure and hydrostatic pressure. Osmotic pressure is the movement of water across the semipermeable membrane from an area of lesser solute concentration to one of greater solute concentration. Hydrostatic pressure forces water from the blood compartment into the dialysate compartment. Cleaned of impurities and excess water, the blood returns to the body through a venous site.

Types of dialyzers

There are three types of dialyzers: the hollow filter, the flat-plate or parallel flow-plate, and the coil. The flat-plate and hollow-filter dialyzers may be used several times on each patient. Heparin is used to prevent clot formation during hemodialysis.

Hollow-filter dialyzer

The hollow-filter dialyzer — the most common type — contains fine capillaries with a semipermeable membrane enclosed in a plastic chamber. Blood flows through these capillaries as the system pumps dialysate in the opposite direction on the outside of the capillaries.

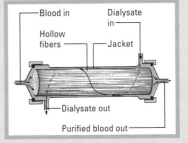

Flat-plate or parallel flow-plate dialyzer

The flat-plate or parallel flow-plate dialyzer has two or more layers of semipermeable membrane bound by a semirigid or rigid structure. Blood ports are located at both ends, between the membranes. Blood flows between the membranes, and dialysate flows in the opposite direction, along the outside of the membranes.

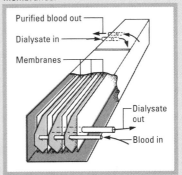

Coil dialyzer

The coil dialyzer, which is no longer widely used, consists of one or more semipermeable membrane tubes supported by mesh and wrapped concentrically around a central core. Blood passes through the coils as dialysate circulates at high speed around the coils and meshwork.

Three system types can be used to deliver dialysate. The batch system uses a reservoir for circulating dialysate. The regenerative system uses sorbents to purify and regenerate recirculating dialysate. The proportioning system — the most common type — mixes concentrate with water to form dialysate, which then circulates through the dialyzer and goes down a drain after a single pass, followed by fresh dialysate.

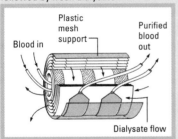

Plastic mesh support

Blood in

Purified blood out

Dialysate flow

needle to the skin with tape to prevent it from dislodging within the vein.

– Perform another venipuncture with the venous needle a few inches above the arterial needle. Flush the needle with heparin flush solution. Clamp the venous needle tubing, and secure the wing tips of the venous needle as with the arterial needle.

– Remove the syringe from the end of the arterial tubing, uncap the arterial line from the hemodialysis machine, and connect the two lines. Tape the connection securely to prevent it from separating during the procedure. Repeat these two steps for the venous line.

– Release the hemostat and start hemodialysis.

■ Discontinue hemodialysis as ordered.

– Wash your hands. Turn the blood pump on the hemodialysis machine to 50 to 100 ml/minute.

– Put on gloves, and remove the tape from the connection site of the arterial lines. Clamp the needle tubing with the hemostat and disconnect the lines. The blood in the machine's arterial line will continue to flow toward the dialyzer, followed by a column of air. Just before the blood reaches the point where the normal saline solution enters the line, clamp the blood line with another hemostat.

– Unclamp the normal saline solution to allow a small amount to flow through the line. Unclamp the hemostat on the machine line. This allows all blood to flow into the dialyzer, where it passes through the

(Text continues on page 442.)

Hemodialysis with a double-lumen catheter or an AV shunt

If the patient has a double-lumen catheter or an arteriovenous (AV) shunt, you'll need to modify the procedure for hemodialysis. Follow the instructions described below.

Beginning hemodialysis with a double-lumen catheter

● Gather the equipment necessary to perform the procedure: povidone-iodine pads or other antiseptic; two sterile 4″ × 4″ gauze pads; two 3-ml and two 5-ml syringes; tape; heparin; bolus syringe; gloves.

● Prepare venous access. If extension tubing isn't already clamped, clamp it to prevent air from entering the catheter. Clean each catheter extension tube, clamp, and luer-lock injection cap with antiseptic pads to remove contaminants. Next, place a sterile 4″ × 4″ gauze pad under the extension tubing and place two 5-ml syringes and two sterile gauze pads on the drape.

● Prepare the anticoagulant regimen as ordered.

● Identify arterial and venous blood lines, and place them near the drape.

● To remove clots and ensure catheter patency, remove catheter caps, attach syringes to each catheter port, open one clamp, and aspirate 1.5 to 3 ml of blood. Close the clamp and repeat the procedure with the other port. Flush each port with 5 ml of heparin flush solution.

● Attach the blood lines to the patient access. First, remove the syringe from the arterial port, and attach the line to the arterial port. Next, administer the heparin according to protocol. This prevents clotting in the extracorporeal circuit.

● Grasp the venous blood line and attach it to the venous port. Open the clamps on the extension tubing, and secure the tubing to the patient's extremity with tape to reduce tension on the tube and minimize trauma to the insertion site.

● Begin hemodialysis according to your facility's protocol.

Discontinuing hemodialysis with a double-lumen catheter

● Gather the necessary equipment: sterile 4″ × 4″ gauze pads; povidone-iodine or other antiseptic pad; precut gauze dressing; clean and sterile gloves; normal saline solution; alcohol pads; heparin flush solution; luer-lock injection caps; optional supplies, such as transparent occlusive dressing, skin barrier preparation, tape, and materials for culturing drainage.

● Wash your hands.

● Clamp the extension tubing to prevent air from entering the catheter. Clean all connection points on the catheter and blood lines as well as the clamps, to reduce the risk of systemic or local infections.

● Place a clean drape under the catheter and place two sterile 4″ × 4″ gauze pads on the drape beneath the catheter lines. Soak the pads with povidone-iodine solution or other antiseptic. Prepare the catheter flush solution with normal saline or heparin flush solution as ordered.

● Put on clean gloves. Grasp each blood line with a gauze pad, and disconnect each line from the catheter.

● Flush each port with normal saline solution to clean the extension tubing and catheter of blood. Administer additional heparin flush solution, as ordered, to ensure catheter patency. Attach luer-lock injection caps to prevent entry of air or loss of blood.

● Clamp the extension tubing.

Re-dressing the catheter insertion site

When hemodialysis is complete, redress the catheter insertion site; also redress it if it's occluded, soiled, or wet.

● Place the patient in a supine position with his face turned away from the in-

Hemodialysis with a double-lumen catheter or an AV shunt *(continued)*

sertion site so that he doesn't contaminate the site by breathing on it.
● Wash your hands and remove the outer occlusive dressing. Put on sterile gloves, remove the old inner dressing, and discard the gloves and the inner dressing.
● Set up a sterile field, and observe the site for drainage. Obtain a drainage sample for culture, if necessary. Notify the physician if the suture appears to be missing.
● Put on sterile gloves, and clean the insertion site with an alcohol pad to remove skin oils. Next, clean the site with a povidone-iodine or other antiseptic pad, and allow it to air-dry.
● Put a precut gauze dressing over the insertion site and under the catheter, and place another gauze dressing over the catheter.
● Apply a skin barrier preparation to the skin surrounding the gauze dressing. Cover the gauze and catheter with a transparent occlusive dressing.
● Apply a 4" to 5" (10- to 12.5 -cm) piece of 2" tape over the cut edge of the dressing to reinforce the lower edge.

Beginning hemodialysis with an AV shunt
● Gather the equipment necessary to perform the procedure: povidone-iodine or other antiseptic pads; alcohol pads; sterile gloves; two sterile shunt adapters; sterile Teflon connector; two bulldog clamps; two 10-ml syringes; normal saline solution; four short strips of adhesive tape; sterile shunt spreader (optional).
● Remove the bulldog clamps, and place them within easy reach of the sterile field. Remove the shunt dressing and clean the shunt, using sterile technique, as you would for daily care. Clean the bulldog clamps with an alcohol pad.
● Assemble the shunt adapters according to the manufacturer's directions.

● Clean the arterial and venous shunt connections with povidone-iodine or other antiseptic pads to remove contaminants. Use a separate pad for each tube and wipe in one direction only, from the insertion site to the connection sites. Allow the tubing to air-dry.
● Put on sterile gloves.
● Clamp the arterial side of the shunt with a bulldog clamp to prevent blood from flowing through it. Clamp the venous side to prevent leakage when the shunt is opened.
● Open the shunt by separating its sides with your fingers or with a sterile shunt spreader, if available. Both sides of the shunt should be exposed. Always inspect the Teflon connector on one side of the shunt to see whether it's damaged or bent, and replace it, if necessary, before proceeding. Note which side contains the connector so you can use the new one to close the shunt after treatment.
● To adapt the shunt to the lines of the machine, attach a shunt adapter and 10-ml syringe filled with about 8 ml of normal saline solution to the side of the shunt containing the Teflon connector. Attach the new Teflon connector to the other side of the shunt with the second adapter. Attach the second 10-ml syringe filled with about 8 ml of normal saline solution to the same side.
● Flush the shunt's arterial tubing by releasing its clamp and gently aspirating it with the normal saline solution-filled syringe. Flush the tubing slowly, observing it for signs of fibrin buildup. Repeat the procedure on the venous side of the shunt.
● Secure the shunt to the adapter connection with adhesive tape to prevent separation during treatment.
● Connect the arterial and venous lines to the adapters, and secure the connections with tape. Tape each line to the pa-

(continued)

Hemodialysis with a double-lumen catheter or an AV shunt *(continued)*

tient's arm to prevent unnecessary strain on the shunt during treatment.
• Begin hemodialysis according to your facility's protocol.

Discontinuing hemodialysis with an AV shunt
• Gather the necessary equipment: sterile gloves; two bulldog clamps; two hemostats; povidone-iodine or other antiseptic solution; sterile 4″ × 4″ gauze pads; alcohol pads; elastic gauze bandages; tape.
• Wash your hands. Turn the blood pump on the hemodialysis machine to 50 to 100 ml/minute.
• Put on the sterile gloves, and remove the tape from the connection site of the arterial lines. Clamp the arterial cannula with a bulldog clamp, and then disconnect the lines. The blood in the machine's arterial line will continue to flow toward the dialyzer, followed by a column of air. Just before the blood reaches the point where the normal saline solution enters the line, clamp the blood line with a hemostat.
• Unclamp the normal saline solution to allow a small amount to flow through the line. Reclamp the normal saline solution line, and unclamp the hemostat on the machine line. This allows all blood to flow into the dialyzer, where it's circulated through the filter and back to the patient through the venous line.

• Just before the last volume of blood enters the patient, clamp the venous cannula with a bulldog clamp and the machine's venous line with a hemostat.
• Remove the tape from the connection site of the venous lines. Turn off the blood pump and disconnect the lines.
• Reconnect the shunt cannula. Remove the older of the two Teflon connectors and discard it. Connect the shunt, taking care to position the Teflon connector equally between the two cannulas. Remove the bulldog clamps.
• Secure the shunt connection with tape to prevent accidental disconnection.
• Clean the shunt and its site with the povidone-iodine or other antiseptic pads. When the cleaning procedure is finished, remove the povidone-iodine (if used) with alcohol pads.
• Make sure blood flows through the shunt adequately.
• Apply a dressing to the shunt site, and wrap it securely (but not too tightly) with elastic gauze bandages. Attach the bulldog clamps to the outside dressing.
• When hemodialysis is complete, assess the patient's weight, vital signs, and mental status. Compare your findings with your predialysis assessment data. Document your findings.
• Disinfect and rinse the delivery system according to the manufacturer's instructions.

filter and back to the patient through the venous line.
– After the blood is retransfused, clamp the venous needle tubing and the machine's venous line with hemostats. Turn off the blood pump.
– Remove the tape from the connection site of the venous lines, and disconnect the lines.

– Remove the venipuncture needle, and apply pressure to the site with a folded 4″ × 4″ gauze pad until bleeding stops, usually within 10 minutes. Apply an adhesive bandage. Repeat the procedure on the arterial line.
■ When hemodialysis is complete, assess the patient's weight, vital signs

(including standing blood pressure), and mental status. Then compare findings with predialysis assessment data, and document your findings.

■ Disinfect and rinse the delivery system according to the manufacturer's instructions or your facility's policy.

Complications
A variety of complications are associated with hemodialysis, including:

■ Bacterial endotoxins in the dialysate may cause fever.

■ Rapid fluid removal and electrolyte changes during hemodialysis can cause early dialysis disequilibrium syndrome. Signs and symptoms include headache, nausea, vomiting, restlessness, hypertension, muscle cramps, backache, and seizures.

■ Excessive removal of fluid during ultrafiltration can cause hypovolemia and hypotension.

■ Diffusion of the sugar and sodium content of the dialysate solution into the blood can cause hyperglycemia and hypernatremia. These conditions, in turn, can cause hyperosmolarity.

■ Cardiac arrhythmias can occur during hemodialysis as a result of electrolyte and pH changes in the blood. They can also develop in patients taking antiarrhythmic drugs because the dialysate removes these drugs during treatment. Angina may develop in patients with anemia or preexisting arteriosclerotic cardiovascular disease because of the physiologic stress on the blood during purification and ultrafiltration.

■ Reduced oxygen levels due to extracorporeal blood flow or membrane sensitivity may require increasing oxygen administration during hemodialysis.

ALERT *Some complications of hemodialysis can be fatal. For example, an air embolism can result if the dialyzer retains air, if tubing connections become loose, or if the saline solution container empties. Symptoms include chest pain, dyspnea, coughing, and cyanosis. Hyperthermia, another potentially fatal complication, can result if the dialysate becomes overheated. Exsanguination can result from separations of the blood lines or from rupture of the blood lines or dialyzer membrane.*

■ Hemolysis can result from obstructed flow of the dialysate concentrate or from incorrect setting of the conductivity alarm limits. Symptoms include chest pain, dyspnea, cherry red blood, arrhythmias, acute decrease in hematocrit, and hyperkalemia.

Nursing considerations
■ Auscultate for bruits and palpate for a thrill to confirm patency of the AV fistula or shunt before beginning and periodically throughout the day; notify the physician if bruits or a thrill is absent.

■ Obtain blood samples from the patient as ordered. Samples are usually drawn before beginning hemodialysis.

ALERT *Always use strict sterile technique to avoid pyrogenic reactions and bacteremia with septicemia resulting from contamination. Discard equipment that has fallen on the floor or that has been disconnected and exposed to the air.*

■ Immediately report any machine malfunction or equipment defect.

■ Avoid unnecessary handling of shunt tubing. However, be sure to inspect the shunt carefully for patency by observing its color. Look for clots and serum and cell separation, and check the temperature of the Silastic tubing. Assess the shunt insertion site for signs of infection, such as purulent drainage, inflammation, and tenderness, which may indicate the body's rejection of the shunt. Check to see if the shunt insertion tips are exposed.

ALERT *Be sure to complete each step in the procedure correctly. Overlooking a single step or performing it incorrectly can cause unnecessary blood loss or inefficient treatment from poor clearances or inadequate fluid removal. For example, never allow a saline solution bag to run dry while priming and soaking the dialyzer because doing so can cause air to enter the patient portion of the dialysate system. Ultimately, failure to perform hemodialysis accurately can lead to patient injury and even death.*

ALERT *If you suspect that air has entered the vascular access, clamp the line immediately and place the patient in the left lateral Trendelenburg position. This position helps to confine the air to the right ventricular apex, preventing its movement to the lungs. Notify the physician immediately, and begin oxygen administration.*

■ If bleeding continues after you remove an AV fistula needle, apply pressure with a sterile, absorbable gelatin sponge. If bleeding persists, apply a similar sponge soaked in topical thrombin solution.

■ Monitor hemoglobin level and hematocrit before each hemodialysis treatment; notify the physician if the patient's hematocrit falls more than 2 percentage points.

■ Throughout hemodialysis, carefully monitor the patient's vital signs. Assess blood pressure at least hourly or as of-

ten as every 15 minutes, if necessary. Monitor the patient's weight before and after the procedure to ensure adequate ultrafiltration during treatment. (Many dialysis units are now equipped with bed scales.)

■ Perform periodic tests for clotting time on the patient's blood samples and samples from the dialyzer. If he receives meals during treatment, make sure they're light.

■ Continue necessary drug administration during dialysis unless the drug would be removed in the dialysate; if so, administer the drug after dialysis.

■ Assess cardiopulmonary status closely, including heart and lung sounds, for signs and symptoms of fluid overload.

ALERT *Headache, nausea, vomiting, decreasing levels of consciousness and, possibly, seizures suggest disequilibrium syndrome that results from fluid shifts in the brain.*

■ Provide care for the vascular access site. Include the patient in teaching how to keep the site clean and dry to prevent infection; clean the site daily until it heals completely and the sutures are removed (usually 10 to 14 days after surgery). Notify the physician if pain, swelling, redness, or drainage is noted in the accessed arm.

■ Explain that after the access site heals, the patient may use the arm freely. In fact, exercise is beneficial because it helps stimulate vein enlargement. Remind him not to allow any treatments or procedures on the accessed arm, including blood pressure monitoring or needle punctures. Tell him to avoid putting excessive pressure on the arm. He shouldn't sleep on it, wear constricting clothing over it, or lift heavy objects or strain with it.

He should also avoid getting wet for several hours after dialysis.

■ Teach the patient exercises for the affected arm to promote vascular dilation and enhance blood flow. Start with squeezing a small rubber ball or other soft object for 15 minutes, when allowed.

■ Document the time treatment began and any problems that occurred, including measures used to alleviate the problem.

■ Record the patient's weight and vital signs before, during, and after treatment.

■ Record the time the treatment was discontinued and the patient's response to the treatment.

■ If blood samples were obtained during the procedure, record the time, the test being performed, and the results.

■ Document any signs and symptoms of complications, treatments instituted, and the patient's response to them.

Peritoneal dialysis

Peritoneal dialysis is indicated for patients with chronic renal failure who have cardiovascular instability, vascular access problems that prevent hemodialysis, fluid overload, or electrolyte imbalances.

In this procedure, dialysate — the solution instilled into the peritoneal cavity by a catheter — draws waste products, excess fluid, and electrolytes from the blood across the semipermeable peritoneal membrane. (See *Principles of peritoneal dialysis*, page 446.)

After a prescribed period, the dialysate is drained from the peritoneal cavity, removing impurities with it. The dialysis procedure is then repeated, using a new dialysate each time, until waste removal is complete and fluid, electrolyte, and acid-base balance has been restored.

The catheter for peritoneal dialysis is inserted in the operating room or at the patient's bedside with a nurse assisting. (See *Comparing peritoneal dialysis catheters*, page 447.) With special preparation, the nurse may perform dialysis, either manually or using an automatic or semiautomatic cycle machine.

Equipment

All equipment must be sterile. Commercially packaged dialysis kits or trays are available.

For catheter placement and dialysis

Prescribed dialysate (in 1-L or 2-L bottles or bags, as ordered) ■ warmer, heating pad, or water bath ■ at least three face masks ■ medication, such as heparin, if ordered ■ dialysis administration set with drainage bag ■ two pairs of sterile gloves ■ I.V. pole ■ fenestrated sterile drape ■ vial of 1% or 2% lidocaine ■ povidone-iodine pads ■ 3-ml syringe with 25G 1″ needle ■ ordered type of multi-eyed, nylon, peritoneal catheter ■ scalpel (with #11 blade) ■ peritoneal stylet ■ sutures or hypoallergenic tape ■ povidone-iodine solution (to prepare abdomen) ■ precut drain dressings ■ protective cap for catheter ■ 4″ × 4″ gauze pads ■ small, sterile plastic clamp ■ optional: 10-ml syringe with 22G 1½″ needle, protein or potassium supplement, specimen container, label, and laboratory request form

Principles of peritoneal dialysis

Peritoneal dialysis works through a combination of diffusion and osmosis.

Diffusion
In diffusion, particles move through a semipermeable membrane from an area of high-solute concentration to an area of low-solute concentration. In peritoneal dialysis, the water-based dialysate being infused contains glucose, sodium chloride, calcium, magnesium, acetate or lactate, and no waste products. Therefore, waste products and excess electrolytes in the blood cross through the semipermeable peritoneal membrane into the dialysate. Removing the waste-filled dialysate and replacing it with fresh solution keeps the waste concentration low and encourages further diffusion.

Osmosis
In osmosis, fluids move through a semipermeable membrane from an areas of low-solute concentration to an area of high-solute concentration. In peritoneal dyalysis, dextrose is added to the dialysate to give it a higher solute concentration than the blood, creating a high osmotic gradient. Water migrates from the blood through the membrane at the beginning of each infusion, when the osmotic gradient is highest.

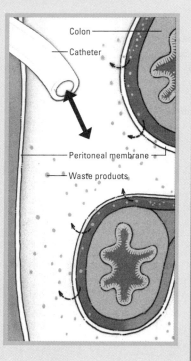

Colon

Catheter

Peritoneal membrane

Waste products

For dressing changes
One pair of sterile gloves ▪ 10 sterile cotton-tipped applicators or sterile 2″ × 2″ gauze pads ▪ povidone-iodine ointment ▪ two precut drain dressings ▪ adhesive tape ▪ povidone-iodine solution or normal saline solution ▪ two sterile 4″ × 4″ gauze pads

Essential steps
▪ Bring all equipment to the patient's bedside.

    ALERT *Make sure the dialysate is at body temperature. This de-*

creases patient discomfort during the procedure and reduces vasoconstriction of the peritoneal capillaries. Dilated capillaries enhance blood flow to the peritoneal membrane surface, increasing waste clearance into the peritoneal cavity. Place the container in a warmer or a water bath, or wrap it in a heating pad set at 98.6° F (37° C) for 30 to 60 minutes to warm the solution.

▪ Explain the procedure to the patient. Assess and record vital signs, weight, and abdominal girth to establish baseline levels.

Comparing peritoneal dialysis catheters

The first step in any type of peritoneal dialysis is the insertion of a catheter to allow instillation of dialyzing solution. The physician may insert one of the three different catheters described here.

Tenckhoff catheter

To implant a Tenckhoff catheter, the physician inserts the first 6¾" (17.1 cm) of the catheter into the patient's abdomen. The next 2¾" (7-cm) segment, which may have a Dacron cuff at one or both ends, is imbedded subcutaneously. Within a few days after insertion, the patient's tissues grow around the cuffs, forming a tight barrier against bacterial infiltration. The remaining 3⅞" (9.8 cm) of the catheter extends outside of the abdomen and is equipped with a metal adapter at the tip that connects to dialyzer tubing.

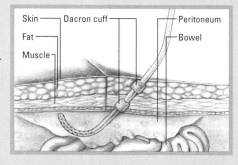

Flanged collar catheter

To insert a flanged collar catheter, the physician positions the collar just below the dermis so that the device extends through the abdominal wall. He keeps the distal end of the cuff from extending into the peritoneum, where it could cause adhesions.

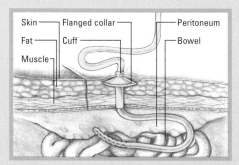

Column disk peritoneal catheter

To insert a column disk peritoneal catheter (CDPC), the physician rolls up the flexible disk section of the implant, inserts it into the peritoneal cavity, and retracts it against the abdominal wall. The implant's first cuff rests just outside the peritoneal membrane, and its second cuff rests just under the skin. Because the CDPC doesn't float freely in the peritoneal cavity, it keeps inflowing dialyzing solution from being directed at the sensitive organs, which increases patient comfort during dialysis.

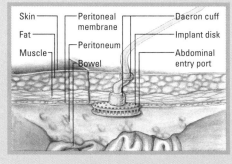

Setup for peritoneal dialysis

The illustration below shows the proper setup for peritoneal dialysis.

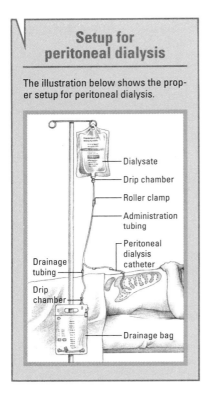

Review recent laboratory values (blood urea nitrogen, serum creatinine, sodium, potassium, and complete blood count).

■ Determine the patient's hepatitis B virus and human immunodeficiency virus status, if known.

■ Have the patient try to urinate to reduce the risk of bladder perforation during insertion of the peritoneal catheter. If he can't urinate and you suspect that his bladder isn't empty, obtain an order for straight catheterization to empty his bladder.

■ Place the patient in the supine position, and have him put on one of the sterile face masks.

■ Wash your hands.

■ Inspect the warmed dialysate, which should appear clear and colorless.

■ Put on a sterile face mask. Prepare to add any prescribed medication to the dialysate, using strict sterile technique to avoid contaminating the solution. Medications should be added immediately before the solution will be hung and used. Disinfect multiple-dose vials by soaking them in povidone-iodine solution for 5 minutes. Heparin is typically added to the dialysate to prevent accumulation of fibrin in the catheter.

■ Prepare the dialysis administration set. (See *Setup for peritoneal dialysis.*)

■ Close the clamps on all lines. Place the drainage bag below the patient to facilitate gravity drainage, and connect the drainage line to it. Connect the dialysate infusion lines to the bottles or bags of dialysate. Hang the bottles or bags on the I.V. pole at the patient's bedside. To prime the tubing, open the infusion lines and allow the solution to flow until all lines are primed, and then close all clamps.

■ Assist with catheter insertion. After putting on a mask and a pair of sterile gloves, the physician cleans the patient's abdomen with povidone-iodine solution and drapes it with a sterile drape.

– Wipe the stopper of the lidocaine vial with povidone-iodine solution, and allow it to dry. Invert the vial, and hand it to the physician so he can withdraw the lidocaine, using the 3-ml syringe with the 25G 1″ needle.

– After anesthetizing a small area of the patient's abdomen below the umbilicus, observe as the physician makes a small incision with the scalpel, inserts the catheter into the peritoneal cavity — using the stylet to guide the catheter — and sutures or tapes the catheter in place.

■ If the catheter is already in place, clean the site with povidone-iodine solution in a circular outward motion, according to your facility's policy, before each dialysis treatment.

■ Connect the catheter to the administration set, using strict sterile technique to prevent contamination of the catheter and the solution, which could cause peritonitis.

■ Open the drain dressing and the 4″ × 4″ gauze pad packages. Put on the other pair of sterile gloves. Apply the precut drain dressings around the catheter. Cover them with the gauze pads, and tape them securely.

■ Unclamp the lines to the patient. Rapidly instill 500 ml of dialysate into the peritoneal cavity to test the catheter's patency.

■ Clamp the lines to the patient. Immediately unclamp the lines to the drainage bag to allow fluid to drain into the bag. Outflow should be brisk.

■ Having established the catheter's patency, clamp the lines to the drainage bag and unclamp the lines to the patient to infuse the prescribed volume of solution over a period of 5 to 10 minutes. As soon as the dialysate container empties, clamp the lines to the patient immediately to prevent air from entering the tubing.

■ Allow the solution to dwell in the peritoneal cavity for the prescribed time (10 minutes to 4 hours). This lets excess fluid, electrolytes, and accumulated wastes move from the blood through the peritoneal membrane and into the dialysate.

■ Warm the solution for the next infusion.

■ At the end of the prescribed dwell time, unclamp the line to the drainage bag and allow the solution to drain from the peritoneal cavity into the drainage bag (normally 20 to 30 minutes).

■ Repeat the infusion-dwell-drain cycle immediately after outflow until the prescribed number of fluid exchanges have been completed.

■ If the physician or your facility's policy requires a dialysate specimen, collect one usually after every 10 infusion-dwell-drain cycles (always during the drain phase), after every 24-hour period, or as ordered. To do this, attach the 10-ml syringe to the 22G 1½″ needle and insert it into the injection port on the drainage line, using strict sterile technique, and aspirate the drainage sample. Transfer the sample to the specimen container, label it appropriately, and send it to the laboratory with a laboratory request form.

■ After completing the prescribed number of exchanges, clamp the catheter and put on sterile gloves. Disconnect the administration set from the peritoneal catheter. Place the sterile protective cap over the catheter's distal end.

■ Dispose of all used equipment appropriately.

■ Change the dressing according to your facility's policy or as ordered.

  – Explain the procedure to the patient and wash your hands.

  – If necessary, carefully remove the old dressings to avoid putting tension on the catheter and accidentally dislodging it and to avoid intro-

ducing bacteria into the tract through movement of the catheter.
– Put on sterile gloves.
– Saturate the sterile applicators or the 2″ × 2″ gauze pads with povidone-iodine or normal saline solution, and clean the skin around the catheter, moving in concentric circles from the catheter site outward. Remove crusted material carefully.
– Inspect the catheter site for drainage and the tissue around the site for redness and swelling.
– Apply povidone-iodine ointment to the catheter site with a sterile gauze pad.
– Place two precut drain dressings around the catheter site. Tape the 4″ × 4″ gauze pads over them to secure the dressings.

Complications

Potential complications of peritoneal dialysis include:
■ Peritonitis, the most common complication, usually follows contamination of the dialysate, but it's also possible if solution leaks from the catheter exit site and flows back into the catheter tract.
■ Respiratory distress secondary to dialysate in the peritoneal cavity increases pressure on the diaphragm, which decreases lung expansion.
■ Protein depletion is possible because of diffusion of protein in the blood into the dialysate solution through the peritoneal membrane. As much as 14 g of protein may be lost daily—more in patients with peritonitis.
■ Constipation is a major cause of inflow-outflow problems.

■ Excessive fluid loss may result from the use of 4.25% solution and may cause hypovolemia, hypotension, and shock.
■ Excessive fluid retention possibly leading to blood volume expansion, hypertension, peripheral edema, and even pulmonary edema and heart failure may occur.
  Other possible complications include electrolyte imbalances and hyperglycemia, which can be identified by frequent blood tests.

Nursing considerations

■ During and after dialysis, monitor the patient and his response to treatment.

ALERT *Peritoneal dialysis is usually contraindicated in patients who have had extensive abdominal or bowel surgery or extensive abdominal trauma, or those who presently have severe vascular disease, obesity, or respiratory distress.*
■ Monitor the patient's vital signs every 10 to 15 minutes for the first 1 to 2 hours of exchanges, then every 2 to 4 hours or more frequently, if necessary. Notify the physician of any abrupt changes in the patient's condition. Assess hemodynamic parameters if a central venous or pulmonary artery catheter is in place.
■ To prevent respiratory distress, position the patient for maximal lung expansion. Promote lung expansion through turning and deep-breathing exercises.

ALERT *If the patient suffers severe respiratory distress during the dwell phase of dialysis, drain the peritoneal cavity and notify the physician. Monitor any patient on peritoneal*

*dialysis who is being weaned from a
ventilator.*

■ To reduce the risk of peritonitis, use strict sterile technique during catheter insertion, dialysis, and dressing changes. Ensure that masks are worn by all personnel in the room whenever the dialysis system is opened or entered. Change the dressing at least every 24 hours or whenever it becomes wet or soiled. Frequent dressing changes will also help prevent skin excoriation from leakage.

■ To prevent protein depletion, expect a high-protein diet or a protein supplement to be ordered, and monitor serum albumin levels as ordered.

■ Remember that dialysate is available in three concentrations — 4.25% dextrose, 2.5% dextrose, and 1.5% dextrose. The 4.25% solution usually removes the largest amount of fluid from the blood because its glucose concentration is highest. If your patient receives this concentrated solution, monitor him carefully to prevent excess fluid loss. Some of the glucose in the 4.25% solution may enter the patient's bloodstream, causing hyperglycemia severe enough to require an insulin injection or an insulin addition to the dialysate.

■ Keep in mind that patients with low serum potassium levels may require the addition of potassium to the dialysate solution to prevent further losses. Anticipate the need for continuous cardiac monitoring to allow for early detection of possible arrhythmias caused by electrolyte imbalances.

■ Monitor fluid volume balance, blood pressure, and pulse to help prevent fluid imbalance. Assess fluid balance at the end of each infusion-dwell-drain cycle. Fluid balance is positive if

less than the amount infused was recovered; it's negative if more than the amount infused was recovered. Notify the physician if the patient retains 500 ml or more of fluid for three consecutive cycles or if he loses at least 1 L of fluid for three consecutive cycles.

■ Weigh the patient daily to help determine how much fluid is being removed during dialysis treatment. Note the time and any variations in the weighing technique next to his weight on his chart.

■ If inflow and outflow are slow or absent, check the tubing for kinks. Try raising the I.V. pole or repositioning the patient to increase the inflow rate. Repositioning the patient or applying manual pressure to the lateral aspects of the patient's abdomen may also help increase drainage. If these maneuvers fail, notify the physician. Improper positioning of the catheter or an accumulation of fibrin may obstruct the catheter.

■ To ensure regular bowel movements, give a laxative or stool softener as needed to avoid constipation, which could interfere with inflow and outflow.

■ Always examine outflow fluid (effluent) for color and clarity. Normally it's clear or pale yellow, but pink-tinged effluent may appear during the first three or four cycles.

ALERT *If the effluent remains pink-tinged, or if it's grossly bloody, suspect bleeding into the peritoneal cavity and notify the physician. Also notify the physician if the outflow contains feces, which suggests bowel perforation, or if it's cloudy, which suggests peritonitis. Obtain a sample for culture and Gram stain. Send the sam-*

ple, in a labeled specimen container, to the laboratory immediately.

■ Expect the patient to complain of discomfort at the start of the procedure. If the patient experiences pain during the procedure, determine when it occurs, its quality and duration, and whether it radiates to other body parts, and then notify the physician.

ALERT *Pain during infusion usually results from a dialysate that's too cool or acidic. Pain may also result from rapid inflow; slowing the inflow rate may reduce the pain. Severe, diffuse pain with rebound tenderness and cloudy effluent may indicate peritoneal infection. Pain that radiates to the shoulder commonly results from air accumulation under the diaphragm. Severe, persistent perineal or rectal pain can result from improper catheter placement.*

■ Assist the patient with activities of daily living. To minimize discomfort, perform daily care during a drain phase in the cycle, when the patient's abdomen is less distended.

■ Record the amount of dialysate infused and drained, any medications added to the solution, and the color and character of effluent. Record the patient's daily weight and fluid balance.

■ Use a peritoneal dialysis flowchart to compute total fluid balance after each exchange. Note the patient's vital signs and tolerance of the treatment and other pertinent observations.

■ Document the condition of the patient's skin at the catheter insertion site, the patient's reports of unusual pain or discomfort, and actions taken.

 MULTISYSTEM DISORDER

Renal transplantation

Ranking among the most commonly performed and most successful of all organ transplants, renal transplant represents an alternative to dialysis for many patients with otherwise unmanageable end-stage renal disease (ESRD). ESRD commonly results from hypertension, diabetes mellitus, and glomerulonephritis. Renal transplantation may also be necessary to sustain life in a patient who has suffered traumatic loss of kidney function or in whom dialysis is contraindicated. Renal transplant, however, isn't performed on all patients who seemingly could benefit from it. For instance, severely debilitated, diabetic, or older adult patients or those with human immunodeficiency virus infection or psychiatric disorders aren't considered good candidates. Contraindications for renal transplant surgery include:

■ cardiopulmonary insufficiency
■ morbid obesity
■ peripheral and cerebrovascular disease
■ hepatic insufficiency
■ other conditions that increase a patient's overall surgical risk.

In some cases, a simultaneous transplant of the kidney and pancreas may be done. This dual organ transplantation is indicated for patients with type 1 diabetes and ESRD or renal insufficiency.

Organs for renal transplantation may be obtained from living donors or cadavers. The prognosis for a patient undergoing a renal transplant is very good. For example, according to the

United Network for Organ Sharing, the 1-year survival rate for patients who received donor kidneys from cadavers is approximately 87% and the 3-year survival rate is 76%. For those patients receiving kidneys from living donors, the 1-year survival rate is increased to 93% and the 3-year survival rate is increased to 86%.

Procedure

With a renal transplant, a healthy kidney harvested from a living relative or cadaver donor is implanted in the recipient's iliac fossa and anastomosed in place. Because the recipient's own kidneys usually secrete erythropoietin fluid, they're typically left in place to increase circulating hematocrit, ease dialysis management, and reduce blood transfusion requirements in case of transplant rejection. The recipient's own kidneys will, however, be removed if they're chronically infected, greatly enlarged, cancerous, or causing intractable hypertension.

With the patient under general anesthesia, the surgeon makes a curvilinear incision in the right or left lower quadrant, extending from the symphysis pubis to the anterior superior iliac spine, and up to just below the thoracic cage. He exposes the iliac fossa with a self-retaining retractor, then performs segmental separation, ligature, and division of perivascular tissue. Next, he clamps the iliac vein and artery in preparation for anastomosis to the donor kidney's renal vein and artery.

Meanwhile, the donor kidney is prepared for transplantation. If a cadaver kidney is being used, it's removed from cold storage or a perfusion preparation machine. Kidneys can be stored for 72 hours, although most transplants are done within 48 hours. If the kidney is from a living donor, it's harvested in an adjacent operating room via nephrectomy and placed in cold lactated Ringer's solution. Historically, a flank incision and possible rib resection were necessary for kidney removal from the donor. However, improved surgical techniques are allowing donor kidney removal by means of laparoscopy or laparoscopy-assisted techniques. Before transplantation, the donor kidney's renal artery is flushed with cold heparinized lactated Ringer's solution to prevent clogging. Then the surgeon positions the kidney in a sling over the implantation site. (He never holds the kidney in his hands because this would warm it and possibly cause necrosis.)

The surgeon then implants the kidney in the retroperitoneal area of the iliac fossa, where it's protected by the hip bone. If a donor's left kidney is being used, the surgeon implants it in the recipient's right side; conversely, he implants a donor's right kidney in the recipient's left side. Doing so permits the renal pelvis to rest anteriorly and allows the new kidney's ureter to rest in front of the iliac artery, where the ureter is more accessible.

When the kidney is in place, the surgeon anastomoses its renal vein to the recipient's iliac vein and the renal artery to the recipient's internal iliac artery. (See *Understanding renal transplantation*, page 454.) He then removes the venous and arterial clamps and checks for patency of the anastomoses. Next, he attaches the donor kidney's ureter to the recipient's bladder, taking care to ensure a watertight closure. Usually, a tunneling technique is used

Understanding renal transplantation

In renal transplantation, the donated organ is implanted in the iliac fossa. The organ's vessels are then connected to the internal iliac vein and internal iliac artery, as shown here. Typically, the patient's own kidneys are left in place.

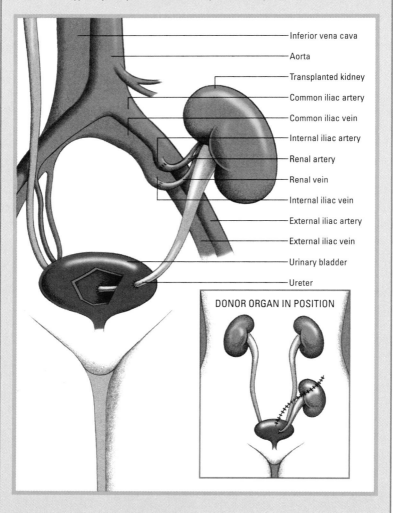

- Inferior vena cava
- Aorta
- Transplanted kidney
- Common iliac artery
- Common iliac vein
- Internal iliac artery
- Renal artery
- Renal vein
- Internal iliac vein
- External iliac artery
- External iliac vein
- Urinary bladder
- Ureter

DONOR ORGAN IN POSITION

Managing transplant rejection

Type of rejection	Pathophysiologic mechanism	Assessment findings	Treatment measures
Hyperacute	Patient's circulating antibodies attack the donor kidney several minutes to hours after transplantation.	• Severe drop in renal perfusion • Ischemia and death of the organ	• Immediate removal of the organ
Acute	Antigen-antibody reaction produces acute tubular necrosis that occurs 1 week to 6 months after transplantation of a living-donor kidney, or 1 week to 2 years after transplantation of a cadaver kidney (most common within 7 to 14 days after transplantation).	• Infection, including fever, rapid pulse, elevated white blood cell count, and lethargy • Oliguria or anuria • Hypertension • Weight gain of more than 3 lb (1.4 kg) in 24 hours • Kidney enlargement and tenderness • Elevated blood urea nitrogen (BUN) and creatinine levels	• Increased dosages of immunosuppressants • Dialysis, if indicated • Removal of the organ, if functioning ceases
Chronic	Long-term antibody destruction of the organ, which may occur from several months to years after transplantation.	• Rising BUN and creatinine levels • Declining glomerular filtration rate • Hypertension • Proteinuria	• Renal scan, renal biopsy, and other tests to determine the extent of damage • Increased dosages of immunosuppressants • Adjustments in diet and fluid regimen • Dialysis or another transplant, if indicated

to connect the ureter to the bladder to prevent urine reflux into the transplanted kidney. When the transplant is complete, the surgeon sutures the incision and sends the patient to the postanesthesia care unit.

Complications

The major impediment to transplantation is rejection of the donated organ. However, careful tissue matching between donor and recipient decreases this risk. (See *Managing transplant rejection.*)

Renal transplantation may also be associated with other complications, including:

■ vascular complications, such as stenosis of the renal artery, vascular leakage, and thrombosis at the surgical site

■ genitourinary tract complications, such as ureteral leakage, ureteral fistula, ureteral obstruction, calculus formation, bladder neck contracture, scrotal swelling, and graft rupture

■ cardiovascular complications, such as hypertension, arrhythmias, heart failure, and increased plasma erythropoietin level

■ respiratory complications, such as pneumonia, pulmonary edema, pulmonary emboli, and reactivated tuberculosis.

Other potential complications include:
■ hepatitis B
■ cirrhosis (associated with azathioprine therapy)
■ peptic ulcers
■ increased histamine levels
■ infection
■ hematomas
■ abscesses
■ lymphoceles
■ steroid-induced diabetes mellitus
■ osteoporosis
■ myopathy
■ aseptic bone necrosis
■ cataracts, glaucoma, and retinitis.

Nursing considerations

When caring for a patient undergoing a kidney transplant, major responsibilities include instructing the patient and monitoring for postoperative complications, including organ rejection.

Before transplantation

■ Prepare the patient thoroughly for transplantation and a prolonged recovery period, and offer him ongoing emotional support.

■ Encourage the patient to express his feelings. If he's concerned about rejection of the donor kidney, explain that if this happens and can't be reversed, he'll resume dialysis and wait for another suitable donor organ. Reassure him that transplant rejection is common and normally isn't life-threatening.

■ Describe routine preoperative measures, such as a thorough physical examination and a battery of laboratory tests to detect infection (followed by antibiotic therapy as treatment), electrolyte studies, abdominal X-rays, an electrocardiogram (ECG), an enema, and hair removal from the operative area if ordered.

■ Tell the patient that he'll undergo dialysis the day before surgery to clean his blood of unwanted fluid and electrolytes. Point out that he may need dialysis for a few days after surgery if his transplanted kidney doesn't start functioning immediately.

■ Review the transplant procedure, supplementing and clarifying the physician's explanation as necessary. Tell the patient that he'll receive a general anesthetic before surgery and that the procedure should take about 4 hours.

■ Explain what the patient can expect after he awakens from anesthesia, including the presence of I.V. lines, an indwelling urinary catheter, an arterial line and, possibly, a mechanical ventilator. Describe routine postoperative care, including frequent checks of vital signs, monitoring of intake and output, and respiratory therapy. Prepare him for postoperative pain, and reassure him that analgesics will be available.

■ Teach the patient the proper methods for performing coughing, turning, deep breathing and, if ordered, incentive spirometry.

■ Discuss the immunosuppressant drugs that the patient will be taking, and explain their possible adverse effects. Point out that these drugs increase his susceptibility to infection.

■ As ordered, begin giving immunosuppressant drugs, such as azathioprine, cyclosporine, muromonab-CD3 (Orthoclone OKT3), and corticosteroids. Oral azathioprine may be started as early as 5 days before surgery.

■ Begin slow I.V. infusion of cyclosporine 4 to 12 hours before surgery; when doing so, closely monitor the patient for anaphylaxis, especially during the first 30 minutes of administration. If anaphylaxis occurs, give epinephrine as ordered.

■ Administer blood transfusions as ordered.

■ Ensure that the patient or a responsible family member has signed an informed consent form.

After transplantation

■ Assess cardiopulmonary and hemodynamic status closely at least every 15 minutes in the immediate postoperative period and then hourly or more frequently, as indicated by the patient's condition. Monitor hemodynamic parameters, including central venous pressure, pulmonary artery pressure, and pulmonary artery wedge pressure for changes indicating changes in fluid volume status.

■ Institute continuous cardiac monitoring, if not already in place, evaluating waveforms frequently for ECG changes indicative of electrolyte balance or ischemia. Watch particularly for signs of hyperkalemia, such as weakness and pulse irregularities and peaked T waves on ECG. If these signs develop, notify the physician and ad-

minister calcium carbonate I.V. as ordered.

■ In the immediate postoperative period, monitor laboratory test results closely, especially blood urea nitrogen (BUN) and creatinine levels.

■ Carefully monitor urine output, at least hourly; promptly report output of less than 100 ml/hour.

ALERT *In a living donor transplant, urine flow usually begins immediately after revascularization and connection of the ureter to the recipient's bladder. In a cadaver renal transplant, however, anuria may persist for anywhere from 2 days to 2 weeks; dialysis will be necessary during this period.*

■ Connect the patient's indwelling urinary catheter to a closed drainage system to prevent overextension of the bladder. Observe urine color; it should be slightly blood-tinged for several days and then should gradually clear. Irrigate the catheter as ordered, using strict sterile technique.

■ If the patient has an endotracheal tube in place and is receiving mechanical ventilation, assist with extubating as soon as possible (usually within 4 to 6 hours) and administer supplemental oxygen as needed, based on mixed venous oxygen saturation or pulse oximetry levels. Encourage coughing and deep breathing and use of incentive spirometer after extubation, splinting, and premedicating for pain as necessary.

■ Assess the patient for pain, and provide analgesics as ordered. Look for a significant decrease in pain after 24 hours; assess for pain related to bladder spasms, which may continue briefly after removal of the catheter, and administer analgesics as ordered.

■ Review daily the results of renal function tests, such as creatinine clearance and BUN, hematocrit, and hemoglobin levels. Review results of tests that assess renal perfusion, such as urine creatinine, urea, sodium, potassium, pH, and specific gravity. Monitor for hematuria and proteinuria.

■ Assess the patient's fluid and electrolyte balance. Weigh the patient daily, and report any rapid gain — a possible sign of fluid retention.

■ Maintain nothing-by-mouth status with nasogastric decompression to low intermittent suction (if appropriate) until bowel sounds return. Administer histamine blockers to suppress gastric acid secretion. Periodically auscultate for bowel sounds, and notify the physician when they return. Begin clear liquids after the patient is extubated and bowel sounds are active. Expect to gradually resume the patient's usual diet, perhaps with some restrictions. For instance, the patient may require a low-sodium diet if he's receiving corticosteroids, to prevent fluid retention.

ALERT *Keep in mind that the patient's immune system has been suppressed by medication and is, therefore, at high risk for infection.*

■ Institute standard precautions and use strict sterile technique when changing dressings and performing catheter care. Limit the patient's contact with staff, other patients, and visitors, and avoid exposing him to persons with any type of infection. Monitor the patient's white blood cell (WBC) count; if it drops precipitously, notify the physician.

■ Watch for signs and symptoms of organ rejection. Observe the transplant site for redness, tenderness, and swelling. Evaluate for fever or an elevated WBC count; decreased urine output with increased proteinuria; sudden weight gain or hypertension; and elevated serum creatinine and BUN levels. Report suspicious signs and symptoms immediately.

■ Change the patient's position at least every 2 hours, getting him out of bed to the chair within 24 hours if his condition is stable. Gradually increase the patient's activity as tolerated.

■ To ease emotional stress, plan care to allow frequent rest periods, and provide as much privacy as possible. Allow family members to visit and comfort the patient as much as possible.

■ Allow family members to express their anxiety and fear.

■ Begin teaching the patient about care after the transplant.

– Advise him to monitor his intake and output and weight; include specific parameters for notifying the physician.

– Teach him to check for signs and symptoms of infection or transplant rejection, including redness, warmth, tenderness, or swelling over the kidney; fever exceeding 100° F (37.8° C); decreased urine output; and elevated blood pressure.

– Review his prescribed medication regimens, and stress the need for compliance with immunosuppressant therapy. Remind him to use antacids (if ordered) immediately before a corticosteroid to combat its ulcerogenic effects.

– Stress the importance of a program of regular, moderate exercise, beginning slowly and increasing gradually.

– Advise him to avoid excessive bending, heavy lifting, or contact sports for at least 3 months or until the physician grants permission for such activities; also advise him to avoid activities or positions that place pressure on the new kidney — for example, long car trips and lap-style seat belts.

– Remind him of the need to wait at least 6 weeks before resuming sexual relations. Because pregnancy poses an added risk to a new kidney, provide the female patient with information on birth control.

– Stress the importance of regular follow-up visits to the physician to evaluate the patient's renal function and transplant acceptance.

6

Endocrine system challenges

Imagine that a patient with diabetes is admitted with a significantly elevated blood glucose level. What would you suspect is happening with the patient? How would you go about determining whether the patient was experiencing diabetic ketoacidosis or hyperglycemic hyperosmolar nonketotic syndrome? What manifestations would support your suspicions? Would the care you give differ depending on which condition was occurring? And if so, how would it be different?

Suppose a patient were diagnosed with diabetes insipidus. What laboratory tests would you expect to monitor? Would you anticipate administering fluids or restricting them? If fluids are to be given, what type of fluid would you expect to use? What if a patient were diagnosed with acute adrenal insufficiency? What fluid and electrolyte imbalances would you expect to find? Why would you continuously monitor the patient's electrocardiogram? How would you determine whether the patient's condition was improving? Worsening?

Another patient is scheduled for a pancreatic transplant. How would you prepare the patient for the surgery? For what posttransplant complications would you be alert? What findings would lead you to suspect that that patient is experiencing acute rejection? In this chapter, you'll find answers to these questions and additional information that will allow you to address the major challenges involving the endocrine system commonly encountered in the critical care area.

 MULTISYSTEM DISORDER

Acute adrenal crisis

Acute adrenal crisis is the result of acute adrenal hypofunction, which is classified as primary or secondary. Primary adrenal hypofunction or insufficiency (Addison's disease) originates within the adrenal gland and is characterized by the decreased secretion of mineralocorticoids, glucocorticoids, and androgens. Addison's disease is relatively uncommon and can occur at any age and in both sexes.

Secondary adrenal hypofunction is caused by impaired pituitary secretion of corticotropin and is characterized by decreased glucocorticoid secretion. The secretion of aldosterone, the major mineralocorticoid, is usually unaffected.

Acute adrenal crisis (also called addisonian crisis) involves a critical deficiency of mineralocorticoids and glucocorticoids. It generally follows acute stress, sepsis, trauma, surgery, or the omission of steroid therapy in patients who have chronic adrenal insufficiency. Adrenal crisis is a medical emergency that needs immediate, vigorous treatment.

Pathophysiology

The most common cause of primary hypofunction is Addison's disease with destruction of more than 90% of both adrenal glands due to an autoimmune process in which circulating antibodies react specifically against the adrenal tissue. Other causes include tuberculosis (at one time the chief cause but now responsible for less than 20% of adult cases), bilateral adrenalectomy, hemorrhage into the adrenal gland, neoplasms, or infections (histoplasmosis or cytomegalovirus). Family history of autoimmune disease may predispose the patient to Addison's disease and other endocrinopathies. Autoimmune Addison's disease is most common in white females, and a genetic predisposition is likely. It's more common in patients with a familial predisposition to autoimmune endocrine diseases. Most persons with Addison's disease are diagnosed in their third to fifth decades.

Addison's disease is a chronic condition that manifests as a clinical syndrome in which the symptoms are associated with deficient production of the adrenocortical hormones, cortisol, aldosterone, and androgens. High levels of corticotropin and corticotropin-releasing hormone accompany the low glucocorticoid levels. Corticotropin acts primarily to regulate the adrenal release of glucocorticoids (primarily cortisol); mineralocorticoids, including aldosterone; and sex steroids that supplement those produced by the gonads. Corticotropin secretion is controlled by corticotropin-releasing hormone from the hypothalamus and by negative feedback control by the glucocorticoids.

Addison's disease involves all zones of the cortex, causing deficiencies of the adrenocortical secretions, glucocorticoids, androgens, and mineralocorticoids. Manifestations of adrenocortical hormone deficiency become apparent when 90% of the functional cells in both glands are lost. In most cases, cellular atrophy is limited to the cortex, although medullary involvement may occur, resulting in catecholamine deficiency. Cortisol deficiency causes decreased liver gluconeogenesis (the formation of glucose from molecules that aren't carbohydrates). The resulting low blood glucose levels can become dangerously low in patients who routinely take insulin.

Aldosterone deficiency causes increased renal sodium loss and enhances potassium reabsorption. Sodium excretion causes a reduction in water volume that leads to hypotension. Patients with Addison's disease may have normal blood pressure when in a supine position but show marked hypotension and tachycardia after standing for several minutes. Low plasma volume and arteriolar pressure stimulate renin release and a resulting increased production of angiotensin II. Androgen deficiency may decrease hair growth in axillary and pubic areas as well as on the extremities of women. The metabolic effects of testicular androgens make such hair growth less noticeable in men.

Secondary adrenal hypofunction occurs when a patient abruptly stops long-term exogenous steroid therapy or when the pituitary is injured by a tumor or by infiltrative or autoimmune processes. These processes occur when circulating antibodies react specifically against adrenal tissue, causing inflammation and infiltration of the cells by lymphocytes. With early diagnosis and adequate replacement therapy, the prognosis for adrenal hypofunction is good.

Causes of secondary hypofunction (glucocorticoid deficiency) include hypopituitarism (causing decreased corticotropin secretion), abrupt withdrawal of long-term corticosteroid therapy (long-term exogenous corticosteroid stimulation suppresses pituitary corticotropin secretion, resulting in adrenal gland atrophy), and removal of a corticotropin-secreting tumor. Adrenal crisis is usually caused by exhausted body stores of glucocorticoids in a person with adrenal hypofunction after trauma, surgery, or other physiologic stress.

Comprehensive assessment

Clinical features vary with the type of adrenal hypofunction. Signs and symptoms of addisonian crisis may include a patient who has profound weakness and fatigue, with nausea, vomiting, dehydration, and hypoglycemia. Blood pressure reveals hypotension, and vital signs show high fever followed by hypothermia (occasionally). After an adrenalectomy, especially a bilateral one, signs and symptoms of acute adrenal crisis may develop. The patient is most prone to acute adrenal crisis during the first 24 to 48 hours after surgery, with the 9th to 12th hours postoperatively being the most common time of onset. If the patient has undergone bilateral adrenalectomy,

he's at lifelong risk for this complication.

The patient may develop the crisis after experiencing marked stress without adjustment in his glucocorticoid replacement therapy or if he abruptly stops his glucocorticoid therapy. If untreated, acute adrenal crisis can ultimately cause vascular collapse, renal shutdown, coma, and death. (See *Understanding acute adrenal crisis*.)

The patient with signs and symptoms of primary hypofunction may exhibit weakness, fatigue, and weight loss. He may complain of nausea, vomiting, and anorexia and have a conspicuous bronze color of the skin, especially in the creases of the hands and over the metacarpophalangeal joints (hand and finger), elbows, and knees. There may be darkening of scars, areas of vitiligo (absence of pigmentation), and increased pigmentation of the mucous membranes, especially the buccal mucosa, due to decreased secretion of cortisol, causing simultaneous secretion of excessive amounts of corticotropin and melanocyte-stimulating hormone by the pituitary gland.

Associated cardiovascular abnormalities may include orthostatic hypotension, decreased cardiac size and output, and weak, irregular pulse. The patient may have decreased tolerance for even minor stress. Fasting hypoglycemia is present because of decreased gluconeogenesis. The patient may have a craving for salty food due to decreased mineralocorticoid secretion (which normally causes salt retention).

Signs and symptoms of secondary hypofunction are similar to primary hypofunction, but without hyperpigmentation because of low corticotropin

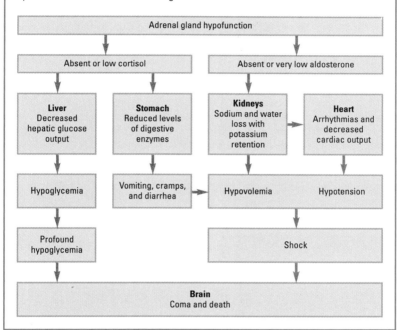

Understanding acute adrenal crisis

Acute adrenal crisis is a life-threatening event that requires prompt assessment and immediate treatment. The flowchart below highlights the underlying mechanisms responsible for the assessment findings.

Adrenal gland hypofunction

Absent or low cortisol

Absent or very low aldosterone

Liver
Decreased hepatic glucose output

Stomach
Reduced levels of digestive enzymes

Kidneys
Sodium and water loss with potassium retention

Heart
Arrhythmias and decreased cardiac output

Hypoglycemia

Vomiting, cramps, and diarrhea

Hypovolemia

Hypotension

Profound hypoglycemia

Shock

Brain
Coma and death

and melanocyte-stimulating hormone levels. In addition, there may possibly be no hypotension and electrolyte abnormalities because of fairly normal aldosterone secretion, and there is usually normal androgen secretion.

Diagnosis

In a patient with typical addisonian symptoms, the following findings strongly suggest acute adrenal insufficiency:

■ decreased plasma cortisol level (less than10 mcg/dl in the morning; less in the evening)

■ decreased serum sodium and fasting blood glucose levels
■ increased serum potassium and blood urea nitrogen levels
■ decreased hematocrit; increased lymphocyte and eosinophil counts
■ X-rays showing adrenal calcification, if the cause is infectious.

In addition, diagnosis of adrenal hypofunction is based on:
■ plasma cortisol levels confirming adrenal insufficiency (corticotropin stimulation test to differentiate between primary and secondary adrenal hypofunction)

- metyrapone test for suspicion of secondary adrenal hypofunction (oral or I.V. metyrapone blocks cortisol production and should stimulate the release of corticotropin from the hypothalamic-pituitary system; in Addison's disease, the hypothalamic-pituitary system responds normally and plasma corticotropin levels are high, but because the adrenal glands are destroyed, plasma concentrations of the cortisol precursor 11-deoxycortisol increase, as do urinary 17-hydroxycorticosteroids)
- rapid corticotropin stimulation test by I.V. or I.M. administration of cosyntropin (Cortrosyn) after baseline sampling for cortisol and corticotropin (samples drawn for cortisol 30 and 60 minutes after injection), to differentiate between primary and secondary adrenal hypofunction.

Collaborations

Care of the patient with acute adrenal insufficiency requires a multidisciplinary approach. Emergency treatment is necessary to manage this life-threatening condition. An endocrinologist may be involved in the management of the patient's adrenal function. As other organ systems become involved, however, the patient may need the assistance of a cardiologist and renal specialist. Respiratory therapists and nutritional consults may also be needed to assist the patient. Spiritual guidance may also be needed for the patient and his family.

Treatment and care

Emergency management includes I.V. bolus of hydrocortisone, 100 mg every 6 hours for 24 hours. Then it may be followed with 50 to 100 mg I.M. or diluted with dextrose in saline solution and given I.V. until the patient's condition stabilizes. Up to 300 mg/day of hydrocortisone and 3 to 5 L of I.V. saline and glucose solutions may be needed during acute adrenal crisis.

With proper treatment, adrenal crisis usually subsides quickly; blood pressure stabilizes, and water and sodium levels return to normal. After the crisis, maintenance doses of hydrocortisone preserve physiologic stability.

Fluids are administered I.V. rapidly to maintain blood pressure. Vasopressors are also used if the patient doesn't respond to initial therapy. These agents are titrated according to the patient's blood pressure.

ALERT *Because of the hormonal deficiencies, patients in acute adrenal crisis have a decreased response to catecholamines, vasopressors, and inotropic agents. Therefore, these agents may not be as effective for these patient as they would for patients with adequate adrenal gland function.*

Vital signs will need to be monitored closely as well as intake and output, electrocardiogram, blood glucose levels, and electrolytes. Replacements for electrolytes and I.V. fluid requirements are adjusted as needed. If fever persists despite hydrocortisone therapy, antipyretics may be administered and cooling procedures initiated.

A nasogastric (NG) tube may be inserted if the patient is vomiting but isn't awake and alert. Respirations may be supported by mechanical ventilation with adjustments made based on assessment and arterial blood gas results. If hypoglycemia becomes profound or persists despite hydrocortisone therapy, I.V. glucose may be administered.

Treatment for adrenal hypofunction may include lifelong corticosteroid replacement, usually with cortisone or hydrocortisone, both of which have a mineralocorticoid effect (primary or secondary adrenal hypofunction). Oral fludrocortisone (Florinef), a synthetic mineralocorticoid, may be used to prevent dangerous dehydration, hypotension, hyponatremia, and hyperkalemia.

Complications
Possible complications of adrenal hypofunction include hyperpyrexia, psychotic reactions, and deficient or excessive steroid treatment. The result is ultimate vascular collapse, renal shutdown, coma, and death (if untreated).

Nursing considerations
■ Assess vital signs every 15 minutes initially and then hourly after the patient is stabilized. Monitor blood pressure with the patient lying and sitting; report any decreases of 10 mm Hg or more on position changes. Institute measures, such as cooling blankets, tepid sponge baths, and antipyretic therapy, as ordered to decrease temperature.

■ Assist with the insertion of a pulmonary artery catheter if one isn't already in place; monitor hemodynamic parameters initially every 15 minutes until stabilized and then every 1 to 2 hours as indicated to evaluate fluid status.

■ Administer hydrocortisone as an I.V. bolus, and repeat every 6 to 8 hours as ordered; alternatively, administer hydrocortisone by continuous I.V. infusion.

ALERT *Hydrocortisone exerts some mineralocorticoid effects. Therefore, emergency replacement of mineralocorticoids, such as fludrocortisone, isn't necessary.*

■ Expect to switch to oral therapy after the patient's condition stabilizes and he's able to ingest fluids.

■ Begin I.V. fluid therapy replacement immediately, initially administering 1 L of solution (usually dextrose 5% and normal saline) in 1 hour, followed by infusion of 1 to 2 L over the next 6 to 8 hours.

■ Assess urinary output hourly; anticipate the need for indwelling urinary catheter insertion to ensure accurate urine outputs. Monitor daily weight and intake and other output sources, including wound drainage, NG tube drainage, and diarrhea.

■ Assess respiratory status frequently. Auscultate breath sounds for the presence of crackles as well as heart sounds for gallops or the presence of an S_3 or S_4, which may indicate fluid overload.

■ Institute continuous cardiac monitoring to evaluate for possible arrhythmias secondary to electrolyte imbalances.

■ Assess level of consciousness frequently, and reorient the patient as needed.

■ Monitor renal function studies and hematocrit and hemoglobin levels regularly as ordered. Review the results of laboratory tests, including serum electrolyte and blood glucose levels. Expect to administer I.V. glucose if hypoglycemia is present; if hyponatremia is present, expect to administer saline, usually in the form of I.V. saline solutions as part of fluid replacement therapy.

■ Assess for and report signs of hypoglycemia (tachycardia, fatigue, nausea, hypotension, diaphoresis, and mental confusion) or electrolyte imbalances.

ALERT *The patient in acute adrenal crisis is at high risk for hyponatremia and hyperkalemia. Be alert for manifestations of hyponatremia, such as headache, malaise, muscle weakness, and abdominal cramps, and manifestations of hyperkalemia, such as lethargy, nausea, vomiting, numbness or tingling of extremities, and hyperactive bowel sounds with diarrhea. Observe the electrocardiogram monitor for evidence of tall, tented T waves, widening QRS complex, prolonged PR interval, and flattened or absent P wave, all findings associated with hyperkalemia.*

■ Minimize the patient's exposure to physiologic and emotional stressors. Maintain a quiet environment. Dim lights and limit visitors as necessary. Provide periods of rest between activities. Use infection control measures during care. Don't allow staff members or visitors with upper respiratory tract infections to come in contact with the patient. Use standard precautions when handling blood and body fluids.

ALERT *Keep in mind that any stress, including infection, can precipitate acute adrenal crisis.*

■ Evaluate and maintain nutritional status. Encourage oral intake as soon as possible after the patient's condition stabilizes. Provide a diet as per nutritional therapy with vitamin supplements as ordered. Give the anorectic patient small, frequent meals.

■ Use appropriate safety measures, such as side rails and restraints, because the patient with central nervous system involvement may become disoriented, light-headed, or confused.

■ Prevent complications of immobility by encouraging frequent coughing and deep breathing and by performing passive range-of-motion exercises. Help the patient walk as soon as possible. Add lubricating lotion to his bath water to combat skin dryness.

■ Assess the patient's ability to resume normal activities of daily living, and plan for the gradual resumption of activity.

■ Provide emotional support to the patient and his family.

Patient teaching

■ Reassure the patient and his family by clearly explaining diagnostic tests, treatments, and procedures.

■ Tell the patient about his prescribed medications, and advise him not to take over-the-counter medications until he has talked with his physician. Stress the importance of complying with the regimen.

■ Stress the importance of following the prescribed diet and fluid allowance, and advise against overexertion.

■ Instruct the patient about preventing infection and avoiding major stress events, which can precipitate a crisis; explain how to recognize signs of infection or stress, urging him to report findings to the physician because adjustments in medication are necessary.

⭐ **MULTISYSTEM DISORDER**

Diabetes insipidus

A disorder of water metabolism, diabetes insipidus results from a deficiency of circulating vasopressin (also called antidiuretic hormone [ADH]) or from renal resistance to this hormone. Pituitary diabetes insipidus is caused by a deficiency of vasopressin, and nephrogenic diabetes insipidus is caused by the resistance of renal tubules to vasopressin. Diabetes insipidus is characterized by excessive fluid intake and hypotonic polyuria. A decrease in ADH levels leads to altered intracellular and extracellular fluid control, causing renal excretion of a large amount of urine.

Causes of diabetes insipidus may be:

■ acquired, familial, idiopathic, neurogenic, or nephrogenic
■ associated with stroke, hypothalamic or pituitary tumors, and cranial trauma or surgery (neurogenic diabetes insipidus)
■ X-linked recessive trait or end-stage renal failure (nephrogenic diabetes insipidus, which is less common)
■ certain drugs, such as lithium (Eskalith), phenytoin (Dilantin), or alcohol (transient diabetes insipidus).

The disorder may start at any age and is slightly more common in men than in women. The incidence is slightly greater today than in the past.

In uncomplicated diabetes insipidus, the prognosis is good with adequate water replacement, and patients usually lead normal lives. However, in patients with an underlying disorder, such as cancer, the prognosis varies.

Pathophysiology

Diabetes insipidus is related to an insufficiency of ADH, leading to polyuria and polydipsia. The three forms of diabetes insipidus are neurogenic, nephrogenic, and psychogenic. Neurogenic, or central, diabetes insipidus is an inadequate response of ADH to plasma osmolarity, which occurs when an organic lesion of the hypothalamus, infundibular stem, or posterior pituitary partially or completely blocks ADH synthesis, transport, or release. The

many organic lesions that can cause diabetes insipidus include brain tumors, hypophysectomy, aneurysms, thrombosis, infections, and immunologic disorders. Neurogenic diabetes insipidus has an acute onset. A three-phase syndrome can occur, which involves:

■ progressive loss of nerve tissue and increased diuresis
■ normal diuresis
■ polyuria and polydipsia, the manifestation of permanent loss of the ability to secrete adequate ADH.

Nephrogenic diabetes insipidus is caused by an inadequate renal response to ADH. The collecting duct permeability to water doesn't increase in response to ADH. Nephrogenic diabetes insipidus is generally related to disorders and drugs that damage the renal tubules or inhibit the generation of cyclic adenosine monophosphate in the tubules, preventing activation of the second messenger. Causative disorders include pyelonephritis, amyloidosis, destructive uropathies, polycystic disease, and intrinsic renal disease. Drugs include lithium (Eskalith), general anesthetics such as methoxyflurane, and demeclocycline (Declomycin). In addition, hypokalemia or hypercalcemia impairs the renal response to ADH. A rare genetic form of nephrogenic diabetes insipidus is an X-linked recessive trait.

Psychogenic diabetes insipidus is caused by an extremely large fluid intake, which may be idiopathic or related to psychosis or sarcoidosis. The polydipsia and resultant polyuria wash out ADH more quickly than it can be replaced. Chronic polyuria may overwhelm the renal medullary concentration gradient, rendering patients partially or totally unable to concentrate urine.

Regardless of the cause, insufficient ADH causes the immediate excretion of large volumes of dilute urine and consequent plasma hyperosmolality. In conscious individuals, the thirst mechanism is stimulated, usually for cold liquids. With severe ADH deficiency, urine output may be greater than 12 L/day, with a low specific gravity. Dehydration develops rapidly if fluids aren't replaced.

Comprehensive assessment

The patient's history shows an abrupt onset of extreme polyuria (usually 2 to 20 L/day of dilute urine, but sometimes as much as 30 L/day), extreme thirst, and polydipsia (5 to 20 L/day). The patient may report weight loss, dizziness, weakness, constipation, slight to moderate nocturia and, in severe cases, fatigue from inadequate rest caused by frequent voiding and excessive thirst.

On inspection, signs of dehydration, such as dry skin and mucous membranes, fever, and dyspnea, may be present. Urine is pale and voluminous. Palpation may reveal poor skin turgor, tachycardia, and decreased muscle strength. Hypotension may be present on blood pressure auscultation.

Diagnosis

To distinguish diabetes insipidus from other types of polyuria, the following tests may be ordered:
- Urinalysis reveals almost colorless urine of low osmolality (50 to 200 mOsm/kg of water, less than that of plasma) and low specific gravity (less than 1.005).
- Dehydration test is a simple, reliable way to diagnose diabetes insipidus and to differentiate vasopressin deficiency from other forms of polyuria by comparing urine osmolality after dehydration with urine osmolality after vasopressin administration. A rise in urine osmolality after vasopressin administration exceeding 9% indicates diabetes insipidus. (Patients with pituitary diabetes insipidus respond to exogenous vasopressin with decreased urine output and increased urine specific gravity. Those with nephrogenic diabetes insipidus show no response to vasopressin.)
- Plasma and urinary vasopressin evaluations (although too expensive and time-consuming to use regularly, these tests may be used occasionally) confirm diagnosis when osmolality measures are inconclusive.

In critically ill patients, diagnosis may be based on the following laboratory values only:
- urine osmolality — below 200 mOsm/kg
- urine specific gravity — below 1.005
- serum osmolality — above 300 mOsm/kg
- serum sodium — above 147 mEq/L.

Collaborations

A multidisciplinary approach to care is necessary. The patient may require consultation with an endocrinologist and other specialists, depending on the underlying cause of the diabetes insipidus. For example, if it's due to a head injury, a neurosurgeon should be consulted as well as a pulmonologist (for mechanical ventilation and airway support as necessary), a cardiologist (for hemodynamic support), and a nutritionist (for dietary support).

Treatment and care

Until the cause of diabetes insipidus is identified and eliminated, administration of vasopressin or a vasopressin stimulant can control fluid balance and prevent dehydration. Medications include:

■ vasopressin aqueous preparation subcutaneously (S.C.) or I.M. several times daily; effective for only 2 to 6 hours (used as a diagnostic agent and, rarely, in acute disease)
■ hypotonic I.V. solution to replace free water lost in urine
■ thiazide diuretics in conjunction with a low-sodium diet for patients with nephrogenic diabetes insipidus
■ transphenoidal hypophysectomy for patients with pituitary tumors.

Complications

Possible complications of diabetes insipidus include:
■ dilatation of the urinary tract
■ severe dehydration
■ shock and renal failure, if dehydration is severe.

Nursing considerations

■ Administer vasopressin as ordered. **ALERT** *Vasopressin can lead to hypertension, angina, or myocardial infarction resulting from the drug's vasoconstrictive effects. The patient with coronary artery disease is particularly at high risk for these effects. Monitor the patient's cardiac status closely.*
■ Begin fluid replacement therapy using hypotonic solutions as ordered. Expect to administer 1 ml of fluid for every 1 ml of urine output; encourage oral fluid intake if appropriate.
■ Monitor vital signs closely, especially heart rate and blood pressure, at least every 15 minutes initially and then less frequently as the patient's condition stabilizes. Note any weak or thready pulse, or hypotension, which may indicate dehydration.
■ Assess hemodynamic status, including central venous pressure, pulmonary artery pressure, mean arterial pressure, and pulmonary artery wedge pressure. Anticipate the need for insertion of a central venous or pulmonary artery catheter if one isn't already in place.
■ Institute continuous cardiac monitoring to assess for arrhythmias, especially after administration of vasopressin.
■ Assess the patient's urinary output and the urine specific gravity to establish as a baseline, and then continue to monitor hourly to evaluate the patient's response to therapy. If necessary, insert an indwelling urinary catheter to ensure accurate urine output measurements.
ALERT *When assessing output, be sure to include output from other sources, such as drainage tubes or emesis. Be sure to include insensible fluid losses because fluid replacement is based on output. Ultimately, the goal is to achieve an equalization of intake with output.*
■ Obtain daily weight, noting any trends in weight loss, and monitor skin turgor.
■ Monitor serum electrolyte levels, especially sodium, blood urea nitrogen levels, and serum osmolality for changes.

ALERT *Hypernatremia is common in patients with diabetes insipidus. It must be corrected slowly to avoid rapid fluid shifts in the brain, which could lead to cerebral edema, seizures, or permanent neurologic damage.*

■ During dehydration testing, watch for signs of hypovolemic shock. Monitor blood pressure, pulse rate, body weight, and changes in mental or neurologic status.

■ Assess the patient receiving vasopressin for signs and symptoms of water intoxication, including drowsiness, light-headedness, headache, seizures and, possibly, coma. Notify the physician immediately.

■ Expect to taper vasopressin therapy, as ordered, to evaluate for resolution of the condition.

ALERT *During tapering, monitor the patient's urine specific gravity and output closely for a return to normal, indicating that diabetes insipidus has resolved. If the patient's urine output increases when vasopressin is tapered or stopped, suspect chronic diabetes insipidus.*

■ If the patient has nephrogenic diabetes insipidus, administer thiazide diuretics and provide a low-sodium diet.

■ Institute safety precautions if the patient experiences alterations in level of consciousness.

■ If the patient is taking chlorpropamide, provide adequate caloric intake and keep orange juice or another carbohydrate handy to treat hypoglycemic episodes. Monitor patients taking chlorpropamide for signs of hypoglycemia. Watch for decreasing urine output and increasing urine specific gravity between doses. Check laboratory values for hyponatremia and hypoglycemia.

■ Prepare the patient for transphenoidal hypophysectomy if the cause of diabetes insipidus is a pituitary tumor; assess neurologic status, including monitoring for signs and symptoms of increased intracranial pressure postoperatively.

■ Urge the patient to verbalize his feelings. Offer encouragement and a realistic assessment of his situation. Reassure him that diabetes insipidus is usually temporary and that he can look for improvement within 5 to 7 days. Inform him, though, that if improvement doesn't occur, chronic diabetes insipidus can result.

Patient teaching

■ Encourage the patient to maintain adequate fluid intake during the day to prevent severe dehydration and to limit fluids in the evening to prevent nocturia.

■ Teach the patient and his family how to monitor daily weight and intake and output and how to measure urine specific gravity.

■ Instruct the patient and his family about signs and symptoms of severe dehydration and impending hypovolemia and the need to report them.

■ Inform the patient and his family about long-term hormone replacement therapy. Inform them that the medication must be taken as prescribed and must not be discontinued abruptly without the physician's advice. Teach them how to give S.C. or I.M. injections and how to use nasal applicators. Discuss the drug's adverse effects and when to report them.

■ Advise the patient to wear a medical identification bracelet and to carry his medication with him at all times.

■ Provide teaching about postoperative care and follow-up, as indicated.

MULTISYSTEM DISORDER

Diabetic ketoacidosis

Diabetic ketoacidosis (DKA) is an acute complication of hyperglycemic crisis that may occur in the patient with diabetes. If not treated properly, it may result in coma or death. Ketoacidosis occurs most commonly in patients with type 1 diabetes; in fact, it may be the first evidence of previously unrecognized type 1 diabetes. However, it also can occur in patients with type 2 diabetes.

The causes of type 1 and type 2 diabetes mellitus remain unknown. Genetic factors may influence the development of both types. Autoimmune disease and viral infections may be risk factors in type 1 diabetes mellitus.

Other risk factors include:
- obesity, which contributes to a resistance to endogenous insulin
- physiologic or emotional stress, which may induce a prolonged elevation of stress hormone levels (cortisol, epinephrine, glucagon, and growth hormone) that subsequently elevates blood glucose and places increased demands on the pancreas
- pregnancy, which causes weight gain and increased estrogen and placental hormone levels
- certain medications, including thiazide diuretics, adrenal corticosteroids, and hormonal contraceptives, which antagonize the effects of insulin.

Pathophysiology

Acute insulin deficiency is absolute in ketoacidosis and can precipitate the condition. Causes include illness, stress, infection, and failure to take insulin. Inadequate insulin hinders glucose uptake by fat and muscle cells. Because the cells can't take in glucose to convert to energy, glucose accumulates in the blood. At the same time, the liver responds to the demands of the energy-starved cells by converting glycogen to glucose and releasing glucose into the blood, further increasing the blood glucose level. When this level exceeds the renal threshold, excess glucose is excreted in the urine.

Still, the insulin-deprived cells can't utilize glucose. Their response is rapid metabolism of protein, which results in loss of intracellular potassium and phosphorus and in excessive liberation of amino acids. The liver converts these amino acids into urea and glucose. As a result of these processes, blood glucose levels are grossly elevated. The aftermath is increased serum osmolarity and glycosuria, leading to osmotic diuresis.

The massive fluid loss from osmotic diuresis causes fluid and electrolyte imbalances and dehydration. Water loss exceeds electrolyte loss, contributing to hyperosmolarity. This in turn perpetuates dehydration, decreasing the glomerular filtration rate and reducing the amount of glucose excreted in the urine. This leads to a deadly cycle: diminished glucose excretion further raises blood glucose levels, producing severe hyperosmolarity and dehydration and finally causing shock, coma, and death.

Absolute insulin deficiency causes cells to convert fats into glycerol and fatty acids for energy. The fatty acids can't be metabolized as quickly as they're released, so they accumulate in the liver, where they're converted into ketones (ketoacids). Acidosis leads to more tissue breakdown, more ketosis, more acidosis, and eventually shock,

Understanding diabetic ketoacidosis

The flowchart below highlights the pathophysiologic events that occur in diabetic ketoacidosis.

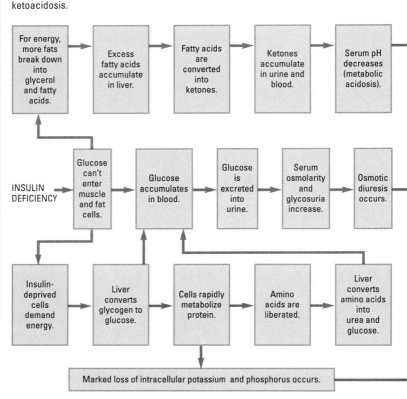

coma, and death. (See *Understanding diabetic ketoacidosis*.)

Comprehensive assessment

The patient may have rapid onset of drowsiness, stupor, and coma. He may have a history of diabetes mellitus. Polyuria and extreme volume depletion may occur, resulting in hypotension, tachycardia, and diaphoresis. Respirations may reveal hyperventila-

tion, and the patient may have an acetone breath odor.

The patient with type 1 diabetes usually reports rapidly developing symptoms. With type 2 diabetes, the patient's symptoms are usually vague and long-standing and develop gradually. Patients with type 2 diabetes generally report a family history of diabetes mellitus, gestational diabetes, or the delivery of a baby weighing more

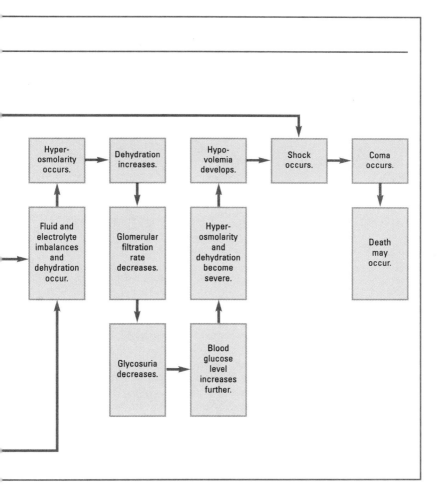

than 9 lb (4.1 kg); a severe viral infection, autoimmune dysfunction, other endocrine disease, or recent stress or trauma; or the use of drugs that increase blood glucose levels.

Patients with type 1 or type 2 diabetes may report symptoms related to hyperglycemia, such as polyuria, polydipsia, polyphagia, weight loss, and fatigue. Or, they may complain of weakness, vision changes, frequent skin infections, sexual problems, vaginal discomfort, or dry, itchy skin — all symptoms of complications.

Inspection may show retinopathy or cataract formation. Skin changes — especially on the legs and feet — represent impaired peripheral circulation. Muscle wasting and loss of subcutaneous fat may be evident in type 1 diabetes; type 2 is characterized by thin, muscular limbs and fat deposits around the face, neck, and abdomen.

Palpation may detect poor skin turgor and dry mucous membranes related to dehydration. Decreased peripheral pulses, cool skin temperature, and decreased reflexes may also be palpable. Auscultation may reveal orthostatic hypotension. Patients with DKA may have a characteristic "fruity" breath odor due to increased acetone production.

Diagnosis

The following findings help diagnose DKA:

■ Blood glucose level is elevated slightly above normal, ranging from 200 to 800 mg/dl.

■ Serum ketone level is elevated.

■ Serum potassium level is normal or elevated initially and then drops.

■ Urine glucose is positive.

■ Urine acetone level is typically high.

■ Serum phosphorus, magnesium, and chloride are decreased.

■ Serum osmolality is slightly elevated, ranging from 300 to 350 mOsm/L.

■ Hematocrit is slightly elevated due to hemoconcentration from osmotic diuresis

■ Arterial blood gas (ABG) studies reveal metabolic acidosis.

■ Electrocardiogram (ECG) may reveal arrhythmias caused by electrolyte imbalances, particularly potassium.

Collaborations

The patient with DKA requires a multidisciplinary approach to care. Care focuses on rehydrating the patient, controlling glucose levels, and restoring electrolyte and acid-base balance. The patient may be managed by an endocrinologist to help control blood glucose levels. Depending on the severity of the symptoms, the patient may require a pulmonologist to assist with ventilatory support. Nutritional therapy also is indicated to assist with dietary needs. A registered dietitian can help the patient meet his needs for a nutritionally planned diet while considering caloric allotment and the glycemic index of foods. A diabetes educator can be extremely valuable in helping the patient learn about his disease and manage it. Additionally, social services may be involved in assisting with follow-up and care at home, including appropriate financial and community resources.

Treatment and care

If the patient is comatose, airway support and mechanical ventilation are indicated. Insulin therapy given I.V. and fluid and electrolyte replacements are ordered based on laboratory test results. Blood glucose and ABGs are monitored carefully, and adjustments are made in I.V. medications and fluids. Cardiac monitoring and frequent vital sign assessment are important. In addition, intake and output are monitored carefully to evaluate the patient's degree of osmotic diuresis. Urine may be tested for glucose and ketones.

Effective treatment of diabetes normalizes the blood glucose level and decreases complications. In type 1 diabetes, goals are achieved with insulin replacement, diet, and exercise. Current forms of insulin replacement therapy include single-dose, mixed-dose, split-mixed-dose, and multiple-dose regimens.

Treatment for both types also requires a diet that's planned to meet nutritional needs, control blood glucose levels, and reach and maintain appropriate body weight. For the obese patient with type 2 diabetes, the calorie allotment may be high, depending on the patient's growth stage and activity level. To be successful, the patient must follow the diet consistently and eat at regular times. Patients with type 2 diabetes may also need oral antidiabetic drugs to stimulate endogenous insulin production, increase insulin sensitivity at the cellular level, suppress hepatic gluconeogenesis, and delay GI absorption of carbohydrates. Combinations of agents may be used.

The long-term goal of treatment is adequate glycemic control and prevention of complications. Vascular complications commonly occur; studies are under way to decrease their occurrence. Treatment for long-term complications may include dialysis or kidney transplantation for renal failure, photocoagulation or vitrectomy for retinopathy, and vascular surgery for large vessel disease. Precise blood glucose control is essential. Pancreas transplantation is available, but this treatment requires chronic immunosuppression. (See "Pancreas transplantation," page 487.)

Complications

Severe hyperosmolarity and dehydration occur, resulting in shock, coma, and death if left untreated. Additionally, patients with diabetes mellitus have a higher risk of various systemic chronic illnesses. The most common chronic complications include cardiovascular and peripheral vascular disease, retinopathy, nephropathy, diabetic dermopathy, and peripheral and autonomic neuropathy. Nearly two-thirds of people with diabetes mellitus die of cardiovascular disease. It's also the leading cause of renal failure and blindness.

Peripheral neuropathy usually affects the hands and feet and may cause numbness or pain. Autonomic neuropathy manifests itself in several ways, including gastroparesis (leading to delayed gastric emptying and a feeling of nausea and fullness after meals), nocturnal diarrhea, sexual dysfunction, and postural hypotension.

Hyperglycemia impairs the patient's resistance to infection because the glucose content of the epidermis and urine encourages bacterial growth. The patient is therefore susceptible to skin and urinary tract infections and vaginitis. Patients with diabetes mellitus also have an increased incidence of cognitive depression.

Nursing considerations

■ Assess the patient's level of consciousness and ability to maintain a patent airway. Monitor respiratory status closely, including respiratory rate and depth and breath sounds. Assess oxygen saturation via pulse oximetry to evaluate for hypoxemia. Anticipate the need for endotracheal intubation and mechanical ventilation if the patient is unable to maintain a patent airway or develops respiratory distress.
■ Monitor vital signs frequently at least every 15 minutes initially and then hourly as indicated. Assess hemodynamic status at least hourly. Assist with the insertion of a central venous or pulmonary artery catheter for hemodynamic monitoring if one isn't already in place.
■ Institute continuous cardiac monitoring to evaluate for possible arrhythmias secondary to electrolyte imbalances.

ALERT *Patients with DKA are at high risk for hyperkalemia prior to treatment due to the movement of potassium out of the cells. Be alert for ECG changes associated with hyperkalemia, such as peaked T waves, widened QRS complexes, prolonged PR intervals, and flattened or absent P waves. After treatment is initiated and potassium begins to move back into the cells, be alert for hypokalemia, evidenced by ST segment depression, flattened T wave, and presence of a U wave. If hypokalemia is severe, the PR interval will be prolonged and the QRS complex will appear widened.*

■ Administer I.V. fluid replacement therapy with normal saline, typically 1 to 2 L during the first hour to correct the fluid deficit secondary to osmotic diuresis; continue fluid replacement therapy with 0.45% saline.

ALERT *When the patient's blood glucose levels approach 250 mg/ dl, anticipate the addition of dextrose to the fluid replacement regimen. Dextrose is necessary to prevent hypoglycemia while also allowing for continued use of insulin to correct the patient's acidosis.*

■ Administer regular insulin I.V. as ordered, usually first as a bolus dose and then by continuous I.V. infusion at a rate of 0.1U/kg/hour. Remember that blood glucose levels must be reduced gradually to prevent cerebral fluid shifting and subsequent cerebral edema.

■ Monitor blood glucose levels and serum electrolyte levels frequently as ordered. Anticipate potassium replacement after insulin therapy is initiated. If the patient has experienced prolonged acidosis or if phosphorus levels are severely decreased, anticipate phosphorus replacement therapy.

ALERT *When phosphorus replacement is required, be sure to institute it gradually and to monitor the patient's serum calcium levels. Remember that calcium and phosphorus have an inverse relationship; therefore, if phosphorus levels rise too quickly, serum calcium levels will fall quickly, predisposing the patient to tetany.*

■ Anticipate the need for nasogastric tube insertion to prevent vomiting and aspiration, if the patient is comatose or obtunded.

■ Monitor the patient for signs and symptoms of infection.

ALERT *Don't rely on temperature or white blood cell (WBC) counts to determine possible infection. Acidosis can mask an elevated temperature; additionally, elevations in WBC counts may be due to dehydration and increased adrenal gland secretion.*

■ Perform meticulous hand washing and use strict sterile technique when caring for any invasive lines (which should be kept to a minimum).

■ Assess for acute complications of diabetic therapy, especially hypoglycemia (shaking, tachycardia, sweating, irritability, anxiety, dizziness, pallor, confusion, headache). Monitor diabetic effects on the cardiovascular, peripheral vascular, and nervous systems.

■ Assess for signs and symptoms of diabetic neuropathy (numbness or pain in the hands and feet, footdrop, and neurogenic bladder). Provide meticulous skin care, especially to the feet and legs. Treat all injuries, cuts, and blisters promptly. Avoid constricting hose, slippers, or bed linens. Refer the patient to a podiatrist.

■ Observe for signs of urinary tract and vaginal infections, and monitor the patient's urine for protein, an early sign of nephropathy.

■ Consult a dietitian to plan a diet with the recommended amounts of calories, protein, carbohydrates, and fats, based on the patient's particular requirements.

■ Encourage the patient to verbalize his feelings about diabetes and its effect on his lifestyle and life expectancy.

■ Consult the services of a diabetes educator to assist with teaching.

Patient teaching

■ Review the prescribed diabetic regimen, and monitor the patient's compliance with it.

■ Stress the importance of strictly complying with the prescribed therapy. Discuss diet, medications, exercise, monitoring techniques, hygiene and foot care, sick day rules, and how to prevent and recognize hypoglycemia and hyperglycemia. Emphasize how blood glucose control affects long-term health.

 MULTISYSTEM DISORDER

Hyperglycemic hyperosmolar nonketotic syndrome

Hyperglycemic hyperosmolar nonketotic syndrome (HHNS) is an acute complication of hyperglycemic crisis that may occur in the diabetic patient. If not treated properly, it may result in coma or death. HHNS occurs most commonly in patients with type 2 diabetes mellitus, but hyperosmolar coma may also occur in anyone whose insulin tolerance is stressed and in pa-

tients who have undergone certain therapeutic procedures, such as peritoneal dialysis, hemodialysis, tube feedings, or total parenteral nutrition.

The causes of type 1 and type 2 diabetes mellitus remain unknown. Genetic factors may influence the development of both types. Autoimmune disease and viral infections may be risk factors in type 1 diabetes mellitus.

Other risk factors include:

■ obesity, which contributes to a resistance to endogenous insulin

■ physiologic or emotional stress, which may induce a prolonged elevation of stress hormone levels (cortisol, epinephrine, glucagon, and growth hormone), subsequently elevating blood glucose and placing increased demands on the pancreas

■ pregnancy, which causes weight gain and increased estrogen and placental hormone levels

■ certain medications, including thiazide diuretics, adrenal corticosteroids, and oral contraceptives, which antagonize the effects of insulin.

Pathophysiology

Acute insulin deficiency is relative in HHNS (rather than absolute, as in diabetic ketoacidosis [DKA]) and can precipitate the condition. Causes include illness, stress, and infection. Inadequate insulin hinders glucose uptake by fat and muscle cells. Because the cells can't take in glucose to convert to energy, glucose accumulates in the blood. At the same time, the liver responds to the demands of the energy-starved cells by converting glycogen to glucose and releasing glucose into the blood, further increasing the blood glucose level. When this level exceeds the renal threshold, excess glucose is excreted in the urine.

Still, the insulin-deprived cells can't utilize glucose. Their response is rapid metabolism of protein, which results in loss of intracellular potassium and phosphorus and in excessive liberation of amino acids. The liver converts these amino acids into urea and glucose. As a result of these processes, blood glucose levels are grossly elevated. The aftermath is increased serum osmolarity and elevated glycosuria leading to osmotic diuresis.

The massive fluid loss from osmotic diuresis causes fluid and electrolyte imbalances and dehydration. Water loss exceeds electrolyte loss, contributing to hyperosmolarity. This in turn perpetuates dehydration, decreasing the glomerular filtration rate and reducing the amount of glucose excreted in the urine. This leads to a deadly cycle: diminished glucose excretion further raises blood glucose levels, producing severe hyperosmolarity and dehydration and finally causing shock, coma, and death.

Comprehensive assessment

The patient may have rapid onset of drowsiness, stupor, and coma. He may have a history of diabetes mellitus. Polyuria and extreme volume depletion may occur, resulting in hypotension, tachycardia, and diaphoresis. Respirations may be slightly rapid, and there's no breath odor. Although the manifestations of HHNS may be similar to those of DKA, there are some subtle differences. (See *Differentiating HHNS and DKA.*)

The onset of HHNS is usually gradual and may not be noticed by the patient. Typically, the patient reports a re-

cent trauma or infection or exhibits an exacerbation of a chronic illness. Patients with type 1 or type 2 diabetes may report symptoms related to hyperglycemia, such as polyuria, polydipsia, polyphagia, weight loss, and fatigue. Or, they may complain of weakness, vision changes, frequent skin infections, sexual problems, vaginal discomfort, or dry, itchy skin — all symptoms of complications.

Inspection may show retinopathy or cataract formation. Skin changes — especially on the legs and feet — represent impaired peripheral circulation. Muscle wasting and loss of subcutaneous fat may be evident in type 1 diabetes; type 2 is characterized by thin, muscular limbs and fat deposits around the face, neck, and abdomen.

Palpation may detect poor skin turgor and dry mucous membranes related to dehydration. Decreased peripheral pulses, cool skin temperature, and decreased reflexes may also be palpable. Auscultation may reveal orthostatic hypotension.

Diagnosis

The following findings help diagnose HHNS:

■ Blood glucose levels are markedly elevated above normal, typically ranging from 800 to 2000 mg/dl.

■ Urine acetone is negative; serum ketones are usually negative.

■ Urine glucose levels are positive.

■ Serum osmolality is elevated, typically above 350 mOsm/L.

■ Serum electrolyte levels reveal hypokalemia, hypophosphatemia, hypomagnesemia, and hypochloremia.

■ Serum creatinine and blood urea nitrogen are typically elevated.

Differentiating HHNS and DKA

Hyperglycemic hyperosmolar nonketotic syndrome (HHNS) and diabetic ketoacidosis (DKA), both acute complications associated with diabetes, share some similarities, but they are two distinct conditions. Use the flowchart below to help determine which condition your patient is experiencing.

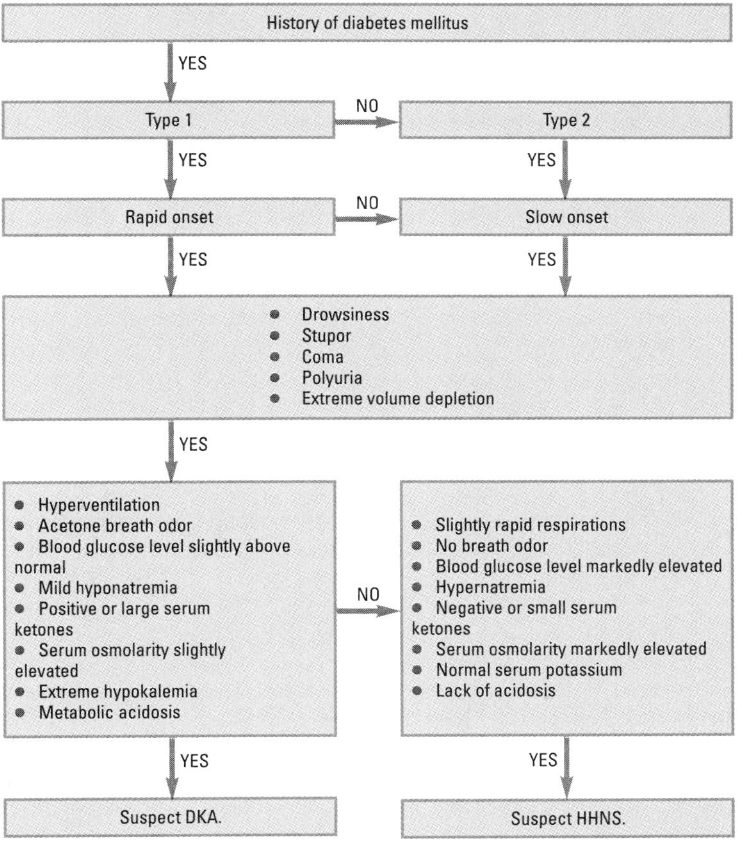
History of diabetes mellitus
YES
Type 1
NO
Type 2
YES
YES
Rapid onset
NO
Slow onset
YES
YES
• Drowsiness
• Stupor
• Coma
• Polyuria
• Extreme volume depletion
YES
• Hyperventilation
• Acetone breath odor
• Blood glucose level slightly above normal
• Mild hyponatremia
• Positive or large serum ketones
• Serum osmolarity slightly elevated
• Extreme hypokalemia
• Metabolic acidosis
NO
• Slightly rapid respirations
• No breath odor
• Blood glucose level markedly elevated
• Hypernatremia
• Negative or small serum ketones
• Serum osmolarity markedly elevated
• Normal serum potassium
• Lack of acidosis
YES
YES
Suspect DKA.
Suspect HHNS.

- Arterial blood gas (ABG) levels are usually normal, without any evidence of acidosis.
- Hematocrit is slightly elevated because of hemoconcentration from osmotic diuresis.

Collaborations

The patient with HHNS requires a multidisciplinary approach to care. The patient may be managed by an endocrinologist to help control blood glucose levels. Depending on the severity of the symptoms, the patient may require a pulmonologist to assist with ventilatory support. Nutritional therapy is also indicated to assist with dietary needs. A registered dietitian can help the patient meet his needs for a nutritionally planned diet while considering caloric allotment and the glycemic index of foods. A diabetes educator can be extremely valuable in helping the patient learn about his disease and manage it. Additionally, social services may be involved in assisting with follow-up and care at home.

Treatment and care

Treatment focuses on correcting the fluid volume deficit and electrolyte imbalances and treating the underlying cause of the problem. The patient with HHNS is typically more ill than the patient with DKA. Additionally, the majority of patients with HHNS experience some type of altered mental status. About one-half of the patients are comatose. If the patient is comatose, airway support and mechanical ventilation may be necessary.

I.V. insulin therapy as well as fluid and electrolyte replacements is administered based on the patient's laboratory test results. Blood glucose and ABGs are monitored carefully, and adjustments are made in I.V. medications and fluids.

Cardiac monitoring and frequent vital sign assessment as well as meticulous intake and output monitoring are also important. Urine may be tested for glucose and ketones. The overall goal is to ensure effective treatment of diabetes to normalize the blood glucose level and reduce complications.

Complications

The patient with HHNS is at risk for the following complications if not treated:
- shock
- coma
- death.

In addition, the patient is also at risk for acute and long-term complications associated with diabetes mellitus. (See "Diabetic ketoacidosis," page 471.)

Nursing considerations

- Assess the patient's level of consciousness and ability to maintain a patent airway. Monitor respiratory status closely, including respiratory rate and depth and breath sounds. Assess oxygen saturation via pulse oximetry to evaluate for hypoxemia. Anticipate the need for endotracheal intubation and mechanical ventilation if the patient can't maintain a patent airway or develops respiratory distress.
- Monitor vital signs frequently at least every 15 minutes initially and then hourly as indicated. Assess hemodynamic status at least hourly. Assist with the insertion of a central venous or pulmonary artery catheter for hemodynamic monitoring if one isn't already in place.

ALERT *Remember that an exacerbation of a chronic disease — usually a cardiac or pulmonary disorder — can precipitate HHNS. When monitoring the patient's hemodynamic parameters, be sure to evaluate them in light of the patient's underlying condition and what's considered normal for that patient.*

- Institute continuous cardiac monitoring to evaluate for possible arrhythmias secondary to electrolyte imbalances.

ALERT *Patients with HHNS commonly have hypokalemia. Be alert for electrocardiogram changes associated with hypokalemia, such as ST segment depression, flattened T wave, and the presence of a U wave. If hypokalemia is severe, the PR interval will be prolonged and the QRS complex will appear widened.*

■ Administer I.V. fluid replacement therapy with isotonic or 0.45% saline, typically giving one-half of the replacement (determined by the extent of fluid deficit) during the first 12 hours, with the remainder of the replacement amount being given over the next 24 hours.

ALERT *When the patient's blood glucose levels approach 250 mg/dl, anticipate the addition of dextrose to the fluid replacement regimen to prevent hypoglycemia.*

■ Administer regular insulin I.V. as ordered by continuous I.V. infusion. Expect to titrate the insulin dosage based on the patient's blood glucose levels. Remember that blood glucose levels must be reduced gradually to prevent cerebral fluid shifting and subsequent cerebral edema.

ALERT *The patient with HHNS has severely elevated glucose levels. However, less insulin is usually needed to reduce the glucose level (when compared to that required for DKA) because the patient typically does secrete some insulin and may be extremely sensitive to additional doses.*

■ Monitor blood glucose levels and serum electrolyte levels frequently as ordered. Administer potassium, phosphate, and magnesium replacement

therapy, as ordered, based on serum levels.

■ Anticipate the need for nasogastric tube insertion to prevent vomiting and aspiration if the patient is comatose or obtunded.

■ Assess peripheral circulation, including pulses, capillary refill, color, temperature, and warmth. Monitor for signs and symptoms of deep vein thrombosis, such as erythema, warmth, tenderness, swelling, or vein prominence. Notify the physician immediately.

ALERT *Patients with HHNS can lose up to 25% of their body water, leading to hyperosmolality. Blood becomes more viscous and flow is slowed, predisposing the patient to possible thromboembolism.*

■ Perform passive range-of-motion exercises every 2 hours, use intermittent pneumatic sequential compression devices as ordered, and change the patient's position frequently.

■ Institute measures to treat the underlying cause. Expect to administer antibiotics if the cause is infection.

■ Assess for acute complications of diabetic therapy, especially hypoglycemia (shaking, tachycardia, sweating, irritability, anxiety, dizziness, pallor, confusion, and headache). Monitor diabetic effects on the cardiovascular, peripheral vascular, and nervous systems.

■ Assess for signs and symptoms of diabetic neuropathy (numbness or pain in the hands and feet, footdrop, and neurogenic bladder). Provide meticulous skin care, especially to the feet and legs. Treat all injuries, cuts, and blisters promptly. Avoid constricting hose, slippers, or bed linens. Refer the patient to a podiatrist.

■ Monitor the patient for signs and symptoms of infection. Observe for signs of urinary tract and vaginal infections, and monitor the patient's urine for protein, an early sign of nephropathy.

■ Consult a dietitian to plan a diet with the recommended amounts of calories, protein, carbohydrates, and fats, based on the patient's particular requirements.

■ Encourage the patient to verbalize his feelings about diabetes and its effect on his lifestyle and life expectancy.

■ Consult the services of a diabetes educator to assist with teaching.

Patient teaching

■ Review the prescribed diabetic regimen, and monitor the patient's compliance with it.

■ Stress the importance of strictly complying with the prescribed therapy. Discuss diet, medications, exercise, monitoring techniques, hygiene and foot care, sick day rules, and how to prevent and recognize hypoglycemia and hyperglycemia. Emphasize how blood glucose control affects long-term health.

 MULTISYSTEM DISORDER

Myxedema coma

Myxedema coma is a life-threatening disorder that progresses from hypothyroidism. Hypothyroidism is classified as primary or secondary. Primary hypothyroidism stems from a disorder of the thyroid gland. Secondary hypothyroidism is caused by a failure to stimu-

late normal thyroid function or by a failure of target tissues to respond to normal blood levels of thyroid hormones. Either type may progress to myxedema coma, which is clinically much more severe and considered a medical emergency.

AGE ISSUE *Hypothyroidism is most prevalent in women. In the United States, the incidence rises significantly in persons between ages 40 and 50.*

Hypothyroidism results from a variety of abnormalities that lead to insufficient synthesis of thyroid hormones. Common causes of hypothyroidism include thyroid gland surgery (thyroidectomy), inflammation from irradiation therapy, chronic autoimmune thyroiditis (Hashimoto's disease), or inflammatory conditions, such as amyloidosis and sarcoidosis.

The disorder may also result from pituitary failure to produce thyroid-stimulating hormone (TSH), hypothalamic failure to produce thyrotropin-releasing hormone, inborn errors of thyroid hormone synthesis, inability to synthesize thyroid hormones because of iodine deficiency (usually dietary), or the use of antithyroid medications such as propylthiouracil.

Pathophysiology

In hypothyroidism, metabolic processes slow down because of a deficiency of the thyroid hormones triiodothyronine (T_3) or thyroxine (T_4). Hypothyroidism may reflect a malfunction of the hypothalamus, pituitary, or thyroid gland, all of which are part of the same negative-feedback mechanism. However, disorders of the hypothalamus and pituitary rarely cause hypothyroidism. Primary hypothyroidism is most common.

Chronic autoimmune thyroiditis, also called chronic lymphocytic thyroiditis, occurs when autoantibodies destroy thyroid gland tissue. Chronic autoimmune thyroiditis associated with goiter is called Hashimoto's thyroiditis. The cause of this autoimmune process is unknown, although heredity has a role, and specific human leukocyte antigen subtypes are associated with greater risk.

Outside the thyroid, antibodies can reduce the effect of thyroid hormone in two ways. First, antibodies can block the TSH receptor and prevent the production of TSH. Second, cytotoxic antithyroid antibodies may attack thyroid cells.

Subacute thyroiditis, painless thyroiditis, and postpartum thyroiditis are self-limited conditions that usually follow an episode of hyperthyroidism. Untreated subclinical hypothyroidism in adults is likely to become overt at a rate of 5% to 20% per year.

Myxedema coma usually occurs gradually. However, when stress aggravates severe or prolonged hypothyroidism, coma may develop abruptly. Stressors may include infection, exposure to severe cold, or trauma. Additionally, withdrawal of thyroid medication or the use of sedatives, narcotics, or anesthetics may precipitate myxedema coma.

Comprehensive assessment

The progression to myxedema coma is usually gradual but may develop abruptly, with stress aggravating severe or prolonged hypothyroidism. The patient exhibits progressive stupor, hypo-

ventilation, hypoglycemia, hyponatremia, hypotension, and hypothermia. Patients in myxedema coma have significantly depressed respirations, so their partial pressure of arterial carbon dioxide levels may rise. Decreased cardiac output and worsening cerebral hypoxia may also occur. The patient is stuporous and hypothermic, and his vital signs reflect bradycardia and hypotension.

The patient's history may reveal signs and symptoms of hypothyroidism, such as vague and varied symptoms that have developed slowly over time. The patient may report energy loss, fatigue, forgetfulness, sensitivity to cold, unexplained weight gain, and constipation. As the disorder progresses, signs and symptoms may include anorexia, decreased libido, menorrhagia, paresthesia, joint stiffness, and muscle cramping.

Inspection reveals characteristic alterations in the patient's overall appearance and behavior. These changes include decreased mental stability (slight mental slowing to severe obtundation) and a thick, dry tongue, causing hoarseness and slow, slurred speech. In addition, inspection may reveal periorbital edema; drooping upper eyelids; dry, flaky, inelastic skin; and puffy face, hands, and feet. Hair may be dry and sparse with patchy hair loss and loss of the outer third of the eyebrow. Nails may be thick and brittle with visible transverse and longitudinal grooves. You may also find ataxia, intention tremor, and nystagmus.

Palpation may detect rough, doughy skin that feels cool, a weak pulse and bradycardia, muscle weakness, sacral or peripheral edema, and delayed reflex relaxation time (especially in the Achilles tendon). The thyroid tissue may not be easily palpable unless a goiter is present. Auscultation may show absent or decreased bowel sounds, hypotension, a gallop or distant heart sounds, and adventitious breath sounds. Percussion and palpation may detect abdominal distention or ascites. The patient may exhibit signs and symptoms of respiratory or cardiac failure.

Diagnosis

Hypothyroidism is confirmed when radioimmunoassay with radioactive iodine (^{131}I) shows low serum levels of thyroid hormones and when a thorough history and physical examination show characteristic signs and symptoms. A differential diagnosis requires additional tests and may reveal the following results:

■ Serum TSH levels determine the primary or secondary nature of the disorder. An increased serum TSH level with hypothyroidism is due to thyroid insufficiency; a decreased TSH level, to hypothalamic or pituitary insufficiency. Thyroid panel differentiates among primary hypothyroidism (thyroid gland hypofunction), secondary hypothyroidism (pituitary hyposecretion of TSH), tertiary hypothyroidism (hypothalamic hyposecretion of TRH), and euthyroid sick syndrome (impaired peripheral conversion of thyroid hormone due to a suprathyroidal illness such as severe infection).

■ Serum cholesterol, alkaline phosphatase, and triglyceride levels are elevated.

■ Normocytic neurochromia anemia is present.

In myxedema coma

■ Laboratory tests also show low sodium and glucose levels, decreased pH, and increased partial pressure of arterial carbon dioxide, indicating respiratory acidosis.

■ Serum cortisol level is typically decreased.

■ Radioisotope scanning of the thyroid tissue identifies ectopic thyroid tissue.

■ Skull X-ray, computed tomography scan, and magnetic resonance imaging help locate pituitary or hypothalamic lesions that may be the underlying cause of hypothyroidism.

Collaborations

Because myxedema coma depresses the metabolic rate, all body systems can be affected, necessitating a multidisciplinary approach to care. Care focuses on increasing thyroid hormone levels, maintaining or improving ventilation and oxygenation, regulating body temperature, and restoring hemodynamic stability. An endocrinologist can help manage the patient's hormonal status. If the patient requires ventilatory support, a pulmonologist and respiratory therapy may be involved. Cardiac specialists may be consulted to help manage hemodynamic status. Additionally, nutritional therapy may be warranted to assist with diet planning. Social services may be involved to assist with financial concerns, follow-up and long term care planning, such as home care or referrals for community support.

Treatment and care

Rapid treatment may be necessary for patients with myxedema coma and those about to undergo emergency surgery (because of sensitivity to central nervous system depression). In these patients, I.V. administration of levothyroxine and hydrocortisone therapy are warranted. If the patient becomes comatose, airway patency with oral or endotracheal intubation and ventilatory support may be necessary. Circulation is maintained with I.V. fluid replacement; fluids and other substances, such as glucose, may require replacement according to serum electrolyte levels. Corticosteroids may be ordered. The patient may require warming by wrapping in warmed blankets; warming blankets aren't recommended as they may increase peripheral vasodilation, causing shock. Sources of infection should be investigated and treated, such as blood, sputum, or urine infections that may have precipitated the coma. After the patient's condition is stabilized, thyroid hormone replacement is necessary.

Complications

A medical emergency, myxedema coma commonly has a fatal outcome. If the patient survives, he's at risk for numerous complications because thyroid hormones affect almost every organ system in the body. Complications of hypothyroidism vary according to the organs involved as well as to the duration and severity of the condition. Cardiovascular complications may include hypercholesterolemia with associated arteriosclerosis and ischemic heart disease. Poor peripheral circulation, heart enlargement, heart failure, and pleural and pericardial effusions may also occur. GI complications include achlorhydria, pernicious anemia, and adynamic colon, resulting in megacolon and intestinal obstruction.

Anemia due to the generalized suppression of erythropoietin may result in bleeding tendencies and iron deficiency anemia. Other complications include conductive or sensorineural deafness, psychiatric disturbances, carpal tunnel syndrome, benign intracranial hypertension, and impaired fertility.

Nursing considerations

■ Assess the patient's level of consciousness and ability to maintain a patent airway. Monitor respiratory status closely, including respiratory rate and depth and breath sounds. Assess oxygen saturation via pulse oximetry to evaluate for hypoxemia. Anticipate the need for endotracheal intubation and mechanical ventilation if the patient can't maintain a patent airway or develops signs and symptoms of respiratory failure.

■ Administer supplemental oxygen as ordered; obtain serial arterial blood gas (ABG) studies as ordered to evaluate oxygenation and acid-base balance. Place the patient in a position to maximize chest expansion. Provide for frequent rest periods to minimize oxygen demand. Use oxygen saturation levels to aid in determining optimal position and evaluate the effect of activities on oxygenation.

■ Assess cardiac status frequently, noting heart rate and rhythm; auscultate heart sounds for changes, such as an S_3 or decreased or muffled heart sounds. Watch for chest pain, dyspnea, or evidence of dependent and sacral edema.

■ Monitor vital signs frequently at least every 15 minutes initially and then hourly as indicated. Assess hemodynamic status at least hourly. Assist with the insertion of a central venous or pulmonary artery catheter for hemodynamic monitoring if one isn't already in place. Monitor central venous pressure, pulmonary artery wedge pressure, and cardiac output and index for changes.

■ Institute continuous cardiac monitoring to evaluate for possible arrhythmias secondary to hypoxemia or electrolyte imbalances.

■ Administer thyroid hormone replacement agents as ordered.

ALERT *Keep in mind that thyroid hormone replacements stimulate metabolic processes, leading to an increase in oxygen consumption and cardiac workload. Assess for tachycardia and monitor the patient's electrocardiogram closely; report any changes in waveform immediately.*

■ Administer I.V. fluid replacement therapy, as ordered, typically to maintain a systolic blood pressure greater than 90 mm Hg. Monitor the patient's fluid status closely for possible overload. If the patient develops or exhibits signs and symptoms of overload, expect to restrict fluids.

ALERT *If the patient's blood pressure fails to respond to fluid replacement therapy, anticipate the use of vasopressors. If used, be ever vigilant for the development of possible lethal arrhythmias.*

■ Assess intake and output every hour. Anticipate the need for insertion of an indwelling urinary catheter to ensure accurate urine measurement. Monitor weight daily, reporting any weight gain of 1 to 2 lb (0.5 to 1 kg) in 24 hours.

■ Evaluate thyroid hormone levels as appropriate. Monitor laboratory test results, including serum sodium and osmolality levels. If the patient has hyponatremia, administer isotonic saline I.V. and institute water restrictions as ordered.

■ Monitor ABGs to detect hypoxemia and subsequent metabolic acidosis secondary to respiratory distress.

■ Monitor core body temperature every 15 minutes initially and then hourly until the temperature is stable. Institute passive warming measures, such as extra blankets, warmed oral fluids (if the patient is alert and has a gag reflex), maintenance of room temperature, and avoidance of drafts.

ALERT *Increase the patient's activity level gradually, and provide frequent rest periods to avoid fatigue and decrease myocardial oxygen demand.*

■ Observe the patient's mental and neurologic status. Check for disorientation, decreased level of consciousness, and hearing loss. Institute safety measures as appropriate to reduce the risk of injury.

■ During thyroid replacement therapy, watch for symptoms of hyperthyroidism, such as restlessness, sweating, tachycardia, hypertension, and tachypnea.

■ Monitor the patient for constipation. Auscultate bowel sounds, check for abdominal distention, and check bowel movement frequency to prevent possible bowel obstruction. Administer cathartics and stool softeners as needed and as ordered.

■ If the patient's serum cortisol is low, expect to administer I.V. hydrocortisone, as ordered, until adrenal gland function stabilizes.

■ Check for possible sources of infection, such as from blood, sputum, or urine, which may have precipitated the coma. Expect to treat infections or any other underlying causative condition.

■ Encourage the patient to cough and breathe deeply to prevent pulmonary complications.

■ If needed, reorient the patient to time, place, and person, and use alternative communication techniques if he has impaired hearing. Explain all procedures slowly and carefully, and avoid sedation, if possible. Provide a consistent environment to decrease confusion and frustration. Offer support and encouragement to the patient and his family.

■ Provide meticulous skin care. Turn and reposition the patient every 2 hours if bed rest is prolonged. Apply antiembolism stockings or intermittent pneumatic sequential compression devices to reduce the risk of thromboembolism. Use alcohol-free skin care products and an emollient lotion after bathing.

■ Encourage the patient to verbalize his feelings and fears about the disorder.

Patient teaching

■ Teach the patient and his family how to identify the signs and symptoms of life-threatening myxedema. Stress the importance of obtaining prompt medical care for respiratory problems and chest pain.

■ Explain the need for long-term hormone replacement therapy. Emphasize that the patient needs lifelong administration if this medication is necessary, that he should take it exactly as prescribed, and that he should never abruptly discontinue it. Advise the patient to always wear a medical identification bracelet and to carry his medication with him.

■ Instruct the patient to eat a well-balanced diet that's high in fiber and fluids to prevent constipation, restrict sodium to prevent fluid retention, and limit calories to minimize weight gain.

■ Help the patient schedule activities to avoid fatigue and to get adequate rest.

MULTISYSTEM DISORDER

Pancreas transplantation

Pancreas transplantation involves the replacement of a person's pancreas with a donor pancreas. It's indicated for patients with end-stage pancreatic disease, primarily type 1 diabetes mellitus. Typically, these patients have serious complications of the disease, including neuropathies, macrovascular disease, and microvascular disease. Thus, the risks associated with transplantation surgery and lifelong immunosuppressive therapy are less than those associated with the complications. Pancreas transplantation aims to restore blood glucose levels to normal and limit the progression of complications.

Pancreas transplantation is contraindicated in the following conditions:
■ heart disease that can't be controlled
■ active infection
■ positive serology for human immunodeficiency virus or hepatitis B surface antigen
■ malignancy within the past 3 years
■ current and active substance abuse
■ history of noncompliance or psychiatric illness
■ active untreated peptic ulcer disease
■ irreversible liver or lung dysfunction

other systemic illness that would delay or prevent recovery.

Most commonly, pancreas transplantation occurs simultaneously with renal transplantation (called simultaneous pancreas-kidney [SPK] transplant). Pancreas transplantation can also be done after renal transplantation (termed pancreas-after-kidney [PAK] transplant) or as a single transplant procedure (termed pancreas transplant alone [PTA]). In patients receiving SPK transplantation, the patient survival rate at 1 year was 95%; the kidney graft survival rate was 92%, while the pancreas graft survival rate was 82%. For patients receiving PAK transplantation, the patient survival rate at 1 year was 94%, while the pancreas graft survival rate was 74%; for PTA transplantation, the patient survival rate at 1 year was 100%, with a pancreas graft survival rate of 76%.

Procedure

Most commonly, an entire pancreas will be transplanted. However, in some instances, such as when a living donor is used, only a segment of the organ will be transplanted. With a PTA, the donor pancreas is typically placed in the right iliac fossa. When SPK or PAK transplant is performed, the donor kidney may be placed in the right iliac fossa or intraperitoneal space and the donor pancreas may be placed in the left iliac fossa or on the side opposite the kidney transplant. Regardless of whether a PTA, SPK, or PAK transplant is being performed, one of two techniques — either systemic bladder or portal enteric technique — is used to connect the pancreas. (See "Renal transplantation," in chapter 5, page 452.)

With the systemic bladder technique, the pancreas and a segment of the donor's duodenum are placed in the iliac fossa. With an SPK or PAK transplant, this side is opposite that of the transplanted kidney. The superior mesenteric and splenic arteries of the donor are connected to the patient's iliac artery. The donor's portal vein is attached to the patient's iliac vein. The segment of duodenum at the head of the donor pancreas is then anastomosed to the patient's bladder (duodenocystostomy) to allow drainage of the pancreatic secretions and enzymes. In this way, urine amylase levels can be used to monitor for graft rejection. (See *SPK transplantation.*)

With the portal enteric technique, the arterial and venous anastomoses are the same as that for the systemic bladder technique. However, instead of the duodenal segment being attached to the bladder, the segment is anastomosed to a portion of the patient's small bowel, usually the jejunum. In this way, pancreatic secretions drain directly into the GI tract for reabsorption, allowing carbohydrates and lipids to be metabolized as normal.

Complications

Surgical complications associated with pancreas transplantation include:
- graft thrombosis (arterial or venous)
- infection
- pancreatitis
- intrapancreatic abscess
- cystitis, urethritis, or urinary tract infection (with systemic bladder technique)
- leakage at the anastomosis (with portal enteric technique)
- rejection (acute or chronic).

SPK transplantation

The illustration below depicts simultaneous pancreas-kidney (SPK) transplant, in which the donor pancreas is anastomosed using the systemic bladder technique.

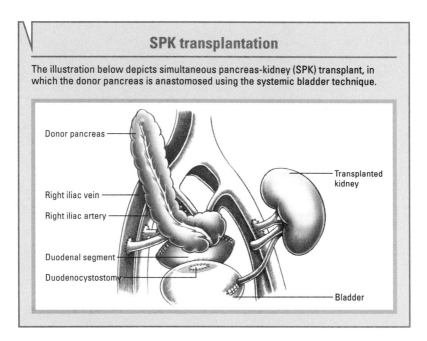

Nursing considerations

When caring for a patient undergoing a pancreas transplant, major responsibilities include instructing the patient and monitoring for postoperative complications, including organ rejection.

Before pancreas transplantation

■ Prepare the patient thoroughly for transplantation and a prolonged recovery period, and offer him ongoing emotional support.

■ Encourage the patient to express his feelings. If he's concerned about rejection, explain what will occur if this happens. Explain that transplant rejection is common.

■ Describe routine preoperative measures, such as a thorough physical examination and a battery of laboratory tests to detect any infection (followed by antibiotic therapy as treatment),

electrolyte studies, abdominal X-rays, an electrocardiogram (ECG), an enema, and hair removal from the operative area, if ordered.

■ If the patient is scheduled for a simultaneous kidney transplant, tell him that he'll undergo dialysis the day before surgery to clean his blood of unwanted fluid and electrolytes. Point out that he may need dialysis for a few days after surgery if the transplanted kidney doesn't start functioning immediately.

■ Review the transplant procedure, supplementing and clarifying the physician's explanation as necessary. Tell the patient that he'll receive a general anesthetic before surgery.

■ Explain to the patient what he can expect after he awakens from anesthesia, including the presence of I.V. lines, an indwelling urinary catheter, an arterial line and, possibly, a mechanical ventilator. Describe routine postoperative care, including frequent checks of vital signs, monitoring of intake and output, and respiratory therapy. Prepare him for postoperative pain, and reassure him that analgesics will be available.

■ Teach the patient the proper methods for performing coughing, turning, deep breathing and, if ordered, incentive spirometry.

■ Discuss the immunosuppressant drugs that the patient will be taking, and explain their possible adverse effects. Point out that these drugs increase his susceptibility to infection.

■ As ordered, begin giving immunosuppressant drugs; expect to administer low-dose aspirin or, possibly, dipyridamole to prevent thrombosis.

■ Ensure that the patient or a responsible family member has signed an informed consent form.

After pancreas transplantation

■ Assess vital signs and cardiopulmonary and hemodynamic status closely at least every 15 minutes in the immediate postoperative period and then hourly or more frequently as indicated by the patient's condition. Monitor hemodynamic parameters, including central venous pressure, pulmonary artery pressure, and pulmonary artery wedge pressure for changes indicating changes in fluid volume status, because the patient is at high risk for fluid shifts and electrolyte imbalance.

■ Institute continuous cardiac monitoring, if not already in place, evaluating waveforms frequently for ECG changes indicative of electrolyte balance or ischemia.

■ Administer fluid replacement therapy, as ordered, to prevent fluid volume depletion. Keep in mind that some patients may require I.V. fluid replacement of 1 to 2 L/day, necessitating insertion of a long-term I.V. access device.

■ Obtain serial arterial blood gases, as ordered, to evaluate oxygenation and acid-base status.

ALERT *Be alert for metabolic acidosis in the patient who has undergone transplantation with systemic bladder technique; pancreatic secretions are highly alkaline and are eliminated along with urine. Some patients increase their respiratory rate to compensate for this imbalance. If metabolic acidosis occurs, expect to administer bicarbonate I.V.*

■ In the immediate postoperative period, monitor laboratory test results closely, especially blood urea nitrogen (BUN) and creatinine levels and serum and urine amylase levels (especially if systemic bladder technique was used or a SPK or PAK transplant was performed); if the patient has a wound drain in place, also monitor amylase level in the wound drainage.

■ Monitor serial blood glucose levels and glycosylated hemoglobin and C-peptide levels to evaluate graft function.

ALERT *In the immediate postoperative period, expect to monitor blood glucose levels every 2 hours to evaluate the endocrine function of the pancreas. If necessary, anticipate administering insulin as ordered. Typically, blood glucose levels begin to decline in about 12 to 24 hours; the patient is euglycemic within several days of the transplant.*

ALERT *Be alert for an acute increase in pain with significant tenderness and swelling at the operative site and a marked rise in blood glucose and amylase levels. These suggest venous graft thrombosis, which is rarely reversible.*

■ Carefully monitor intake and output, including urine and any drainage from a nasogastric tube or wound, at least hourly; maintain urinary catheter drainage for at least 5 days following use of the systemic bladder technique.

■ Administer anticoagulation therapy as ordered, such as subcutaneous or I.V. heparin therapy, for patients who have had a PTA transplant. Administer prophylactic antibiotic, antifungal, and antiviral agents as ordered; expect patient to continue these after discharge.

■ Weigh the patient daily, and report any rapid gain (a possible sign of fluid retention).

■ Maintain nothing-by-mouth status with nasogastric decompression to low intermittent suction (if appropriate) until bowel sounds return. Administer histamine blockers to suppress gastric acid secretion. Periodically auscultate for bowel sounds, and notify the physician when they return. Begin clear liquids after the patient is extubated and bowel sounds are active. Institute measures to prevent constipation, which can lead to reflux pancreatitis.

ALERT *Keep in mind that the patient's immune system has been suppressed by medication and, therefore, is at high risk for infection. Institute standard precautions and use strict sterile technique when changing dressings and performing catheter care; limit the patient's contact with staff, other*
patients, and visitors; and avoid exposing him to persons with any type of infection. Monitor the patient's white blood cell (WBC) count; if it drops precipitously, notify the physician.

■ Assess the patient for pain, and provide analgesics as ordered. Look for a significant decrease in pain after 24 hours.

■ If the patient has an endotracheal tube in place and is receiving mechanical ventilation, assist with extubating as soon as possible (usually within 4 to 6 hours) and administer supplemental oxygen, as needed, based on mixed venous oxygen saturation or pulse oximetry levels. Encourage coughing and deep breathing and the use of an incentive spirometer after extubation, splinting, and premedicating for pain as necessary.

■ Change the patient's position at least every 2 hours, getting him out of bed to the chair within 24 hours if his condition is stable. Gradually increase the patient's activity as tolerated; assess him for signs and symptoms of complications related to immobility.

■ Monitor the patient for signs and symptoms of rejection, including low-grade fever, elevated WBC count, swelling of the graft area, and increasing serum amylase, lipase, and glucose levels (late appearing).

ALERT *Elevations in serum amylase and lipase may also suggest pancreatitis and thus aren't specific indicators for rejection. However, when the systemic bladder technique is used, watch for a decrease in urinary amylase levels. This decline typically occurs before hyperglycemia occurs and thus can be a useful marker for identifying acute rejection. The only true* way to confirm rejection is through a pancreatic biopsy.

 ALERT *In patients having undergone SPK transplantation, monitor serum creatinine and BUN levels because rejection of the kidney and pancreas occur simultaneously and kidney function begins to deteriorate before pancreatic function does.*

■ To ease emotional stress, plan care to allow frequent rest periods and provide as much privacy as possible. Allow family members to visit and comfort the patient as much as possible.

■ Allow the family to express their anxiety and fear.

■ Begin teaching the patient about care after the transplant, including:
 – signs and symptoms of infection or transplant rejection.
 – prescribed medication regimens and need for compliance with immunosuppressant therapy; the use of an antacid (if ordered) immediately before a corticosteroid to combat its ulcerogenic effects and prophylactic anti-infective therapy
 – the importance of regular follow-up to evaluate the pancreatic function (and renal function, if appropriate) and transplant acceptance.

MULTISYSTEM DISORDER

Syndrome of inappropriate antidiuretic hormone

Syndrome of inappropriate antidiuretic hormone (SIADH) results when excessive antidiuretic hormone (ADH) secretion is triggered by stimuli other than increased extracellular fluid osmolarity and decreased extracellular fluid volume, reflected by hypotension. SIADH is a relatively common complication of surgery or critical illness.

Usually, SIADH results from oat cell carcinoma of the lung, which secretes excessive ADH or vasopressor-like substances. Other neoplastic diseases (such as pancreatic and prostatic cancers, Hodgkin's disease, and thymoma) may also trigger SIADH.

Additionally, SIADH may result from:

■ central nervous system (CNS) disorders, including brain tumor or abscess, stroke, head injury, and Guillain-Barré syndrome

■ pulmonary disorders (such as pneumonia, tuberculosis, lung abscess) and positive-pressure ventilation

■ drugs (for example, chlorpropamide, tolbutamide, vincristine, cyclophosphamide, haloperidol, carbamazepine, clofibrate, morphine, and thiazides)

■ endocrine disorders, such as adrenal insufficiency, myxedema, and anterior pituitary insufficiency

■ other conditions such as psychosis.

The prognosis varies with the degree of disease and the speed at which it develops. SIADH usually resolves within 3 days of effective treatment.

Pathophysiology

In the presence of excessive ADH, excessive water reabsorption from the distal convoluted tubule and collecting ducts causes hyponatremia and normal to slightly increased extracellular fluid volume. (See *Understanding SIADH.*)

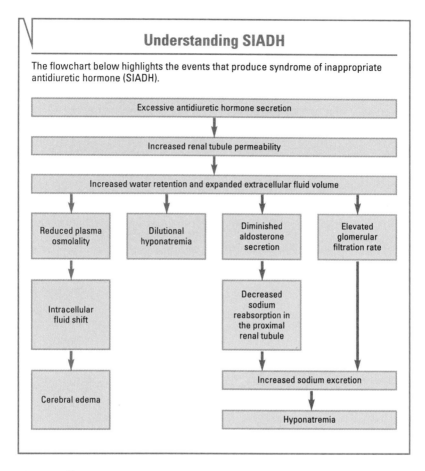

Understanding SIADH

The flowchart below highlights the events that produce syndrome of inappropriate antidiuretic hormone (SIADH).

Excessive antidiuretic hormone secretion

Increased renal tubule permeability

Increased water retention and expanded extracellular fluid volume

Reduced plasma osmolality

Dilutional hyponatremia

Diminished aldosterone secretion

Elevated glomerular filtration rate

Intracellular fluid shift

Decreased sodium reabsorption in the proximal renal tubule

Cerebral edema

Increased sodium excretion

Hyponatremia

Comprehensive assessment

The patient's medical and medication histories may provide a clue to the cause of SIADH. A history of cerebrovascular disease, cancer, pulmonary disease, or recent head injury is especially significant. Most commonly, a patient with SIADH complains of anorexia, nausea, and vomiting. Despite these symptoms, the patient may report weight gain. The patient or family may also report CNS symptoms, such as lethargy, headaches, and emotional and behavioral changes.

Inspection usually fails to reveal edema because much of the free water excess is within cellular boundaries. Palpation may detect tachycardia associated with increased fluid volume. Neurologic assessment may detect disorientation, which may progress to seizures and coma. Examination findings may also include sluggish deep tendon reflexes and muscle weakness.

Other signs and symptoms of SIADH include:

■ thirst and fatigue, followed by vomiting and intestinal cramping due to hyponatremia and electrolyte imbalance manifestations

■ water retention and decreased urinary output due to hyponatremia

■ additional neurologic symptoms (such as restlessness, confusion, irritability, and decreasing reflexes) caused by electrolyte imbalances and worsening with the degree of water intoxication.

Diagnosis

SIADH is diagnosed by the following laboratory results:

■ serum osmolarity less than 280 mOsm/kg of water

■ hyponatremia (serum sodium less than 135 mEq/L); lower values indicating worse condition

■ elevated urinary sodium level (more than 20 mEq/day)

■ elevated serum ADH level.

Renal function tests are normal, with no evidence of dehydration in SIADH.

Collaborations

The patient with SIADH requires a multidisciplinary approach to care. Care focuses on restricting fluids and treating the underlying cause. An endocrinologist can help manage the patient's hormonal control. Depending on the severity of the symptoms, the patient may require other specialists. Additionally, social services may be involved in assisting with follow-up and care at home.

Treatment and care

Based primarily on the patient's symptoms, treatment begins with restricted fluid intake (500 to 1,000 ml/day). Some patients who continue to have symptoms are given a high-salt, high-protein diet or urea supplements to enhance fluid excretion. Other patients may receive demeclocycline or lithium to help block the renal response to ADH, especially if fluid restriction is ineffective.

Rarely, with severe fluid intoxication, administration of 200 to 300 ml of 3% to 5% sodium chloride solution may be necessary to raise the serum sodium level. A loop diuretic may also be prescribed to reduce the risk of heart failure after the excess fluid load and the administration of the hypertonic sodium chloride solution. When possible, treatment should include correction of the underlying cause of SIADH. If SIADH is due to cancer, the use of surgery, irradiation, or chemotherapy may alleviate fluid retention.

Complications

Complications of SIADH include:

■ cerebral edema

■ brain herniation

■ central pontine myelinosis.

Nursing considerations

■ Assess the patient's level of consciousness and ability to maintain a patent airway. Monitor respiratory status closely, including respiratory rate and depth and breath sounds. Assess oxygen saturation via pulse oximetry to evaluate for hypoxemia. Anticipate the need for endotracheal intubation and mechanical ventilation if the patient can't maintain a patent airway or develops signs and symptoms of respiratory distress.

■ Administer supplemental oxygen as ordered; obtain serial arterial blood gas values, as ordered, to evaluate oxygenation and acid-base balance.

■ Assess cardiac status frequently, noting heart rate and rhythm; auscultate heart sounds for changes, such as an S_3 or decreased or muffled heart sounds. Monitor for signs and symptoms of heart failure.

■ Monitor vital signs frequently at least every 15 minutes initially and then hourly as indicated. Assess hemodynamic status at least hourly. Assist with the insertion of a central venous or pulmonary artery catheter for hemodynamic monitoring if one isn't already in place. Monitor central venous pressure, pulmonary artery wedge pressure, and cardiac output and index for changes. Institute continuous cardiac monitoring to evaluate for possible arrhythmias, as appropriate.

■ Institute fluid restrictions as ordered, typically 1,000 ml/24 hours. Remove any liquids from the patient's bedside, explaining the rationale for their removal. Keep strict records of intake.

ALERT *For the patient with SIADH, meticulously monitor the patient's fluid intake, including the amount of ice chips given. Always remember that when measuring ice chips as fluid intake, record the fluid as one-half of the amount of ice chips. For example, if 4 oz ice chips are given and the patient ingests the entire amount, then record 2 oz fluid intake. Although sometimes minimal in amount, ice chips can be significant for a patient whose fluids are being restricted.*

■ Administer I.V. fluids as ordered and at the specified rate. Expect to use normal or hypertonic saline if the patient's serum sodium level is severely depleted. Anticipate administering furosemide or mannitol I.V. in conjunction with additional I.V. fluids to promote water excretion.

■ Obtain serial specimens for serum and urine sodium levels and osmolarity and urine specific gravity, evaluating for trends.

ALERT *Monitor serum sodium levels closely because these are used to determine the rate of I.V. fluid therapy with saline. If serum sodium levels are raised too quickly, the patient is at risk for neurologic damage (central pontine myelinosis). The goal is to raise the serum sodium level less than 12 mEq/L in 24 hours.*

■ Assess intake and output every hour. Anticipate the need for insertion of an indwelling urinary catheter to ensure accurate urine measurement. Monitor weight daily, reporting any weight gain of 1 to 2 lb (0.5 to 1 kg) in 24 hours; monitor hydration status, including skin turgor.

■ Administer demeclocycline or lithium, as ordered, to inhibit ADH action on the kidneys, thereby promoting fluid excretion.

■ Perform frequent mouth care, and offer oral rinses and lozenges as appropriate to help with thirst.

■ Expect to treat the underlying cause of the patient's condition; if medication is suspected as the cause, withhold as ordered.

■ Elevate the head of the bed approximately 10 to 20 degrees to promote venous return. Remember that decreased venous return is a stimulus for ADH release.

- Institute seizure and safety precautions as appropriate to reduce the risk of injury.
- Minimize the amount of stress to which the patient is exposed as much as possible because stress can stimulate ADH release. Obtain an order for an analgesic if the patient complains of pain. Pain is a stressor that also leads to ADH secretion.
- If needed, reorient the patient to time, place, and person. Explain all procedures slowly and carefully. Provide a consistent environment to decrease confusion and frustration. Offer support and encouragement to the patient and his family.

Patient teaching

Explain to the patient and his family the need for fluid restrictions, and review ways to decrease the patient's discomfort from thirst.

- If drug therapy is prescribed, teach the patient and his family about the regimen, including dosage, action, and possible adverse effects.
- Discuss self-monitoring techniques for fluid retention, including measurement of intake and output and daily weight. Teach the patient to recognize signs and symptoms that require immediate medical intervention.

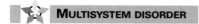 **MULTISYSTEM DISORDER**

Thyroid storm

Thyroid storm, also known as thyrotoxic crisis, is an acute manifestation of hyperthyroidism, usually occurring in patients with preexisting (though commonly unrecognized) thyrotoxicosis. Left untreated, it's invariably fatal.

Thyroid hormone overproduction results in the metabolic imbalance hyperthyroidism, which is also called thyrotoxicosis. There are several forms of this disease. The most common form of hyperthyroidism is Graves' disease, which increases thyroxine (T_4) production, enlarges the thyroid gland (goiter), and causes multiple systemic changes. Other forms include toxic adenoma (Plummer's disease), toxic multinodular goiter, thyrotoxicosis factitia, functioning metastatic thyroid carcinoma, thyroid-stimulating hormone (TSH)–secreting pituitary tumor, and subacute thyroiditis.

Hyperthyroidism can result from genetic and immunologic factors. In Graves' disease, thyroid-stimulating antibodies bind to and then stimulate the TSH receptors of the thyroid gland. The trigger for this autoimmune disease is unclear. Increased incidence in monozygotic twins suggests an inherited factor, probably a polygenic inheritance pattern. Graves' disease occasionally coexists with abnormal iodine metabolism and other endocrine abnormalities, such as diabetes mellitus, thyroiditis, and hyperparathyroidism. It's also associated with production of autoantibodies (long-acting thyroid stimulator [LATS], LATS-protector, and human thyroid adenylate cyclase stimulators), possibly caused by a defect in suppressor-T-lymphocyte function that allows the formation of these autoantibodies.

Thyrotoxic crisis is almost always abrupt in onset, evoked by a stressful event, such as trauma, surgery, or infection. Other less common precipitators include:

- insulin-induced hypoglycemia or diabetic ketoacidosis

- stroke
- myocardial infarction
- pulmonary embolism
- sudden discontinuation of antithyroid drug therapy
- initiation of radioactive iodine (^{131}I) therapy
- subtotal thyroidectomy with excess intake of synthetic thyroid hormone.

With treatment, most patients can lead normal lives. However, thyrotoxic crisis or thyroid storm — an acute exacerbation of hyperthyroidism — is a medical emergency that may lead to life-threatening cardiac, hepatic, or renal failure.

Pathophysiology

The thyroid gland secretes the thyroid hormones, triiodothyronine (T_3) and T_4. When it overproduces them in response to precipitating factors, systemic adrenergic activity increases. This results in epinephrine overproduction and severe hypermetabolism, leading rapidly to cardiac, GI, and sympathetic nervous system decompensation.

Comprehensive assessment

The patient presenting in thyrotoxic crisis initially may have marked tachycardia, vomiting, and stupor. Other findings may include irritability and restlessness; visual disturbance such as diplopia; tremor and weakness; angina; or shortness of breath, a cough, and swollen extremities. Palpation may disclose warm, moist flushed skin and a high fever, typically above 100.4° F (38° C), that begins insidiously and rises rapidly to a lethal level. Untreated, he may experience vascular collapse, hypotension, coma, and death.

The patient's history may disclose that the onset of symptoms followed a period of acute physical or emotional stress. A family history of Graves' disease is also common. The patient may report classic symptoms of nervousness, heat intolerance, weight loss despite increased appetite, excessive sweating, diarrhea, tremor, and palpitations. The patient may complain of difficulty concentrating, trouble climbing stairs, dyspnea on exertion and possibly at rest, anorexia, nausea, and vomiting. The female patient may also report menstrual abnormalities.

On inspection, the patient typically appears anxious and restless. Fine tremors of the fingers and tongue, shaky handwriting, clumsiness, emotional instability, and mood swings (occasional outbursts to overt psychosis) may be noted. The skin appears flushed, and the hair is fine and soft. Premature graying and increased hair loss occur commonly in both sexes. The nails appear fragile, and the distal nail may be separated from the nail bed (onycholysis). Inspection also reveals pretibial myxedema over the dorsum of the legs or feet, which produces raised, thickened skin that may be itchy, hyperpigmented, and usually well demarcated from normal skin. Lesions typically appear plaquelike or nodular. Generalized or localized muscle atrophy and acropachy (soft-tissue swelling with underlying bone changes where new bone formation occurs) may also be seen.

Inspection of the eyes detects infrequent blinking, a characteristic stare, and lid lag, resulting from sympathetic overstimulation. Another characteristic finding is exophthalmos, which results from accumulated mucopolysaccharides and fluids in the retro-orbital tissues that force the eyeball outward. The conjunctiva and cornea may appear reddened. The patient may have an impaired upward gaze, convergence, and strabismus due to ocular muscle weakness (exophthalmic ophthalmoplegia).

On palpation, the thyroid gland may feel asymmetrical, lobular, and enlarged to three or four times its normal size. The liver may also feel enlarged. The skin is warm and moist with a velvety texture, and tachycardia with a full bounding pulse is palpable. Hyperreflexia is present. Auscultation of the heart may detect paroxysmal supraventricular tachycardia and atrial fibrillation (especially in elderly patients) and, occasionally, a systolic murmur at the left sternal border. Wide pulse pressures may be audible when taking blood pressure readings. Auscultation of the abdomen may detect increased bowel sounds. In Graves' disease, an audible bruit over the thyroid gland indicates thyrotoxicity but, occasionally, it may also be present in other disorders associated with a hyperplastic thyroid.

Diagnosis

The following laboratory test results confirm the diagnosis of hyperthyroidism:

■ Radioimmunoassay shows increased serum T_3 and T_4 concentrations.

ALERT *Radioimmunoassay is contraindicated in pregnant patients.*

■ Thyroid scan reveals increased uptake of ^{131}I.

■ Thyrotropin-releasing hormone (TRH) stimulation test indicates hyperthyroidism if TSH level fails to rise

within 30 minutes after administration of TRH.

Other supportive test results show increased serum protein-bound iodine and decreased serum cholesterol and total lipid levels.

Collaborations

Because thyrotoxic crisis increases the metabolic rate, all body systems can be affected, necessitating a multidisciplinary approach to care. Care focuses on decreasing thyroid hormone levels; maintaining or improving ventilation, oxygenation, and cardiac function; regulating body temperature; and restoring hemodynamic stability. An endocrinologist can help manage the patient's hormonal status. If the patient requires ventilatory support, a pulmonologist and respiratory therapy may be involved. Cardiac specialists may be consulted to help manage hemodynamic status and arrhythmias. Additionally, nutritional therapy may be warranted to assist with diet planning. Social services may be involved to assist with financial concerns, follow-up, and long-term care planning, such as home care or referrals for community support.

Treatment and care

The patient requires monitoring of vital signs, electrocardiogram (ECG), and cardiopulmonary status continuously. Medications, such as an antithyroid drug (propylthiouracil [PTU]) or beta-adrenergic blockers (propranolol), are administered to block sympathetic effects, a corticosteroid may be given to inhibit the conversion of T_3 and T_4 and to replace depleted cortisol, and an iodide to block the release of the thyroid hormones.

Cooling measures with close monitoring of the patient's temperature are indicated. Acetaminophen may also be administered, but not aspirin, because it may further increase the patient's metabolic rate. In addition, supportive care, such as vitamins, nutrients, fluids, and sedatives, is administered as necessary. (See *Nursing care in thyrotoxic crisis,* pages 500 and 501.)

Treatment for hyperthyroidism may include ^{131}I consisting of a single oral dose and is the treatment of choice for women past reproductive age or men and women not planning to have children. During treatment, the thyroid gland picks up the radioactive element as it would regular iodine. The radioactivity destroys some of the cells that normally concentrate iodine and produce thyroxine, thus decreasing thyroid hormone production and normalizing thyroid size and function. In most patients, hypermetabolic symptoms diminish within 6 to 8 weeks after such treatment. However, some patients may require a second dose.

Subtotal (partial) thyroidectomy is indicated for the patient under age 40 who has a very large goiter and whose hyperthyroidism has repeatedly relapsed after drug therapy. This surgery removes part of the thyroid gland, decreasing its size and capacity for hormone production. Preoperatively, the patient may receive iodides (Lugol's solution or potassium iodide oral solution), antithyroid drugs, or high doses of propranolol to help prevent thyroid storm. If euthyroidism isn't achieved, surgery should be delayed and propranolol should be given to decrease cardiac arrhythmias caused by hyperthyroidism.

Therapy for hyperthyroid ophthalmopathy includes local applications of topical medications but may require high doses of corticosteroids. A patient with severe exophthalmos that causes pressure on the optic nerve may require surgical decompression to lessen the pressure on the orbital contents.

Complications

Because thyroid hormones have widespread effects on almost all body tissues, the complications of hypersecretion may be far-reaching and varied, including:

- muscle weakness and atrophy
- paralysis
- osteoporosis
- vitiligo; skin hyperpigmentation
- corneal ulcers
- myasthenia gravis
- impaired fertility
- decreased libido
- gynecomastia in male patients.

AGE ISSUE *Cardiovascular complications are most common in elderly patients and include arrhythmias, especially atrial fibrillation, cardiac insufficiency, cardiac decompensation, and resistance to the usual therapeutic dose of cardiac glycosides.*

Nursing considerations

- Assess the patient's level of consciousness and ability to maintain a patent airway. Monitor respiratory status closely, including respiratory rate and depth and breath sounds. Assess oxygen saturation via pulse oximetry to evaluate for hypoxemia. Anticipate the need for endotracheal intubation and mechanical ventilation if the patient can't maintain a patent airway or

(Text continues on page 502.)

Nursing care in thyrotoxic crisis

When a patient is experiencing thyrotoxic crisis, prompt intervention is needed. Use the flowchart shown below to guide your care.

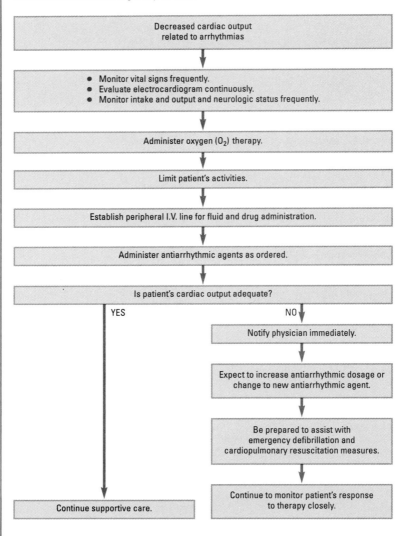

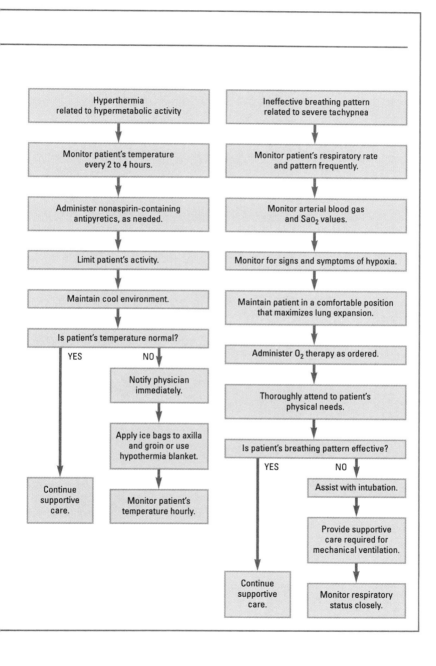

develops signs and symptoms of respiratory distress.

■ Administer supplemental oxygen as ordered; obtain serial arterial blood gas (ABG) studies, as ordered, to evaluate oxygenation and acid-base balance. Place the patient in a position to maximize chest expansion. Provide for frequent rest periods to minimize oxygen demand. Use oxygen saturation levels to aid in determining optimal position and evaluate the effect of activities on oxygenation.

■ Assess cardiac status frequently, noting heart rate and rhythm. Auscultate heart sounds for changes, such as an S_3 or decreased or muffled heart sounds, indicative of heart failure. Watch for chest pain or dyspnea, suggesting possible myocardial ischemia.

■ Monitor vital signs at least every 15 minutes for the first hour and then hourly as indicated. Monitor blood pressure continuously. Assess hemodynamic status at least hourly. Assist with the insertion of a central venous or pulmonary artery catheter for hemodynamic monitoring if one isn't already in place. Monitor mean arterial pressure, central venous pressure, pulmonary artery wedge pressure, and cardiac output and index for changes.

ALERT *Maintain mean arterial pressure at 70 mm Hg because a mean arterial pressure less than this can interfere with cerebral and renal perfusion.*

■ Institute continuous cardiac monitoring to evaluate for possible arrhythmias; be alert for ST-segment changes.

■ Administer thyroid hormone replacement agents as ordered.

ALERT *Keep in mind that thyroid hormone replacements stim-*

ulate metabolic processes, leading to an increase in oxygen consumption and cardiac workload. Assess for tachycardia, monitor the patient's ECG closely, and report any changes in waveform immediately.

■ Administer beta-adrenergic blockers, such as propranolol, to control tachycardia and hypertension; be alert for possible hypotension secondary to the medication and also from fever.

■ Administer I.V. fluid replacement therapy as ordered. Monitor the patient's fluid status closely for possible overload. If the patient develops or exhibits signs and symptoms of overload or heart failure, expect to administer cardiac glycosides and diuretics such as furosemide.

ALERT *Monitor the patient's serum electrolyte levels, especially potassium levels, if the patient is receiving diuretics. Hypokalemia predisposes the patient to numerous complications, including arrhythmias and digoxin toxicity.*

■ Administer antithyroid agents, such as PTU, iodide, or methimazole, as ordered. When administering PTU, monitor complete blood count results periodically to detect leukopenia, thrombocytopenia, and agranulocytosis. Anticipate administering dexamethasone, as ordered, to help suppress T_3 and T_4 conversion and also to replace cortisol being rapidly metabolized because of the patient's hypermetabolic state.

ALERT *If PTU and iodide are ordered, give iodide at least 1 hour after giving PTU to enhance effectiveness.*

■ Evaluate laboratory tests results, including thyroid hormone levels, to evaluate the effectiveness of therapy.

■ Assess the patient for signs and symptoms of hyperglycemia, and monitor blood glucose levels closely.

ALERT *When thyroid hormones are excessive, glycogenolysis increases and insulin levels decrease. Therefore, the patient is at risk for hyperglycemia. Anticipate the need for insulin therapy if the patient develops hyperglycemia.*

■ Assess intake and output every hour. Anticipate the need for insertion of an indwelling urinary catheter to ensure accurate urine measurement. Monitor weight daily, reporting any weight gain of 1 to 2 lb (0.5 to 1 kg) in 24 hours. Assess hydration status, including skin turgor, mucous membranes, and complaints of thirst; a fluid deficit can adversely affect the patient's cardiac output.

■ Monitor serial ABGs as ordered to detect hypoxemia and acid-base balance.

■ Monitor core body temperature every 15 minutes for the first hour, and then every 30 minutes to 1 hour until stable. Institute cooling measures such as a cooling blanket. Administer antipyretics, such as acetaminophen, as ordered.

ALERT *Don't use aspirin to lower the patient's temperature. Aspirin increases circulating thyroid hormones, thus exacerbating the patient's already hyperthyroid state.*

■ Provide comfort measures, such as keeping the room cool and changing the patient's gown and sheets as necessary should they become wet with diaphoresis.

■ Assess the patient's GI status, including auscultating for bowel sounds; assist with nutritional therapy, including small frequent feedings and calorie counts as indicated. Anticipate the need for total parenteral nutrition if the patient can't consume adequate calories and protein.

■ Institute safety measures as appropriate to reduce the risk of injury.

■ Provide frequent rest periods to avoid fatigue and decrease myocardial oxygen demand.

■ During antithyroid therapy, watch for symptoms of hypothyroidism, such as weakness, fatigue, sensitivity to cold, weight gain, decreasing level of consciousness, and bradycardia.

■ Check for possible sources of infection, such as from blood, sputum or urine, which may have precipitated the crisis. Expect to treat infections or any other underlying causative condition.

■ Encourage the patient to verbalize his feelings and fears about the disorder.

Patient teaching

■ Teach the patient and his family how to identify the signs and symptoms of life-threatening thyrotoxic crisis. Stress the importance of obtaining prompt medical care if any occur.

■ Explain the need for long-term therapy, emphasizing the need to take the medication exactly as prescribed and to never abruptly discontinue it. Advise the patient to always wear a medical identification bracelet and carry his medication with him.

■ Stress the importance of regular medical follow-up because hypothyroidism may develop 2 to 4 weeks postoperatively and after ^{131}I therapy.

■ Stress the need for repeated measurement of thyroid hormone levels.

■ Instruct the patient taking PTU and methimazole to take these drugs with meals to minimize GI distress and to avoid over-the-counter cough preparations because many contain iodine.

■ Tell the patient taking propranolol to rise slowly after sitting or lying down to prevent a feeling of faintness; instruct the patient taking antithyroid drugs or radioisotope therapy how to identify and report symptoms of hypothyroidism.

Imagine you have a patient who develops disseminated intravascular coagulation. For what precipitating factors and assessment findings would you be alert? How would you best intervene? What type of blood component therapy would you expect to administer? What if the patient suddenly developed a fever, chills, and a back pain during the transfusion? Is this a transfusion reaction or is it related to the patient's underlying disorder? What would you do first?

A patient is admitted to the critical care unit with major burns. How would you determine the extent and type of burns? What would your priorities be when caring for such a patient? What if the patient was a child? Would your assessment differ? Would your priorities change?

Another patient suffered a near drowning and is hypothermic. How would you care for him? What rewarming methods would you expect to use? In this chapter, you'll find answers to these questions and additional information that will allow you to address the major challenges involving multisystem issues encountered in the critical care area.

 MULTISYSTEM DISORDER

Anaphylaxis

Anaphylaxis is an acute, potentially life-threatening type I (immediate) hypersensitivity reaction marked by the sudden onset of rapidly progressive urticaria (vascular swelling in skin accompanied by itching) and respiratory distress.

Anaphylaxis usually results from ingestion of, or other systemic exposure to, sensitizing drugs or other substances. Such substances may include:
- serums (usually horse serum)
- vaccines
- allergen extracts
- enzymes such as L-asparginase
- hormones
- penicillin or other antibiotics (Antibiotics induce anaphylaxis in 1 to 4 of every 10,000 patients treated; most likely after parenteral administration or prolonged therapy and in patients with an inherited tendency to food or drug allergy, or atopy.)
- sulfonamides
- local anesthetics
- salicylates
- polysaccharides
- diagnostic chemicals, such as sulfobromophthalein, sodium dehydrocholate, and radiographic contrast media

- food proteins, such as those in legumes, nuts, berries, seafood, and egg albumin
- food additives containing sulfite
- insect venom.

With prompt recognition and treatment, the prognosis is good. However, a severe reaction may precipitate vascular collapse, leading to systemic shock and, sometimes, death. The reaction typically occurs within minutes but can occur up to 1 hour after reexposure to the antigen.

Pathophysiology

Anaphylaxis requires previous sensitization or exposure to the specific antigen, resulting in immunoglobulin (Ig) E production by plasma cells in the lymph nodes and enhancement by helper T cells. IgE antibodies then bind to basophils and to membrane receptors on mast cells in connective tissue.

On reexposure, the antigen binds to adjacent IgE antibodies or cross-linked IgE receptors, activating a series of cellular reactions that trigger mast cell degranulation. With degranulation, powerful chemical mediators, such as histamine, eosinophil chemotactic factor of anaphylaxis, and platelet-activating factor, are released from the mast cells. IgG or IgM enters into the reaction and activates the complement cascade, leading to the release of the complement fractions.

At the same time, two other chemical mediators, bradykinin and leukotrienes, induce vascular collapse by stimulating contraction of certain groups of smooth muscles and increasing vascular permeability. These substances, together with the other chemical mediators, cause vasodilation, smooth muscle contraction, enhanced vascular permeability, and increased mucus production.

Continued release, along with the spread of these mediators through the body by way of the basophils in the circulation, triggers the systemic responses. Increased vascular permeability leads to decreased peripheral resistance and plasma leakage from the circulation to the extravascular tissues. Consequent reduction of blood volume causes hypotension, hypovolemic shock, and cardiac dysfunction. (See *Understanding anaphylaxis*.)

Comprehensive assessment

An anaphylactic reaction produces sudden physical distress within seconds or minutes after exposure to an allergen. A delayed or persistent reaction may occur up to 24 hours later. The severity of the reaction is inversely related to the interval between exposure to the allergen and the onset of symptoms.

The patient, a relative, or another responsible person will report the patient's exposure to an antigen. Immediately after exposure, the patient may complain of a feeling of impending doom or fright, weakness, sweating, sneezing, dyspnea, nasal pruritus, and urticaria. He may appear extremely anxious. Keep in mind that the sooner signs and symptoms begin after exposure to the antigen, the more severe the anaphylaxis.

On inspection, the patient's skin may display well-circumscribed, discrete cutaneous wheals with erythematous, raised, serpiginous borders and blanched centers. They may coalesce to form giant hives. Angioedema may cause the patient to complain of a

Understanding anaphylaxis

An anaphylactic reaction occurs following previous sensitization or exposure to a specific antigen. The sequence of events in anaphylaxis is described here.

Response to the antigen

Immunoglobulin (Ig) M and IgG recognize the antigen as a foreign substance and attach to it. Destruction of the antigen by the complement cascade begins but remains unfinished, either because of insufficient amounts of the protein catalyst or because the antigen inhibits certain complement enzymes. The patient has no signs and symptoms at this stage.

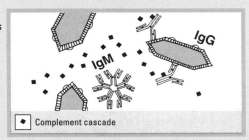

Complement cascade

Released chemical mediators

The antigen's continued presence activates IgE on basophils. The activated IgE promotes the release of mediators, including histamine, serotonin, and leukotriene. The sudden release of histamine causes vasodilation and increases capillary permeability. The patient begins to have signs and symptoms, including sudden nasal congestion, itchy and watery eyes, flushing, sweating, weakness, and anxiety.

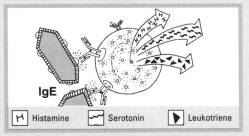

Histamine   Serotonin   Leukotriene

Intensified response

The activated IgE also stimulates mast cells in connective tissue along the venule walls to release more histamine and eosinophil chemotactic factor of anaphylaxis (ECF-A). These substances produce disruptive lesions that weaken the venules. Now, red and itchy skin, wheals, and swelling appear, and signs and symptoms worsen.

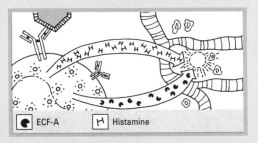

ECF-A   Histamine

(continued)

Understanding anaphylaxis *(continued)*

Distress

In the lungs, histamine causes endothelial cells to burst and endothelial tissue to tear away from surrounding tissue. Fluids leak into the alveoli, and leukotriene prevents the alveoli from expanding, thus reducing pulmonary compliance. Tachypnea, crowing, use of accessory muscles, and cyanosis signal respiratory distress. Resulting neurologic signs and symptoms include changes in level of consciousness, severe anxiety and, possibly, seizures.

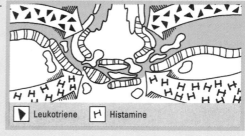

Leukotriene   H Histamine

Deterioration

Basophils and mast cells begin to release prostaglandins and bradykinin along with histamine and serotonin. These substances increase vascular permeability, causing fluids to leak from the vessels. Shock, confusion, cool and pale skin, generalized edema, tachycardia, and hypotension signal rapid vascular collapse.

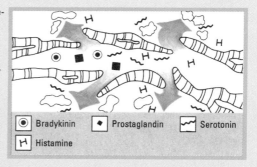

Bradykinin   Prostaglandin   Serotonin

H Histamine

Failed compensatory mechanisms

Damage to the endothelial cells causes basophils and mast cells to release heparin. Additional substances are also released to neutralize the other mediators— eosinophils release arylsulfatase B to neutralize leukotriene, phospholipase D to neutralize heparin, and cyclic adenosine monophosphate and the prostaglandins E_1 and E_2 to increase the metabolic rate. These events can't reverse anaphylaxis. Hemorrhage, disseminated intravascular coagulation, and cardiopulmonary arrest result.

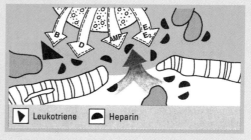

Leukotriene   Heparin

"lump" in his throat, or you may hear hoarseness or stridor. Wheezing, dyspnea, and complaints of chest tightness suggest bronchial obstruction. These are early signs of impending, potentially fatal respiratory failure.

Other effects may follow rapidly. The patient may report GI and genitourinary effects, including severe stomach cramps, nausea, diarrhea, and urinary urgency and incontinence. Neurologic effects include dizziness, drowsiness, headache, restlessness, and seizures. Cardiovascular effects include hypotension, shock, and cardiac arrhythmias, which may precipitate vascular collapse if untreated.

Diagnosis

No single diagnostic test can identify anaphylaxis. Anaphylaxis can be diagnosed by the rapid onset of severe respiratory or cardiovascular symptoms after ingestion or injection of a drug, vaccine, diagnostic agent, food, or food additive, or after an insect sting. If these symptoms occur without a known allergic stimulus, other possible causes of shock (such as acute myocardial infarction, status asthmaticus, or heart failure) must be ruled out.

The following test results may provide some clues to the patient's risk for anaphylaxis:
■ skin tests showing hypersensitivity to a specific allergen
■ elevated serum IgE levels.

Collaborations

The patient experiencing anaphylaxis requires multidisciplinary care to prevent vascular collapse and death. Respiratory and cardiovascular specialists may be needed to assist with measures to assist with and maintain lung and

heart function. Respiratory therapy may be involved if the patient requires supplemental oxygen, tracheotomy, or endotracheal (ET) intubation and mechanical ventilation. A specialist in allergy or immunology may be needed to assist with identifying the precipitating agent. Nutritional therapy may be involved if the patient's triggering event was a food substance. Social services may be helpful with long-term planning, support, and referrals to community resources.

Treatment and care

Treatment focuses on maintaining a patent airway, ensuring adequate oxygenation, restoring vascular volume, and controlling and counteracting the effects of the chemical mediators released. Treatment includes:
■ immediate administration of epinephrine 1:1,000 aqueous solution to reverse bronchoconstriction and cause vasoconstriction, I.M. or subcutaneously if the patient hasn't lost consciousness and is normotensive, or I.V. if the reaction is severe (repeating dosage every 5 to 20 minutes as needed)
■ tracheostomy or ET intubation and mechanical ventilation to maintain a patent airway
■ oxygen therapy to increase tissue perfusion
■ longer-acting epinephrine, corticosteroids, and diphenhydramine (Benadryl) to reduce the allergic response (long-term management)
■ albuterol mini-nebulizer treatment
■ Tagamet or another histamine-2 (H_2) blocker
■ aminophylline to reverse bronchospasm

- volume expanders to maintain and restore circulating plasma volume
- I.V. vasopressors, such as norepinephrine (Levophed) and dopamine (Intropin), to stabilize blood pressure
- cardiopulmonary resuscitation to treat cardiac arrest.

Complications

Complications of anaphylaxis include:
- respiratory obstruction
- systemic vascular collapse
- death.

Nursing considerations

- Administer epinephrine as ordered.

ALERT *Check the patient's history for medication use. Epinephrine may be ineffective in patients taking beta-adrenergic blocking agents. Instead, anticipate administering glucagon as a 1 mg I.V. bolus as ordered.*

- When administering epinephrine I.M., expect to give doses of 0.3 to 0.5 mg and repeat after 5 to 10 minutes if no improvement is seen. Remember that I.V. administration of epinephrine is limited to profound, immediately life-threatening situations (such as the patient who is in shock or experiencing airway obstruction); in these cases, expect to give a dose of 0.1 to 0.5 mg I.V. over 5 minutes. If the patient is in cardiac arrest, give high-dose epinephrine (1 mg) I.V. push and repeat every 3 to 5 minutes.
- Assess the patient's airway, breathing, and circulation. If the patient is in cardiac arrest, begin cardiopulmonary resuscitation and provide appropriate care based on the asystole algorithm.
- To reverse hypoxemia, administer supplemental oxygen as ordered at appropriate concentrations (usually start-

ing at 6 L/minute) to maintain partial pressure of arterial oxygen (PaO_2).

- Assess the patient's vital signs and respiratory status initially every 5 to 15 minutes and then less frequently as the patient's condition improves. Note continued evidence of hypotension and report immediately. Auscultate lungs for decreases in adventitious breath sounds.

ALERT *Decreased wheezing may signal an improvement in the patient's airflow. However, it also could indicate worsening of bronchoconstriction and obstruction. To determine what's happening, auscultate air movement throughout the lung fields. If decreased wheezing is a result of worsening bronchoconstriction, airflow will be decreased.*

- Observe for a positive response to oxygen therapy, such as improved breathing, color, and oximetry and ABG values.
- Monitor oxygen saturation levels and ABG results for changes. Anticipate the need for ET intubation and mechanical ventilation if PaO_2 continues to fall or partial pressure of arterial carbon dioxide rises.

ALERT *Expect ET intubation if the patient exhibits hoarseness, lingual edema, or posterior or oropharyngeal swelling. However, keep in mind that tracheal intubation may be difficult or impossible because it can result in increased laryngeal edema, bleeding, and further narrowing of the glottic opening. Fiberoptic tracheal intubation, needle cricothyrotomy (followed by transtracheal ventilation), or cricothyrotomy may be necessary.*

- Institute continuous cardiac monitoring to evaluate for arrhythmias and

Fluid replacement

Fluid replacement is essential for the patient with burns because of the massive fluid shifts that occur. However, extreme caution is necessary because of the risk of overreplacement. Numerous formulas may be used to determine the amount of fluid replacement to be administered during the first 24 hours after a burn injury. Typically, these formulas use body weight and the percentage of body surface area (BSA) burned. One of the most common formulas used is the Parkland formula:

2 to 4 ml of lactated Ringer's solution/kg
percentage of BSA burned

Typically, one-half of the calculated amount is administered during the first 8 hours following the injury. (Note that the time of injury — not the time of the patient's arrival in the emergency department — is used as the initial start time of the 8-hour duration.) The remaining half of the amount is then administered over the next 16 hours.

During the first 24 hours, crystalloid solutions are commonly used because capillary permeability is greatly increased, allowing proteins to leak into the interstitial tissues. After the first 24 hours, colloidal solutions can be included. Giving colloids before the initial 24-hour period would supply additional protein that could leak into the interstitial tissue.

During fluid replacement, always be alert for indications of overreplacement and underreplacement. Signs and symptoms of heart failure and pulmonary edema suggest overreplacement. Assessment findings of hypovolemic shock suggest underreplacement.

---

prepare to treat as ordered should any occur.

■ Assist with insertion of a central venous or pulmonary artery catheter for hemodynamic monitoring, if indicated. Monitor parameters at least every 15 to 30 minutes initially, and then every hour as the patient's condition improves.

■ Begin I.V. fluid replacement therapy with crystalloids such as lactated Ringer's or normal saline solution and colloids, such as albumin and plasma protein fraction, as ordered. Monitor the patient's hemodynamic status for changes indicating improved cardiac output. (See *Fluid replacement.*)

■ Assess the patient closely for signs and symptoms of fluid overload, such as crackles, S_3 heart sounds, jugular vein distention, and increases in hemodynamic parameters.

■ If the patient doesn't respond to fluid replacement therapy, expect to administer vasopressors to raise blood pressure.

■ Monitor intake and output closely, checking urine output every hour. Insert an indwelling urinary catheter as indicated and ordered to ensure accurate measurements. Notify the physician if urine output is less than 30 ml/hour.

■ Administer additional pharmacotherapy as ordered, including antihistamines such as diphenhydramine, H_2-receptor antagonists such as cimetidine, inhaled beta$_2$-adrenergic agonists such as albuterol, and high-dose corticosteroids.

ALERT *If the patient's history reveals use of beta-adrenergic blocking agents, anticipate administration of inhaled anticholinergic agent,* such as ipratropium instead of a beta$_2$-adrenergic agonist agent.

■ Monitor level of consciousness for changes indicating decreased cerebral perfusion.

■ Evaluate peripheral tissue perfusion, including skin color, temperature, pulses, and capillary refill.

■ Institute measures to control itching, such as cool compresses, avoidance of scratching, using finger pads instead of nails.

■ Reassure the patient and stay with him. Help him to relax as much as possible.

■ Encourage the patient to express his fears and concerns about his illness. Answer his questions honestly. Encourage him to identify and comply with care measures and activities that promote relaxation.

Patient teaching

■ Teach the patient about the offending allergen and ways to avoid future exposure.

■ Urge the patient to obtain an emergency anaphylaxis kit and teach him how to use it.

■ Advise the patient to obtain and consistently wear medical alert identification that lists the offending allergens.

Bone marrow transplantation

Bone marrow transplantation, which is the treatment of choice for aplastic anemia and severe combined immunodeficiency diseases, involves the infusion of fresh or stored bone marrow. The procedure may also be used to treat acute and chronic myeloid leukemia, acute lymphocytic leukemia, lymphoma, multiple myeloma, and certain solid tumors. Recently, bone marrow transplantation has been useful in the treatment of sickle cell anemia.

The bone marrow used in the transplantation may be obtained by autologous, syngeneic, or allogeneic means. In an *autologous* donation, the bone marrow is harvested from the patient before he receives chemotherapy or radiation therapy, or while he's in remission, and then frozen for later use.

In a *syngeneic* donation, bone marrow is taken from the patient's identical twin. Obviously, syngeneic donations are rare; but when possible, they're the ideal type. That's because an identical twin has healthy bone marrow that's histologically identical to the patient's own tissue.

The most common type of transplantation involves an *allogeneic* donation. For this procedure, bone marrow is obtained from a histocompatible individual. This is usually a sibling, although it's possible for an unrelated donor to meet the requirements. Because the donor's and patient's tissue don't match perfectly, the patient must receive medications to suppress his immune system. Even then, the procedure isn't always successful.

Peripheral stem cell transplantation involves the collection of stem cells harvested from peripheral blood. The donor may be the patient or someone else. Typically the donor receives hemopoietic growth factors to stimulate the production of circulating stem cells. The cells, removed in a process called *apheresis,* are collected and then processed and stored for later infusion into the patient after high-dose chemotherapy and, possibly, radiotherapy.

Procedure

If the patient will be receiving his own bone marrow, the donation will have been made 2 weeks earlier and frozen. For a syngeneic or allogeneic transplantation, physicians will obtain the donor bone marrow in the operating room the same day as the transplantation.

The transplantation procedure itself will occur at the patient's bedside. Just before the procedure, an antihistamine or analgesic is administered to minimize adverse reactions. In the case of an allogeneic or syngeneic donation, someone will bring the bone marrow to the patient's room as soon as it's obtained. For an autologous donation, the marrow will be allowed to thaw. Then, as soon as the marrow has been made available or has thawed, the physician will infuse it into the patient through a central venous catheter.

The rate of infusion varies, depending on the volume of marrow being infused. Once infused, the marrow cells will migrate to the patient's marrow cavity, where they'll begin to proliferate. This process, called *engraftment,* takes from 10 days to 4 weeks.

Complications

During infusion, potential complications include volume overload, anaphylaxis, and pulmonary fat emboli. After infusion, the patient may develop an infection or abnormal bleeding. If the bone marrow was obtained from an allogeneic donor, the patient may develop graft-versus-host disease (GVHD; see "Graft-versus-host-disease," page 542). This serious complication can occur anywhere from a few days to years after transplantation. Other complications include renal insufficiency and veno-occlusive disease.

Nursing considerations

When caring for a patient receiving bone marrow transplantation, nursing responsibilities focus on educating the patient and on protecting him from potential complications.

Before bone marrow transplantation

- Reinforce the physician's explanation of bone marrow transplantation.
- Provide the patient and his family time to discuss the procedure fully to be sure they understand its risks and benefits. Make sure they know that, if the transplantation fails, the patient may die.
- Ensure that the patient or a responsible family member has signed a consent form.
- Inform the patient that, because his white blood cells will be depleted, he'll be at high risk for infection immediately after the procedure and may remain in protective isolation for several weeks. Explain that contact with his family will be limited during this time.
- Prepare the patient for the pretransplantation regimen, including chemotherapy or radiation therapy (or both) to kill any residual cancer cells.
- During this pretransplantation regimen, monitor for adverse reactions, such as bone marrow suppression, diarrhea, fever, cystitis, nausea, vomiting, and mucositis. Administer prophylactic antiemetics as ordered. Monitor intake and output and administer

fluids to prevent fluid and electrolyte imbalances and cystitis.

■ Before the procedure begins, make sure that diphenhydramine and epinephrine are readily available to manage transfusion reactions.

■ Begin an I.V. line for hydration if one isn't already in place. Obtain an administration set (without a filter, which can trap the marrow cells) for the bone marrow infusion.

■ Obtain baseline vital signs.

During bone marrow transplantation

■ When the transfusion has begun, take the patient's vital signs at least every 15 minutes for 1 hour, every 30 minutes for the next 2 hours, and then every hour for another 4 hours. Be alert for fever, dyspnea, and hypotension.

■ Monitor the patient for other reactions, such as bronchospasm, urticaria, erythema, chest pain, and back pain. Administer ordered medications to relieve these symptoms.

After bone marrow transplantation

■ Continue to monitor the patient's vital signs closely and assess the patient every 4 hours for any signs or symptoms of infection, such as fever or chills.

ALERT *Because the patient is already pancytopenic from the pretransplantation regimen, he's at risk for hemorrhage and infection. Maintain strict asepsis when caring for him and take measures to protect him from injury. Prepare to administer blood or platelet transfusions (or both) as ordered.*

■ If necessary, anticipate the need to place the patient in a room with laminar flow to further reduce the possibility of infection.

■ Obtain specimens for laboratory analysis as ordered and monitor the patient's hematologic status. Notify the physician immediately of any changes.

■ On the seventh day after the transplantation, begin to watch for signs of GVHD, such as dermatitis, hepatitis, hemolytic anemia, and thrombocytopenia.

■ Teach the patient and his family about infection control measures and bleeding precautions, caring for central venous catheter, medication regimen and signs and symptoms of possible complications.

■ Stress the importance of contacting the physician immediately if any danger signs should occur.

■ Emphasize the need for continued follow-up.

MULTISYSTEM DISORDER

Burns

Burns, tissue injury resulting from contact with fire, a thermal chemical, or an electrical source, can cause cellular skin damage and a systemic response that leads to altered body function.

Thermal burns, the most common type, frequently result from:
■ residential fires
■ automobile accidents
■ playing with matches
■ improper handling of firecrackers
■ scalding accidents and kitchen accidents (such as a child climbing on top of a stove or grabbing a hot iron)

■ parental abuse (in children or elders)

■ clothes that have caught on fire.

Chemical burns result from contact, ingestion, inhalation, or injection of acids, alkalis, or vesicants.

Electrical burns usually result from contact with faulty electrical wiring or high-voltage power lines. Sometimes young children chew electrical cords. Friction or abrasion burns occur when the skin rubs harshly against a coarse surface. Sunburn results from excessive exposure to sunlight.

Burns are classified as first degree, second-degree superficial partial-thickness, second-degree deep partial-thickness, third-degree full-thickness, and fourth degree. A first-degree burn is limited to the epidermis. The most common example of a first-degree burn is sunburn, which results from exposure to the sun. In a second-degree burn, the epidermis and part of the dermis are damaged. A third-degree burn damages the epidermis and dermis, and vessels and tissue are visible. In fourth-degree burns, the damage extends through deeply charred subcutaneous tissue to muscle and bone. A major burn affects every body system and organ; it usually requires painful treatment and a long period of rehabilitation.

Each year in the United States, about 2 million people receive burn injuries. Of these, 300,000 are burned seriously, and more than 6,000 die, making burns the nation's third leading cause of accidental death. About 60,000 people are hospitalized each year for burns. Most significant burns occur in the home; home fires account for the highest burn fatality rate.

In victims younger than age 4 and older than age 60, there's a higher incidence of complications and thus a higher mortality. Immediate, aggressive burn treatment increases the patient's chance for survival. Later, supportive measures and strict sterile technique can minimize infection. Meticulous, comprehensive burn care can make the difference between life and death. Survival and recovery from a major burn are more likely once the burn wound is reduced to less than 20% of the total body surface area (BSA).

Pathophysiology

The injuring agent denatures cellular proteins. Some cells die because of traumatic or ischemic necrosis. Loss of collagen cross-linking also occurs with denaturation, creating abnormal osmotic and hydrostatic pressure gradients that cause the movement of intravascular fluid into interstitial spaces. Cellular injury triggers the release of mediators of inflammation, contributing to local and, in the case of major burns, systemic increases in capillary permeability. Specific pathophysiologic events depend on the cause and classification of the burn. (See *Burn classifications,* page 516.)

A *first-degree* burn causes localized injury or destruction to the skin (epidermis only) by direct (such as chemical spill) or indirect (such as sunlight) contact. The barrier function of the skin remains intact, and these burns aren't life-threatening.

A *second-degree superficial partial-thickness* burn involves destruction to the epidermis and some dermis. Thin-walled, fluid-filled blisters develop within a few minutes of the injury. As

Burn classifications

The depth of skin and tissue damage determines burn classification. The following illustration shows the four degrees of burn classification.

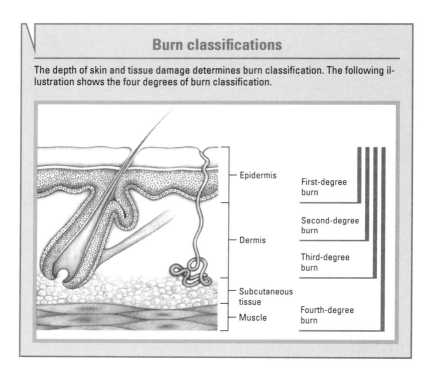

these blisters break, the nerve endings become exposed to the air. Because pain and tactile responses remain intact, subsequent treatments are very painful. The barrier function of the skin is lost.

A *second-degree deep partial-thickness* burn involves destruction of the epidermis and dermis, producing blisters and mild-to-moderate edema and pain. The hair follicles are still intact, so hair will grow again. Compared with a second-degree superficial partial-thickness burn, there's less pain sensation with this burn because the sensory neurons have undergone extensive destruction. The areas around the burn injury remain very sensitive to pain because the barrier function of the skin is lost.

A *third-degree full-thickness* burn extends through the epidermis and dermis and into the subcutaneous tissue layer. A *fourth-degree* burn involves muscle, bone, and interstitial tissues. Within only hours, fluids and protein shift from capillary to interstitial spaces, causing edema. There's an immediate immunologic response to a burn injury, making burn wound sepsis a potential threat. Finally, an increase in calorie demand after a burn injury increases the metabolic rate.

Comprehensive assessment

The patient's history usually reveals the cause of the burn. It may also disclose a preexisting medical condition — such as a cardiac or pulmonary problem, diabetes mellitus, peripheral vascular disease, chronic alcohol or drug abuse, or a psychiatric disorder — that could complicate burn treatment and recovery. If the patient is under age 5 or over age 65, there's a higher incidence of complications and, consequently, a higher risk of death. Obtain the patient's history as soon as possible because medications, confusion resulting from the injury, or the use of an endotracheal tube may prevent the patient from giving an accurate history later.

Overall assessment provides a general idea of burn severity. First, determine the depth of tissue damage. A partial-thickness burn damages the epidermis and part of the dermis; a full-thickness burn also affects the subcutaneous tissue. The more traditional method is to gauge burns by degree. Most burns include a combination of degrees and thicknesses.

Signs and symptoms depend on the type of burn, and may include:
■ localized pain and erythema, usually without blisters in the first 24 hours (first-degree burn)
■ chills, headache, localized edema, and nausea and vomiting (more severe first-degree burn)
■ thin-walled, fluid-filled blisters appearing within minutes of the injury, with mild-to-moderate edema and pain (second-degree superficial partial-thickness burn)
■ white, waxy appearance to damaged area (second-degree deep partial-thickness burn)
■ white, brown, or black leathery tissue and visible thrombosed vessels due to destruction of skin elasticity (dorsum of hand, most common site of thrombosed veins), without blisters (third-degree burn)

■ silver-colored, raised area, usually at the site of electrical contact (electrical burn)
■ singed nasal hairs, mucosal burns, voice changes, coughing, wheezing, soot in mouth or nose, and darkened sputum (with smoke inhalation and pulmonary damage).

Inspection reveals other characteristics of the burn as well, including location and extent. Keep in mind that burns on the face, hands, feet, and genitalia are most serious because of a possible loss of function or severe impact on body image. Note the burn's configuration. If the patient has a circumferential burn, he runs the risk of edema totally occluding circulation in his extremity. If he has burns on his neck, he may suffer airway obstruction; burns on the chest can lead to restricted respiratory excursion.

Inspect the patient for other injuries that may complicate his recovery. In particular, look for signs of pulmonary damage from smoke inhalation — singed nasal hairs, mucosal burns, voice changes, coughing, wheezing, soot in the mouth or nose, and darkened sputum. Look for respiratory distress and cyanosis — signs of systemic complications from noxious fumes such as cyanide from burning carpets.

Palpation reveals edema and alteration in pulse rate, strength, and regularity, which can signify vascular compromise.

Lung auscultation may reveal respiratory distress, including stridor, wheezing, crackles, and rhonchi. Heart auscultation may reveal adventitious heart sounds, such as S_3, or S_4, gallop or murmur, which is a sign of myocardial injury or decompensation. The

Using the Rule of Nines and the Lund-Browder classification

Quickly estimate the extent of an adult patient's burn by using the Rule of Nines, which divides an adult's body surface area (BSA) into percentages. To use this method, mentally transfer the patient's burns to the body chart shown here, then add up the corresponding percentages for each burned body section. The total, an estimate of the extent of the patient's burn, enters into the formula to determine his initial fluid replacement needs.

You can't use the Rule of Nines for infants and children because their body section percentages differ from those of adults. For example, an infant's head accounts for about 17% at the total BSA compared with 7% for an adult. Instead, use the Lund-Browder classification.

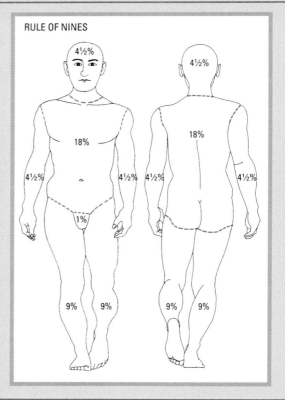

RULE OF NINES

4½% · 4½% · 18% · 18% · 4½% · 4½% · 4½% · 4½% · 1% · 9% · 9% · 9% · 9%

patient with severe burns may be hypotensive, indicating hypovolemia and, possibly, shock.

ALERT *To obtain a blood pressure even if all extremities are burned, place a 4" × 4" sterile gauze pad or sterile towel on the extremity before applying the blood pressure cuff.*

Abdominal auscultation may disclose absent bowel sounds if the patient has an ileus, which usually accompanies a burn that covers more than 25% of total BSA.

Diagnosis

Diagnosis involves determining the size and classifying the wound. The following methods are used to determine size:

■ percentage of BSA covered by the burn using the Rule of Nines chart
■ Lund-Browder classification (more accurate because it allows BSA changes

LUND-BROWDER CLASSIFICATION

To determine the extent of an infant's burns or those of a child, use the Lund-Browder classification shown here.

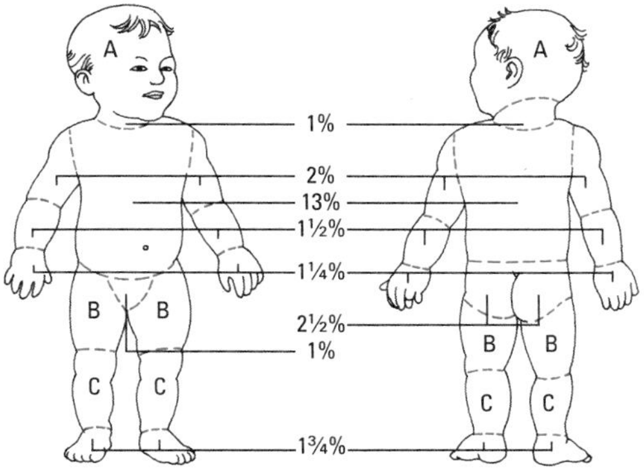

1%
2%
13%
1½%
1¼%
2½%
1%
1¾%

RELATIVE PERCENTAGES OF AREAS AFFECTED BY GROWTH

At birth	0 to 1 yr	1 to 4 yr	5 to 9 yr	10 to 15 yr	15 yr to adult
A: Half of head					
9½%	8½%	6½%	5½%	4½%	3½%
B: Half of thigh					
2¾%	3¼%	4%	4¼%	4½%	4¾%
C: Half of leg					
2½%	2½%	2¾%	3%	3¼%	3½%

with age); correlation of the burn's depth and size to estimate its severity. (See *Using the Rule of Nines and the Lund-Browder classification*.)

Major burns are classified as:
■ third-degree burns on more than 10% of BSA
■ second-degree burns on more than 25% of BSA in adults (over 20% of BSA in children)
■ burns of hands, face, feet, or genitalia
■ burns complicated by fractures or respiratory damage
■ electrical burns
■ all burns in poor-risk patients.

Moderate burns are classified as:
■ third-degree burns on 2% to 10% of BSA
■ second-degree burns on 15% to 25% of BSA in adults (10% to 20% of BSA in children).

Minor burns are classified as:

- third-degree burns on less than 2% of BSA
- second-degree burns on less than 15% of BSA in adults (10% of BSA in children).

Additional diagnostic tests may include the following:
- Arterial blood gas (ABG) levels may be normal early on but may reveal hypoxemia and metabolic acidosis later.
- Carboxyhemoglobin level may reveal the extent of smoke inhalation due to the presence of carbon monoxide.
- Complete blood count (CBC) may reveal a decreased hemoglobin (due to hemolysis), increased hematocrit secondary to hemoconcentration, and leukocytosis resulting from a systemic inflammatory response or possible development of sepsis.
- Electrolyte levels may show hyponatremia from massive fluid shifting and hyperkalemia from fluid shifting and cell lysis; other laboratory tests may reveal elevated blood urea nitrogen (BUN) levels secondary to fluid loss or increased protein breakdown, and decreased total protein and albumin resulting from leakage of plasma proteins into the interstitial spaces.
- Creatine kinase (CK) level may be elevated.

ALERT *Keep in mind that CK is a helpful indicator of muscle damage. Therefore, the more significant or greater the elevation of CK level is, the greater or more extensive the muscle damage is.*

Collaborations
The patient with a serious burn needs the attention of a skilled burn care facility and burn care team. Additional specialists are consulted as needed to manage pulmonary and nutritional needs. In addition, if the patient experiences renal failure, a renal care specialist is necessary. Physical therapy and occupational therapy may be warranted as the patient's condition improves. Depending on the degree of burn injury, rehabilitation may be required. Social services may be consulted for assistance with rehabilitation and long term care planning, follow-up care and referrals and supportive services. The patient and his family may also benefit from spiritual counseling and support.

Treatment and care
Initial burn treatments are based on the type of burn and may include:
- immersion of the burned area in cool water (55°F [12.8°C]) or applying cool compresses (minor burns)
- pain medication as needed or anti-inflammatory medications
- coverage of the area with an antimicrobial agent and a nonstick bulky dressing (after debridement); prophylactic tetanus injection as needed
- maintenance of an open airway; assessing airway, breathing, and circulation; checking for smoke inhalation immediately on receipt of the patient; assisting with endotracheal intubation; and giving 100% oxygen (first immediate treatment for moderate and major burns)
- control of active bleeding
- coverage of partial-thickness burns over 30% of BSA or full-thickness burns over 5% of BSA with a clean, dry, sterile bed sheet (Because of drastic reduction in body temperature, *don't* cover large burns with saline-soaked dressings.)

■ removal of smoldering clothing (first soaking in saline solution if clothing is stuck to the patient's skin), rings, and other constricting items

■ immediate I.V. therapy (with lactated Ringer's solution or a fluid replacement formula) to prevent hypovolemic shock and maintain cardiac output (CO) (Additional I.V. lines or central line placement may be needed; monitor intake and output closely.)

■ antimicrobial therapy (all patients with major burns)

■ laboratory tests, such as CBC, electrolyte, glucose, BUN, and serum creatinine levels; ABG analysis; typing and crossmatching; urinalysis for myoglobinuria and hemoglobinuria

■ close monitoring of intake and output with frequent vital signs (every 15 minutes), possibly inserting indwelling urinary catheter

■ nasogastric (NG) tube to decompress the stomach and avoid aspiration of stomach contents

■ wound irrigation with copious amounts of normal saline solution (chemical burns)

■ surgical intervention, including skin grafts and more thorough surgical debridement for major burns (Tetanus prophylaxis is administered as ordered.)

■ nontreatment of the burn wound itself for a patient being transferred to a specialty facility within 4 hours (Wrap the patient in a sterile sheet and blanket for warmth, elevate the burned extremity, and prepare him for transport.)

■ nutritional therapy to promote healing and recovery.

Complications

Possible complications of burns include:

■ loss of function (burns to face, hands, feet, and genitalia)

■ total occlusion of circulation in extremity (due to edema from circumferential burns)

■ airway obstruction (neck burns) or restricted respiratory expansion (chest burns)

■ pulmonary injury (from smoke inhalation or pulmonary embolism)

■ adult respiratory distress syndrome (due to left-sided heart failure or myocardial infarction)

■ greater damage than indicated by the surface burn (electrical and chemical burns) or internal tissue damage along the conduction pathway (electrical burns)

■ cardiac arrhythmias (due to electrical shock)

■ infected burn wound

■ stroke, heart attack, or pulmonary embolism (due to formation of blood clots resulting from slower blood flow)

■ burn shock (due to fluid shifts out of the vascular compartments, possibly leading to kidney damage and renal failure)

■ peptic ulcer disease (due to decreased blood supply in the abdominal area)

■ disseminated intravascular coagulation in patients with more severe burn states (See "Disseminated intravascular coagulation," page 528.)

■ added pain, depression, and financial burden (due to psychological component of disfigurement).

Nursing considerations

■ Immediately assess the patient's airway, breathing, and circulation. Institute emergency resuscitative measures as necessary.

![icon] **ALERT** *If the patient experienced an electrical burn, be alert for ventricular fibrillation and cardiac and respiratory arrest due to the electrical shock; begin cardiopulmonary resuscitation at once. Get an estimate of the voltage that caused the injury. Tissue damage from an electrical burn is difficult to assess because internal destruction along the conduction pathway usually is greater than the surface burn would indicate. An electrical burn that ignites the patient's clothes may cause thermal burns as well.*

- If the patient has a chemical burn, do the following:
  - Irrigate the wound with copious amounts of water or normal saline solution. Using a weak base (such as sodium bicarbonate) to neutralize hydrofluoric acid, hydrochloric acid, or sulfuric acid on skin or mucous membranes is controversial, particularly in the emergent phase, because the neutralizing agent can produce more heat and tissue damage.
  - If the chemical entered the patient's eyes, flush them with large amounts of water or normal saline solution for at least 30 minutes. In an alkali burn, irrigate until the pH of the conjunctival cul-de-sacs returns to 7.0. Have the patient close his eyes and cover them with a dry, sterile dressing. Note the type of chemical that caused the burn and any noxious fumes. If necessary, refer the patient for an ophthalmologic examination.
- Monitor cardiac and respiratory status closely, at least every 15 minutes, or more frequently, depending on the patient's condition. Assess level of con-

sciousness for changes, such as increasing confusion, restlessness, or decreased responsiveness.
- Auscultate lung sounds for crackles, rhonchi, or stridor. Observe for any signs of laryngeal edema or tracheal obstruction, including labored breathing, severe hoarseness, and dyspnea.
- Administer supplemental humidified oxygen as ordered.

![icon] **ALERT** *Adjust the fraction of inspired oxygen (FIO_2) as soon as possible because carboxyhemoglobin levels generally are reduced within 30 to 60 minutes of receiving 1.0 FIO_2.*

  - Monitor oxygen saturation via continuous pulse oximetry and serial ABG analyses for evidence of hypoxemia and anticipate the need for endotracheal intubation and mechanical ventilation should the patient's respiratory status deteriorate.

![icon] **ALERT** *If the patient has facial or neck burns, anticipate the need for early intubation to reduce the risk of airway obstruction.*

- Place the patient in semi-Fowler's position to maximize chest expansion. Keep the patient as quiet and comfortable as possible to minimize oxygen demands. Administer bronchodilators and mucolytics as ordered to aid in removal of secretions.
- Prepare the patient for an emergency escharotomy of the chest and neck for deep burns or circumferential injuries, if necessary, to promote lung expansion and decrease pulmonary compromise.
- Perform oropharyngeal or tracheal suctioning as indicated by the patient's inability to clear the airway or evidence of abnormal breath sounds.
- Administer rapid fluid replacement therapy as ordered using a large bore

peripheral catheter or central venous catheter as indicated. (See *Fluid replacement,* page 511.)

■ Monitor vital signs continuously for changes indicating hypovolemic shock or evidence of overreplacement. Observe skin color and check capillary refill. Notify the physician if capillary refill is greater than 2 seconds. Maintain core body temperature by covering patient with a sterile blanket and exposing only small areas of his body at a time.

■ Assist with insert of pulmonary artery catheter, if indicated, to evaluate hemodynamic status. Monitor hemodynamic parameters, including central venous pressure, pulmonary artery wedge pressure, and CO, frequently — as often as every 15 to 30 minutes — to evaluate the patient's status and response to treatment.

■ Institute continuous cardiac monitoring to evaluate for possible arrhythmias, myocardial injury or ischemia, or adverse effects of treatment.

■ Assess intake and output every hour; insert an indwelling urinary catheter as indicated to ensure accurate urine measurement. Monitor for urine output of 1 ml/kg/hour in children, 30 to 50 ml/hour for adults, and 75 to 100 ml/hour for those with electrical burns. Check urine specific gravity; if elevated, anticipate the need for additional fluids.

■ Assess patient's level of pain including nonverbal indicators, and administer analgesics such as morphine sulfate I.V. as ordered.

ALERT *Expect to administer analgesics I.V. rather than I.M., because tissue damage associated with the burn injury may impair absorption of the drug when given I.M.*

■ Keep the patient calm, provide periods of uninterrupted rest in between procedures, and use nonpharmacologic pain relief measures as appropriate.

■ Monitor result of serial laboratory testing such as hematocrit and hemoglobin, serum sodium, and potassium levels. Expect hematocrit to return to normal levels as fluid volume is restored.

ALERT *Be alert for hypokalemia, which may occur 3 to 4 days after the initial burn injury. Potassium levels (initially elevated due to cell lysis, increased cell permeability, and fluid shifts) may decrease during this time due to restoration of cell membrane integrity and subsequent decrease in cell permeability and diuresis. Monitor serum levels and electrocardiogram waveform closely for changes.*

■ Assess abdomen for distention and presence of bowel sounds; report any decrease or absent bowel sounds, which may suggest ileus (possible secondary to splanchnic constriction from hypovolemia). Insert or assist with insertion of a NG tube and attach to intermittent suction as ordered. Maintain tube patency and position. Keep the patient on nothing by mouth (NPO) status until bowel sounds return.

■ Administer histamine-2 receptor antagonists as ordered to reduce the risk of ulcer formation.

■ Obtain daily weights and monitor intake including daily calorie counts. Provide high calorie, high protein diet. If the patient is on NPO status, administer enteral feedings as ordered; anticipate the need for parenteral nutrition if the patient develops a paralytic ileus or can't tolerate enteral feedings.

■ Assess patient for signs and symptoms of infection, including fever, ele-

Positioning the burn patient to prevent deformity

Burned area	Potential deformity	Preventive positioning	Nursing considerations
Neck	• Flexion contraction of neck	• Extension	• Remove pillow from bed.
	• Extensor contraction of neck	• Prone with head slightly elevated	• Place pillow or rolled towel under upper chest to flex cervical spine, or apply cervical collar.
Axilla	• Adduction and internal rotation	• Shoulder joint in external rotation and 100- to 103-degree abduction	• Use an I.V. pole, bedside table, or sling to suspend arm.
	• Adduction and external rotation	• Shoulder in forward flexion and 100- to 130-degree abduction	• Use an I.V. pole, bedside table, or sling to suspend arm.
Pectoral region	• Shoulder protraction	• Shoulders abducted and externally rotated	• Remove pillow from bed.
Chest or abdomen	• Kyphosis	• Same as for pectoral region, with hips neutral (not flexed)	• Use no pillows under head or legs.
Lateral trunk	• Scoliosis	• Supine; affected arm abducted	• Put pillows or blanket roll at sides.
Elbow	• Flexion and pronation	• Arm extended and supinated	• Use an elbow splint, arm board, or bedside table.
Wrist	• Flexion	• Splint in 15-degree extension	• Apply a hand splint.
	• Extension	• Splint in 15-degree flexion	• Apply a hand splint.
Fingers	• Adhesions of the extensor tendons; loss of plantar grip	• Metacarpophalangeal joints in maximum flexion; interphalangeal joints in slight flexion; thumb in maximum abduction	• Apply a hand splint; wrap fingers separately.

Positioning the burn patient to prevent deformity *(continued)*

Burned area	Potential deformity	Preventive positioning	Nursing considerations
Hip	• Internal rotation, flexion, and adduction; possible joint subluxation if contracture is severe	• Neutral rotation and abduction; extension by prone position	• Put a pillow under buttocks (if supine) or use trochanter rolls or knee or long leg splints.
Knee	• Flexion	• Extension	• Use a knee splint with no pillows under legs.
Ankle	• Plantar flexion if foot muscles are weak or their tendons are divided	• 90-degree dorsiflexion	• Use a footboard or ankle splint.

vated white blood cell count, changes in burn wound appearance or drainage. Obtain a wound culture and administer antipyretic and antimicrobial agents as ordered.

■ Administer tetanus prophylaxis, if indicated.

■ Perform burn wound care as ordered. Prepare patient for possible grafting as indicated.

■ Assess neurovascular status of the injured area including pulses, reflexes, paresthesia, color and temperature of the injured area at least every 2 to 4 hours, or more frequently, if indicated.

■ Assist with splinting, positioning, compression therapy, and exercise to the burned area as indicated. Maintain burned area in a neutral position to prevent contractures and minimize deformity. (See *Positioning the burn patient to prevent deformity*.)

■ Explain all procedures to the patient before performing them. Speak calmly and clearly to help alleviate his anxiety.

Encourage him to actively participate in his care as much as possible.

■ Provide opportunities for patient to voice his concerns, especially about altered body image. If appropriate, arrange for him to meet a patient with similar injuries. When possible, show the patient how his bodily functions are improving. If necessary, refer him for mental health counseling.

Patient teaching

■ Review treatment course with patient and his family including procedures, such as wound care and cleansing and medications ordered and their intended effects, dosage, and adverse effects to report. Answer questions honestly and provide information as needed.

■ Teach the patient and his family about the signs and symptoms of infection; include instructions to notify the physician should any occur.

- Instruct in measures to promote mobility and maintain function, including splinting and exercise; review measures for wound care.
- Provide preoperative teaching for grafting procedures as indicated.
- Emphasize the need for continued follow-up and care.

Care of the organ donor

Since the mid 1950s, when the first kidney transplant took place, organ transplant has steadily increased and yielded successful results for organ recipients. As a result, the demand for donor organs has greatly increased.

Many factors have contributed to the improved survival of organ recipients. These include refined criteria for donor and recipient selection, development of tissue biopsy as a diagnostic tool, better organ preservation, advances in immunosuppression therapy, definitive treatment of immunosuppressive complications and advances in the education of health care personnel caring for transplant patients.

The majority of organs available for transplant come from cadavers. Once brain death has been determined for the donor, organ function is maintained with specific treatment. Research has shown that time from determination of brain death until organ procurement directly influences the number and severity of complications that develop in the donor, thus affecting the overall success of the transplant. Therefore, specific care is needed to preserve the donor's hemodynamic status, protect the organs to be donated, and avoid possible complications associated with brain death. (See complications, later in this section.)

Essential steps

- Identify patient as potential organ donor and ensure that explicit informed consent is obtained.
- Notify transplant coordinator of possible organ donor.
- Assist with determination of brain death, including monitoring for the following: early indicators such as hemodynamic lability, heart rate instability, and decreased bronchial secretion, absence of brainstem reflexes and lack of respiratory effort, and EEG and transcranial Doppler study results.
- Obtain laboratory and diagnostic tests as ordered such as complete blood count, electrolytes, arterial blood gas studies, ABO blood typing, human leukocyte antigen typing, blood cultures, sputum gram stain, culture and sensitivities, urinalysis, urine culture and sensitivity, viral serology (human immunodeficiency virus, Epstein-Barr virus, cytomegalovirus, human T-cell leukemia type 1, and hepatitis B and C), and Venereal Disease Research Laboratories test or rapid plasma regain.

ALERT *Expect more specialized diagnostic testing for specific organ donation such as the heart — for example, electrocardiogram, chest X-ray, echocardiogram, isoenzymes of creatine kinase (CK-MB) and troponin levels, and cardiac catheterization if the patient is over age 45.*

- Assist with insertion of central venous catheter or pulmonary artery catheter if one isn't already in place. Monitor hemodynamic parameters at least hourly. Maintain central venous pressure (CVP) at approximately 8 to 12 mm Hg. Anticipate the need for fluid therapy to maintain CVP.

■ Monitor pulse rate, CVP and pulse oximetry levels every hour or more frequently, if necessary. Maintain mechanical ventilation and regulate settings as ordered; use the least amount of FIO_2 to maintain an arterial oxygen concentration of 100 mm Hg.

■ Assess temperature every 2 hours; maintain temperature between 97° F to 100° F (36.1° C to 37.8° C). Use cooling or warming blankets as necessary to maintain temperature.

■ Assess blood pressure every hour; expect to administer inotropic agents such as dopamine as ordered but in the smallest dose possible to maintain systolic blood pressure above 100 mm Hg; if systolic blood pressure is greater than 200 mm Hg, expect to administer nitroprusside.

■ Monitor urine output hourly; insert an indwelling urinary catheter if not already in place; report any urine output below 100 ml/hour. Expect to maintain a urine output of approximately 100 to 300 ml/hour. Anticipate administration of diuretics to increase urine output if the patient's blood pressure and hydration status is within acceptable parameters.

■ Ensure adequate volume replacement. Administer I.V. fluid therapy, adjusting infusion to a rate that's at least 50 ml/hour greater than that of urine output.

■ Monitor renal functions studies and serum electrolyte levels and expect to correct electrolyte imbalances as ordered.

■ If the patient develops diabetes insipidus, administer pitressin as ordered, titrating it to maintain urine

output within the desired range of 100 to 300 ml/hour.

■ Administer corticosteroids and antimicrobial agents as ordered.

■ Prepare to transfuse blood and blood products to correct any coagulopathies; monitor hemoglobin level and hematocrit; maintain hematocrit above 30%.

■ Prepare the patient for surgical removal of the organs.

Complications
The following complications may develop in organ donor patients who are brain dead:
■ diabetes insipidus
■ adrenal insufficiency
■ disseminated intravascular coagulation
■ cardiac arrhythmias
■ pulmonary edema
■ hypoxia
■ positive bacterial cultures
■ seizures
■ metabolic acidosis
■ hypothermia
■ respiratory arrest.

Nursing considerations
■ Check your facility's policy for specific requirements for organ donation.

■ Be sure to monitor all aspects of the patient's condition closely. The success of the transplant is influenced by the status of the donated organs.

■ Provide comfort for the patient's family; ensure that the family understands what's happening; explain all treatments, procedures, and equipment being used.

■ Allow the family to visit with the patient before he's taken to surgery.

■ Document all assessments and monitoring parameters; ensure that necessary laboratory and diagnostic test results are on the patient's medical record.

■ Record abnormal findings, including the time they occurred, notification of the physician, and measures instituted.

■ Document the time that the patient was taken to surgery.

ALERT *Provide the donor's family with a private area for grieving. Assist them with arrangements, as necessary, following organ donation. Arrange for social services or pastoral care to provide additional emotional support.*

⭐ MULTISYSTEM DISORDER

Disseminated intravascular coagulation

Disseminated intravascular coagulation (DIC) occurs as a complication of diseases and conditions that accelerate clotting, causing small blood vessel occlusion, organ necrosis, depletion of circulating clotting factors and platelets, activation of the fibrinolytic system, and consequent severe hemorrhage. Clotting in the microcirculation usually affects the kidneys and extremities but may occur in the brain, lungs, pituitary and adrenal glands, and GI mucosa. DIC, also called *consumption coagulopathy* or *defibrination syndrome,* is generally an acute condition but may be chronic in cancer patients.

Causes of DIC include:

■ infection, including gram-negative or gram-positive septicemia and viral, fungal, rickettsial, or protozoal infection

■ obstetric complications, including abruptio placentae, amniotic fluid embolism, retained dead fetus, septic abortion, eclampsia

■ neoplastic disease, including acute leukemia, metastatic carcinoma, aplastic anemia

■ disorders that produce necrosis, including extensive burns and trauma, brain tissue destruction, transplant rejection, hepatic necrosis

■ other conditions, including heatstroke, shock, poisonous snakebite, cirrhosis, fat embolism, incompatible blood transfusion, cardiac arrest, surgery requiring cardiopulmonary bypass, giant hemangioma, severe venous thrombosis, and purpura fulminans.

Prognosis depends on early detection and treatment, the severity of the hemorrhage, and treatment of the underlying disease.

Pathophysiology

It isn't clear why certain disorders lead to DIC or whether they use a common mechanism. In many patients, the triggering mechanisms may be the entrance of foreign protein into the circulation and vascular endothelial injury.

Regardless of how DIC begins, the typical accelerated clotting results in generalized activation of prothrombin and a consequent excess of thrombin. The thrombin converts fibrinogen to fibrin, producing fibrin clots in the microcirculation. This process uses huge amounts of coagulation factors (especially fibrinogen, prothrombin, platelets, and factors V and VIII), causing hypofibrinogenemia, hypoprothrombinemia, thrombocytopenia, and deficiencies in factors V and VIII. Circulating thrombin also activates the fibrinolytic system, which dissolves fibrin clots into fibrin degradation products. Hemorrhage may be mostly the result of the anticoagulant activity of fibrin degradation products and the depletion of plasma coagulation factors.

Comprehensive assessment

The most significant clinical feature of DIC is abnormal bleeding without a history of a hemorrhagic disorder. Signs and symptoms are related to bleeding and thrombosis. Bleeding problems are usually more common than thrombotic problems unless coagulation occurs to a greater extent than fibrinolysis.

The patient history may include one of the causes of DIC. In addition, although bleeding may occur from any site, the patient may report signs of bleeding into the skin, such as cutaneous oozing, petechiae, ecchymoses, and hematomas. If the patient is receiving treatment for another disorder when this problem occurs, he may also have bleeding from surgical or invasive procedure sites, such as incisions or venipuncture sites.

Other reported signs and symptoms may include nausea; vomiting; severe muscle, back, and abdominal pain; chest pain; hemoptysis; epistaxis; seizures; and oliguria. Inspection may reveal petechiae and other signs of bleeding into the skin, acrocyanosis, and dyspnea. On palpation, peripheral pulses may be diminished. Auscultation may disclose decreased blood pressure, and neurologic assessment may reveal mental status changes, including confusion.

Diagnosis

Diagnosis of DIC is based on the following:

- decreased platelet count, usually less than 100,000/µl, because platelets are consumed during thrombosis
- fibrinogen less than 150 mg/dl because fibrinogen is consumed in clot formation (levels possibly normal if elevated by hepatitis or pregnancy)
- prothrombin time (PT) greater than 15 seconds
- partial thromboplastin time (PTT) greater than 60 seconds
- increased fibrin degradation products, often greater than 45 mcg/ml, due to excess fibrinolysis by plasmin
- D-dimer test (presence of an asymmetrical carbon compound fragment formed in the presence of fibrin split products) positive at less than 1:8 dilution
- positive fibrin monomers, diminished levels of factors V and VIII, fragmentation of red blood cells (RBCs), and hemoglobin less than 10 g/dl
- reduced urine output (less than 30 ml/hour), elevated blood urea nitrogen (greater than 25 mg/dl), and elevated serum creatinine (greater than 1.3 mg/dl).

Collaborations

Because DIC is a multisystem disorder, a multidisciplinary approach to care is essential. Care focuses on reestablishing the coagulation process, that is, controlling bleeding and accelerated clotting. Numerous health care personnel are usually involved in the patient's care. The patient with DIC is very ill and requires the expertise of a hematologist and other skilled physicians and specialists depending on the cause and extent of the situation. Respiratory therapy may be consulted to assist with maintaining optimal respiratory function. The severity of the illness makes this an extremely stressful time for the patient and his family members. As needed, enlist the aid of a social worker, spiritual counselor, and other members of the health care team in providing such support.

Treatment and care

Successful management of DIC requires prompt recognition and adequate treatment of the underlying disorder. Treatment may be supportive (when the underlying disorder is self-limiting, for example) or highly specific. If the patient isn't actively bleeding, supportive care alone may reverse DIC. Active bleeding may require administration of blood, fresh frozen plasma (FFP), platelets, or packed RBCs to support hemostasis.

Heparin therapy is controversial. It may be used early in the disease to prevent microclotting but may be considered a last resort in the patient who is actively bleeding. If thrombosis occurs, heparin therapy is usually mandatory. In most cases, it's administered in combination with transfusion therapy. (See *Understanding DIC and its treatment.*)

Complications

Complications of DIC include:
■ acute tubular necrosis
■ shock
■ multiple organ failure.

Nursing considerations

■ Ensure a patent airway and assess breathing and circulation. Monitor cardiac and respiratory status closely, at least every 30 minutes, or more fre-

quently, depending on the patient's condition.
■ Monitor vital signs frequently (at least every 30 minutes) for changes indicating hypovolemic shock. Observe skin color and check peripheral circulation, including color, temperature, and capillary refill. Notify the physician if capillary refill is greater than 2 seconds.
■ Administer supplemental oxygen as ordered. Monitor oxygen saturation via continuous pulse oximetry and serial arterial blood gas studies for evidence of hypoxemia and anticipate the need for endotracheal intubation and mechanical ventilation should the patient's respiratory status deteriorate. Place the patient in semi-Fowler's position to maximize chest expansion. Keep the patient as quiet and comfortable as possible to minimize oxygen demands.

ALERT *Be especially alert for signs and symptoms of pulmonary embolism, including sudden onset of severe, sharp chest pain, dyspnea, tachypnea, restlessness, anxiety, pallor, and cyanosis. Notify the physician immediately if any occurs. (See "Pulmonary embolism" in chapter 2, page 229.)*
■ Assess the patient's level of consciousness and neurologic status frequently — at least every hour, or more often, if indicated — for changes, such as decreased sensorium, confusion, lethargy, or somnolence, indicating decreased cerebral perfusion or intracranial bleeding.
■ Assess the patient for the extent of blood loss and begin fluid replacement as ordered. Obtain a type and cross-match for blood component therapy.

ALERT *When bleeding is severe, lactated Ringer's solution is pre-*

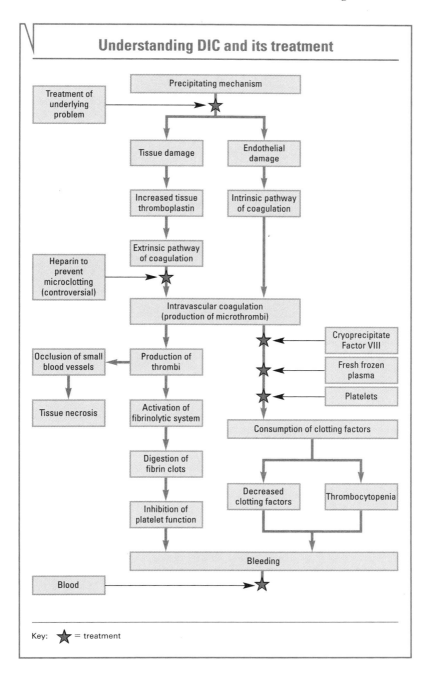

Understanding DIC and its treatment

Precipitating mechanism

Treatment of underlying problem →★

Tissue damage

Endothelial damage

Increased tissue thromboplastin

Intrinsic pathway of coagulation

Extrinsic pathway of coagulation

Heparin to prevent microclotting (controversial) →★

Intravascular coagulation (production of microthrombi)

★← Cryoprecipitate Factor VIII

★← Fresh frozen plasma

★← Platelets

Occlusion of small blood vessels ← Production of thrombi

Tissue necrosis

Activation of fibrinolytic system

Consumption of clotting factors

Digestion of fibrin clots

Decreased clotting factors

Thrombocytopenia

Inhibition of platelet function

Bleeding

Blood →★

Key: ★ = treatment

ferred for fluid volume replacement because its use minimizes the risk of electrolyte imbalances. If the patient becomes severely hypotensive, expect to administer vasoactive drugs such as amrinone, dobutamine, dopamine, epinephrine, and nitroprusside, as ordered.

■ Assist with insert of central venous or pulmonary artery catheter to evaluate hemodynamic status. Monitor hemodynamic parameters, including central venous pressure, pulmonary artery wedge pressure, and cardiac output and input, frequently — as often as every 15 minutes — to evaluate the patient's status and response to treatment.

ALERT *The patient with DIC, while at risk for hemorrhage, is also at risk for pulmonary emboli due to accelerated clotting. Watch hemodynamic parameters closely; decreased values suggest hemorrhage while increased values suggest emboli.*

■ Institute continuous cardiac monitoring to evaluate for possible arrhythmias, myocardial ischemia, or adverse effects of treatment.

■ As soon as possible, begin blood component therapy as ordered. Typically, packed RBCs, clotting factors, and FFP are used for replacement. Adhere to facility's guidelines for blood administration; be alert for signs and symptoms of transfusion reactions.

ALERT *FFP administration allows for replacement of clotting factors and inhibitors. Cryoprecipitate is the drug of choice if the patient's fibrinogen levels are significantly decreased. Cryoprecipitate provides 5 to 10 times the amount of fibrinogen when compared with that of plasma.*

■ Obtain serial hemoglobin and hematocrit levels; monitor results of coagulation studies including PTT, PT, fibrinogen levels, fibrin split/degradation products, and platelet counts; notify the physician of any levels below prescribed parameter.

■ Administer heparin in low doses via I.V. infusion as ordered.

ALERT *Although the patient is at risk for thrombus and emboli, thrombolytic agents such as urokinase, streptokinase, and tissue plasminogen activator aren't used because they can lead to excessive bleeding.*

■ Administer antifibrinolytic agents cautiously as ordered.

ALERT *Although antifibrinolytic agents, such as epsilon-aminocaproic acid, are useful in inhibiting fibrinolysis, they must be given cautiously to patients with DIC because of the risk of thrombosis. Therefore, expect to administer these agents in conjunction with heparin to reduce this risk.*

■ Expect to administer vitamin K and folate as ordered to correct deficiencies.

■ Monitor intake and output, at least hourly as indicated; expect to insert an indwelling urinary catheter to assess urine output hourly. Check all stools and drainage for occult blood.

■ Inspect skin and mucous membranes for signs of bleeding; assess all invasive insertion sites and dressings for evidence of frank bleeding or oozing. Weigh the dressings that are wet or saturated to aid in determining extent of blood loss. Watch for bleeding from the GI and genitourinary tracts. If you suspect intra-abdominal bleeding, measure the patient's abdominal girth at least every 4 hours and observe closely for signs of shock.

■ Institute bleeding precautions. Limit all invasive procedures, such as venipunctures and intramuscular injections, as much as possible. Apply pressure for 3 to 5 minutes over venous insertion sites and for 10 to 15 minutes over arterial sites.

■ Institute safety precautions to minimize the risk of injury.

■ Provide emotional support and reassurance as appropriate.

Patient teaching

■ Explain the disorder to the patient and his family, including early recognition of signs of abnormal bleeding, prompt treatment of the underlying disorders, and prevention of further bleeding.

■ Review ordered treatments and medications and their intended effects, dosage, and adverse effects to report. Answer questions honestly and provide information as needed.

 MULTISYSTEM DISORDER

Drug overdose, poisoning

Drug overdose and poisoning usually involve overdoses of common prescription or over-the-counter (OTC) medications. Other commonly ingested substances that can cause toxicity include illegal drugs, chemicals in the home or workplace, plants, and food.

Toxicity usually results from ingestion; however, other sources of exposure include inhalation, injection, and direct absorption through the skin and mucous membranes. In the United States, about 1 million people are poisoned annually, 800 of them fatally.

AGE ISSUE *Because of their curiosity and ignorance, children are the most common poison victims. In fact, accidental poisoning, usually from the ingestion of salicylates (aspirin), cleaning agents, insecticides, paints, cosmetics, and plants, is the fourth leading cause of death in children.*

In adults, poisoning is most common among chemical company employees, particularly those in companies that use chlorine, carbon dioxide, hydrogen sulfide, nitrogen dioxide, and ammonia, and in companies that ignore safety standards. Other causes of poisoning in adults include improper cooking, canning, and storage of food; ingestion of or skin contamination from plants (for example, dieffenbachia, mistletoe, azalea, and philodendron); and accidental or intentional drug overdose (usually barbiturates) or chemical ingestion.

Several factors influence the signs and symptoms noticed after an accidental or intentional toxic ingestion. These include:

■ type of substance ingested
■ amount of substance ingested
■ patient's tolerance to the toxin
■ number of toxins ingested
■ time between ingestion and treatment.

When one or more toxic substances have been ingested, the effect may be synergistic or antagonistic. Synergistic effects occur when drug combinations produce an effect that's greater than the sum of the effect of the two drugs. Antagonistic effects occur when a drug combination produces an effect that's less than the sum of the drugs acting alone.

Pathophysiology

Changes produced by toxic ingestion usually result from an exaggeration of the toxin's normal therapeutic and side effects. For example, depressed level of consciousness (LOC) and hypoventilation typically occur after ingestion of sedatives and opiates, while hypotension and arrhythmias occur after ingestion of beta and calcium channel blockers. Some toxins such as acetaminophen and ethylene glycol, have organ specific toxic effects. (See *Understanding specific drug toxicities.*)

Comprehensive assessment

Assessment of the patient with a toxic ingestion must include a simultaneous history, assessment of airway, breathing, and circulation, and initiation of life support as indicated.

The patient's history whether from the patient or significant others should reveal the source of poison and the form of exposure (ingestion, inhalation, injection, or skin contact). Assessment findings vary with the poison. (See *Assessing drug overdose,* pages 537 to 540.)

The patient will present with a history related to the specific poison. It's important to determine what substance was taken, when it was taken and how much, the time since it was taken, and the route (ingested, injected, inhaled, and so forth). In addition, information related to any measures used and their results is important. The substance may be a prescription or an OTC medication or other substance and may be legal or illegal. The substance may also have been taken on purpose as directed under a physician's care, or may be an unsuccessful suicide or an accidental occurrence.

The patient may be alert and able to respond to questions, or he may be agitated, delirious, obtunded, and unresponsive. He may also present with constricted or dilated pupils. He may have tremors or seizures; he may be in a coma, or exhibit posturing neurologically. He may have rapid respirations, Kussmaul's respirations, or no respirations at all; he may present in cardiac arrest.

Skin may be diaphoretic, tinged pink, or cyanotic. He may have accompanying dry mouth, diarrhea, nausea, vomiting, or hematemesis.

Diagnosis

Toxicologic studies (including drug screens) determine levels of poison in the mouth, vomitus, urine, or stool. Blood on the patient's hands or clothing may also confirm the diagnosis. Drug screens identify the toxin and amount. If possible, have the family or patient bring the container holding the poison to the facility for a comparable study.

These diagnostic tests may also be used:
■ Chest X-ray may reveal pulmonary infiltrates or edema in petroleum distillate inhalation or aspiration pneumonia (with inhalation poisoning).
■ Abdominal X-rays may reveal iron pills or other radiopaque substances, such as calcium, enteric coated aspirin, and phenothiazines.
■ Arterial blood gas (ABG) analyses aid in ruling out hypoxia, hypercapnia and metabolic acidosis as the cause of the patient's altered LOC.
■ Blood glucose level aids in ruling out hypoglycemia as the cause of the patient's altered LOC.

Understanding specific drug toxicities

Acetaminophen

Acetaminophen, the active ingredient in many over-the-counter analgesics and antipyretics, is the most commonly reported pharmaceutical ingestion in adults and children. The drug is rapidly absorbed and metabolized in the liver. Normally, a small amount of acetaminophen (less than 5%) is metabolized to a toxic intermediate metabolite, N-acetyl-para-benzoquinoneimine (NAPQI), which is further metabolized by glutathione to nontoxic products.

NAPQI is a powerful oxidizing agent that leads to cell death by bonding to cellular proteins. After an acute single toxic dose (7.5 g in an adult), the glutathione is used up and can't regenerate fast enough to detoxify all of the intermediate metabolite. Consequently, the NAPQI builds up, causing liver damage. Evidence of liver damage may not be apparent until 24 to 36 hours after ingestion.

Alcohols

All alcohols, including ethanol, ethylene glycol, methanol, and isopropanol, are rapidly absorbed from the GI tract and metabolized by the liver enzyme alcohol dehydrogenase. Isopropanol and methanol also are easily absorbed through the skin and mucous membranes and can result in toxicity. Ethylene glycol and methanol are the most toxic alcohols. Ethylene glycol commonly is found in antifreeze and cleaning solutions; methanol is found in windshield washer fluid and solvents. Both are minimally toxic prior to metabolism but, in addition of their inebriating effects, have specific organ toxicity once metabolized. Both alcohols are metabolized in the liver, and blood levels above 20 mg/dl are considered toxic for both.

Metabolism of ethylene glycol produces glycolaldehyde, glycolic acid, glyoxylic acid, and oxalic acid. Symptoms result from the direct effects of these toxins and progress through three stages. Symptoms in stage I (first 12 hours) include altered mental status, seizures, and severe anion-gap metabolic acidosis. Cardiac toxicity occurs in stage II (12 to 36 hours). Stage III, renal failure, the hallmark of ethylene glycol toxicity, occurs at 36 to 48 hours.

Metabolism of methanol produces formaldehyde and formic acid. Folic acid is required for further metabolism to nontoxic products. Symptoms of methanol toxicity appear 12 to 24 hours after ingestion and result primarily from the effects of formic acid. Formic acid damages the optic nerve. Hemorrhages also have been found in a portion of the basal ganglia called the putamen. Symptoms include severe anion-gap metabolic acidosis caused by acid production, hypotension, visual changes that can progress to blindness, coma, and sudden respiratory arrest.

Cocaine

Cocaine blocks the reuptake of norepinephrine, epinephrine, and dopamine, causing excesses at the postsynaptic receptor sites. This leads to central and peripheral adrenergic stimulation and to a generalized vasoconstriction that affects multiple organs. These effects may include hypertension, hyperthermia, tachycardia, excited delirium, and seizures. Hyperthermia can cause rhabdomyolysis and later renal failure. Direct effects on the heart include increased myocardial oxygen consumption, coronary artery spasm, ischemia, myocardial infarction, depressed myocardial contractility, acute heart failure, sudden death from arrhythmias, and dilated cardiomyopathy. Recent studies also have shown that cocaine increases platelet aggregation and thrombus formation. I.V. drug users also are at risk for endocarditis.

(continued)

Understanding specific drug toxicities *(continued)*

Cyclic antidepressants

Cyclic antidepressants are responsible for almost half of all overdose-related adult admissions to critical care units and are the leading cause of overdose-related deaths in emergency departments. Cyclic drugs include the older tricyclics, such as amitriptyline and nortriptyline, and such newer agents as maprotiline (Ludiomil). These drugs are rapidly absorbed from the GI tract, although absorption may be delayed in large overdoses because of anticholinergic adverse effects. They are metabolized in the liver.

In an overdose, the enzymes responsible for metabolism become saturated, and some of the drug and its metabolites are secreted into the bile and gastric fluid and are later reabsorbed. Toxicity results from central and peripheral blockage of norepinephrine reuptake, anticholinergic effects, and quinidine-like effects on the heart. Central nervous system (CNS) effects may include initial agitation followed rapidly by lethargy, coma, and seizures. Anticholinergic effects include tachycardia, mydriasis, dry and flushed skin, hypoactive bowel sounds, and urine retention. Cardiovascular effects include hypotension, arrhythmias, and quinidine-like changes on the electrocardiogram with widening of the QRS complex.

Organophosphates and carbamates

Organophosphates and carbamates commonly are found in pesticides and account for 80% of pesticide-related hospital admissions. They are highly lipid-soluble and easily absorbed through skin and mucous membranes. The primary mechanism of toxicity is cholinesterase inhibition. This leads to excess acetylcholine at muscarinic, nicotinic, and CNS receptors. The effects of excessive acetylcholine include excessive salivation and lacrimation, muscle fasciculations and weakness, constricted pupils, decreased level of consciousness, and seizures. Bradycardia is typically present, but tachycardia has also been reported.

■ Electrocardiogram reveals ischemia, arrhythmias, and widened QRS complexes associated with cyclic antidepressant therapy.
■ Serum electrolyte levels reveal high anion gap (associated with methanol, ethylene glycol, iron, and salicylate toxicity), low anion gap (associated with lithium toxicity), hyperkalemia (associated with ethylene glycol and methanol toxicity), hypokalemia (associated with loop diuretics and salicylate toxicity), or hypocalcemia (associated with ethylene glycol toxicity).
■ Complete blood count may reveal leukocytosis secondary to ethylene glycol toxicity.

■ Coagulation studies may reveal prolonged coagulation times, suggesting toxicity of warfarin.

Collaborations

Because a multidisciplinary approach to care is needed, numerous health care personnel may be involved in caring for the patient with a drug overdose. Cardiac, renal, neurologic, and hepatic specialists may be consulted depending on the organs affected by the toxic ingestion. Respiratory therapy may be involved to assist with maintaining ventilation and perfusion. Renal care personnel may be needed to

(Text continues on page 540.)

Assessing drug overdose

Drug	Assessment findings
Acetaminophen	● Plasma levels greater than 300 µg/ml 4 hours after ingestion; 50 µg/ml 12 hours after ingestion (suggestive of hepatoxicity) ● Nausea, vomiting, diaphoresis, and anorexia 12 to 24 hours after ingestion ● Cyanosis ● Anemia ● Jaundice ● Skin eruptions ● Fever ● Emesis ● Delirium ● Methemoglobinemia progressing to central nervous system (CNS) depression, coma, vascular collapse, seizures, and death
Amphetamines, cocaine	● Abdominal cramps ● Aggressiveness ● Arrhythmias ● Confusion ● Diarrhea ● Fatigue ● Hallucinations ● Hyperreflexia ● Nausea, vomiting ● Restlessness ● Seizures ● Tachypnea ● Tremor ● Coma ● Death
Anticholinergics	● Blurred vision ● Decreased or absent bowel sounds ● Dilated, nonreactive pupils ● Dry mucous membranes ● Dysphagia ● Flushed, hot, dry skin ● Hypertension ● Hyperthermia ● Increased respiratory rate ● Tachycardia ● Urine retention
Anticoagulants	● Hematuria ● Internal or external bleeding ● Skin necrosis

(continued)

538 Multisystem challenges

Assessing drug overdose *(continued)*	
Drug	**Assessment findings**
Antihistamines	• Drowsiness • Moderate anticholinergic symptoms (selected histamine-1 antagonists) • Respiratory depression • Seizures • Coma
Barbiturates	• Areflexia • Confusion • Pulmonary edema • Respiratory depression • Slurred speech • Sustained nystagmus • Somnolence • Unsteady gait • Coma
Benzodiazepines	• Bradycardia • Confusion • Dyspnea • Hypoactive reflexes • Hypotension • Impaired coordination • Labored breathing • Slurred speech • Somnolence
CNS depressants	• Absent pupillary reflexes • Apnea • Dilated pupils • Hypotension • Hypothermia followed by fever • Inadequate ventilation • Loss of deep tendon reflexes • Tonic muscle spasms • Coma
Iron supplements	• GI irritation with epigastric pain, nausea, vomiting • Diarrhea (initially green, then tarry, then melena) • Hematemesis • Metabolic acidosis • Hepatic dysfunction • Renal failure • Bleeding diathesis • Circulatory failure • Coma • Death

Assessing drug overdose *(continued)*

Drug	Assessment findings
Nonsteroidal anti-inflammatory agents	• Abdominal pain • Apnea • Cyanosis • Dizziness • Drowsiness • Headache • Nausea, vomiting • Nystagmus • Paresthesia • Sweating
Opiates	• Respiratory depression with or without CNS depression and miosis • Hypotension • Bradycardia • Hypothermia • Shock • Cardiopulmonary arrest • Circulatory collapse • Pulmonary edema • Seizures
Phenothiazines	• Abnormal involuntary muscle movements • Agitation • Arrhythmias • Autonomic nervous system dysfunction • Deep unarousable sleep • Extrapyramidal symptoms • Hypotension • Hypothermia or hyperthermia • Seizures
Salicylates	• Hyperpnea • Metabolic acidosis • Respiratory alkalosis • Tachypnea

Tricyclic antidepressants	• CNS stimulation (first 12 hours after ingestion)
	  – Agitation
	  – Confusion
	  – Constipation, ileus
	  – Dry mucous membranes
	  – Hallucinations
	  – Hyperthermia
	  – Irritation
	  – Parkinsonism
	  – Pupillary dilation
	  – Seizures
	  – Urine retention

(continued)

Assessing drug overdose *(continued)*

Drug	Assessment findings
Tricyclic antidepressants (continued)	• CNS depression – Cardiac irregularities – Cyanosis – Decreased or absent reflexes – Hypotension – Hypothermia – Sedation

assist with removal of the toxin via dialysis. Social services and psychological specialists may be necessary to assist with coping mechanisms and provide therapy if it's determined that the ingestion was intentional. Social services may also assist with community and financial support services and arrangements for follow-up.

Treatment and care
Initial treatment includes emergency resuscitation, support for the patient's airway, breathing, and circulation, prevention of further absorption of poison, administration of the antidote, if available, enhancement of drug's elimination, and prevention of metabolism of the toxin and complications. (See *Common antidotes,* in Part II, page 615.) Continued treatment focuses on supportive or symptomatic care.

Measures to reduce drug absorption include induced emesis, gastric lavage, and administration of activated charcoal. Inducing emesis contraindicated when corrosive acid poisoning is suspected, if the patient is unconscious or has seizures, or if the gag reflex is impaired even in a conscious patient. Gastric lavage is recommended only for patients who have ingested a potentially lethal amount of drug or toxin and present within 1 hour of ingestion.

Methods used to enhance the drug's elimination include:
■ cathartics such as sorbitol, magnesium citrate, or magnesium sulfate
■ repeated multiple doses of activated charcoal
■ whole bowel irrigation with a solution such as a balanced electrolyte solution
■ forced diuresis
■ dialysis.

Complications
Complications of poisoning or drug overdose vary widely depending on the type of substance and type of exposure, but can include hypotension, cardiac arrhythmias, seizures, coma, and death.

Nursing considerations
■ Immediately assess the patient's airway, breathing, and circulation. Institute emergency resuscitative measures as necessary.
■ Monitor neurologic, cardiac and respiratory status closely, at least every 15 minutes or more frequently depending on the patient's condition. As-

sess LOC for changes such as increasing confusion, restlessness, or decreased responsiveness.

ALERT *Be vigilant when assessing the patient because his status can deteriorate quickly depending on the type and amount of drug ingested. Institute seizure precautions as appropriate.*

■ Auscultate lung sounds for crackles, rhonchi, or stridor. Observe for any signs of airway obstruction, including labored breathing, severe hoarseness, and dyspnea.

■ Administer supplemental humidified oxygen as ordered. Monitor oxygen saturation via continuous pulse oximetry and serial ABG studies for evidence of hypoxemia, and anticipate the need for endotracheal intubation and mechanical ventilation should the patient's respiratory status deteriorate.

ALERT *Monitor ABG levels for increasing partial pressure of arterial carbon dioxide and decreasing pH, which suggest respiratory acidosis.*

■ Administer I.V. fluid therapy as ordered. Obtain laboratory specimens to assess for drug, electrolytes, and glucose levels. Anticipate administering normal saline solution and vasopressors if the patient is hypotensive; administering dextrose 5% and water if the patient is hypoglycemic.

ALERT *For the patient who has a history of chronic alcohol abuse, use of dextrose solutions may precipitate Wernicke-Korsakoff syndrome, a thiamine deficiency with severe neurologic impairment. This results because the carbohydrates in the dextrose solution increase the body's demand for thiamine, which is depleted in patients with chronic alcohol use. Therefore, expect to administer thiamine first — before administering the dextrose solution.*

■ Place the patient in semi-Fowler's position to maximize chest expansion. Keep the patient as quiet and comfortable as possible to minimize oxygen demands. Administer bronchodilators as ordered.

■ Perform oropharyngeal or tracheal suctioning as indicated by the patient's inability to clear the airway or evidence of abnormal breath sounds.

■ Monitor vital signs continuously for changes. Assess for signs and symptoms of hyperthermia such as a temperature above 101° F (38.3° C), pallor, lack of perspiration, and skin that's warm to the touch; institute cooling measures such as cool packs to the axilla and groin, cooling bath, and cooling blanket.

■ Assist with insert of pulmonary artery catheter if indicated to evaluate hemodynamic status. Monitor hemodynamic parameters, including central venous pressure, pulmonary artery wedge pressure, and cardiac output and input, frequently (at least every 30 minutes).

■ Institute continuous cardiac monitoring to evaluate for possible arrhythmias or effects of drug ingestion. If the patient develops heart block, prepare for cardiac pacing. Administer antiarrhythmic agents as ordered.

■ Assess intake and output every hour; insert an indwelling urinary catheter as indicated to ensure accurate urine measurement.

■ Administer antidote as ordered and available.

ALERT *When administering flumazenil and naloxone, watch for signs of withdrawal. Flumazenil may precipitate seizures especially in* *patients who have ingested cyclic anti-depressants or have been on long-term sedation with benzodiazepines. Assess the patient for return of overdose symptoms because the drug may last longer than the dose of antidote.*

■ Institute measures to prevent drug absorption as ordered. If gastric lavage is ordered, instill 30 ml of fluid by a nasogastric tube; then aspirate the liquid. Repeat until the aspirate is clear. Save vomitus and aspirate for analysis.

ALERT *To prevent aspiration in the unconscious patient, an endotracheal tube should be in place before lavage.*

■ Monitor laboratory test results, such as electrolyte levels, blood urea nitrogen, and serum and urine osmolality for changes indicating fluid volume deficit or renal failure.

■ Anticipate the need for dialysis to aid in removal of the absorbed drug.

■ Institute safety precautions; reorient patient as necessary. Explain all procedures to the patient before performing them. Speak calmly and clearly to help alleviate his anxiety.

■ Provide opportunities for patient to voice his concerns. Assess patient's potential for self-harm or violence toward others. Institute suicide precautions as indicated. If necessary, apply restraints as ordered. Anticipate referral to mental health professional if the toxic ingestion was intentional.

Patient teaching

■ Explain about the effects of drug overdose and necessary treatments.
■ Ensure that the patient understands any prescribed drug therapy.
■ Caution patient about excessive use of OTC medications.

■ To prevent accidental poisoning, instruct the patient to read the label before he takes medication. Tell him to store all medications and household chemicals properly, keep them out of reach of children, and discard old medications. Warn him not to take medications prescribed for someone else, not to transfer medications from their original containers to other containers without labeling them properly, and never to transfer poisons to food containers.

■ Warn parents to avoid taking medication in front of their young children or calling medication "candy" to get children to take it. Urge the use of childproof caps.

■ Make sure the patient understands the importance of using toxic sprays only in well-ventilated areas and of following instructions carefully and that household chemicals should never be mixed as a harmful chemical reaction can occur.

MULTISYSTEM DISORDER

Graft-versus-host disease

Graft-versus-host disease (GVHD) can occur when an immunologically impaired recipient receives a graft from an immunocompetent donor. GVHD can be acute or chronic. *Acute GVHD* occurs within the first 100 days after a transplant. *Chronic GVHD* occurs after day 100 of a transplant and involves an autoimmune response that affects multiple organs. Older patients and those who have suffered previous acute GVHD face the greatest risk of chronic GVHD.

GVHD disease usually develops after a patient with impaired immune function — from congenital immunodeficiency, radiation treatment, or immunosuppressant therapy — receives a bone marrow transplantation from an incompatible donor. It also can occur following solid organ transplants, most commonly liver transplants. Additionally, GVHD may result from the transfusion of a blood product containing viable lymphocytes. This means that patients may develop GVHD during the transfusion of whole blood or transplant of fetal thymus, liver, or bone marrow. The risk of GVHD disease transmission also exists during maternal-fetal blood transfusions and intrauterine transfusions.

Fewer than one-half of recipients with histocompatibility identical to the donor develop GVHD. This incidence increases to greater than 60% when there's one antigen mismatch. Development of acute GVHD is a major contributing factor for mortality following bone marrow transplantation. Death with GVHD is commonly due to sepsis. Patients who develop chronic GVHD immediately following acute GVHD have the highest mortality rates.

Pathophysiology

Three criteria are necessary for the development of GVHD: immunologically competent cells in the graft; graft recognition of the host as foreign; and inability of the host to react to the graft. If donor and recipient cells aren't histocompatible, the foreign or graft cells may launch an attack against the host cells, which can't reject them. This process begins when graft cells become sensitized to the recipient's class II antigens. The exact mechanism by which this occurs remains unclear, although biopsy of active GVHD lesions usually reveals infiltration by mononuclear cells, eosinophils, and phagocytic and histiocytic cells.

Comprehensive assessment

Signs of acute GVHD include skin rash, severe diarrhea, and jaundice. Rash usually develops 10 to 30 days after transplant. It typically begins as a diffuse erythematous macular rash on the palms, soles, and scalp and may spread to the trunk and, possibly, the extremities. In severe GVHD, the rash can become desquamative. As the disease progresses, the erythematous macules may develop into papules. Abdominal cramps and, in severe cases, GI bleeding may accompany watery diarrhea. Jaundice results from the hyperbilirubinemia caused by inflammation of the small bile ducts.

Chronic GVHD is commonly manifested by skin changes that resemble scleroderma that can ultimately lead to ulcerations, joint contractures, and impaired esophageal motility.

Diagnosis

Although graft survival typically hinges on early detection of transplant rejection, no single test or combination of tests proves definitive. Tests reveal only nonspecific evidence, which may easily be attributed to other causes, especially infection. Diagnosis commonly becomes a matter of exclusion and depends on careful evaluation of signs and symptoms along with results from specific organ function tests, standard laboratory studies, and tissue biopsy.

Tissue biopsy provides the most accurate, reliable diagnostic information, especially in heart, liver, and kidney transplants. Biopsy usually reveals immunocompetent T cells along with the extent of lymphocytic infiltration and tissue damage.

Repeat biopsies help identify early histologic changes characteristic of rejection, determine the degree of change from previous biopsies, and monitor the course and success of treatment. Liver function studies reveal elevated levels of bilirubin, serum alkaline phosphatase, alanine aminotransferase, and aspartate aminotransferase.

Collaborations

GVHD a multisystem disorder that requires multidisciplinary care involving numerous members of the health care team. Transplant specialists along with hematologic, dermatologic, and gastroenterologic specialists may be necessary to aid in guiding treatment. Infection control personnel may be consulted to reduce the patient's risk for infection. Other disciplines, including neurologists and nephrologists, may be consulted for assistance depending on the involvement of the patient's organs and prognosis. The patient and his family could benefit from supportive counseling and a referral for social services.

Treatment and care

Because GVHD can be fatal, initial interventions must focus on prevention. Most patients receive immunosuppressant therapy with methotrexate, with or without prednisone, antithymocyte globulin, cyclosporine, cyclophosphamide, or tacrolimus for the first 3 to 12 months after a transplant. Other strategies to decrease the incidence of GVHD involve attempting to deplete donor marrow of T cells. This technique has been shown to reduce the severity and incidence of GVHD; however, patients have experienced an increase in graft failure and recurrent leukemia.

Once a diagnosis of GVHD is confirmed, immunosuppressive therapy continues along with the addition of methylprednisolone.

Complications

Complications associated with acute GVHD include:

■ sepsis
■ electrolyte imbalances secondary to diarrhea
■ liver dysfunction
■ hepatorenal syndrome.
    With chronic GVHD, complications may include:
■ joint contractures
■ skin atrophy and ulceration
■ esophageal strictures
■ lichen planus
■ widespread immune impairment.

Nursing considerations

■ Institute measures appropriate following bone marrow transplantation or organ transplant. (See "Bone marrow transplantation," page 512, and sections on specific organ transplantation in previous chapters.)
■ Inspect the patient's skin closely for development of skin erythema. Pay special attention to the soles and palms. Provide meticulous skin care if erythema occurs.
■ Assess the patient's skin color for evidence of jaundice, especially the sclera of the eyes. Report any darkened urine or clay-colored stools.

■ Monitor the patient's vital signs at least every 4 hours. Notify the physician of any temperature elevation.

■ Assess fluid balance status. Monitor intake and output frequently. Maintain hydration status with I.V. fluids as ordered. Anticipate the need for hemodynamic monitoring to assess the patient's status.

■ Administer immunosuppressive agents as ordered.

■ Monitor liver function study results closely for changes in enzyme levels.

■ Assess the patient's bowel elimination pattern and auscultate bowel sounds. Be alert for severe diarrhea.

ALERT *Be alert for the development of electrolyte and acid-base imbalances secondary to losses from diarrhea. Expect to administer fluid electrolyte replacement therapy based on laboratory results. Keep in mind that potassium is a major electrolyte that's lost with diarrhea; anticipate the need for continuous cardiac monitoring to detect possible arrhythmias secondary to hypokalemia.*

■ Obtain blood and stool cultures as ordered to evaluate for possible sources of infection.

■ Assess the patient for signs and symptoms of sepsis. (See "Septic shock," page 569.)

Patient teaching

■ Teach the patient about the disease course and its treatment.

■ Instruct the patient in the need for continued immunosuppressive therapy and ways to minimize exposure to infection.

■ Review danger signs and symptoms with the patient, emphasizing the need to notify the physician should any occur.

 MULTISYSTEM DISORDER

Human immunodeficiency virus infection

Human immunodeficiency virus (HIV) infection may cause acquired immunodeficiency syndrome (AIDS). Although it's characterized by gradual destruction of cell-mediated (T-cell) immunity, it also affects humoral immunity and even autoimmunity because of the central role of the CD4+ (helper) T lymphocyte in immune reactions. The resulting immunodeficiency makes the patient susceptible to opportunistic infections, cancers, and other abnormalities that define AIDS. Because transmission is similar, AIDS shares epidemiologic patterns with hepatitis B and sexually transmitted diseases.

AIDS is more prevalent in large urban areas with a high incidence of I.V. drug use and high-risk sexual practices.

AGE ISSUE *HIV is predominantly an infection in young people, with most cases involving those between ages 17 and 55. However, it has also been reported in elderly men and women. In the United States, AIDS is the leading cause of death among women ages 25 to 44.*

The incidence is increasing faster among women than men, and heterosexual transmission of HIV is the major mode of transmission. The majority of women with heterosexually transmitted HIV infection report having had sexual contact with an I.V. drug user, often during adolescence. An increase of AIDS in this childbearing age group is expected to cause an increase in the number of children with HIV infection.

The HIV-I retrovirus is the primary etiologic agent. Transmission occurs by contact with infected blood or body fluids and is associated with identifiable high-risk behaviors. It's disproportionately represented in:

■ homosexual and bisexual men
■ I.V. drug users
■ neonates of infected women
■ recipients of contaminated blood or blood products (dramatically decreased since mid-1985)
■ heterosexual partners of persons in the former groups.

Pathophysiology

The natural history of AIDS begins with infection by the HIV retrovirus, which is detectable only by laboratory tests, and ends with death. Twenty years of data strongly suggest that HIV isn't transmitted by casual household or social contact. The HIV virus may enter the body by any of several routes involving the transmission of blood or body fluids, for example:

■ direct inoculation during intimate sexual contact, especially associated with the mucosal trauma of receptive rectal intercourse
■ transfusion of contaminated blood or blood products (a risk diminished by routine testing of all blood products)
■ sharing contaminated needles
■ transplacental or postpartum transmission from infected mother to fetus (by cervical or blood contact at delivery and in breast milk).

HIV strikes helper T cells bearing the CD4+ antigen. Normally a receptor for major histocompatibility complex

molecules, the antigen serves as a receptor for the retrovirus and allows it to enter the cell. Viral binding also requires the presence of a co-receptor on the cell surface. The virus may also infect CD4+ antigen-bearing cells of the GI tract, uterine cervix, and neuroglia.

Like other retroviruses, HIV copies its genetic material in a reverse manner compared with other viruses and cells. Through the action of reverse transcriptase, HIV produces deoxyribonucleic acid (DNA) from its viral ribonucleic acid (RNA). Transcription is commonly poor, leading to mutations, and some such mutations make HIV resistant to antiviral drugs. The viral DNA enters the nucleus of the cell and is incorporated into the host cell's DNA, where it's transcribed into more viral RNA. If the host cell reproduces, it duplicates the HIV DNA along with its own and passes it on to the daughter cells. Thus, if activated, the host cell carries this information and, if activated, replicates the virus. Viral enzymes, proteases, arrange the structural components and RNA into viral particles that move out to the periphery of the host cell, where the virus buds and emerges from the host cell. Thus, the virus is now free to travel and infect other cells.

HIV replication may lead to cell death or it may become latent. HIV infection leads to profound pathology, either directly through destruction of CD4+ cells, other immune cells, and neuroglial cells, or indirectly through the secondary effects of CD4+ T-cell dysfunction and resulting immunosuppression.

The HIV infectious process takes three forms:

■ immunodeficiency (opportunistic infections and unusual cancers)

■ autoimmunity (lymphoid interstitial pneumonitis, arthritis, hypergammaglobulinemia, and production of autoimmune antibodies)

■ neurologic dysfunction (AIDS dementia complex, HIV encephalopathy, and peripheral neuropathies).

Comprehensive assessment

HIV infection manifests in many ways. After a high-risk exposure and inoculation, the infected person usually experiences a mononucleosis-like syndrome, which may be attributed to flu or another virus and then may remain asymptomatic for years. In this latent stage, the only sign of HIV infection is laboratory evidence of seroconversion.

When symptoms appear, they may take many forms, including:

■ persistent generalized lymphadenopathy secondary to impaired function of CD4+ cells

■ nonspecific symptoms, including weight loss, fatigue, night sweats, fevers related to altered function of CD4+ cells, immunodeficiency, and infection of other CD4+ antigen-bearing cells

■ neurologic symptoms resulting from HIV encephalopathy and infection of neuroglial cells

■ opportunistic infection or cancer related to immunodeficiency.

AGE ISSUE *In children, HIV infection has a mean incubation time of 17 months. Signs and symptoms resemble those in adults, except for findings related to sexually transmitted diseases. Children have a high incidence of opportunistic bacterial infections: otitis media, sepsis, chronic salivary gland enlargement, lymphoid interstitial pneumonia,* Mycobacterium avium–intracellulare *complex function, and pneumonias, including* Pneumocystis carinii.

Diagnosis

The Centers for Disease Control and Prevention (CDC) has developed an HIV/AIDS classification matrix that defines AIDS as an illness characterized by one or more indicator diseases, coexisting with laboratory evidence of HIV infection and other possible causes of immunosuppression. Diagnosis of AIDS includes one or more of the following:

■ confirmed presence of HIV infection

■ CD4+ T-cell count of less than 200 cells/ml

■ the presence of one or more conditions specified by the CDC as Categories A, B, or C. (See *Conditions associated with AIDS,* page 548.)

Antibody tests, the most commonly performed tests, indicate HIV infection indirectly by revealing HIV antibodies (initial screening with an enzyme-linked immunosorbent assay [ELISA]; if positive, ELISA is repeated, and then confirmed by an alternative method, usually the Western blot or an immunofluorescence assay).

Additional tests to support the diagnosis help evaluate the severity of immunosuppression, including CD4+ and CD8+ T-lymphocyte subset counts, erythrocyte sedimentation rate, complete blood count, anergy testing, and serum beta$_2$-microglobulin, p24 antigen, and neopterin levels. Because many opportunistic infections in AIDS patients are reactivations of previous infections, patients are also tested for syphilis, hepatitis B, tuberculosis, tox-

Conditions associated with AIDS

The Centers for Disease Control and Prevention (CDC) lists diseases associated with acquired immunodeficiency syndrome (AIDS) under three categories. From time to time, the CDC adds to these lists.

Category A
- Persistent generalized lymph node enlargement
- Acute primary human immunodeficiency virus (HIV) infection with accompanying illness
- History of acute HIV infection

Category B
- Bacillary angiomatosis
- Oropharyngeal or persistent vulvovaginal candidiasis, fever or diarrhea lasting longer than 1 month
- Idiopathic thrombocytopenic purpura
- Pelvic inflammatory disease, especially with a tubulo-ovarian abscess
- Peripheral neuropathy

Category C
- Candidiasis of the bronchi, trachea, lungs, or esophagus
- Invasive cervical cancer
- Disseminated or extrapulmonary coccidiomycosis
- Extrapulmonary cryptococcosis
- Chronic interstitial cryptosporidiosis
- Cytomegalovirus (CMV) disease affecting organs other than the liver, spleen, or lymph nodes
- CMV retinitis with vision loss
- Encephalopathy related to HIV
- Herpes simplex infection with chronic ulcers or herpetic bronchitis, pneumonitis, or esophagitis
- Disseminated or extrapulmonary histoplasmosis
- Chronic intestinal isopsoriasis
- Kaposi's sarcoma
- Burkitt's lymphoma or its equivalent
- Immunoblastic lymphoma or its equivalent
- Primary brain lymphoma
- Disseminated or extrapulmonary *Mycobacterium avium-intracellulare* complex or *M. kansasii*
- Pulmonary or extrapulmonary *M. tuberculosis*
- Disseminated or extrapulmonary infection with any other species of *Mycobacterium*
- *Pneumocystis carinii pneumoniae*
- Recurrent pneumonia
- Progressive multifocal leukoencephalopathy
- Recurrent *Salmonella* septicemia
- Toxoplasmosis of the brain
- Wasting syndrome caused by HIV

oplasmosis and, in some areas, histoplasmosis.

Collaborations

The patient requires the skill of an immunologist specializing in HIV disease. He may also need the assistance of pulmonary specialists, if his respiratory system is compromised, and nutritional therapy to optimize his condition. There are support groups available to the patient and his family to help meet his needs, and spiritual counseling is also an option. Home health care agencies and social services can also meet specific care needs regarding his condition.

Treatment and care

No cure has yet been found for AIDS. Primary therapy includes the use of various combinations of three different types of antiretroviral agents to try to gain the maximum benefit of inhibiting HIV viral replication with the fewest adverse reactions. Current recommendations include the use of two nucleosides plus one protease inhibitor, or two nucleosides and one non-nucleoside to help inhibit the production of resistant, mutant strains. The drugs include:

■ protease inhibitors to block replication of virus particle formed through the action of viral protease (reducing the number of new virus particles produced)

■ nucleoside reverse-transcriptase inhibitors to interfere with the copying of viral RNA into DNA by the enzyme reverse transcriptase

■ nonnucleoside reverse-transcriptase inhibitors to interfere with the action of reverse transcriptase.

Additional treatment may include:

■ immunomodulatory agents to boost the immune system weakened by AIDS and retroviral therapy

■ human granulocyte colony-stimulating growth factor to stimulate neutrophil production (retroviral therapy causes anemia, so patients may receive epoetin alfa)

■ anti-infective and antineoplastic agents to combat opportunistic infections and associated cancers (some prophylactically to help resist opportunistic infections)

■ supportive therapy, including nutritional support, fluid and electrolyte replacement therapy, pain relief, and psychological support.

Complications

Complications of AIDS include repeated, opportunistic infections. (See *Opportunistic infections in AIDS,* page 550.)

Nursing considerations

■ Adhere to standard precautions at all times. Anticipate the need for transmission based precautions if patient develops other infection.

■ Assess cardiopulmonary status frequently — at least every 2 to 4 hours — including heart and lung sounds. Report any cough, sore throat or adventitious sounds that might suggest a respiratory infection such as pneumonia. Monitor oxygen saturation via pulse oximetry and arterial blood gases. Administer supplemental oxygen as indicated and ordered.

ALERT *Be alert for changes in the patient's respiratory status. Anticipate the need for airway insertion or endotracheal intubation and mechanical ventilation if the patient's respiratory status deteriorates. Encourage coughing and deep breathing and incentive spirometry every 2 hours.*

■ Assess vital signs every 2 to 4 hours, or more frequently, if indicated. Report any evidence of fever. Administer antipyretics and employ cooling measures as ordered.

■ Monitor hemodynamic status for changes. If indicated, assist with insertion of central venous or pulmonary artery catheter for monitoring.

■ Assess the patient's neurologic status frequently — at least every 4 hours — including level of consciousness, pupillary response, and reflexes. Reorient patient as necessary. Report any changes suggesting a decrease in neurologic function.

■ Auscultate bowel sounds and monitor abdomen for distention.

■ Administer I.V. fluid therapy as ordered. Monitor intake and output closely. Report urine output less than 30 ml/hour.

Opportunistic infections in AIDS

This chart shows the complicating infections that may occur in acquired immunodeficiency syndrome (AIDS).

Microbiological agent	Organism	Condition
Protozoa	*Pneumocystis carinii*	Pneumocystosis
	Cryptosporidium	Cryptosporidiosis
	Toxoplasma gondii	Toxoplasmosis
	Histoplasma	Histoplasmosis
Fungi	*Candida albicans*	Candidiasis
	Cryptococcus neoformans	Cryptococcosis
Viruses	Herpes	Herpes simplex 1 and 2
	Cytomegalovirus (CMV)	CMV retinitis
Bacteria	*Mycobacterium tuberculosis*	Tuberculosis
	M. avium	*M. avium* complex

Note: Other opportunistic conditions include Kaposi's sarcoma, wasting syndrome, and AIDS dementia complex.

■ Assess nutritional status, including hydration. Check skin turgor and mucous membranes. Obtain daily weights. Offer small frequent meals with increased fluids as appropriate. Monitor calorie counts as ordered. Anticipate the need for enteral or parenteral nutrition if the patient can't tolerate oral feedings.

■ Use strict sterile technique when providing care to catheter insertion and other invasive monitoring sites. Monitor sites for erythema, swelling, or drainage and report immediately.

■ Monitor for signs and symptoms of opportunistic infections or signs of disease progression, and treat infections as ordered.

■ Provide meticulous skin care especially if the patient is severely debilitated or is experiencing diarrhea. Turn the patient every 2 hours.

ALERT *If the patient experiences diarrhea, be sure to include stool as part of the patient's output. In addition, monitor laboratory test results and be alert for signs and symptoms of possible acid-base and electrolyte imbalances such as hyponatremia, hypokalemia, and metabolic acidosis that may result from prolonged or profuse diarrhea. If electrolyte imbalances are present, anticipate continuous car-*

diac monitoring to evaluate for possible arrhythmias that may result from these imbalances.

■ Recognize that a diagnosis of AIDS is profoundly distressing because of the disease's social impact and the discouraging prognosis. Offer support to the patient and significant others. Assist with referral to social service as ordered.

■ Encourage the patient to maintain as much physical activity as he can tolerate. Ensure time for adequate rest periods. Arrange for physical therapy as ordered to assist with energy conservation and exercises.

Patient teaching

■ Teach the patient about medication regimen and need for compliance, which, if lacking, may lead to resistance and treatment failure.

■ Urge the patient to inform potential sexual partners and health care workers that he has HIV infection.

■ Teach the patient how to identify the signs of impending infection, and stress the importance of reporting these signs immediately.

 MULTISYSTEM DISORDER

Hyperthermia

Hyperthermia refers to an elevation in body temperature over 99° F (37.2° C). Normally, humans adjust to excessive temperatures through complex cardiovascular and neurologic changes, which are coordinated by the hypothalamus. Heat loss offsets heat production to regulate the body temperature. It does this by evaporation (of sweat) or vasodilation, which cools the body's surface by radiation, conduction, and convection.

Sometimes, environmental and internal factors can increase heat production or decrease heat loss beyond the body's ability to compensate. When this happens, hyperthermia, also known as *heat syndrome,* results. There are three categories of heat syndrome: heat cramps, heat exhaustion, and heatstroke.

Pathophysiology

Heat syndrome may result from conditions that increase heat production, such as excessive exercise, infection, and drugs (for example, amphetamines). It also can stem from factors that impair heat dissipation. These include high temperatures or humidity, lack of acclimatization, excess clothing, cardiovascular disease, obesity, dehydration, sweat gland dysfunction, and drugs, such as phenothiazines and anticholinergics.

■ **AGE ISSUE** *Heatstroke is commonly seen in elderly people during excessively hot summer days, particularly when they're inside with windows and doors closed and have no air conditioning. They might not open windows and doors because they're afraid someone may break in and injure them.*

If the body temperature remains elevated, fluid loss becomes excessive leading to hypovolemic shock. If untreated, the patient's thermoregulatory mechanisms can fail.

Comprehensive assessment

Assessment findings vary with the degree of hyperthermia or type of heat syndrome. (See *Understanding heat syndrome,* page 552.)

Understanding heat syndrome

Hyperthermia, also known as *heat syndrome,* may be classified as mild (heat cramps), moderate (heat exhaustion), or critical (heat stroke). This table highlights the major assessment findings associated with each classification.

Classification	Assessment findings
Mild hyperthermia (heat cramps)	• Mild agitation; central nervous system findings otherwise normal • Mild hypertension • Moist, cool skin and muscle tenderness; involved muscle groups possibly hard and lumpy • Muscle twitching and spasms • Nausea, abdominal cramps • Report of prolonged activity in a very warm or hot environment, without adequate salt intake • Tachycardia • Temperature ranging from 99° to 102° F (37.2° to 38.9° C)
Moderate hyperthermia (heat exhaustion)	• Dizziness • Headache • Hypotension • Muscle cramping • Nausea, vomiting • Oliguria • Pale, moist skin • Rapid thready pulse • Syncope or confusion • Temperature elevated up to 104° F (40° C) • Thirst • Weakness
Critical hyperthermia (heat stroke)	• Atrial or ventricular tachycardia • Confusion, combativeness, delirium • Fixed, dilated pupils • Hypertension followed by hypotension • Hot, dry, reddened skin • Loss of consciousness • Seizures • Tachypnea • Temperature greater than 106° F (41.1° C)

Diagnosis

Several diagnostic tests can help to confirm the diagnosis:

■ Serum electrolyte levels may reveal hyponatremia, hypokalemia, hypocalcemia, and hypophosphatemia.

■ Arterial blood gas (ABG) studies may reveal respiratory alkalosis.

■ Blood studies reveal leukocytosis, elevated blood urea nitrogen levels, hemoconcentration, thrombocytopenia, increased bleeding and clotting times, fibrinolysis, and consumption coagulopathy.

■ Urinalysis results show concentrated urine, with elevated protein levels, tubular casts, and myoglobinuria.

Collaborations

A multidisciplinary approach to care is crucial. Depending upon the severity of the condition, other specialists may need to be consulted. If the patient requires mechanical ventilation, respiratory therapy and a pulmonary specialist may be needed. If an underlying neurologic condition is involved, a neurosurgeon may be consulted.

Treatment and care

For mild hyperthermia (heat cramps), treatment consists of moving the patient to a cool environment, providing rest, and administering oral or I.V. fluid and electrolyte replacement. Salt tablets aren't recommended because the body absorbs them slowly when compared with other methods.

Treatment for moderate hyperthermia (heat exhaustion) involves moving the patient to a cool environment, providing rest, and administering oral fluid and electrolyte replacement. If I.V. fluid replacement is necessary, laboratory test results determine the choice of I.V. solution — usually saline or isotonic glucose solution.

Treatment for critical hyperthermia (heatstroke) focuses on lowering the body temperature as rapidly as possible. The patient's clothing is removed, and cool water is applied to the skin, followed by fanning with cool air. Shivering is controlled with diazepam or chlorpromazine. Application of hypothermia blankets and ice packs to the groin and axillae also helps lower

body temperature. Treatment continues until the body temperature drops to 102.2° F (39° C). Supportive measures include oxygen therapy, central venous pressure and pulmonary artery wedge pressure monitoring and, if necessary, endotracheal intubation. Observe the patient closely for complications.

Complications

Heatstroke, a medical emergency, can lead to hypovolemic or cardiogenic shock, cardiac arrhythmias, and renal failure caused by rhabdomyolysis, disseminated intravascular coagulation, and hepatic failure.

Nursing considerations

■ Assess the patient's airway, breathing, and circulation and initiate emergency resuscitative measures as indicated. Remove as much of the patient's clothing as possible.

■ Assess oxygenation status via pulse oximetry and ABG studies; administer supplemental oxygen as indicated and ordered. Monitor the patient's pulmonary status closely, including respiratory rate and depth and lung sounds; anticipate the need for endotracheal intubation and mechanical ventilation if respiratory status deteriorates.

■ Monitor vital signs continuously, especially core body temperature.

ALERT *Although the goal is to reduce the patient's temperature rapidly, too rapid a reduction can lead to vasoconstriction, which can cause shivering.*

■ Assess cardiac status closely, including heart rate and rhythm. Institute continuous cardiac monitoring to evaluate for arrhythmias secondary to electrolyte imbalances.

■ Monitor peripheral circulation, including skin color, peripheral pulses, and capillary refill.

■ Assess neurologic status for changes.

■ Assist with insertion of central venous or pulmonary artery catheter to assess patient's hemodynamic status.

■ Place the patient in a cool environment (approximately 70° F [21° C]). Apply tepid water to the patient's skin and allow cool air, such as that generated by fans, to blow over him to aid in evaporative heat loss.

■ Monitor the patient for shivering.

ALERT *Shivering increases metabolic demand and oxygen consumption and should be avoided. Observe the patient for jaw muscle tightening or clenching, an early indicator of shivering. Monitor electrocardiogram waveform for an artifact that may be associated with a muscle tremor suggesting shivering.*

■ Employ external cooling measures, such as cool wet sheets, tepid baths, and cooling blankets.

ALERT *When using a cooling blanket, be sure to precool the blanket if possible before applying it to the patient. Use only a single blanket to absorb the patient's perspiration. Turn the patient every 2 hours, making sure that the blanket stays in contact with the patient at all times. If the patient's temperature remains elevated, apply ice packs to the axillae and groin to aid in cooling.*

■ Expect to discontinue the cooling blanket when the patient's temperature reaches 102.2° F (39° C) to prevent overcooling even with the blanket turned off.

■ If the patient's temperature remains elevated, anticipate the use of internal cooling methods such as iced saline lavage, or cool saline bladder or rectal irrigations as ordered.

■ Monitor laboratory test results including serum electrolyte levels and ABG levels for changes. Assess renal function studies to evaluate for possible rhabdomyolysis.

■ If the patient is alert and the gag reflex is intact offer oral fluids. Supply additional I.V. fluids as ordered.

Patient teaching

■ Explain the disease course and treatments to the patient and his family.

■ Teach patient and his family about preventative measures, including avoiding strenuous activity with excessive heat and need for adequate fluid replacement.

■ Instruct patient and his family in danger signs and symptoms.

⭐ **MULTISYSTEM DISORDER**

Hypothermia

Hypothermia — core body temperature below 95° F (35° C) — affects chemical changes in the body. It may be classified as mild (89.6° to 95° F [32° to 35° C]), moderate (86° to 89.6° F [30° to 32° C]), or severe (77° to 86° F [25° to 30° C]). Hypothermia commonly results from cold-water near drowning and prolonged exposure to cold temperatures. It also can occur in normal temperatures if disease or debility alters the patient's homeostasis. The administration of large amounts of cold blood or blood products can cause hypothermia.

Severe hypothermia can be fatal. The risk of serious cold injury, especially hypothermia, increases with youth, old age, lack of insulating body fat, wet or inadequate clothing, drug abuse, cardiac disease, smoking, fatigue, malnutrition and depletion of caloric reserves, and excessive alcohol intake.

Pathophysiology

In hypothermia, metabolic changes slow the functions of most major organ systems, resulting in decreased renal blood flow and decreased glomerular filtration, for example.

Hypothermia has a physiologic effect on vital organs. Severe hypothermia results in depression of cerebral blood flow, diminished oxygen requirements, reduced cardiac output, and decreased arterial pressure.

Comprehensive assessment

The history of a patient with a cold injury reveals the cause, the temperature to which the patient was exposed, and the length of exposure.

Assessment findings in a patient with hypothermia vary with the patient's body temperature. A patient with mild hypothermia shows severe shivering, slurred speech, and amnesia. A patient with moderate hypothermia is unresponsive, with peripheral cyanosis and muscle rigidity. If the patient was improperly rewarmed, he may show signs of shock.

ALERT *If a patient has hypothermia, use an esophageal or rectal probe that reads as low as 77° F (25° C) to determine an accurate core body temperature. Core body temperature also can be determined using a pulmonary artery catheter.*

A patient with severe hypothermia appears dead, with no palpable pulse and no audible heart sounds. His pupils may be dilated, and he may appear to be in a state of rigor mortis. Ventricular fibrillation and a loss of deep tendon reflexes commonly occur. A patient with a body temperature below is at risk for cardiopulmonary arrest.

Diagnosis

■ Technetium-99m pertechnetate scanning shows perfusion defects and deep tissue damage and can be used to identify nonviable bone.
■ Doppler and plethysmographic studies help determine pulses and the extent of frostbite after thawing.

Essential laboratory tests during treatment of moderate or severe hypothermia include a complete blood count, coagulation profile, urinalysis, and serum amylase, electrolyte, hemoglobin, glucose, liver enzyme, blood urea nitrogen, creatinine, and arterial blood gas levels.

Collaborations

Because hypothermia is a multisystem problem, a multidisciplinary approach to care is needed. Depending upon the severity of the patient's condition, the patient may require the services of a pulmonary specialist (for mechanical ventilation), neurosurgeon (if he remains obtunded when rewarmed), or a cardiologist (for cardiac involvement).

Treatment and care

Treatment for hypothermia consists of supportive measures and specific rewarming techniques, including:
■ passive rewarming (the patient rewarms on his own)

■ active external rewarming with heating blankets, warm water immersion, heated objects such as water bottles, and radiant heat
■ active core rewarming with heated I.V. fluids, genitourinary tract irrigation, extracorporeal rewarming, hemodialysis, and peritoneal, gastric, and mediastinal lavage.

Any arrhythmias that develop usually convert to normal sinus rhythm with rewarming. If the patient has no pulse or respirations, cardiopulmonary resuscitation (CPR) is needed until rewarming raises the core temperature to at least 89.6° F (32° C).

Administration of oxygen, endotracheal intubation, controlled ventilation, I.V. fluids, and treatment of metabolic acidosis depend on test results and careful patient monitoring.

Complications
Common complications associated with hypothermia include severe infection, aspiration pneumonia, cardiac arrhythmias, hypoglycemia or hyperglycemia, metabolic acidosis, pancreatitis, and renal failure.

Nursing considerations
■ Assess airway, breathing, and circulation. Follow hypothermia algorithm. (See *Treating hypothermia*.)

ALERT *Keep in mind that drug metabolism is decreased, necessitating longer than usual intervals between dosing of I.V. medications. In addition, as the patient is rewarmed, be alert for a boluslike effect that can occur with medications due to vasodilation that occurs during rewarming.*

■ Continue CPR until the patient's core body temperature increases to at least 89.6° F (32° C).

ALERT *Keep in mind that hypothermia helps protect the brain from anoxia, which normally accompanies prolonged cardiopulmonary arrest. So even if the patient has been unresponsive for a long time, CPR may resuscitate him, especially after a cold-water near drowning.*

■ Assist with rewarming techniques as necessary. In moderate to severe hypothermia, only experienced personnel should attempt aggressive rewarming.
■ During rewarming, provide supportive measures as ordered, including mechanical ventilation and heated, humidified therapy to maintain tissue oxygenation, and I.V. fluids that have been warmed with a warming coil to correct hypotension and maintain urine output.
■ Insert an indwelling urinary catheter and assess urine output hourly.
■ Continuously monitor the patient's core body temperature and other vital signs during and after initial rewarming. Continuously monitor his cardiac status, including continuous cardiac monitoring for evidence of arrhythmias.
■ If the patient's core temperature is below 89.6° F, use internal and external warming methods to raise the patient's body core and surface temperatures 1° to 2° F (0.6° to 1.1° C) per hour. (See *Rewarming methods*, page 558.)
■ If the patient's temperature is 86° to 93° F (30° to 33.9° C), limit active rewarming to the neck, axilla, or groin areas. Using these techniques in peripheral areas can contribute to a continued drop in core temperature as cold blood from the periphery is mobilized.

Treating hypothermia

Assess responsiveness, breathing, and pulse.

Pulse and breathing present | Pulse or breathing absent

If the patient's core temperature is 93.2° to 96.8° F (34° to 36° C), initiate passive rewarming and active external rewarming.

- Initiate cardiopulmonary resuscitation (CPR).
- Defibrillate ventricular fibrillation (VF) or pulseless ventricular tachycardia (VT) with up to a maximum of three shocks.
- Secure the patient's airway.
- Ventilate with warm, humidified oxygen (108° to 115° F).
- Establish I.V. access, and infuse warm normal saline solution (110° F).

If the patient's core temperature is 86° to 93° F (30° to 38.9° C), initiate passive rewarming and active external rewarming of truncal areas only.

If the patient's core temperature is less than 86° F, continue CPR, and withhold I.V. medications.

If the patient's core temperature is greater than 86° F but less than 95° F, continue CPR, administer I.V. medications spaced at longer-than-standard ACLS intervals, and repeat defibrillation for VF or VT as core temperature rises.

If the patient's core temperature is less than 86° F, initiate active internal rewarming by warming I.V. fluids (110° F [43.3° C]); administering warm, humidified oxygen (108° to 115° F [42.2° to 46.1° C]); performing peritoneal lavage; using extracorporeal rewarming; and inserting esophageal rewarming tubes.

Continue internal rewarming until core temperature is higher than 95° F (35° C) or spontaneous circulation returns or resuscitative efforts cease.

Rewarming methods

Passive and active methods may be used to rewarm a patient. Active methods may be external or internal; passive methods are external only.

Passive rewarming methods
- Use of a warm environment
- Application of warmed blankets

Active external rewarming methods
- Forced hot air
- Warm baths
- Warm packs
- Hypothermia blanket

Active internal rewarming methods
- Humidified oxygen warmed to a temperature between 108° to 115° F (42.2° to 46.1° C)
- Centrally administered I.V. fluids warmed to 110° F (43.3° C) at a rate of 150 to 200 ml/hour
- Peritoneal lavage using potassium-free solution (2 L at a time) warmed to 100° F (37.8° C)
- Pleural lavage using warmed normal saline instilled into the patient's chest tube
- Extracorporeal blood warming with partial bypass

ALERT *Be sure to rewarm the patient internally and externally at the same time; rewarming the surface first could cause rewarming shock with potentially fatal ventricular fibrillation.*

■ If using a hyperthermia blanket, discontinue the warming when the core body temperature is within 1° to 2° F (0.6° to 1.1° C) of the desired temperature. The patient's temperature will continue to rise even with the device turned off.

■ If the patient has been hypothermic for longer than 45 to 60 minutes, administer additional fluids as ordered to compensate for the expansion of the vascular space that occurs during vasodilation in rewarming. Monitor the patient's heart rate and hemodynamic parameters closely to evaluate fluid needs and response to treatment.

■ Monitor serum electrolyte levels closely, especially potassium. Be alert for signs and symptoms of hyperkalemia. If hyperkalemia occurs, administer calcium chloride, sodium bicarbonate, glucose and insulin as ordered. Anticipate the need for sodium polystyrene sulfonate enemas. If potassium levels are extremely elevated, prepare the patient for dialysis or exchange transfusion.

■ Offer warm oral fluids if the patient is alert and has an intact gag reflex. Otherwise, administer warmed I.V. fluids.

Patient teaching

■ Explain the disease course and treatments to the patient and his family.

■ Reinforce measures to prevent hypothermia.

 MULTISYSTEM DISORDER

Hypovolemic shock

Hypovolemic shock most commonly results from acute blood loss — about 20% of total volume. Massive blood loss may result from GI bleeding, internal or external hemorrhage, or any condition that reduces circulating intravascular volume or other body fluids. Other causes include intestinal obstruction, peritonitis, acute pancreatitis, ascites and dehydration from excessive perspiration, severe diarrhea or protracted vomiting, diabetes insipidus, diuresis, and inadequate fluid intake. Without sufficient blood or fluid replacement, hypovolemic shock may lead to irreversible damage to organs and systems.

Pathophysiology

Potentially life-threatening, hypovolemic shock stems from reduced intravascular blood volume, which leads to decreased cardiac output (CO) and inadequate tissue perfusion. The subsequent tissue anoxia prompts a shift in cellular metabolism from aerobic to anaerobic pathways. This results in an accumulation of lactic acid, which produces metabolic acidosis.

When compensatory mechanisms fail, hypovolemic shock occurs in the following sequence:
- decreased intravascular fluid volume
- diminished venous return, which reduces preload and decreases stroke volume
- reduced CO
- decreased mean arterial pressure
- impaired tissue perfusion
- decreased oxygen and nutrient delivery to cells
- multisystem organ failure.

Comprehensive assessment

The specific signs and symptoms exhibited by the patient depend on the amount of fluid loss. (See *Estimating fluid loss*.)

Typically, the patient's history will include conditions that reduce blood

Estimating fluid loss

The following assessment parameters indicate the severity of fluid loss.

Minimal fluid loss
Intravascular volume loss of 10% to 15% is regarded as minimal. Signs and symptoms include:
- slight tachycardia
- normal supine blood pressure
- positive postural vital signs, including a decrease in systolic blood pressure > 10 mm Hg or an increase in pulse rate > 20 beats/minute
- increased capillary refill time > 3 seconds
- urine output > 30 ml/hour
- cool, pale skin on arms and legs
- anxiety.

Moderate fluid loss
Intravascular volume loss of about 25% is regarded as moderate. Signs and symptoms include:
- rapid, thready pulse
- supine hypotension
- cool truncal skin
- urine output 10 to 30 ml/hour
- severe thirst
- restlessness, confusion, or irritability.

Severe fluid loss
Intravascular volume loss of 40% or more is regarded as severe. Signs and symptoms include:
- marked tachycardia
- marked hypotension
- weak or absent peripheral pulses
- cold, mottled, or cyanotic skin
- urine output < 10 ml/hour
- unconsciousness.

volume, such as GI hemorrhage, trauma, and severe diarrhea and vomiting. A patient with cardiac disease may report anginal pain.

Inspection may reveal pale skin, decreased sensorium, and rapid, shallow respirations. Urine output usually falls below 25 ml/hour. Palpation may disclose rapid, thready peripheral pulses and cold, clammy skin.

Auscultation of blood pressure usually detects a mean arterial pressure below 60 mm Hg and a narrowing pulse pressure. In patients with chronic hypotension, the mean pressure may fall below 50 mm Hg before signs of shock appear. Orthostatic vital signs and the tilt test may also detect shock. Central venous pressure (CVP), right atrial pressure, pulmonary artery wedge pressure (PAWP), and CO will all be decreased.

AGE ISSUE *Suspect hypovolemia in the infant or child who has a capillary return greater than 2 seconds and accompanying history and signs of hypovolemic shock (such as tachycardia, altered level of consciousness [LOC], pale skin, lack of tears, and depressed fontanels).*

Diagnosis
No single diagnostic test confirms the hypovolemic shock, but the following tests help to support the diagnosis:
■ low hematocrit and decreased hemoglobin level and red blood cell and platelet counts
■ elevated serum potassium, sodium, lactate dehydrogenase, creatinine, and blood urea nitrogen levels
■ increased urine specific gravity (greater than 1.020) and urine osmolality; urine sodium levels less than 50 mEq/L
■ decreased urine creatinine levels
■ decreased pH and partial pressure of arterial oxygen and increased partial pressure of arterial carbon dioxide

■ gastroscopy, X-rays, aspiration of gastric contents through a nasogastric tube, and tests for occult blood
■ coagulation studies for coagulopathy from disseminated intravascular coagulation (DIC).

Collaborations
Hypovolemic shock is a multisystem problem that requires a multidisciplinary approach to care. Medical and nursing care focus on maintaining all body functions. Specialists may become involved in the patient's case, depending on the cause of the hypovolemic shock. For example, a cardiologist may manage problems associated with an underlying cardiac problem or one that develops from hypovolemic shock or its treatment. A GI specialist or internist may manage problems relating to the GI tract. Respiratory therapy may be involved to assist with measures to ensure a patent airway and improve respiratory functioning. Nutritional support is indicated to assist ensuring adequate nutrients for maximum tissue healing. Physical therapy may be involved to help minimize the risks of bed rest. Surgical intervention may be necessary to the underlying problem, such as repairing a bleeding source or treating the reason for peritonitis as the cause of hypovolemic shock. Social services may be involved to assist with emotional support for the patient and his family and follow-up care issues.

Treatment and care
Emergency treatment relies on prompt and adequate fluid and blood replacement to restore intravascular volume and to raise blood pressure and maintain it above 60 mm Hg. Rapid infu-

sion of normal saline or lactated Ringer's solution and, possibly, albumin or other plasma expanders may expand volume adequately until whole blood can be matched.

AGE ISSUE *Fluid replacement for an infant and a child is generally crystalloid at a volume of 20 ml/kg of body weight for a fluid bolus. This bolus may be repeated for a total of three times while monitoring capillary refill as response.*

Treatment may also include application of a pneumatic antishock garment (although controversial), oxygen administration, control of bleeding, dopamine or another inotropic drug and, possibly, surgery. To be effective, dopamine or other inotropic drugs must be used with vigorous fluid replacement.

Complications

Without immediate treatment, hypovolemic shock can cause adult respiratory distress syndrome, acute tubular necrosis and renal failure, DIC, multisystem organ failure, and death.

Nursing considerations

■ Assess the patient for the extent of fluid loss and begin fluid replacement as ordered. Obtain a type and crossmatch for blood component therapy.

ALERT *If hypovolemic shock is caused by massive bleeding, lactated Ringer's solution is preferred for fluid volume replacement because its use minimizes the risk of electrolyte imbalances.*

■ Assess airway, breathing, and circulation. If the patient experiences cardiac or respiratory arrest, start cardiopulmonary resuscitation.

■ Administer supplemental oxygen as ordered. Monitor oxygen saturation via continuous pulse oximetry and serial arterial blood gas studies for evidence of hypoxemia and anticipate the need for endotracheal intubation and mechanical ventilation should the patient's respiratory status deteriorate. Place the patient in semi-Fowler's position to maximize chest expansion. Keep the patient as quiet and comfortable as possible to minimize oxygen demands.

■ Monitor vital signs continuously for changes. Observe skin color and check capillary refill. Notify the physician if capillary refill is greater than 2 seconds.

ALERT *If the patient's systolic blood pressure drops below 80 mm Hg, increase the oxygen flow rate and notify the physician immediately because systolic blood pressure below 80 mm Hg usually results in inadequate coronary artery blood flow, cardiac ischemia, arrhythmias, and further complications of low CO. Alert the physician and increase the infusion rate if the patient experiences a progressive drop in blood pressure accompanied by a thready pulse. This usually signals inadequate CO from reduced intravascular volume.*

■ Assist with insert of central venous or pulmonary artery catheter to evaluate hemodynamic status. Monitor hemodynamic parameters, including CVP, PAWP, and CO and input, frequently — as often as every 15 minutes — to evaluate the patient's status and response to treatment.

■ Institute continuous cardiac monitoring to evaluate for possible arrhythmias, myocardial ischemia, or adverse effects of treatment.

■ Assess LOC frequently — approximately every 30 minutes until the patient stabilizes, and then every 2 to 4 hours, as indicated by the patient's status.

■ Monitor intake and output closely. Insert an indwelling urinary catheter and assess urine output hourly. If bleeding from the GI tract is suspected as the cause, check all stools, emesis, and gastric drainage for occult blood. If output falls below 30 ml/hour in an adult, expect to increase the I.V. fluid infusion rate, but watch for signs of fluid overload such as elevated PAWP. Notify the physician if urine output doesn't increase.

■ Administer blood component therapy as ordered; monitor serial hemoglobin values and hematocrit to evaluate effects of treatment.

■ Administer dopamine or norepinephrine I.V., as ordered, to increase cardiac contractility and renal perfusion.

■ During therapy, assess skin color and temperature and note any changes.

ALERT *Cold, clammy skin may signal continuing peripheral vascular constriction, indicating progressive shock. Notify the physician at once.*

■ Watch for signs of impending coagulopathy (such as petechiae, bruising, bleeding or oozing from gums or venipuncture sites) and report them immediately.

■ Provide emotional support and reassurance appropriately in the wake of massive fluid losses.

■ Prepare the patient for surgery as appropriate.

Patient teaching

■ Review disease course with the patient and his family, including treatments and medications ordered and their intended effects, dosage, and adverse effects to report. Answer questions honestly and provide information as needed.

■ Explain the risks associated with transfusions if they're to be used.

■ Provide preoperative teaching as indicated.

 MULTISYSTEM DISORDER

Near drowning

In near drowning, the victim survives (at least temporarily) the physiologic effects of submersion in fluid. Hypoxemia and acidosis are the primary problems in victims of near drowning.

Near drowning typically results from an inability to swim. In swimmers, it can result from panic, a boating accident, sudden acute illness (seizure or myocardial infarction) or a blow to the head while in the water, venomous stings from aquatic animals, excessive alcohol consumption before swimming, a suicide attempt, or decompression sickness from deep-water diving.

Pathophysiology

Near drowning occurs in three forms. In *dry* near drowning, the victim doesn't aspirate fluid but suffers respiratory obstruction or asphyxia (10% to 15% of patients). In *wet* near drowning, the victim aspirates fluid and suffers from asphyxia or secondary changes from fluid aspiration (about 85% of patients). In *secondary* near drowning, the victim suffers recurrence of respiratory distress (usually aspiration pneumonia or pulmonary edema) within minutes or 1 to 2 days after a near-drowning incident.

Regardless of the tonicity of the fluid aspirated, hypoxemia is the most serious consequence of near drowning, followed by metabolic acidosis. Other consequences depend on the kind of water aspirated. After freshwater aspiration, changes in the character of lung surfactant result in exudation of protein-rich plasma into the alveoli. This, plus increased capillary permeability, leads to pulmonary edema and hypoxemia.

After saltwater aspiration, the hypertonicity of seawater exerts an osmotic force, which pulls fluid from pulmonary capillaries into the alveoli. The resulting intrapulmonary shunt causes hypoxemia. The pulmonary capillary membrane may be injured and may induce pulmonary edema. In wet and secondary near drownings, pulmonary edema and hypoxemia occur secondary to aspiration.

Regardless of the type of near drowning (freshwater or saltwater), aspiration of contaminants can occur. The victim may aspirate chlorine, mud, algae, weeds, and other foreign material. Saltwater aspiration is considered more dangerous because saltwater contains more types of disease-causing bacteria. These contaminants may lead to obstruction, aspiration pneumonia, and pulmonary fibrosis.

A protective effect may be seen in cold water submersion (exposure to temperatures 69.8° F [21° C]). Rapid body cooling results in cardiac arrest and decreased tissue oxygen demand. The protective effect is most pronounced in children and may be due to the large ration of body surface area to mass. Because water rapidly conducts heat away from the body, even persons who drown in warm water may suffer from hypothermia. (See *Physiologic changes in near drowning,* page 564.)

Comprehensive assessment
The patient's history (obtained from a family member, friend, or emergency personnel, if necessary) reveals the cause of the near drowning. The patient may display any of a host of signs and symptoms. If he's conscious, he may complain of a headache or substernal chest pain.

The initial assessment of the patient's vital signs may detect fever, confusion, seizures, rapid, slow, or absent pulse, and shallow, gasping, or absent respirations. If the patient was exposed to cold temperatures, he may experience hypothermia.

On initial observation, the patient may be unconscious, semiconscious, or awake. If he's awake, he usually appears apprehensive, irritable, restless, or lethargic, and he may vomit. Inspection may reveal cyanosis or pink, frothy sputum (indicating pulmonary edema). Palpation of the abdomen may disclose abdominal distention.

Auscultation of the lungs may reveal crackles, rhonchi, wheezing, or apnea. You may note tachycardia, an irregular heartbeat (arrhythmias), or cardiac arrest. The patient may also be hypotensive.

Diagnosis
Supportive tests include:
■ arterial blood gas (ABG) analysis to show the degree of hypoxia, intrapulmonary shunt, and acid-base imbal-

Physiologic changes in near drowning

The diagram below shows the primary cellular alterations that occur during near drowning. Separate pathways are shown for saltwater and freshwater incidents. Hypothermia presents a separate pathway that may preserve neurologic function by decreasing the metabolic rate. All pathways lead to diffuse pulmonary edema.

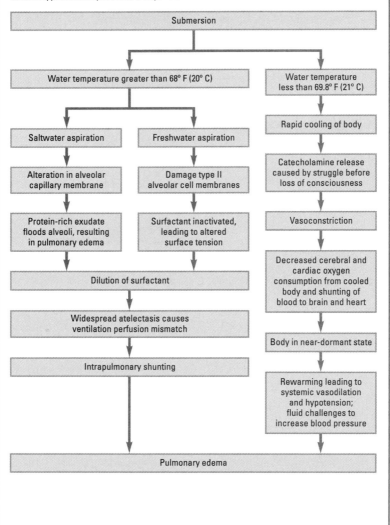

ance and to identify hypoxemia, hypercapnia, and a combined respiratory and metabolic acidosis

■ serum electrolyte levels to reveal hyperkalemia secondary to acidosis or red blood cell hemolysis.

■ complete blood count to identify hemolysis if the patient aspirated large amounts of fluid; elevated white blood cell (WBC) count secondary to alveolar inflammation; and decreased WBC count if the patient is hypothermic

■ blood urea nitrogen and creatinine levels and urinalysis to identify renal function

■ cervical spine X-ray to rule out fracture

■ serial chest X-rays to reveal inflammation, fluid accumulation, excess air accumulation, fractures, and foreign objects; pulmonary infiltrates suggesting pulmonary edema

■ electrocardiogram to reveal myocardial ischemia.

Collaborations

Near drowning is a multisystem problem that requires a multidisciplinary approach to care. Medical and nursing care focus on maintaining all body functions. Specialists may become involved, depending upon the patient's needs. For example, a pulmonologist and respiratory therapy may be involved to manage the ventilatory needs of the patient. As other systems become involved, specialists for those systems may be consulted. Social services may be involved to assist with emotional support for the patient and his family and follow-up care issues.

Treatment and care

Care before transport includes stabilizing the patient's neck and spine to pre-vent further injury, cardiopulmonary (CPR) as needed, and supplemental oxygen. After the patient reaches the facility, resuscitation continues. His oxygenation and circulation are maintained. X-rays confirm cervical spine integrity, and the patient's blood pH and electrolyte imbalances are corrected. If he's hypothermic, steps are taken to rewarm him.

ABG results help guide pulmonary therapy and determine the need for sodium bicarbonate to treat metabolic acidosis. If the patient can't maintain an open airway, has abnormal ABG levels and pH, or doesn't have spontaneous respirations, he may need endotracheal intubation and mechanical ventilation. If he develops bronchospasm, he may need bronchodilators. Hemodynamic monitoring, specifically, central venous pressure (CVP) or pulmonary artery wedge pressure (PAWP) help to guide fluid replacement and cardiac drug therapy. The patient may also require standard treatment for pulmonary edema. A nasogastric (NG) tube may be inserted to prevent vomiting and reduce the risk of further aspiration; an indwelling urinary catheter allows monitoring of urine output.

Complications

Near drowning may result in neurologic impairment; seizure disorders; pulmonary edema; renal damage, including acute renal failure; bacterial aspiration; and pulmonary or cardiac complications, such as arrhythmias and decreased blood pressure, disseminated intravascular coagulation, and death.

Nursing considerations

■ Assess airway, breathing, and circulation. If the patient experiences cardiac or respiratory arrest, start CPR and advanced cardiac life support.

🖎 **ALERT** *If the patient is hypothermic, keep in mind that drug metabolism is decreased, necessitating longer than usual intervals between dosing of I.V. medications. In addition, as the patient is rewarmed, be alert for a boluslike effect that can occur with medications due to vasodilation that occurs during rewarming.*

■ Administer supplemental oxygen as ordered.

🖎 **ALERT** *If the patient is hypothermic, be sure to use warm humidified oxygen to prevent additional cooling.*

■ Monitor oxygen saturation via continuous pulse oximetry and serial ABG analyses for evidence of hypoxemia and anticipate the need for endotracheal intubation and mechanical ventilation should the patient's respiratory status deteriorate. Anticipate using positive end-expiratory pressure (PEEP) if the patient continues to demonstrate hypoxia or pulmonary edema and doesn't respond to increasing levels of oxygen.

🖎 **ALERT** *PEEP is especially helpful for patients who experienced freshwater near drowning because alveoli remain open due to the pressure even without adequate surfactant. Keep in mind that the patient may experience low levels of surfactant for 2 to 3 days after aspirating freshwater; therefore, discontinue PEEP carefully and monitor the patient closely for a deterioration in his respiratory status during discontinuation.*

■ Auscultate lung sounds every hour for changes, such as crackles, rhonchi or friction rubs. Suction as necessary; send sputum for culture as ordered.

■ Place the patient in semi-Fowler's position to maximize chest expansion. Keep the patient as quiet and comfortable as possible to minimize oxygen demands.

■ Assess for signs of worsening hypoxemia, including use of accessory muscles, stridor, nasal flaring, grunting retractions, tachypnea, tachycardia, and cyanosis.

■ Obtain serial ABG analyses as ordered and monitor for changes indicating a deterioration or improvement in the patient's condition.

■ Monitor vital signs continuously for changes. Observe skin color and check capillary refill. Notify the physician if capillary refill is greater than 2 seconds. Continuously monitor the patient's core temperature.

■ Assist with insert of central venous or pulmonary artery catheter to evaluate hemodynamic status. Monitor hemodynamic parameters, including CVP, PAWP, and cardiac output and input, frequently — as often as every 15 minutes — to evaluate the patient's status and response to treatment.

■ Institute continuous cardiac monitoring to evaluate for possible arrhythmias, myocardial ischemia, or adverse effects of treatment.

■ Assess level of consciousness (LOC) frequently — approximately every 30 to 60 minutes for the first 24 hours. Monitor for signs and symptoms of increased intracranial pressure (ICP), including decreasing LOC, irritability, nausea or vomiting, altered pupillary response, altered motor response, or disconjugate gaze. Administer osmotic diuretics as ordered to control ICP. Anticipate the need for ICP monitoring.

ALERT *Be alert for signs and symptoms of brain herniation, such as bradycardia, hypertension, widening pulse pressure, and altered respiratory rate and pattern.*

■ Ensure I.V. access and administer I.V. fluids as ordered. Monitor intake and output closely. Insert an indwelling urinary catheter and assess urine output hourly. Monitor serum electrolyte levels and renal function studies for changes.

■ Assess abdomen for distention and presence of bowel sounds every 2 to 4 hours.

ALERT *Bowel ischemia and necrosis may occur from prolonged periods of hypoxemia and hypotension secondary to shunting of blood to more vital organs.*

■ Insert an NG tube as indicated to remove swallowed water and reduce the risk of vomiting and aspiration.

■ Institute rewarming measures as ordered. (See "Hypothermia," page 554.)

■ Administer pharmacologic agents as ordered, for example, sodium bicarbonate if the patient has metabolic acidosis or aerosolized bronchodilators for bronchospasm.

■ Watch for signs of impending coagulopathy (such as petechiae, bruising, bleeding or oozing from gums or venipuncture sites) and report them immediately. Monitor results of coagulation studies.

■ Provide emotional support and reassurance appropriately in the wake of this potentially fatal episode.

Patient teaching

■ Explain the disease course and treatments to the patient and his family.

■ Teach the patient and his family about measures to prevent future episodes, such as avoidance of alcohol or drugs when in the water and observance of safety swimming rules.

Plasmapheresis

Plasmapheresis, also called *plasma exchange,* consists of a therapeutic removal of plasma from withdrawn blood and the reinfusion of formed blood elements. By removing and replacing the plasma, plasmapheresis cleans the blood of harmful substances, such as toxins, and of disease mediators, such as immune complexes and autoantibodies. Consequently, plasmapheresis has several neurologic applications, such as in Guillain-Barré syndrome, multiple sclerosis, and especially myasthenia gravis. In myasthenia gravis, plasmapheresis removes circulating anti-acetylcholine receptor antibodies. If successful, treatment may relieve symptoms for months; however, results vary. Used most commonly in patients with long-standing neuromuscular disease, plasmapheresis may also treat acute exacerbations. Acutely ill patients may undergo this procedure as often as four times a week; others about once every 2 weeks.

Procedure

Blood removed from the patient flows into a cell separator, where it's divided into plasma and formed elements. The plasma is separated out and filtered to remove a specific disease mediator. The cellular blood components are then retransfused using fresh frozen plasma or albumin in place of the removed plasma. During the procedure, frequent blood samples are taken to monitor calcium and potassium levels.

Complications

Plasmapheresis risks several possible complications, including a hypersensitivity reaction to the ingredients of the replacement solution and hypocalcemia from excessive binding of circulating calcium to the citrate solution used as an anticoagulant in the replacement solution. Hypokalemia can follow plasmapheresis, producing severe muscle cramps and tetany. In addition, because large amounts of fluid are removed during treatment, hypotension and other complications of hypovolemia may occur. Myasthenic crisis is possible due to the removal of circulating anticholinesterase drugs. Additionally, cholinergic crisis may occur because antibodies are removed and there's a decrease in the need for anticholinesterase drugs after the procedure.

Nursing considerations

Before plasmapheresis

■ Briefly discuss the treatment and its purpose with the patient. Urge the patient to report any paresthesias during the procedure because these could indicate hypocalcemia or hypokalemia.

■ If the patient is taking oral foods, allow him to eat lightly before treatment and to drink milk before and during treatment to help reduce the risk of hypocalcemia.

■ Ensure that the patient's bladder is empty before the procedure. A full bladder may lead to mild hypotension as a result of fluid shift or a vasovagal reaction.

■ Obtain baseline vital signs and hemodynamic parameters as appropriate.

■ Institute continuous cardiac monitoring if not already in place.

■ Obtain blood samples for tests to determine baseline levels of hemoglobin, hematocrit, and other blood substances.

■ If medications are ordered, administer them after treatment instead of before, if possible, to prevent their removal from the blood.

During and after plasmapheresis

■ As plasmapheresis begins, observe the patient for signs of hypersensitivity, such as respiratory distress, hives, diaphoresis, hypotension, or thready pulse and report immediately.

■ During treatment, monitor vital signs every 15 to 30 minutes. (Don't take blood pressure readings in the arm being used for blood withdrawal and reinfusion, however.)

■ Pay particular attention to temperature; reinfusion of blood that has cooled while in the cell separator can produce hypothermia.

■ Observe the electrocardiogram and report any serious arrhythmias. Because arrhythmias can result from electrolyte imbalance or volume depletion, monitor blood levels of calcium and potassium and replace electrolytes as ordered.

ALERT *Patients who are receiving prednisone or digoxin therapy have a greater risk of developing hypokalemia. Monitor closely.*

■ Administer electrolyte replacements and antiarrhythmic agents as ordered during reinfusion.

■ Administer fluids as ordered throughout the procedure. Monitor intake and output hourly to ensure adequate hydration. Watch for signs of circulatory compromise. Compare levels of hematocrit, hemoglobin, electrolytes, antibody titers, and immune complexes with pretreatment levels.

■ Weigh the patient after the procedure for changes suggesting fluid loss.

■ If the patient is undergoing plasmapheresis for unstable myasthenia gravis, keep emergency equipment and medications readily available; monitor blood pressure and pulse rate closely.

ALERT *Observe for symptoms of myasthenic or cholinergic crisis, which may occur due to removal of anticholinesterase drugs or antibodies from the blood. Be prepared for endotracheal intubation and mechanical ventilation if the patient experiences crisis.*

■ After completion of treatment and removal of needles, apply direct pressure on the puncture sites for at least 10 minutes, then apply pressure dressings. Frequently (at least every 30 minutes) assess the dressings for drainage and the puncture sites for signs of extravasation.

■ Monitor coagulation studies, including prothrombin time, partial thromboplastin time, and platelet levels for increases that suggest impaired clotting. Patients undergoing repeated treatments may require transfusions of fresh frozen plasma to replace normal clotting factors lost in removed plasma.

■ Allow the patient to rest because fatigue is common after plasmapheresis.

(If he's undergoing repeated treatments, he may develop chronic fatigue.)

■ Provide a high-protein diet and administer multivitamin with iron as ordered.

■ Because plasmapheresis can cause immunosuppression, institute appropriate infection control precautions.

★ MULTISYSTEM DISORDER

Septic shock

Low systemic vascular resistance and an elevated cardiac output (CO) characterize septic shock. The disorder is thought to occur in response to infections that release microbes or one of the immune mediators.

Any pathogenic organism can cause septic shock. Gram-negative bacteria, such as *Escherichia coli, Klebsiella pneumoniae, Serratia, Enterobacter,* and *Pseudomonas* rank as the most common causes and account for up to 70% of all cases. Opportunistic fungi cause about 3% of cases. Rare causative organisms include mycobacteria and some viruses and protozoa.

Many organisms that are normal flora on the skin and in the intestines are beneficial and pose no threat unless they spread throughout the body by way of the bloodstream. Organisms that gain entry through an alteration in the body's normal defenses, or through artificial devices that penetrate the body, such as I.V., intra-arterial, and urinary catheters, or knife or bullet wounds, can cause overwhelming infection unless body defenses destroy them.

Septic shock can occur in any person with impaired immunity, but el-

Understanding septic shock

An immune response is triggered when bacteria release endotoxins. In response, macrophages secrete tumor necrosis factor (TNF) and interleukins. These mediators, in turn, are responsible for increase release of platelet-activating factor (PAF), prostaglandins, leukotrienes, thromboxane A_2, kinins, and complement. The consequences are vasodilation and vasoconstriction, increased capillary permeability, reduced systemic vascular resistance, microemboli, and an elevated cardiac output (CO). Endotoxins also stimulate the release of histamine, further increasing capillary permeability. Moreover, myocardial depressant factor, TNF, PAF, and other factors depress myocardial function. CO falls, resulting in multisystem organ failure.

derly people are at greatest risk. About two-thirds of septic shock cases occur in hospitalized patients, most of whom have underlying diseases. Those at high risk include patients with burns, diabetes mellitus, immunosuppression, malnutrition, stress, excessive antibiotic use, and chronic cardiac, hepatic, or renal disorders. Also at risk are patients who have had invasive diagnostic or therapeutic procedures, surgery, or traumatic wounds.

Pathophysiology
Septic shock is a type of distributive shock. (See *Understanding Septic shock.*)

Comprehensive assessment
The patient's history may include a disorder or treatment that can cause immunosuppression, or it may include a history of invasive tests or treatments, surgery, or trauma. At onset, the patient may have fever and chills, although 20% of patients may be hypothermic.

The patient's signs and symptoms will reflect either the hyperdynamic (warm) phase of septic shock or the hypodynamic (cold) phase. The *hyperdynamic phase* is characterized by increased CO, peripheral vasodilation, and decreased systemic vascular resistance. The patient's skin may appear pink and flushed. Altered level of consciousness (LOC) is reflected in agitation, anxiety, irritability, and shortened attention span. Respirations are rapid and shallow. Urine output is below normal. Palpation of peripheral pulses may detect a rapid, full, bounding pulse. The skin may feel warm and dry. Blood pressure may be normal or slightly elevated.

The *hypodynamic phase* is characterized by decreased CO, peripheral vasoconstriction, increased systemic vascular resistance, and inadequate tissue perfusion. The patient's skin may appear pale and possibly cyanotic. Peripheral areas may be mottled. His LOC may be decreased; obtundation and coma may be present. Respirations are rapid and shallow, and urine output may be less than 25 ml/hour or absent.

Palpation of peripheral pulses may reveal no pulse or a rapid pulse that's weak or thready. Peripheral pulses may also be irregular if arrhythmias are present. The skin may feel cold and clammy.

Auscultation of blood pressure may reveal hypotension, usually with a systolic pressure below 90 mm Hg or 50 to 80 mm Hg below the patient's previous level. Auscultation of the lungs may reveal crackles or rhonchi if pulmonary congestion is present.

The pulmonary artery wedge pressure (PAWP) is likely to be reduced or normal, and CO is almost always moderately to severely increased or normal. Rarely, CO is decreased.

Diagnosis

The following findings aid in the diagnosis of septic shock:

■ Blood cultures are positive for the offending organism.

■ Complete blood count shows the presence or absence of anemia and leukopenia, severe or absent neutropenia, and usually the presence of thrombocytopenia.

■ Arterial blood gas (ABG) studies may reveal metabolic acidosis, hypoxemia, and low partial pressure of arterial carbon dioxide ($PaCO_2$) early on that progresses to increased $PaCO_2$ (thereby indicating respiratory acidosis).

■ Blood urea nitrogen and creatinine levels are increased and creatinine clearance is decreased.

■ Prothrombin time, partial thromboplastin time, and bleeding time are increased; platelets are decreased and fibrin split products are increased.

■ Electrocardiogram shows ST depression, inverted T waves, and arrhythmias resembling myocardial infarction.

■ Amylase and lipase levels may show pancreatic insufficiency.

■ Hepatic enzyme levels are elevated due to liver ischemia.

■ Blood glucose levels are initially elevated, and then decrease.

■ Chest X-rays reveal evidence of pneumonia (as the underlying infec-

tion) or adult respiratory distress syndrome (indicating progression of septic shock).

■ Computed tomography reveals abscesses or sources of possible infection.

Collaborations

The patient with septic shock is usually extremely ill, requiring the efforts of a multidisciplinary team of professionals. Because the source of the infection may be unknown, an infectious disease specialist can help coordinate and determine antimicrobial treatment. In addition, the patient may require a nutritionist to meet metabolic needs through parenteral nutrition. A renal care specialist and other specialists may be required if organs begin to fail. The patient may require a pulmonary specialist for pulmonary involvement and a cardiologist to assist with hemodynamic management. A physical therapist can assist if the patient requires splinting and range-of-motion exercises to maintain mobility. The patient and the family may also benefit from a referral to social services and for spiritual counseling and support.

Treatment and care

Location and treatment of the underlying sepsis is essential to treating septic shock. If any I.V., intra-arterial, or urinary drainage catheters are in place, they should be removed. Aggressive antimicrobial therapy appropriate for the causative organism must be initiated immediately. Culture and sensitivity tests help determine the most effective antimicrobial drug. Surgery may be necessary for example, to repair a bowel perforation, drain an abscess, or debride a wound, if either is the cause of the infection.

For patients who are immunosupressed because of drug therapy, drugs should be discontinued or reduced. Granulocyte transfusions may be used in patients with severe neutropenia. Oxygen therapy should be initiated to maintain arterial oxygen saturation greater than 95%. Mechanical ventilation may be required if respiratory failure occurs.

Colloid or crystalloid infusions are given to increase intravascular volume and raise blood pressure. After sufficient fluid volume has been replaced, diuretics such as furosemide can be given to maintain urine output above 20 ml/hour. If fluid replacement fails to increase blood pressure, a vasopressor such as dopamine can be started. Blood transfusion may be needed if anemia is present.

Complications

Septic shock is usually a complication of another disorder or invasive procedure and has a mortality as high as 25%. In septic shock, complications include disseminated intravascular coagulation, renal failure, heart failure, GI ulcers, and abnormal liver function. In early sepsis, a generalized systemic inflammatory response syndrome (SIRS) occurs. If this uncontrolled SIRS continues, affecting two or more vital organs, multiple organ dysfunction syndrome results. (See *Multisystem organ dysfunction syndrome*.)

Nursing considerations

■ Assess airway, breathing, and circulation. Assess cardiopulmonary status closely.

■ Administer supplemental oxygen as ordered. Monitor oxygen saturation via continuous pulse oximetry and serial

ABGs for evidence of hypoxemia and anticipate the need for endotracheal intubation and mechanical ventilation should the patient's respiratory status deteriorate. Place the patient in semi-Fowler's position to maximize chest expansion. Keep the patient as quiet and comfortable as possible to minimize oxygen demands.

■ Monitor vital signs continuously for changes. Observe skin color and check capillary refill. Notify the physician if capillary refill is greater than 2 seconds.

ALERT *Keep in mind that the temperature is usually elevated in the early stages of septic shock and the patient commonly experiences shaking chills. As the shock progresses, temperature typically drops and the patient experiences diaphoresis.*

ALERT *If the patient's systolic blood pressure drops below 80 mm Hg, increase the oxygen flow rate, and notify the physician immediately because systolic blood pressure below 80 mm Hg usually results in inadequate coronary artery blood flow, cardiac ischemia, arrhythmias, and further complications of low CO. Alert the physician and increase the infusion rate if the patient experiences a progressive drop in blood pressure accompanied by a thready pulse. This usually signals inadequate CO from reduced intravascular volume.*

■ Remove I.V., intra-arterial, or urinary drainage catheters and send them to the laboratory to culture for the presence of the causative organism (prepare to reinsert or assist with reinsertion of new devices). Obtain blood cultures as ordered and begin antimicrobial therapy as ordered. Monitor

Multisystem organ dysfunction syndrome

Multisystem organ dysfunction syndrome (MODS) is a condition that occurs when two or more organs or organ systems become affected and are unable to function in their role of maintaining homeostasis. Intervention is necessary to support and maintain organ function. MODS isn't an illness itself. Rather, it's a manifestation of another progressive underlying condition.

MODS develops when widespread systemic inflammation, a condition known as *systemic inflammatory response syndrome* (SIRS) overtaxes a patient's compensatory mechanisms. Infection, ischemia, trauma of any sort, reperfusion injury, or multisystem injury can trigger SIRS. If allowed to progress, SIRS can lead to organ inflammation and ultimately, MODS.

Typically, MODS is classified as primary or secondary. In primary MODS, organ or organ system failure is due to a direct injury, such as trauma or a primary disorder, usually involving the lungs, such as pneumonia, aspiration, near drowning, or pulmonary embolism. The organ failure can be positively linked to the direct injury. Typically, adult respiratory distress syndrome (ARDS) develops and progresses, leading to encephalopathy and coagulopathy due to hepatic involvement. As the syndrome continues, other organ systems are affected.

In secondary MODS, organ or organ system failure is due to sepsis. Typically, the infection source isn't associated with the lungs. The most common infection sources include intra-abdominal sepsis, extensive blood loss, pancreatitis, or major vascular injuries. With secondary MODS, ARDS develops sooner and progressive involvement of other organs and organ systems occurs more rapidly.

Regardless of the type of MODS or triggering event, the overall underlying problem is inadequate perfusion.

Assessment findings
The assessment findings associated with MODS typically reveal an acutely ill patient with signs and symptoms associated with SIRS. Early findings may include:

- fever, usually greater than 101° F (38.3° C) (early indicator)
- tachycardia
- narrowed pulse pressure
- tachypnea
- decreased pulmonary artery pressure, decreased pulmonary artery wedge pressure (PAWP), decreased central venous pressure, and increased cardiac output (CO) (due to tachycardia).

As SIRS progresses, findings reflect impaired perfusion of the tissues and organs, such as decreasing level of consciousness, respiratory depression, diminished bowel sounds, jaundice, oliguria, or anuria. Pulmonary artery pressure increases (due to pulmonary edema). PAWP increases and CO decreases with the development of heart failure.

Organ dysfunction is determined by specific criteria. For example, pulmonary organ dysfunction is identified by the development of ARDS requiring positive end–expiratory pressure greater than 10 cm H_2O and fraction of inspired oxygen less then 0.5. Hepatic dysfunction is evidenced by jaundice with a serum bilirubin level of 8 to 10 mg/dl. Oliguria of less than 500 ml/day or an increasing serum creatinine level indicate mild renal system dysfunction while the need for dialysis suggests severe organ involvement. Development of disseminated intravascular coagulation typically indicates severe hematologic system dysfunction.

Treatment
Treatment focuses on supporting respiratory and circulatory function with the use of mechanical ventilation, supplemental oxygen, hemodynamic monitoring, and

(continued)

Multisystem organ dysfunction syndrome *(continued)*

fluid infusion to expand and maintain the intravascular compartment. Renal function is closely monitored, including hourly urine output measurements and serial laboratory tests to evaluate for trends indicating acute renal failure. Dialysis ultimately may be necessary.

Numerous pharmacologic agents may be used:
● antimicrobial agents to treat underlying infection
● vasopressors, such as dopamine and norepinephrine
● isotonic crystalloid solutions, such as normal saline and lactated Ringer's solution, to expand the intravascular fluid spaces
● colloids such as albumin to help expand plasma volume without the added risk of causing fluid overload.

Some experimental agents are being used, such as antitumor necrosis factor (TNF), endotoxin, and anti-interleukin-1 antibodies. However, evidence supporting the effectiveness of these agents is currently unavailable.

Nursing care
Nursing care for the patient with MODS is primarily supportive. The patient is acutely ill and requires close, often extensive monitoring. Emotional support also is crucial because the mortality rate for a patient with MODS is directly proportional to the number of organs or organ systems affected. For example, the mortality rate is 85% when three organs are involved; it jumps to 95% when four organs are involved and up to 99% with five-organ involvement.

---

the patient for possible adverse effects of therapy.

■ Assist with insertion of central venous or pulmonary artery catheter to evaluate hemodynamic status. Monitor hemodynamic parameters, including central venous pressure, PAWP, and CO and input, frequently — as often as every 15 minutes — to evaluate the patient's status and response to treatment.

■ Institute continuous cardiac monitoring to evaluate for possible arrhythmias, myocardial ischemia, or adverse effects of treatment.

■ Assess LOC frequently, approximately every 30 minutes until the patient stabilizes, and then every 2 to 4 hours as indicated by the patient's status.

■ Monitor intake and output closely. Insert an indwelling urinary catheter if one isn't already in place and assess

urine output hourly. Notify the physician if the urine output is less than 30 ml/hour.

■ Administer I.V. fluid therapy as ordered, usually normal saline or lactated Ringer's solution. If the patient has suffered abdominal trauma, avoid using I.V. sites in the lower extremities. Infused fluid may escape through the ruptured vessel into the abdomen. Monitor hemodynamic parameters to determine response to therapy.

ALERT *Be alert for signs and symptoms of possible fluid overload, such as dyspnea, tachypnea, crackles, peripheral edema, jugular vein distention, and increased pulmonary artery pressures.*

■ Administer positive inotropic agents as ordered to assist in improving cardiac contractility and maintaining CO despite the widespread vasodilation and vasopressors as ordered to maintain perfusion.

■ Allow for frequent rest periods to minimize oxygen demands.

■ Institute infection control precautions; use strict aseptic technique for all invasive procedures.

ALERT *Assess the patient for the development of adult respiratory distress syndrome (ARDS). For the patient receiving mechanical ventilation, suspect ARDS if the patient needs increasing fraction of inspired oxygen in conjunction with increasing levels of positive end-expiratory pressure to maintain partial pressure of arterial oxygen above 60 mm Hg. (See "Adult respiratory distress syndrome" in chapter 2, page 172.)*

■ Assist with nutritional support therapy, including administration of short and medium chain fatty acid and branched chain amino acids (usually via intralipid therapy) to halt protein metabolism.

■ Monitor laboratory test results, especially coagulation and studies and hepatic enzyme levels, for changes indicative of disseminated intravascular coagulopathy and hepatic failure, respectively.

■ Provide emotional support to the patient and his family. Prepare the patient for surgery as appropriate.

Patient teaching

■ Explain the disease course and treatments to the patient and his family.

■ Provide preoperative teaching as appropriate.

■ Review the danger signs and symptoms to report, emphasizing the need to report them immediately.

Trauma, multiple

Multiple trauma as the name implies refers to injuries to more than one body area or organ. The type of trauma determines the extent of injury, whether blunt or penetrating. Trauma is the leading cause of death in people younger than age 45. It's the third leading cause of death in the United States.

A patient experiencing multiple trauma has many needs, requiring a multidisciplinary team approach. The patient may have a head injury accompanied by chest and cardiac trauma. Or the patient may have experienced a spinal cord injury along with numerous fractures and contusions to other body areas. Prompt, efficient, organized care, is the key. Usually assessment, treatment, and care occur simultaneously. As always, airway, breathing, and circulation take priority. (For additional information on each of the major types of trauma, see the system-specific chapters.)

Wound care, traumatic

Traumatic wounds include abrasions, lacerations, puncture wounds, and amputations. In an abrasion, the skin is scraped, with partial loss of the skin surface. In a laceration, the skin is torn, causing jagged, irregular edges; the severity of a laceration depends on its size, depth, and location. A puncture wound occurs when a pointed object, such as a knife or glass fragment, penetrates the skin. Traumatic amputation refers to removal of part of the body, a limb, or part of a limb.

Initial management concentrates on controlling bleeding, usually by applying firm, direct pressure and elevating the extremity. If bleeding continues, you may need to compress a pressure point. Assess the condition of the wound. Management and cleaning technique usually depend on the specific type of wound and degree of contamination.

Equipment

Sterile basin ■ normal saline solution ■ sterile 4″ × 4″ gauze pads ■ sterile gloves ■ clean gloves ■ dry sterile dressing, nonadherent pad, or petroleum gauze ■ linen-saver pad ■ optional: scissors, sterile towel, goggles, mask, gown, 50-ml catheter-tip syringe, surgical scrub brush, antibacterial ointment, sterile porous tape, sutures and suture set, hydrogen peroxide

Essential steps

■ Prepare the equipment.
  – Place a linen-saver pad under the area to be cleaned. Remove any clothing covering the wound. If necessary, cut hair around the wound with scissors to promote cleaning and treatment.
  – Assemble needed equipment at the patient's bedside. Fill a sterile basin with normal saline solution. Make sure the treatment area has enough light to allow close observation of the wound. Depending on the nature and location of the wound, wear sterile or clean gloves to avoid spreading infection.
■ Check the patient's medical history for previous tetanus immunization and, if needed and ordered, arrange for immunization.
■ Administer pain medication, if ordered.
■ Wash your hands and wear appropriate protective equipment, such as a gown, a mask, and goggles, if spraying or splashing of body fluids is possible.
■ If the wound is an abrasion, follow these steps:
  – Flush the scraped skin with normal saline solution.
  – Remove dirt or gravel with a sterile 4″ × 4″ gauze pad moistened with normal saline solution. Rub in the opposite direction from which the dirt or gravel became embedded.
  – If the wound is extremely dirty, use a surgical brush to scrub it.
  – With a small wound, allow it to dry and form a scab. With a larger wound, cover it with a nonadherent pad or petroleum gauze and a light dressing if appropriate. Apply antibacterial ointment if ordered.
■ If the wound is a laceration, follow these steps:
  – Moisten a sterile 4″ × 4″ gauze pad with normal saline solution. Clean the wound gently, working outward from its center to about 2″ (5 cm) beyond its edges. Discard the soiled gauze pad and use a fresh one as necessary. Continue until the wound appears clean.
  – If the wound is dirty, irrigate it with a 50-ml catheter-tip syringe and normal saline solution.
  – Assist the physician in suturing the wound edges using the suture kit, or apply sterile strips of porous tape.

– Apply the prescribed antibacterial ointment to help prevent infection.

– Apply a dry sterile dressing over the wound to absorb drainage and help prevent bacterial contamination.

■ If the wound is a puncture, follow these steps:

– If the wound is minor, allow it to bleed for a few minutes before cleaning it.

– For a larger puncture wound, possibly irrigate it before applying a dry dressing.

– Stabilize any embedded foreign object until the physician can remove it. After removal and the bleeding is stabilized, clean the wound as that for a laceration or deep puncture wound.

■ If the wound is a traumatic amputation, follow these steps:

– Apply a gauze pad moistened with normal saline solution to the amputation site. Elevate the affected part and immobilize it for surgery.

– Recover the amputated part and prepare it for transport to a facility where microvascular surgery is performed.

Complications

Cleaning and care of traumatic wounds may temporarily increase the patient's pain. Excessive, vigorous cleaning may further disrupt tissue integrity.

Nursing considerations

■ When irrigating a traumatic wound, avoid using more than 8 psi of pressure. High-pressure irrigation can seriously interfere with healing, kill cells, and allow bacteria to infiltrate the tissue.

■ To clean the wound, use hydrogen peroxide if appropriate; its foaming action facilitates debris removal.

ALERT *However, hydrogen peroxide should never be instilled into a deep wound because of the risk of embolism from the evolving gases. Be sure to rinse hands well after using hydrogen peroxide.*

■ After a wound has been cleaned, anticipate the possible need for debridement to remove dead tissue and reduce the risk of infection and scarring. If this is necessary, pack the wound with gauze pads soaked in normal saline solution until debridement.

■ Observe for signs and symptoms of infection, such as warm red skin at the site or purulent discharge. Be aware that infection of a traumatic wound can delay healing, increase scar formation, and trigger systemic infection such as septicemia.

■ Observe all dressings. If edema is present, adjust the dressing to avoid impairing circulation to the area.

■ Document the date and time of the procedure, wound size and condition, medication administration, specific wound care measures, and patient teaching.

Wound dehiscence and evisceration

Although surgical wounds typically heal without incident, occasionally the edges of a wound may fail to join or may separate even after they seem to be healing normally. This develop-

Recognizing dehiscence and evisceration

In wound dehiscence, the layers of the surgical wound separate. In evisceration, the viscera (in this case, a loop of bowel) protrude through the surgical incision.

WOUND DEHISCENCE

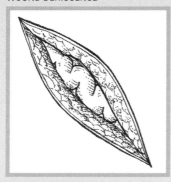

EVISCERATION OF BOWEL LOOP

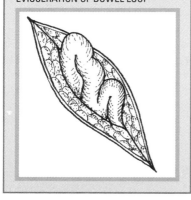

ment, called *wound dehiscence,* may lead to an even more serious complication: evisceration, in which a portion of the viscera (usually a bowel loop) protrudes through the incision. Evisceration, in turn, can lead to peritoni-

tis and septic shock. (See *Recognizing dehiscence and evisceration.*)

Equipment

Sterile towel ▪ 1 L of sterile normal saline solution ▪ sterile irrigation set, including a basin, solution container, and 50-ml catheter-tip syringe ▪ several large abdominal dressings ▪ sterile, waterproof drape ▪ linen-saver pads ▪ sterile gloves

If the patient will return to the operating room, also gather the following equipment: I.V. administration set and I.V. fluids ▪ equipment for nasogastric intubation ▪ preoperative medications as ordered ▪ suction apparatus.

Essential steps

▪ Provide reassurance and support to ease the patient's anxiety.

▪ Assess the patient's vital signs to establish a baseline.

▪ Keep the patient in bed and stay with him while someone else notifies the physician and collects the necessary equipment.

▪ Place a linen-saver pad under the patient to keep the sheets dry when the exposed viscera is moistened.

▪ Using sterile technique, unfold a sterile towel to create a sterile field. Open the package containing the sterile irrigation set and place the basin, solution container, and 50-ml syringe on the sterile field.

▪ Open the bottle of sterile normal saline solution and pour about 400 ml into the solution container. Pour about 200 ml into the sterile basin.

▪ Open several large abdominal dressings and place them on the sterile field.

▪ Put on the sterile gloves and place one or two of the large abdominal dressings into the basin to saturate them with saline solution.

■ Place the moistened dressings over the exposed viscera. Then place a sterile, waterproof drape over the dressings to prevent the sheets from getting wet.

■ Moisten the dressings every hour by withdrawing saline solution from the container through the syringe and then gently squirting the solution on the dressings.

ALERT *When moistening the dressings, inspect the color of the viscera. If it appears dusky or black, notify the physician immediately. With its blood supply interrupted, a protruding organ may become ischemic and necrotic.*

■ Maintain the patient on absolute bed rest in low Fowler's position (elevated no more than 20 degrees) with his knees flexed. This prevents injury and reduces stress on an abdominal incision.

■ Institute nothing by mouth in preparation for surgery to decrease the risk of aspiration during surgery.

■ Monitor the patient's pulse, respirations, blood pressure, and temperature every 15 minutes to detect shock.

■ Prepare the patient to return to the operating room.

■ Make sure the patient has signed a consent form and that the operating room staff has been informed about the procedure.

Complications

Infection, which can lead to peritonitis and, possibly, septic shock, is the most severe and most common complication of wound dehiscence and evisceration. Caused by bacterial contamination or by drying of normally moist abdominal contents, infection can impair circulation and lead to necrosis of the affected organ.

Nursing considerations

■ Keep in mind that the best treatment is prevention. When caring for a postoperative patient who is at risk for poor healing, make sure he gets an adequate supply of protein, vitamins, and calories. Monitor his dietary deficiencies and discuss any problems with the physician and the dietitian.

■ When changing wound dressings, always use sterile technique. Inspect the incision with each dressing change; be alert for early signs of infection and report immediately. Begin treatment as ordered before dehiscence or evisceration can occur.

■ Document when the problem occurred, the patient's activity preceding the problem, his condition, and the time the physician was notified.

■ Record the appearance of the wound or eviscerated organ; amount, color, consistency, and odor of any drainage; and nursing actions taken.

■ Record the patient's vital signs, his response to the incident, and the physician's actions.

Agents used to control postoperative bleeding

Drug	Indications	Adverse effects*
Aminocaproic acid (Amicar)	• Excessive acute bleeding from hyper-fibrinolysis • Chronic bleeding tendency • Antidote for excessive thrombolysis resulting from administration of strepto-kinase or urokinase	• Seizures • Bradycardia, arrhythmias (with rapid I.V. infusion) • Acute renal failure
Aprotinin (Trasylol)	• Prophylactic reduction of periopera-tive blood loss and the need for blood transfusion in patients undergoing cardio-pulmonary bypass during repeat coronary artery bypass graft surgery	• Cerebral embolism, stroke • Cardiac arrest, heart failure, ven-tricular tachycardia, MI, heart block, atrial fibrillation, atrial flutter, hypo-tension, supraventricular tachycar-dia • Nephrotoxicity, renal failure • Hemolysis • Apnea • Anaphylaxis, shock, sepsis
Desmopressin acetate (DDAVP, Stimate)	• Hemophilia A, von Willebrand's dis-ease • Central cranial diabetes insipidus, tem-porary polyuria, polydipsia related to pitu-itary trauma	• Headache • Flushing, slight rise in blood pres-sure at high dosage

*Common or life-threatening only

Special considerations

- Contraindicated in patients with active intravascular clotting or presence of disseminated intravascular coagulation unless heparin is used concomitantly.
- Use cautiously in patients with cardiac, renal, or hepatic disease.
- May increase BUN, creatinine, CK, AST, ALT, and potassium levels.
- To prepare an I.V. infusion, use normal saline solution, D_5W, or lactated Ringer's injection for dilution. Dilute doses up to 5 g with 250 ml of solution, doses of 5 g or greater with at least 500 ml.
- Avoid rapid I.V. infusion to minimize risk of cardiovascular adverse reactions, such as hypotension, bradycardia, and arrhythmias.

- Contraindicated in patients hypersensitive to beef because drug is prepared from bovine lung.
- May increase AST, ALT, creatinine, CK, and glucose levels; may increase PTT and ACT (celite activation clotting time); may decrease potassium levels.
- Administer by I.V. injection and I.V. infusion through a central venous line; drug also is added to the priming fluid of the cardiopulmonary bypass circuit. No other drug should be administered concomitantly with aprotinin. Rapid I.V. administration of large (loading) doses of aprotinin should be avoided because of the potential for hypotension or anaphylactoid reactions.
- Monitor closely even after uneventful administration of the test dose; the full therapeutic dose of aprotinin may cause anaphylaxis.

- Contraindicated in patients with type IIB von Willebrand's disease.
- Not indicated for patients with hemophilia B, patients with hemophilia A who have factor VIII levels up to 5%, patients with factor VIII antibodies, or patients with severe von Willebrand's disease.
- If using preoperatively, administer 30 minutes before procedure.
- Monitor the patient for early signs of water intoxication — drowsiness, listlessness, headache, confusion, anuria, and weight gain.
- Weigh the patient daily and observe for edema.
- Monitor urine volume and osmolarity of urine and plasma in patients with diabetes insipidus.

Antibiotics (guidelines for the use of antimicrobials)

This table provides guidelines for the first-line (denoted by the numeral 1) and second-line (numeral 2) management of selected organisms and should be used as a general reference

	Aminoglycosides				Cephalosporins									Miscellaneous					
	Amikacin	Gentamicin	Netilmicin	Tobramycin	Cefazolin	Cefepime	Cefixime	Cefotaxime	Cefoxitin	Ceftazidime	Ceftizoxime	Ceftriaxone	Cefuroxime	Azithromycin	Aztreonam	Chloramphenicol	Clarithromycin	Clindamycin	Eyrthromycin
Acinetobacter	1	2	2	2															
Bacillus anthracis																	2		2
Bacteroides fragilis									2									2	
Borrelia burgdorferi (skin)												2	2	2			2		2
Campylobacter jejuni														2			2	2	1
Chlamydia pneumoniae														2			2		2
Chlamydia psittaci																2			
Chlamydia trachomatis														1					2
Citrobacter freundii		1		1											2				
Clostridium difficile																			
Clostridium perfringens					2			2	2		2	2						2	
Enterobacter sp.	1	1	1	1		2													
Enterococcus faecalis																			
Enterococcus faecium																2			
Escherichia coli	2	2	2	2	1		1	1	1	1	1	1	1		2				
Haemophilus influenzae †							1			1	1				2				
Haemophilus influenzae ‡								2				2	2	2			2		
Klebsiella pneumoniae (UTI)					1		1	1	1		1	1	1		2				
Klebsiella pneumoniae (pneumonia)	2	2	2	2			1	1	1	1	1	1	1		2				
Legionella pneumophila														1			2		2
Listeria monocytogenes		1		1															
Moraxella catarrhalis						2	2	2	2	2	2	2	2	2			2		
Mycoplasma pneumoniae														2			2		1
Neisseria gonorrhoeae							1					1							
Nocardia asteroides																			
Pneumocystis carinii																			
Proteus mirabilis					2	2	2	2	2	2	2	2	2		2				
Proteus vulgaris							1	1		1	1	1							
Pseudomonas aeruginosa	2	2	2	1		2				1							2		
Serratia marcescens	2	2	2	2				1		2	2	1			2				
Shigella sp.																			
Staphylococcus aureus					1													2	
Staphylococcus saprophyticus																		2	
Streptococcus pneumoniae								2				2							
Streptococcus pyogenes (group A)					1	1	1	1	1		1	1	1	2			2	2	2
Streptococcus (anaerobic sp.)																		2	
Streptococcus (viridans group)		1										2		2			2	2	2
Vibrio cholerae																			

† life-threatening   ‡ non-life-threatening

only. Use patient condition, sensitivities, facility policies, and recent research when initiating new therapy.

Miscellaneous							Penicillins							Combinations with ß-lactamase inhibitors				Tetracyclines		Fluoroquinolones			
Imipenem/Cilastatin	Meropenem	Metronidazole	Pentamidine	Rifampin	Trimethoprim/Sulfamethoxazole	Vancomycin	Amoxicillin	Ampicillin	Mezlocillin	Nafcillin	Penicillin G	Piperacillin	Ticarcillin	Amoxicillin/Clavulanic acid	Ampicillin/Sulbactam	Piperacillin/Tazobactam	Ticarcillin/Clavulanic acid	Doxycycline	Minocycline	Ciprofloxacin	Levofloxacin	Norfloxacin	Ofloxacin
1	1				2									2						2			2
											1							1					
2	2	1												2	2	2	2						
								1			2							1					
																				2			2
																		1			2		
																		1					
																		1					2
1	1																			1			
		1				2																	
											1												
1	1																			1			
						2	1	1			1												
						1												2					
2	2				2											2				2	2	2	2
2	2														1	2	2			1	1		1
					1									1	1					2	2		2
					2									2			2			1	2	2	2
2	2				2									2	2	2	2			2	2		2
				2														2		1	1		1
					2			1			1												
					1									1	1					2	2		2
																			1		2		
																				2			2
					1														2				
			2		1																		
					1																		
					1									2						1	1	1	1
2	2								1			1	1							2			
	2				1															2	2		2
					1					2								2		1		1	1
			2	2		1				1				2	2	2	2			2	2		2
																				2		1	2
						1	1	1			1							1			1		
						1					1												
											1												
											1												
					2															1		1		1

Antiarrhythmics

Drug	Indications	Adverse effects*
Type IA **Disopyramide** **(Norpace,** **Norpace CR)**	• PVCs (unifocal, multifocal, or coupled); ventricular tachycardia; conversion of atrial fibrillation, atrial flutter, and paroxysmal atrial tachycardia to normal sinus rhythm	• Hypotension, heart failure, heart block, arrhythmias • Blurred vision, dry eyes or nose • Cholestatic jaundice
Procainamide **(Procanbid,** **Pronestyl,** **Pronestyl-SR)**	• Symptomatic PVCs; life-threatening ventricular tachycardia • Maintenance of normal sinus rhythm after conversion of atrial flutter • Prevention of atrial fibrillation or paroxysmal atrial tachycardia • Treatment of malignant hyperthermia	• Seizures • Hypotension, ventricular asystole, bradycardia, AV block, ventricular fibrillation (after parenteral use) • Thrombocytopenia, neutropenia (especially with sustained-release forms), agranulocytosis • Maculopapular rash, urticaria, pruritus, flushing, angioneurotic edema • Lupuslike syndrome (especially after prolonged administration)
Quinidine **gluconate** **(Quinaglute** **Dura-Tabs,** **Quinalan);** **quinidine** **sulfate** **(Quinidex** **Extentabs,** **Quinora)**	• Atrial flutter or fibrillation conversion • PSVT • Premature atrial contractions, PVCs, paroxysmal AV junctional rhythm or atrial or ventricular tachycardia, maintenance of cardioversion • Malaria (when quinine dihydrochloride is unavailable)	• Vertigo, headache, ataxia • PVCs, ventricular tachycardia, atypical ventricular tachycardia (torsades de pointes), hypotension, complete AV block, tachycardia, ECG changes (particularly widening of QRS complex and QT and PR intervals) • Tinnitus • Diarrhea, nausea, vomiting • Hemolytic anemia, thrombocytopenia, agranulocytosis • Hepatotoxicity • Acute asthmatic attack, respiratory arrest • Angioedema, cinchonism
Type IB **Lidocaine** **hydrochloride** **(LidoPen Auto-** **Injector, Xylo-** **caine HCL IV)**	• Ventricular arrhythmias from MI, cardiac manipulation, or cardiac glycosides • Status epilepticus	• Confusion, tremor, stupor, restlessness, light-headedness, hallucinations • Bradycardia, cardiac arrest, hypotension, new or worsened arrhythmias, asystole • Tinnitus, blurred or double vision • Respiratory arrest, status asthmaticus • Anaphylaxis

*Common or life-threatening only

Special considerations

• Contraindicated in patients with cardiogenic shock or second- or third-degree heart block in the absence of an artificial pacemaker, in congenital QT prolongation, and in sick sinus syndrome.
• Monitor serum electrolyte and drug levels; may decrease serum potassium and glucose levels and increase cholesterol and triglyceride levels.
• Patients with atrial flutter or fibrillation should be digitalized before disopyramide administration to ensure that enhanced AV conduction doesn't lead to ventricular tachycardia.
• Monitor for signs of developing heart block, such as QRS complex widening by more than 25% or QT interval lengthening by more than 25% above baseline.

• Contraindicated in patients with complete, second-, or third-degree heart block in the absence of an artificial pacemaker; and in patients with myasthenia gravis or systemic lupus erythematosus. Also contraindicated in patients with atypical ventricular tachycardia (torsades de pointes) because procainamide may aggravate this condition.
• Administer cardiac glycoside before beginning procainamide therapy when treating atrial fibrillation and flutter because ventricular rate may accelerate because of vagolytic effects on the AV node.
• Monitor blood pressure and ECG continuously during I.V. administration. Watch for prolonged QT interval and QRS complex (50% or greater widening), heart block, or increased arrhythmias. When these ECG signs appear, stop drug and monitor the patient closely.

• Contraindicated in patients with intraventricular conduction defects, cardiac glycoside toxicity when AV conduction is grossly impaired, abnormal rhythms caused by escape mechanisms, and a history of drug-induced torsades de pointes or QT syndrome.
• When drug is used to treat atrial tachyarrhythmias, ventricular rate may be accelerated from anticholinergic effects of drug on AV node. Previous treatment with a cardiac glycoside will prevent this.
• Monitor ECG, especially when giving large doses. Quinidine-induced cardiotoxicity causes conduction defects (50% widening of the QRS complex), ventricular tachycardia or flutter, frequent PVCs, and complete AV block. When these signs appear, stop drug and monitor the patient closely.

• Repeat administration of initial I.V. bolus every 5 to 10 minutes until arrhythmia subsides; simultaneously, begin constant infusion of 1 to 4 mg/minute. If single bolus has been given, repeat smaller bolus (usually one-half initial bolus) 5 to 10 minutes after start of infusion to maintain therapeutic serum level. After 24 hours of continuous infusion, decrease rate by one-half.
• Contraindicated in patients hypersensitive to amide-type local anesthetics, and in those with Stokes-Adams syndrome, Wolff-Parkinson-White syndrome, and severe degrees of SA, AV, or intraventricular block in absence of artificial pacemaker. Also contraindicated in patients with inflammation or infection in puncture region, septicemia, severe hypertension, spinal deformities, and neurologic disorders.

(continued)

Antiarrhythmics *(continued)*

Drug	Indications	Adverse effects*
Lidocaine hydrochloride *(continued)*		
Mexiletine (Mexitil)	• Treatment of documented life-threatening arrhythmias	• New or worsened cardiac arrhythmias • Nausea, vomiting, diarrhea, heartburn • Rash • Tremors • Visual disturbances
Tocainide (Tonocard)	• Treatment of life-threatening ventricular arrhythmias	• Light-headedness, tremor, vertigo • Hypotension, new or worsened arrhythmias, heart failure, bradycardia • Nausea, vomiting • Blood dyscrasia • Hepatitis • Respiratory arrest, pulmonary fibrosis, pneumonitis
Type IC ***Flecainide (Tambocor)***	• Sustained ventricular tachycardia • PSVT, paroxysmal atrial fibrillation or flutter in patients without structural heart disease	• Headache, light-headedness, syncope • New or worsened arrhythmias, heart failure, cardiac arrest, palpitations • Blurred vision and other visual disturbances • Dyspnea
Propafenone (Rythmol)	• Suppression of documented life-threatening ventricular arrhythmias	• Drowsiness • Bradycardia, heart failure, proarrhythmic events (ventricular tachycardia, PVCs, ventricular fibrillation) • Nausea, vomiting

*Common or life-threatening only

Antiarrhythmics 589

Special considerations

● In many severely ill patients, be alert for seizures, which may be the first sign of toxicity. However, severe reactions are usually preceded by somnolence, confusion, and paresthesia. Regard all signs and symptoms of toxicity as serious, and promptly reduce dosage or discontinue therapy. Continued infusion could lead to seizures and coma. Give oxygen through nasal cannula, if not contraindicated. Keep oxygen and CPR equipment handy.

● Monitor the patient for signs of excessive depression of cardiac conductivity (such as sinus node dysfunction, PR-interval prolongation, QRS complex widening, and appearance or exacerbation of arrhythmias). If they occur, reduce dosage or discontinue drug.

● Contraindicated in patients with heart failure, cardiogenic shock, hypotension, or second- or third-degree heart block.

● Be alert for fine tremor, usually in the hand. This is an early sign of toxicity that can progress to dizziness and later to ataxia and nystagmus as blood levels increase.

● When changing from lidocaine to mexiletine, stop the infusion with the first dose of mexiletine. Keep the infusion line open until the arrhythmia appears to be satisfactorily controlled.

● Monitor drug levels; therapeutic levels range from 0.75 to 2 µg/ml.

● Contraindicated in patients hypersensitive to lidocaine or other amide-type local anesthetics and in those with second- or third-degree AV block in the absence of a pacemaker.

● Drug is considered an oral lidocaine and may be used to ease transition from I.V. lidocaine to oral antiarrhythmic therapy.

● Monitor blood levels; therapeutic levels range from 4 to 10 µg/ml.

● Observe the patient for tremors, a possible sign that the maximum safe dose has been reached.

● Contraindicated in patients with cardiogenic shock, second- or third-degree AV block, or right bundle-branch block with a left hemiblock (in the absence of an artificial pacemaker). Drug has proarrhythmic effects in patients with atrial fibrillation or flutter; therefore, it isn't recommended for these patients.

● Drug has been linked to excessive mortality or nonfatal cardiac arrest rate in national multicenter trials. Restrict use to those patients in whom benefits outweigh risks.

● Drug is a strong negative inotrope and may cause or worsen heart failure, especially in those with cardiomyopathy, heart failure, or low ejection fraction.

● Before giving drug, correct any hypokalemia or hyperkalemia, which may alter drug effects.

● Monitor serum levels; adverse effects increase when trough serum levels exceed 0.7 µg/ml.

● Drug may increase acute and chronic endocardial pacing thresholds and may suppress ventricular escape rhythms.

● Contraindicated in patients with severe or uncontrolled heart failure; cardiogenic shock; SA, AV, or intraventricular disorders of impulse conduction in the absence of a pacemaker; bradycardia; marked hypotension; bronchospastic disorders; or electrolyte imbalance.

● Be prepared to individualize dosage because propafenone pharmacokinetics are complex.

(continued)

Antiarrhythmics *(continued)*

Drug	Indications	Adverse effects*
Type II **Esmolol hydrochloride (Brevibloc)**	• SVT • Intraoperative and postoperative tachycardia and hypertension • Acute myocardial ischemia	• Dizziness • Hypotension • Nausea • Bronchospasm
Propranolol hydrochloride (Inderal)	• Hypertension • Management of angina pectoris • Supraventricular, ventricular, and atrial arrhythmias; tachyarrhythmias caused by excessive catecholamine action during anesthesia, hyperthyroidism, and pheochromocytoma • Reduction in post-MI mortality • Hypertrophic subaortic stenosis	• Fatigue, lethargy • Bradycardia, hypotension, heart failure, worsening of AV block • Agranulocytosis • Bronchospasm
Type III **Amiodarone hydrochloride (Cordarone, Pacerone)**	• Recurrent ventricular fibrillation and unstable ventricular tachycardia; atrial fibrillation; angina; hypertrophic cardiomyopathy • Supraventricular arrhythmias	• Malaise, fatigue • Bradycardia, hypotension, arrhythmias, heart failure, heart block, sinus arrest, asystole • Corneal microdeposits • Nausea, vomiting • Coagulation abnormalities, pancytopenia, neutropenia • Hepatic failure • Severe pulmonary toxicity (pneumonitis, alveolitis), organizing pneumonia, pleuritis • Photosensitivity
Dofetilide (Tikosyn)	• Maintenance of normal sinus rhythm in patients with symptomatic atrial fibrillation or atrial flutter for more than 1 week; conversion of atrial fibrillation and atrial flutter to normal sinus rhythm	• Headache, dizziness, syncope, stroke • Ventricular fibrillation, ventricular tachycardia, torsades de pointes, bradycardia, cardiac arrest, sudden death, MI • Angioedema
Ibutilide fumarate (Corvert)	• Rapid conversion of atrial fibrillation or atrial flutter of recent onset to sinus rhythm	• Sustained ventricular tachycardia, AV block, QT-interval prolongation, bradycardia

*Common or life-threatening only

Special considerations

- Contraindicated in patients with sinus bradycardia, heart block greater than first-degree, cardiogenic shock, or overt heart failure.
- Don't use the 2,500-mg ampule for direct I.V. injection.
- Don't mix the drug with 5% sodium bicarbonate injection USP; they're incompatible.
- Diluted solutions of esmolol hydrochloride are stable for at least 24 hours at room temperature.
- To convert to other antiarrhythmic therapy after control has been achieved with esmolol, reduce esmolol infusion rate by half 30 minutes after giving first dose of other drug. If, after the second dose of the other drug, a satisfactory response is maintained for 1 hour, discontinue esmolol.

- Contraindicated in patients with bronchial asthma, sinus bradycardia and heart block greater than first-degree, cardiogenic shock, and heart failure (unless failure is secondary to a tachyarrhythmia that can be treated with propranolol).
- Monitor serum glucose level; drug may mask signs of hypoglycemia.

- Contraindicated in patients with severe SA node disease resulting in bradycardia. Unless an artificial pacemaker is present, drug is contraindicated in patients with second- or third-degree AV block and in those in whom bradycardia has caused syncope.
- Use with caution in patients already receiving antiarrhythmics, beta blockers, and calcium channel blockers. Use of amiodarone and ritonavir is contraindicated. Use cautiously with amprenavir.
- Decrease digoxin, quinidine, phenytoin, and procainamide doses during amiodarone therapy to avoid toxicity.
- When mixed in D_5W, be aware that amiodarone is incompatible with aminophylline, cefamandole nafate, cefazolin sodium, mezlocillin, heparin sodium, and sodium bicarbonate.
- Administer solutions containing 2 mg/ml or more via a central venous catheter. Use an in-line filter. Infusions are administered in a three-step process: a rapid loading dose, a slow loading dose, and a maintenance infusion.
- Administer amiodarone I.V. infusions exceeding 2 hours in glass or polyolefin bottles containing D_5W.

- Contraindicated in patients with creatinine clearance less than 20 ml/minute and in those with congenital or acquired long QT interval syndrome. Don't use in patients with baseline QT interval greater than 440 msec (500 msec in patients with ventricular conduction abnormalities).
- The patient must be in a facility equipped with ECG monitoring and a staff trained in managing ventricular arrhythmias for at least 3 days; or, the patient must be monitored for a minimum of 12 hours after pharmacologic or electrical conversions to normal sinus rhythm, whichever is longer.
- Withhold class I or III antiarrhythmics for at least three half-lives before starting drug.

- Contraindicated in patients with a history of polymorphic ventricular tachycardia such as torsades de pointes.
- Correct hypokalemia and hypomagnesemia before therapy begins to reduce the potential for proarrhythmia.
- Admixtures of the product, with approved diluents, are chemically and physically stable for 24 hours at room temperature and for 48 hours at refrigerated temperatures.

(continued)

Antiarrhythmics *(continued)*

Drug	Indications	Adverse effects*
Ibutilide fumarate *(continued)*		
Sotalol (Betapace, Betapace AF)	• Documented, life-threatening ventricular arrhythmias (Betapace) • Maintenance of normal sinus rhythm (delay in time to recurrence of atrial fibrillation/atrial flutter [AFIB/AFL]) in patients with symptomatic AFIB/AFL who are currently in sinus rhythm (Betapace AF)	• Bradycardia, palpitations, chest pain, arrhythmias, heart failure, AV block, proarrhythmic events (ventricular tachycardia, PVCs, ventricular fibrillation) • Nausea, vomiting • Dyspnea, bronchospasm
Type IV **Verapamil hydrochloride (Calan, Calan SR, Covera-HS, Isoptin, Isoptin SR, Verelan, Verelan PM)**	• Management of Prinzmetal's or variant angina or unstable or chronic stable angina pectoris • SVTs • Control of ventricular rate in digitalized patients with chronic atrial flutter or fibrillation • Prophylaxis of repetitive paroxysmal supraventricular tachycardia • Hypertension	• Dizziness • Transient hypotension, heart failure, pulmonary edema, bradycardia, AV block, ventricular asystole, ventricular fibrillation • Constipation
Miscellaneous **Adenosine (Adenocard)**	• Conversion of PSVT to sinus rhythm	• Facial flushing • Blurred vision, throat tightness • Groin pressure • Chest pressure, dyspnea, shortness of breath, hyperventilation
Digoxin (Lanoxin)	• Heart failure, atrial fibrillation and flutter, paroxysmal atrial tachycardia	• Fatigue, generalized muscle weakness, agitation, hallucinations, dizziness • Arrhythmias (most commonly, conduction disturbances with or without AV block, PVCs, and supraventricular arrhythmias) that may lead to increased severity of heart failure and hypotension • Yellow-green halos around visual images, blurred vision, light flashes, photophobia, diplopia • Anorexia, nausea

*Common or life-threatening only

Special considerations

● Monitor the patient's ECG continuously throughout drug administration and for at least 4 hours afterward or until QT interval has returned to baseline, because drug can induce or worsen ventricular arrhythmias in some patients. Longer monitoring is required if arrhythmic activity is noted.

● Contraindicated in patients with severe sinus node dysfunction, sinus bradycardia, second- and third-degree AV block in the absence of an artificial pacemaker, congenital or acquired long-QT syndrome, cardiogenic shock, uncontrolled heart failure, and bronchial asthma.
● Monitor serum electrolyte levels regularly, especially if the patient is receiving diuretics. Electrolyte imbalances, such as hypokalemia or hypomagnesemia, may enhance QT interval prolongation and increase risk of serious arrhythmias such as torsades de pointes.
● Adjust dosage slowly, allowing 3 days (or five to six doses if the patient is receiving once-daily doses) between dose increments for adequate monitoring of QT intervals and for drug plasma levels to reach steady state.

● Contraindicated in patients with severe left ventricular dysfunction, cardiogenic shock, second- or third-degree AV block or sick sinus syndrome except in presence of functioning pacemaker, atrial flutter or fibrillation and accessory bypass tract syndrome, severe heart failure (unless secondary to verapamil therapy), and severe hypotension. In addition, I.V. verapamil is contraindicated in patients receiving I.V. beta blockers and in those with ventricular tachycardia.
● If verapamil is added to therapy of the patient receiving digoxin, anticipate a reduction in digoxin dosage by half and monitor subsequent serum drug levels.
● Stop disopyramide 48 hours before starting verapamil, and don't resume until 24 hours after verapamil has been stopped.

● Contraindicated in patients with second- or third-degree heart block or sick sinus syndrome, unless an artificial pacemaker is present, because adenosine decreases conduction through the AV node and may produce first-, second-, or third-degree heart block. These effects are usually transient; however, patients in whom significant heart block develops after a dose of adenosine shouldn't receive additional doses.
● Don't use in atrial fibrillation or atrial flutter.
● Don't use solutions that aren't clear.
● Use Adenocard cautiously in patients with previous history of ventricular fibrillation or those taking digoxin and verapamil.
● Monitor ECG rhythm during administration; drug may cause short-lasting first-, second-, or third-degree heart block or asystole.
● Don't confuse adenosine phosphate with adenosine (Adenocard).

● Contraindicated in patients with digoxin-induced toxicity, ventricular fibrillation, or ventricular tachycardia unless caused by heart failure.
● Watch for ECG changes, including increased PR interval and depression of ST segment; drug may cause false-positive ST-T changes on an ECG during exercise testing.

Antiseizure agents

Drug	Indications	Adverse effects*
Carbamazepine (Carbatrol, Epitol, Tegretol)	• Generalized tonic-clonic, complex-partial, mixed seizure patterns • Bipolar affective disorder • Trigeminal neuralgia	• Vertigo, drowsiness, worsening of seizures • Heart failure, arrhythmias, AV block • Nausea, vomiting • Aplastic anemia, agranulocytosis, thrombocytopenia • Hepatitis • Erythema multiforme, Stevens-Johnson syndrome
Clonazepam (Klonopin, Rivotril)	• Absence and atypical absence seizures, akinetic and myoclonic seizures, generalized tonic-clonic seizures • Parkinsonian dysarthria • Acute manic episodes • Neuralgia	• Drowsiness, ataxia • Palpitations • Leukopenia, thrombocytopenia • Respiratory depression
Diazepam (Apo-Diazepam, Diastat, Novodipam, Valium, Vivol, Zetran)	• Anxiety • Acute alcohol withdrawal • Adjunct to seizure disorders • Adjunct to anesthesia, endoscopic procedures • Cardioversion • Status epilepticus	• Drowsiness, transient amnesia • Hypotension, cardiovascular collapse, bradycardia, phlebitis (at injection site) • Neutropenia • Respiratory depression • Acute withdrawal syndrome after sudden discontinuation in physically dependent persons
Ethosuximide (Zarontin)	• Absence seizures	• Drowsiness, headache, fatigue, dizziness, irritability • Nausea, vomiting, diarrhea, weight loss, cramps, anorexia, epigastric and abdominal pain • Leukopenia, agranulocytosis, pancytopenia, aplastic anemia • Urticaria, pruritic and erythematous rash, Stevens-Johnson syndrome

*Common or life-threatening only

Special considerations

- Contraindicated in patients with history of previous bone marrow suppression, and in patients who have taken an MAO inhibitor within 14 days of therapy.
- Use cautiously in patients with mixed-type seizure disorders.
- For administration through a nasogastric tube, mix with an equal volume of diluent (D_5W or normal saline solution) and administer; then flush with 100 ml of diluent.
- Monitor hematologic and liver function studies.
- Drug may activate latent psychosis, confusion, or agitation in elderly patients; use with caution.

- Contraindicated in patients with significant hepatic disease, in those with sensitivity to benzodiazepines, and in patients with acute angle-closure glaucoma.
- Use cautiously in patients with mixed-type seizures, respiratory disease, or glaucoma.
- Abrupt withdrawal may precipitate status epilepticus.
- Monitor CBC and liver function test results.
- Monitor the patient for oversedation.
- Elderly patients may require lower doses because of diminished renal function and are at greater risk for oversedation from CNS depressants.

- Contraindicated in patients with angle-closure glaucoma; and patients experiencing shock, coma, or acute alcohol intoxication (parenteral form). Also contraindicated in administration with ketoconazole and itraconazole.
- Use cautiously in elderly or debilitated patients and in patients with impaired hepatic or renal function.
- Don't discontinue drug suddenly.
- To enhance taste, mix oral solution with liquids or semisolid foods, such as applesauce or pudding, immediately before administration.
- When prescribed with opiates for endoscopic procedures, expect to reduce opiate dose by at least one-third.
- Dilute parenteral forms of diazepam in normal saline solution.
- Diazepam interacts with plastic. Don't store it in plastic syringes or use plastic administration sets because doing so decreases drug availability.
- For I.V. administration, infuse drug slowly, directly into a large vein, at no more than 5 mg/minute for adults. Don't inject diazepam into small veins, to avoid extravasation into subcutaneous tissue. Observe infusion site for phlebitis.
- Don't mix diazepam with other drugs in a syringe or infusion container.
- Elderly patients are more sensitive to the CNS depressant effects of diazepam. Use cautiously. Parenteral administration of this drug in the elderly is more likely to cause apnea, hypotension, and bradycardia.

- Contraindicated in patients hypersensitive to succinimide derivatives.
- Use cautiously in patients who have hepatic or renal disease.
- Administer ethosuximide with food to minimize GI distress.
- Ethosuximide may cause false-positive Coombs' test results. It also may cause abnormal results in renal function tests.
- Avoid abrupt discontinuation of drug, which may precipitate absence seizures.
- Observe the patient for skin reactions, joint pain, unexplained fever, or unusual bruising or bleeding (which may signal hematologic or other severe adverse reactions).
- Obtain CBC, liver function tests, and urinalysis periodically.
- Monitor plasma levels as ordered; therapeutic plasma levels range from 40 to 100 µg/ml.
- Use cautiously in geriatric patients.

(continued)

Antiseizure agents *(continued)*

Drug	Indications	Adverse effects*
Fosphenytoin sodium (Cerebyx)	• Status epilepticus • Prevention and treatment of seizures during neurosurgery • Short-term substitution for oral phenytoin therapy	• Intracranial hypertension, cerebral hemorrhage, dizziness, somnolence • Hypertension, cardiac arrest, palpitations, bradycardia, QT interval prolongation, ventricular extrasystoles, vasodilation, tachycardia, hypotension • Taste changes • Hypokalemia • Pruritus, rash
Gabapentin (Neurontin)	• Adjunctive treatment of partial seizures with and without secondary generalization • Neuropathic pain	• Fatigue, somnolence, dizziness • Peripheral edema, vasodilation • Diplopia, rhinitis, amblyopia, nystagmus • Leukopenia
Lamotrigine (Lamictal)	• Adjunct therapy for partial seizures caused by epilepsy and Lennox-Gastaut syndrome • Adjunct treatment of Lennox-Gastaut syndrome in patients receiving hepatic enzyme–inducing anticonvulsants with or without concomitant valproic acid therapy	• Dizziness, headache, seizures, suicide attempts • Palpitations, peripheral edema • Diplopia, blurred vision • Stevens-Johnson syndrome, rash, photosensitivity
Phenobarbital (Bellatal, Solfoton); phenobarbital sodium (Luminal Sodium)	• All forms of epilepsy except febrile seizures in children or absence seizures • Status epilepticus • Sedation • Insomnia • Preoperative sedation • Drug withdrawal	• Drowsiness, lethargy, hangover • Bradycardia, hypotension • Respiratory depression, apnea • Rash, erythema multiforme, Stevens-Johnson syndrome • Angioedema, physical and psychological dependence

*Common or life-threatening only

Special considerations

● Contraindicated in patients with sinus bradycardia, SA block, second- and third-degree AV block, and Adams-Stokes syndrome because of the effect of parenteral phenytoin on ventricular automaticity.

● Use cautiously in patients with hypotension, severe myocardial insufficiency, impaired renal or hepatic function, hypoalbuminemia, porphyria, diabetes mellitus, and history of hypersensitivity to similarly structured drugs, such as barbiturates and succinimides.

● Drug is always prescribed and dispensed in PE units. Don't make adjustments in the recommended doses when substituting fosphenytoin for phenytoin and vice versa.

● Administer dose of I.V. fosphenytoin used to treat status epilepticus at a maximum of 150 mg PE/minute.

● Discontinue drug in patients with acute hepatotoxicity.

● Monitor the patient's ECG, blood pressure, and respiration continuously throughout the period of maximum serum phenytoin levels, about 10 to 20 minutes after the end of fosphenytoin infusion.

● Severe cardiovascular complications are most common in elderly or gravely ill patients. Reduction in rate of administration or discontinuation of dosing may be needed.

● Discontinue drug if rash appears. If rash is exfoliative, purpuric, or bullous or if lupus erythematosus, Stevens-Johnson syndrome, or toxic epidermal necrolysis is suspected, don't resume drug; give alternative therapy.

● Following drug use, don't expect to monitor phenytoin levels until conversion to phenytoin is essentially complete — about 2 hours after the end of an I.V. infusion or 4 hours after I.M. administration.

● Use cautiously in patients with altered renal function due to drug accumulation.

● Don't withdraw other anticonvulsants suddenly in patients starting gabapentin therapy. Discontinue drug therapy or substitute alternative drug gradually over at least 1 week to minimize risk of seizures.

● Don't confuse Neurontin with Noroxin (norfloxacin).

● Use cautiously in patients with impaired renal, hepatic, or cardiac function.

● Administer drug without regard to meals.

● Don't stop drug abruptly, because of increased risk of seizures. Instead, expect to taper drug over at least 2 weeks.

● Stop drug immediately if drug-induced rash appears.

● Contraindicated in patients with a history of manifest or latent porphyria, hepatic dysfunction, respiratory disease with dyspnea or obstruction, or nephritis.

● Use cautiously in elderly or debilitated patients and in those with acute or chronic pain, depression, suicidal tendencies, history of drug abuse, blood pressure alterations, cardiovascular disease, shock, or uremia.

● Mix oral solution with water or juice to improve taste. Don't crush or break extended-release form.

● Use a larger vein for I.V. administration to prevent extravasation.

● Avoid I.V. administration at more than 60 mg/minute to prevent hypotension and respiratory depression. It may take up to 30 minutes after I.V. administration to achieve maximum effect.

● Administer parenteral dose within 30 minutes of reconstitution because drug hydrolyzes in solution and on exposure to air.

● Keep emergency resuscitation equipment on hand when administering phenobarbital I.V.

(continued)

Antiseizure agents *(continued)*

Drug	Indications	Adverse effects*
Phenytoin (Dilantin)	• Generalized tonic-clonic seizures, status epilepticus, nonepileptic seizures (post–head trauma, Reye's syndrome) • Neuritic pain (migraine, trigeminal neuralgia, Bell's palsy) • Skeletal muscle relaxant • Prophylactic control of seizures during neurosurgery	• Ataxia, slurred speech, mental confusion, decreased coordination • Hypotension • Nystagmus, diplopia • Thrombocytopenia, leukopenia, agranulocytosis, pancytopenia • Toxic hepatitis • Exfoliative or purpuric dermatitis; Stevens-Johnson syndrome, hirsutism; toxic epidermal necrolysis; photosensitivity
Primidone (Mysoline)	• Generalized tonic-clonic seizures, focal seizures, complex-partial (psychomotor) seizures • Benign familial tremor (essential tremor)	• Drowsiness, ataxia • Diplopia • Thrombocytopenia • Morbilliform rash
Valproic acid (Depakene); divalproex sodium (Depakote, Depakote Sprinkle, Depakote ER); valproate sodium (Depacon)	• Complex partial seizures • Simple and complex absence seizures • Status epilepticus refractory to I.V. diazepam • Mania	• Sedation, headache, dizziness, asthenia, tremor • Vomiting, indigestion, diarrhea, pancreatitis • Thrombocytopenia, hemorrhage, leukopenia, bone marrow suppression • Toxic hepatitis • Erythema multiforme

*Common or life-threatening only

Special considerations

- Contraindicated in patients with sinus bradycardia, SA block, second- or third-degree AV block, or Adams-Stokes syndrome.
- Use cautiously in elderly or debilitated patients; in those with hepatic dysfunction, hypotension, myocardial insufficiency, diabetes, or respiratory depression; and in those receiving hydantoin derivatives.
- Monitor laboratory test results; drug may increase alkaline phosphatase, GGT, and glucose levels and may decrease hemoglobin, hematocrit, and platelet, WBC, RBC, and granulocyte counts.
- Oral or nasogastric feeding may interfere with absorption of oral suspension; separate dosing and feeding times as much as possible, but by no less than 1 hour. During continuous tube feeding, tube should be flushed before and after dose.
- Avoid I.M. administration; it's painful, and drug absorption is erratic.
- Mix I.V. doses in normal saline solution and use within 30 minutes; mixtures with D_5W will precipitate. Don't refrigerate solution, and don't mix with other drugs. In-line filter is recommended.
- If using I.V. bolus, use slow (50 mg/minute) I.V. push or constant infusion; too-rapid I.V. injection may cause hypotension and circulatory collapse. Don't use I.V. push in veins on back of hand; larger veins are needed to prevent discoloration caused by purple glove syndrome.
- When giving I.V., monitor ECG, blood pressure, and respiratory status continuously.
- Monitor serum drug levels because of dose-dependent excretion.
- Abrupt withdrawal may precipitate status epilepticus.

- Contraindicated in patients with porphyria.
- Abrupt withdrawal of drug may cause status epilepticus; reduce dosage gradually.
- Administer a reduced dosage in elderly patients; many have decreased renal function.

- Use cautiously in the elderly and in patients with history of hepatic dysfunction.
- Don't give valproate sodium injection to patients with hepatic disease, significant hepatic dysfunction, or acute head trauma.
- Administer drug with food to minimize GI irritation.
- Administer I.V. as 60-minute infusion at no more than 20 mg/minute.
- Use of valproate sodium injection for periods of more than 14 days hasn't been studied. Switch patients to oral products as soon as clinically feasible.
- Don't withdraw drug abruptly.
- Monitor plasma level; therapeutic range of drug is 50 to 100 µg/ml.
- Watch for tremors; they may indicate need for dosage reduction.
- Evaluate liver function, platelet count, and PT at baseline.

Arterial blood gas interpretation

This chart compares abnormal arterial blood gas values and their significance for patient care.

Disorder	pH	Paco$_2$ (mm Hg)	HCO$_3^-$ (mEq/L)	Compensation
Normal	7.35 to 7.45	35 to 45	22 to 26	
Respiratory acidosis	< 7.35	> 45	• Acute: may be normal • Chronic: > 26	• Renal: increased secretion and excretion of acid; compensation takes 24 hours to begin • Respiratory: rate increases to expel CO_2
Respiratory alkalosis	> 7.45	< 35	• Acute: normal • Chronic: < 22	• Renal: decreased H + secretion and active secretion of HCO$_3^-$ into urine • Respiratory: lungs expel more CO_2 by increasing rate and depth of respirations
Metabolic acidosis	< 7.35	< 35	< 22	• Respiratory: hypoventilation is immediate but limited because of ensuing hypoxemia
Metabolic alkalosis	> 7.45	> 45	> 26	• Renal: more effective but slow to excrete less acid and more base

Assessing abnormal breath sounds

	Description	**Cause**
Crackles	Light crackling, popping, nonmusical sound, like hairs being rubbed together; further classified by pitch: high, medium, or low	Air passing through moisture, especially in the small airways and alveoli, with pulmonary edema; also, alveoli "popping open" in atelectasis
Wheezes	Whistling sound; can be described as sonorous, bubbling, moaning, musical, sibilant and rumbling, crackling, or groaning	Fluid or secretions in the large airways or in airways narrowed by mucus, bronchospasm, or tumor
Rhonchi	Bubbling sound	Air passing through fluid-filled airways, as in upper respiratory tract infection
Pleural friction rub	Superficial squeaking or grating sound, like pieces of sandpaper being rubbed together	Inflamed parietal and visceral pleural linings rubbing together
Grunting	Grunting noise	Physiologic retention of air in lungs to prevent alveolar collapse
Stridor	Crowing noise	Forced movement of air through edematous upper airway (in adults, laryngoedema as in allergic reaction or smoke inhalation; laryngospasm, as in tetany)

Beta-adrenergic blocking agents

Drug	Indications	Adverse effects*
Acebutolol (Sectral)	• Hypertension • Ventricular arrhythmias • Angina	• Bradycardia, heart failure • Bronchospasm
Atenolol (Tenormin)	• Hypertension • Chronic stable angina pectoris • To reduce risk of cardiovascular mortality in patients with acute MI • To slow rapid ventricular response to atrial tachyarrhythmias following acute MI without left-ventricular dysfunction and AV block	• Fatigue, dizziness • Bradycardia, heart failure • Renal impairment, dysuria, nocturia • Agranulocytosis, nonthrombocytopenic or thrombocytopenic purpura, thrombocytopenia • Bronchospasm • Hypoglycemia
Betaxolol hydrochloride (Kerlone)	• Management of hypertension (alone or with other antihypertensives)	• Bradycardia, heart failure • Bronchospasm
Bisoprolol fumarate (Zebeta)	• Hypertension (used alone or with other antihypertensives)	• Headache, hypesthesia, vivid dreams, depression, insomnia • Bradycardia • Leukopenia, thrombocytopenia • Hypoglycemia, hyperkalemia
Carteolol hydrochloride (Cartrol)	• Hypertension • Angina	• Asthenia, paresthesia • Conduction disturbances • Muscle cramps
Labetalol hydrochloride (Normodyne, Trandate)	• Hypertension, pheochromocytoma • Severe hypertension and hypertensive emergencies, hypertension due to clonidine withdrawal • Controlled hypotension during anesthesia	• Orthostatic hypotension, dizziness, ventricular arrhythmias • Bronchospasm • Toxic myopathy

*Common or life-threatening only

Special considerations

● Contraindicated in patients with persistent severe bradycardia, second- and third-degree heart block, overt cardiac failure, and cardiogenic shock.
● Use cautiously in patients at risk for heart failure, those with impaired hepatic function, and those with bronchospastic disease, diabetes, hyperthyroidism, and peripheral vascular disease.
● Carefully monitor blood pressure during dosage adjustment.

● Contraindicated in patients with sinus bradycardia, greater than first-degree heart block, overt cardiac failure, or cardiogenic shock.
● Use cautiously in patients at risk for heart failure and in those with bronchospastic disease, diabetes, and hyperthyroidism.
● I.V. atenolol affords a rapid onset of the protective effects of beta blockade against reinfarction.
● Patients who can't tolerate I.V. atenolol after an MI may be candidates for oral atenolol therapy. Some evidence suggests that gastric absorption of atenolol may be delayed in the early phase of MI. This may result from the physiologic changes that accompany MI or from the effects of morphine, which is commonly administered to treat chest pain. However, oral therapy alone may still provide benefits.
● Administer I.V. atenolol undiluted or diluted at no more than 1 mg/minute.

● Contraindicated in patients hypersensitive to drug and those with severe bradycardia, greater than first-degree heart block, cardiogenic shock, or uncontrolled heart failure.
● Monitor serum glucose level; signs of hypoglycemia may be masked in patients taking beta blockers.

● Contraindicated in patients with cardiogenic shock, overt cardiac failure, marked sinus bradycardia, or second- or third-degree AV block.
● Use cautiously in patients with bronchospastic disease.
● Patients with renal or hepatic dysfunction or bronchospastic disease unresponsive to or intolerant of other antihypertensive therapies should start therapy at low daily doses. Have a $beta_2$-adrenergic agonist (bronchodilator) readily available for patients with bronchospastic disease. Taper bisoprolol therapy over 1 week while carefully observing the patient. Worsening of angina pectoris, MI, and ventricular arrhythmia has been observed in patients with coronary artery disease after abrupt cessation of therapy with beta blockers. If withdrawal symptoms occur, restart bisoprolol therapy, at least temporarily.
● Monitor serum glucose level; signs of hypoglycemia may be masked in patients taking beta blockers.

● Contraindicated in patients with bronchial asthma, severe COPD, sinus bradycardia, second- or third-degree AV block, overt cardiac failure, or cardiogenic shock.
● Monitor the patient for signs and symptoms of heart failure. Discontinue drug at first sign of cardiac failure.

● Contraindicated in patients with severe and prolonged hypotension, patients with a history of obstructive airway disease such as bronchial asthma, and patients with overt cardiac failure, greater than first-degree heart block, cardiogenic shock, or severe bradycardia.
● Keep patients receiving I.V. labetalol infusion in the supine position during the infusion and for 3 hours after the infusion.

(continued)

Beta-adrenergic blocking agents *(continued)*

Drug	Indications	Adverse effects*
Metoprolol succinate (Toprol XL); metoprolol tartrate (Lopressor)	• Mild to severe hypertension • Early and late intervention in acute MI • Atrial tachyarrhythmias following acute MI • Angina • Stable, symptomatic heart failure of ischemic, hypertensive, or cardiomyopathic origin	• Fatigue, dizziness • Bradycardia, hypotension, heart failure, arrhythmias • Bronchospasm
Nadolol (Corgard)	• Hypertension • Long-term prophylactic management of chronic stable angina pectoris • Arrhythmias	• Bradycardia, heart failure • Increased airway resistance
Pindolol (Visken)	• Hypertension • Angina	• Insomnia, fatigue, vertigo, nervousness • Edema, bradycardia, heart failure • Nausea • Muscle pain, joint pain • Increased airway resistance, dyspnea
Sotalol (Betapace, Betapace AF)	• Documented, life-threatening ventricular arrhythmias (Betapace) • Maintenance of normal sinus rhythm (delay in time to recurrence of atrial fibrillation/atrial flutter [AFIB/AFL]) in patients with symptomatic AFIB/AFL who are currently in sinus rhythm (Betapace AF)	• Bradycardia, palpitations, chest pain, arrhythmias, heart failure, AV block, proarrhythmic events (ventricular tachycardia, PVCs, ventricular fibrillation) • Nausea, vomiting • Dyspnea, bronchospasm
Timolol maleate (Blocadren)	• Hypertension • Reduction of risk of cardiovascular mortality and reinfarction after MI • Angina	• Stroke, arrhythmias, bradycardia, heart failure • Bronchospasm, pulmonary edema • Pruritus

*Common or life-threatening only

Special considerations

● Contraindicated in patients with sinus bradycardia, heart block greater than first-degree, cardiogenic shock, or overt cardiac failure when used to treat hypertension or angina. When used to treat MI, drug also is contraindicated in patients with heart rate less than 45 beats/minute, second- or third-degree heart block, PR interval of 0.24 second or longer with first-degree heart block, systolic blood pressure less than 100 mm Hg, or moderate to severe cardiac failure.

● When this drug is used for angina, it's used only if AV block and left ventricular dysfunction aren't present.

● If heart failure worsens, expect an increase in diuretic doses and possible lowered dose of Toprol-XL or temporary discontinuation. Dose isn't increased until symptoms of worsening heart failure are stabilized. Monitor heart rate closely, and expect to decrease dose of Toprol XL if the patient experiences symptomatic bradycardia.

● Contraindicated in patients with bronchial asthma, sinus bradycardia, greater than first-degree heart block, overt cardiac failure, and cardiogenic shock.

● Use cautiously in patients with hyperthyroidism, heart failure, diabetes, chronic bronchitis, emphysema, or impaired renal or hepatic function, and in heart failure unless secondary to tachyarrhythmia that's treatable with beta blockers.

● Monitor the patient for reflex bradycardia, which may be treated with atropine.

● Contraindicated in patients with bronchial asthma, severe bradycardia, heart block greater than first-degree, cardiogenic shock, or overt cardiac failure. Also contraindicated in patients taking thioridazine.

● Always check patient's apical pulse rate before giving drug. If extremes in pulse rate are detected, withhold drug and reevaluate drug therapy.

● Keep in mind that beta blockers may mask tachycardia caused by hyperthyroidism. In patients with suspected thyrotoxicosis, withdraw beta blocker gradually to avoid thyroid storm.

● Monitor glucose levels in diabetic patients closely. Drug masks certain signs and symptoms of hypoglycemia.

● Contraindicated in patients with severe sinus node dysfunction, sinus bradycardia, second- and third-degree AV block in the absence of an artificial pacemaker, congenital or acquired long-QT syndrome, cardiogenic shock, uncontrolled heart failure, or bronchial asthma.

● Monitor serum electrolyte levels regularly, especially if the patient is receiving diuretics. Electrolyte imbalances, such as hypokalemia or hypomagnesemia, may enhance QT interval prolongation and increase risk of serious arrhythmias such as torsades de pointes.

● Adjust dosage slowly, allowing 3 days (or five to six doses, if the patient is receiving once-daily doses) between dose increments for adequate monitoring of QT intervals and for drug plasma levels to reach steady state.

● Contraindicated in patients with bronchial asthma, severe COPD, sinus bradycardia and heart block greater than first-degree, cardiogenic shock, heart failure, or overt cardiac failure.

● Use cautiously in patients with diabetes, hyperthyroidism, or respiratory disease (especially nonallergic bronchospasm or emphysema).

● Use oral form cautiously in patients with compensated heart failure and hepatic or renal disease.

Blood compatibility

Precise typing and crossmatching of donor and recipient blood can avoid transfusions of incompatible blood, which can be fatal. RBCs are classified as type A, B, or AB, depending on the antigen detected on the cell, or type O, which has no detectable A or B antigens. Similarly, blood plasma has or lacks anti-A or anti-B antibodies.

A person with type O blood is a universal donor. Because his blood lacks A or B antigens, it can be transfused in an emergency in limited amounts to any patient regardless of blood type and with little risk of reaction. A person with AB blood is a universal recipient. Because his blood lacks A and B antibodies, he can receive types A, B, or O blood (given as packed RBCs). This chart shows ABO compatibility at a glance.

Blood group	Antibodies in plasma	Compatible RBCs	Compatible plasma
Recipient			
O	Anti-A and Anti-B	O	O, A, B, AB
A	Anti-B	A, O	A, AB
B	Anti-A	B, O	B, AB
AB	Neither Anti-A nor Anti-B	AB, A, B, O	AB
Donor			
O	Anti-A and Anti-B	O, A, B, AB	O
A	Anti-B	A, AB	A, O
B	Anti-A	B, AB	B, O
AB	Neither Anti-A nor Anti-B	AB	AB, A, B, O

Body surface area nomogram

HEIGHT **BODY SURFACE AREA** **WEIGHT**

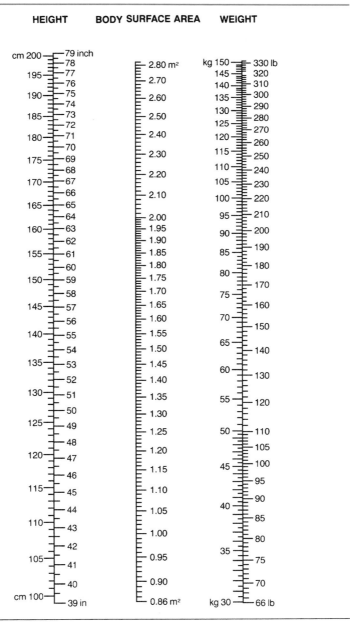

Source: Geigy Scientific Tables; 1990, 8th ed., Vol 5, p. 105 ©Novartis.

Brain injury location

This chart highlights the deficits that may be noted when a patient experiences a brain injury to the lobes of the cerebrum or cerebellum.

Area of injury	Possible associated deficits
Cerebrum	
Frontal lobe	• Concentration • Abstract thought • Memory • Motor function • Word formulation (if Broca's area [located on dominant side] is injured) • Affect • Judgment • Personality • Inhibitions
Parietal lobe	• Sensory function, including texture, size, and shape • Awareness of one's body in space, orientation in space • Spatial (three-dimensional) relations • Taste perception
Temporal lobe	• Auditory reception • Integration of somatization, vision, and hearing • Speech (if Wernicke's area is injured)
Occipital lobe	• Visual interpretation
Cerebellum	• Orderly sequencing of skilled movements • Prediction of speed or distance • Voluntary movement • Equilibrium • Integration of sensations • Sense of position

Calcium correction formula

Calcium occurs in the body in two forms: ionized or protein-bound. As a result, serum calcium levels must be evaluated in light of the patient's serum albumin level. If albumin levels are decreased, the amount of protein-bound calcium is also reduced, causing a significant decrease in the total serum calcium level. To adjust for this, several formulas may be used to calculate a corrected calcium level. (The formula used depends on the laboratory.) Three examples are shown here.

1.
Corrected calcium mg/dl =
Measured total calcium level mg/dl + 0.8
(4.4 [which represents an average serum albumin level] – serum albumin gm/dl)

2.
Corrected calcium mg/dl = Calcium level mg/dl – 0.8 (albumin g/dl – 4)

3.
Multiply the change in albumin by 0.8 (constant),
and then add the results to the patient's serum calcium level.

Central venous access devices

Device and description	Use
Short-term central venous (CV) catheter	• Short-term CV access • Emergency access
Groshong catheter	• Long-term CV access
Hickman catheter	• Long-term CV access • Home I.V. therapy
Broviac catheter	• Long-term CV access • Patients, such as children and elderly, with small central vessels
Hickman-Broviac catheter	• Long-term CV access • Patients in need of multiple infusions
Peripherally inserted central catheter	• Long-term CV access • Patients with poor CV access or at risk for fatal complications from CV catheter insertion • Patients who need CV access but are having or have had head and neck surgery

Nursing considerations

- Catheter may be single or multilumen.
- Assist with percutaneous placement.
- Expect catheter to be changed every 3 to 7 days or according to your facility's policy.
- Minimize patient movement.
- Apply dressing and change it according to your facility's policy (for example, change transparent dressing every 5 to 7 days; change gauze dressings on alternate days or with catheter change).
- Flush catheter (each lumen) with heparin, 2 to 3 ml per day.
- Use saline to flush the catheter before and after medication administration.
- Monitor insertion site for signs and symptoms of infection and clot formation.
- Use the same lumen each time for the same task.

- Catheter requires surgical insertion and is tunneled.
- Catheter has a closed end with a pressure-sensitive two-way valve, eliminating the need for frequent heparin flushes.
- Change surgical sites' dressings after catheter insertion.
- Handle catheter carefully.
- Check the external portion of the catheter frequently for kinks and leaks.
- Have a repair kit readily available.
- Flush with normal saline, 5 to 10 ml per week, to maintain patency.
- Flush catheter with enough saline solution to clear it after drawing or administering blood.
- Apply dressing and change it according to your facility's policy (for example, change transparent dressing every 5 to 7 days; change gauze dressings on alternate days).

- Catheter requires surgical insertion and is tunneled.
- Change surgical sites' dressings after catheter insertion.
- Handle catheter carefully.
- Observe the catheter frequently for kinks and tears.
- Have a repair kit readily available.
- Clamp the catheter with a nonserrated clamp anytime it becomes disconnected or open.
- Apply dressing and change it according to your facility's policy (for example, change transparent dressing every 5 to 7 days; change gauze dressings on alternate days)
- Flush with normal saline before and after administration of medications.
- Routinely flush with 3 ml heparin every 1 to 2 days while in use and at least weekly when not in use.

- The lumen of this catheter is smaller than that of the Hickman catheter.
- Follow the same measures as for a Hickman catheter.
- Check facility's policy before drawing blood or administering blood or blood products (smaller lumen may limit catheter's uses).

- Double-lumen Hickman catheter allows for sampling and administration of blood.
- Use Broviac lumen to administer I.V. fluids, including total parenteral nutrition.
- Label each lumen with its use to prevent confusion.
- Follow the same measures as for single-lumen Hickman catheter.

- Assist with insertion (above the antecubital fossa) at bedside, or insert (if specially trained to do so).
- The basilic vein is preferred over the cephalic vein.
- The lumen is smaller than that of tunneled catheters.
- Check frequently for signs and symptoms of phlebitis and thrombus formation.
- Use an armboard as necessary.
- Because of the length of the catheter, CV pressure measurements may be altered.

(continued)

Central venous access devices *(continued)*

Device and description	Use
Peripherally inserted central catheter *(continued)*	
Implanted ports	● Long-term CV access for intermittent infusions

Nursing considerations

- Flush with normal saline before and after medication administration.
- Flush with heparin (100 U/ml), 3 ml per day; alternatively, flush with heparin (10 U/ml), 3 ml three times per week
- Change dressing at insertion site 24 hours after insertion; thereafter, change according to your facility's policy (for example, change transparent dressing every 5 to 7 days; change gauze dressings on alternate days).

- Insertion occurs in the operating room or radiology; port is placed subcutaneously with attached catheter threaded into the superior vena cava.
- May be single-lumen, double-lumen, or low-profile ports.
- Use special noncoring needle (Huber needle) to access port; change needle every 7 days if kept in place for continuous infusions.
- Apply topical anesthetics, such as EMLA cream, over the port area for 1 hour prior to needle insertion to minimize discomfort when accessing port.
- Flush with normal saline before and after medication administration.
- Flush every 4 weeks with normal saline and heparin when not in use.
- When in use, change transparent dressing every week or gauze dressing on alternate days.

Cincinnati prehospital stroke scale

If any one of the three signs described here is abnormal, the probability of a stroke is 72%.

Facial droop
Tell the patient to show his teeth or smile. If he hasn't had a stroke, both sides of his face will move equally. If he has had a stroke, one side of his face won't move as well as the other side.

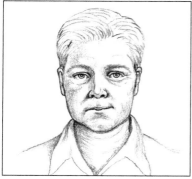

NORMAL

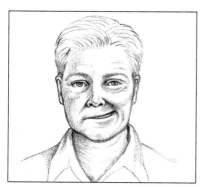

STROKE PATIENT WITH FACIAL DROOP ON RIGHT SIDE OF FACE

Arm drift
Tell the patient to close her eyes and hold both arms straight out in front of her for 20 seconds. If she hasn't had a stroke, her arms won't move or, if they do move, they'll move the same amount. Other findings, such as pronator grip, may be helpful.

If the patient has had a stroke, one arm won't move or one arm will drift down compared with the other arm.

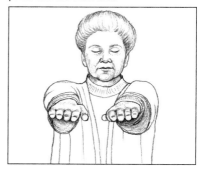

NORMAL RESPONSE

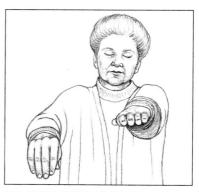

ONE-SIDED MOTOR WEAKNESS (RIGHT ARM)

Abnormal speech
Have the patient say "You can't teach an old dog new tricks." If he hasn't had a stroke, he'll use correct words and his speech won't be slurred. If he has had a stroke, his words will be slurred, he may use the wrong words, or he may be unable to speak at all.

Adapted with permission from Kothari, R., et al. "Early Stroke Recognition: Developing an Out-of-Hospital NIH Stroke Scale," *Academy of Emergency Medicine* 4(10):986-90, October 1997.

Common antidotes

Drug or toxin	Antidote
Acetaminophen	Acetylcysteine (Mucomyst)
Anticholinergics	Physostigmine (Antilirium)
Benzodiazepines	Flumazenil (Romazicon)
Calcium channel blockers	Calcium chloride
Cyanide	Amyl nitrate, sodium nitrate, and sodium thiosulfate (Cyanide Antidote Kit); methylene blue; hydroxocobalamin (Fromnitroprusside)
Digoxin, cardiac glycosides	Digoxin immune fab (Digibind)
Ethylene glycol	Ethanol
Heparin	Protamine sulfate
Insulin-induced hypoglycemia	Glucagon
Iron	Deferoxamine mesylate (Desferal)
Lead	Edetate calcium disodium (Calcium Disodium Versenate)
Opioids	Naloxone (Narcan), nalmefene (Revex), naltrexone (ReVia)
Organophosphates, anticholinesterases	Atropine, pralodixime (Protopam)

Compatibility in a syringe

KEY

Y = compatible for at least 30 minutes
P = provisionally compatible; administer within 15 minutes
P(5) = provisionally compatible; administer within 5 minutes
N = not compatible
* = conflicting data
(A blank space indicates no available data.)

	atropine sulfate	butorphanol tartrate	chlorpromazine HCl	cimetidine HCl	codeine phosphate	dexamethasone sodium phosphate	dimenhydrinate	diphenhydramine HCl	droperidol	fentanyl citrate	glycopyrrolate	heparin Na	hydromorphone HCl	hydroxyzine HCl	meperidine HCl	metoclopramide HCl
atropine sulfate	■	Y	P	Y			P	P	P	P	Y	P(5)	Y	P*	P	P
butorphanol tartrate	Y	■	Y	Y			N	Y	Y	Y				Y	Y	Y
chlorpromazine HCl	P	Y	■	N			N	P	P	P	Y	N	Y	P	P	P
cimetidine HCl	Y	Y	N	■			Y	Y	Y	Y	P(5)*		Y	Y	Y	
codeine phosphate					■						Y			Y		
dexamethasone sodium phosphate						■		N*			N		N*			Y
dimenhydrinate	P	N	N				■	P	P	P	N	P(5)	Y	N	P	P
diphenhydramine HCl	P	Y	P	Y		N*	P	■	P	P	Y		Y	P	P	Y
droperidol	P	Y	P	Y			P	P	■	P	Y	N		P	P	P
fentanyl citrate	P	Y	P	Y			P	P	P	■		P(5)	Y	P	P	P
glycopyrrolate	Y		Y	Y	Y	N	N	Y	Y		■		Y	Y	Y	
heparin Na	P(5)		N	P(5)*			P(5)		N	P(5)		■			N	P(5)*
hydromorphone HCl	Y		Y	Y		N*	Y	Y		Y	Y		■	Y		
hydroxyzine HCl	P*	Y	P	Y	Y		N	P	P	P	Y		Y	■	P	P
meperidine HCl	P	Y	P	Y			P	P	P	P	Y	N		P	■	P
metoclopramide HCl	P	Y	P			Y	P	Y	P	P	P(5)*		P	P		■
midazolam HCl	Y	Y	Y	Y			N	Y	Y	Y	Y		Y	Y	Y	Y
morphine sulfate	P	Y	P	Y			P	P	P	P	Y	N*		P	N	P
nalbuphine HCl	Y			Y			Y	Y		Y			Y			
pentazocine lactate	P	Y	P	Y			P	P	P	P	N	N	Y	P	P	P
pentobarbital Na	P	N	N	N			N	N	N	N	N		Y	N	N	
perphenazine	Y	Y	Y	Y			Y	Y	Y	Y				Y	Y	P*
phenobarbital Na												P(5)				
prochlorperazine edisylate	P	Y	P	Y			N	P	P	P	Y		N*	P	P	P
promazine HCl	P		P	Y			N	P	P	P	Y			P	P	P
promethazine HCl	P	Y	P	Y			N	P	P	P	Y	N	Y	P	P	P*
ranitidine HCl	Y		N*		Y	Y	Y		Y	Y			Y	N	Y	Y
scopolamine HBr	P	Y	P	Y			P	P	P	P	Y		Y	P	P	P
sodium bicarbonate												N				N
thiethylperazine maleate		Y												Y		
thiopental Na			N				N	N			N				N	

midazolam HCl	morphine sulfate	nalbuphine HCl	pentazocine lactate	pentobarbital Na	perphenazine	phenobarbital Na	prochlorperazine edisylate	promazine HCl	promethazine HCl	ranitidine HCl	scopolamine HBr	sodium bicarbonate	thiethylperazine maleate	thiopental Na	
Y	P	Y	P	P	Y		P	P	P	Y	P				atropine sulfate
Y	Y		Y	N	Y		Y		Y		Y		Y		butorphanol tartrate
Y	P		P	N	Y		P	P	P	N*	P			N	chlorpromazine HCl
Y	Y	Y	Y	N	Y		Y	Y	Y		Y				cimetidine HCl
															codeine phosphate
											Y				dexamethasone sodium phosphate
N	P		P	N	Y		N	N	N	Y	P			N	dimenhydrinate
Y	P	Y	P	N	Y		P	P	P	Y	P			N	diphenhydramine HCl
Y	P	Y	P	N	Y		P	P	P		P				droperidol
Y	P		P	N	Y		P	P	P	Y	P				fentanyl citrate
Y	Y	Y	N	N			Y	Y	Y	Y	Y	N		N	glycopyrrolate
	N*		N			P(5)		N							heparin Na
Y		Y	Y				N*		Y	Y	Y		Y		hydromorphone HCl
Y	P	Y	P	N	Y		P	P	P	N	P				hydroxyzine HCl
Y	N		P	N	Y		P	P	P	Y	P			N	meperidine HCl
Y	P		P	P*			P	P	P*	Y	P	N			metoclopramide HCl
	Y	Y		N	N		N	Y	Y	N	Y		Y		midazolam HCl
Y			P	N*	Y		P*	P	P*	Y	P			N	morphine sulfate
Y				N			Y		N*	Y	Y		Y		nalbuphine HCl
	P			N	Y		P	P*	P*	Y	P				pentazocine lactate
N	N*	N	N		N		N	N	N	N	P	Y		Y	pentobarbital Na
N	Y		Y	N			Y		Y	Y	Y		N		perphenazine
										N					phenobarbital Na
N	P*	Y	P	N	Y			P	P	Y	P			N	prochlorperazine edisylate
Y	P		P*	N			P		P		P				promazine HCl
Y	P*	N*	P*	N	Y		P	P		Y	P			N	promethazine HCl
N	Y	Y	Y	N	Y	N	Y		Y		Y		Y		ranitidine HCl
Y	P	Y	P	P	Y		P	P	P	Y				Y	scopolamine HBr
		Y												N	sodium bicarbonate
Y		Y		N						Y				N	thiethylperazine maleate
	N			Y			N		N		Y	N			thiopental Na

Conversion factors

Weight conversion
To convert a patient's weight in pounds to kilograms, divide the number of pounds by 2.2 kg; to convert a patient's weight in kilograms to pounds, multiply the number of kilograms by 2.2 lbs.

Temperature conversion
To convert Fahrenheit to Celsius, subtract 32 from the temperature in Fahrenheit and then multiply that number by 5/9; to convert Celsius to Fahrenheit, multiply the temperature in Celsius by 9/5 and then add 32.

$$(F - 32) \times 5/9 = C \text{ degrees}$$

$$(C \times 9/5) + 32 = F \text{ degrees}$$

Pounds	Kilograms
10	4.5
20	9
30	13.6
40	18.1
50	22.7
60	27.2
70	31.8
80	36.3
90	40.9
100	45.4
110	49.9
120	54.4
130	59
140	63.5
150	68
160	72.6
170	77.1
180	81.6
190	86.2
200	90.8

Fahrenheit degrees (F°)	Celsius degrees (C°)	Fahrenheit degrees (F°)	Celsius degrees (C°)
89.6	32	101	38.3
91.4	33	101.2	38.4
93.2	34	101.4	38.6
94.3	34.6	101.8	38.8
95.0	35	102	38.9
95.4	35.2	102.2	39
96.2	35.7	102.6	39.2
96.8	36	102.8	39.3
97.2	36.2	103	39.4
97.6	36.4	103.2	39.6
98	36.7	103.4	39.7
98.6	37	103.6	39.8
99	37.2	104	40
99.3	37.4	104.4	40.2
99.7	37.6	104.6	40.3
100	37.8	104.8	40.4
100.4	38	105	40.6
100.8	38.2		

Solid equivalents

Milligram (mg)	Gram (g)	Grain (gr)
1,000	1	15
600 (or 650)	0.6	10
500	0.5	7.5
300 (or 325)	0.3	5
200	0.2	3
100	0.1	1.5
60 (or 65)	0.06	1
30	0.03	½
15	0.15	¼

Liquid equivalents

Metric (ml)	Apothecary	Household
—	1 minim = 1 drop (gtt)	—
1	16 minims	—
4	1 dram	—
5	—	1 teaspoon (tsp)
15	4 drams or ½ ounce	1 tablespoon (tbsp, or T)
30	8 drams or 1 ounce	1 ounce or 2 tbsp
50	—	1 pint
1,000	—	1 quart or 2 pints

Coumadin reversal protocol

This protocol identifies the steps for correcting excess anticoagulation from the drug warfarin (Coumadin).

● Assess the International Normalized Ratio (INR) and, if elevated beyond accepted levels, stop the warfarin and notify the physician.

● If the INR ranges from 4 to 10:
1. Administer vitamin K 1 to 2 mg orally (dilute the parenteral form in a flavored drink).
2. If the patient isn't able to take the drug orally, administer vitamin K 0.5 to 1 mg I.V.

● If the INR is greater than 10 and the patient exhibits no signs or symptoms of bleeding:
1. Administer vitamin K 3 mg subcutaneously or by slow I.V. infusion.
2. Recheck the INR in 6 hours.
3. Repeat vitamin K administration if INR remains unchanged.

● If the INR is elevated to any level and the patient is exhibiting signs and symptoms of severe bleeding:
1. Administer vitamin K 10 mg subcutaneously or by slow I.V. infusion.
2. Administer fresh frozen plasma 15 ml/kg.
3. Administer prothrombin complex concentrate 50 U/kg.
4. Recheck INR in 6 hours.

Crisis values of laboratory tests

The abnormal laboratory test values listed here have immediate life-or-death significance to the patient. Report such values to the patient's physician immediately.

Test	Low value	Common causes and effects	High value	Common causes and effects
Ammonia	< 15 µg/dl	Renal failure	> 50 µg/dl	Severe hepatic disease: hepatic coma, Reye's syndrome, GI hemorrhage, heart failure
Calcium, serum	< 7 mg/dl	Vitamin D or parathyroid hormone deficiency: tetany, seizures	> 12 mg/dl	Hyperparathyroidism: coma
Carbon dioxide and bicarbonate, blood	< 10 mEq/L	Complex pattern of metabolic and respiratory factors	> 40 mEq/L	Complex pattern of metabolic and respiratory factors
Creatine kinase isoenzymes (CK-MB)			> 5%	Acute myocardial infarction (MI)
Creatinine, serum			> 4 mg/dl	Renal failure: coma
D-dimer, serum or cerebrospinal fluid (CSF)			> 250 µg/ml	Disseminated intravascular coagulation (DIC), pulmonary embolism, arterial or venous thrombosis, subarachnoid hemorrhage (CSF only), secondary fibrinolysis
Glucose, blood	< 40 mg/dl	Excessive insulin administration: brain damage	> 300 mg/dl (with ketonemia and electrolyte imbalance)	Diabetes: diabetic coma
Gram stain, CSF			Gram-positive or gram-negative	Bacterial meningitis

(continued)

Crisis values of laboratory tests *(continued)*

Test	Low value	Common causes and effects	High value	Common causes and effects
Hemoglobin	< 8 g/dl	Hemorrhage or vitamin B_{12} or iron deficiency: heart failure	> 18 g/dl	Chronic obstructive pulmonary disease: thrombosis, polycythemia vera
International Normalized Ratio			> 3.0	DIC, uncontrolled oral anticoagulation
Partial pressure of carbon dioxide, in arterial blood	< 20 mm Hg	Complex pattern of metabolic and respiratory factors	> 70 mm Hg	Complex pattern of metabolic and respiratory factors
Partial pressure of oxygen, in arterial blood	< 50 mm Hg	Complex pattern of metabolic and respiratory factors		
Partial thromboplastin time			> 40 seconds (> 70 seconds for patient on heparin)	Anticoagulation factor deficiency: hemorrhage
pH, arterial blood	< 7.2	Complex pattern of metabolic and respiratory factors	> 7.6	Complex pattern of metabolic and respiratory factors
Platelet count	< 50,000/µl	Bone marrow suppression: hemorrhage	> 500,000/µl	Leukemia, reaction to acute bleeding: hemorrhage
Potassium, serum	< 3 mEq/L	Vomiting and diarrhea, diuretic therapy: cardiotoxicity, arrhythmia, cardiac arrest	> 6 mEq/L	Renal disease, diuretic therapy: cardiotoxicity, arrhythmia
Prothrombin time			> 14 seconds (> 20 seconds for patient on warfarin)	Anticoagulant therapy, anticoagulation factor deficiency: hemorrhage

Crisis values of laboratory tests *(continued)*

Test	Low value	Common causes and effects	High value	Common causes and effects
Sodium, serum	< 120 mEq/L	Diuretic therapy: cardiac failure	> 160 mEq/L	Dehydration: vascular collapse
Troponin I			> 2 µg/ml	Acute MI
White blood cell (WBC) count	< 2,000/µl	Bone marrow suppression: infection	> 20,000/µl	Leukemia: infection
WBC count, CSF			> 10/µl	Meningitis, encephalitis: infection

Dialyzable drugs

The amount of a drug removed by dialysis differs among patients and depends on several factors, including the patient's condition, the drug's properties, length of dialysis and dialysate used, rate of blood flow or dwell time, and purpose of dialysis. This table indicates the effect of hemodialysis on selected drugs.

Drug	Level reduced by hemodialysis	Drug	Level reduced by hemodialysis
Acetaminophen	Yes (may not influence toxicity)	Cefepime	Yes
		Cefonicid	Yes (only by 20%)
Acyclovir	Yes	Cefoperazone	Yes
Allopuril	Yes	Cefotaxime	Yes
Alprazolam	No	Cefotetan	Yes (only by 20%)
Amikacin	Yes	Cefoxitin	Yes
Amiodarone	No	Ceftazidime	Yes
Amitriptyline	No	Ceftizoxime	Yes
Amoxicillin	Yes	Ceftriaxone	No
Amoxicillin/Clavulanate potassium	Yes	Cefuroxime	Yes
Amphotericin B	No	Cephalexin	Yes
Ampicillin	Yes	Cephalothin	Yes
Ampicillin/Clavulanate potassium	Yes	Cephradine	Yes
		Chloral hydrate	Yes
Aspirin	Yes	Chlorambucil	No
Atenolol	Yes	Chlordiazepoxide	No
Azathioprine	Yes	Chloroquine	No
Aztreonam	Yes	Chlorpheniramine	No
Captopril	Yes	Chlorpromazine	No
Carbamazepine	No	Chlorthalidone	No
Carbenicillin	Yes	Cimetidine	Yes
Carmustine	No	Ciprofloxacin	Yes (only by 20%)
Cefaclor	Yes	Cisplatin	No
Cefadroxil	Yes	Clindamycin	No
Cefamandole	Yes	Clofibrate	No
Cefazolin	Yes	Clonazepam	No

Dialyzable drugs *(continued)*

Drug	Level reduced by hemodialysis	Drug	Level reduced by hemodialysis
Clonidine	No	Flucytosine	Yes
Clorazepate	No	Fluorouracil	Yes
Cloxacillin	No	Fluoxetine	No
Codeine	No	Flurazepam	No
Colchicine	No	Fosinopril	No
Cortisone	No	Furosemide	No
Co-trimoxazole	Yes	Gabapentin	Yes
Cyclophosphamide	Yes	Ganciclovir	Yes
Diazepam	No	Gemfibrozil	No
Diclofenac	No	Gentamicin	Yes
Dicloxacillin	No	Glipizide	No
Digoxin	No	Glutethimide	Yes
Diltiazem	No	Glyburide	No
Diphenhydramine	No	Guanfacine	No
Dipyridamole	No	Haloperidol	No
Disopyramide	Yes	Heparin	No
Doxazosin	No	Hydralazine	No
Doxepin	No	Hydrochlorothiazide	No
Doxorubicin	No	Hydroxyzine	No
Doxycycline	No	Ibuprofen	No
Enalapril	Yes	Imipenem/Cilastatin	Yes
Erythromycin	Yes (only by 20%)	Imipramine	No
Ethambutol	Yes (only by 20%	Indapamide	No
Ethchlorvynol	Yes	Indomethacin	No
Ethosuximide	Yes	Insulin	No
Famotidine	No	Irbesartan	No
Fenoprofen	No	Iron dextran	No
Flecainide	No	Isoniazid	Yes
Fluconazole	Yes	Isosorbide	No

(continued)

Dialyzable drugs *(continued)*

Drug	Level reduced by hemodialysis	Drug	Level reduced by hemodialysis
Isradipine	No	Minocycline	No
Kanamycin	Yes	Minoxidil	Yes
Ketoconazole	No	Misoprostol	No
Ketoprofen	Yes	Morphine	No
Labetalol	No	Nabumetone	No
Levofloxacin	No	Nadolol	Yes
Lidocaine	No	Nafcillin	No
Lithium	Yes	Naproxen	No
Lomustine	No	Nelfinavir	Yes
Loracarbef	Yes	Netilmicin	Yes
Loratadine	No	Nifedipine	No
Lorazepam	No	Nimodipine	No
Mechlorethamine	No	Nitrofurantoin	Yes
Mefenamic acid	No	Nitroglycerin	No
Meperidine	No	Nitroprusside	Yes
Mercaptopurine	Yes	Nizatidine	No
Methadone	No	Nofloxacin	No
Methicillin	No	Notriptyline	No
Methotrexate	Yes	Ofloxacin	Yes
Methyldopa	Yes	Olanzapine	No
Methylprednisolone	No	Omeprazole	No
Metoclopramide	No	Oxazepam	No
Metolazone	No	Paroxetine	No
Metoprolol	No	Penicillin G	Yes
Metronidazole	Yes	Pentamidine	No
Mexiletine	Yes	Pentazocine	Yes
Mezlocillin	Yes	Phenobarbital	Yes
Miconazole	No	Phenylbutazone	No
Midazolam	No	Phenytoin	No

Dialyzable drugs *(continued)*

Drug	Level reduced by hemodialysis	Drug	Level reduced by hemodialysis
Piperacillin	Yes	Sulbactam	Yes
Piroxicam	No	Sulindac	No
Prazosin	No	Temazepam	No
Prednisone	No	Theophylline	Yes
Primidone	Yes	Ticarcillin	Yes
Procainamide	Yes	Timolol	No
Promethazine	No	Tobramycin	Yes
Propoxyphene	No	Tocainide	Yes
Propranolol	No	Tolbutamide	No
Protriptyline	No	Topirimate	Yes
Quinidine	Yes	Trazodone	No
Ramipril	No	Triazolam	No
Ranitidine	Yes	Trimethoprim	Yes
Rifampin	No	Valacyclovir	Yes
Rofecoxib	No	Valproic acid	No
Sertraline	No	Valsartan	No
Sotalol	Yes	Vancomycin	No
Stavudine	Yes	Verapamil	No
Streptomycin	Yes	Warfarin	No
Sucralfate	No		

Diuretics

Use cautiously in patients with impaired renal or hepatic function. Obtain baseline serum electrolyte levels before starting therapy and at periodic intervals during therapy. Be alert for excess diuresis, which promotes orthostatic hypotension, dehydration, hypovolemia, hyponatremia, hypomagnesemia, and hypokalemia.

Drug	Indications	Adverse effects*
Thiazide-like or thiazide diuretics *Chlorthalidone (Hygroton, Thalitone)*	• Edema • Hypertension	• Pancreatitis, • Aplastic anemia, agranulocytosis, leukopenia, thrombocytopenia • Hypersensitivity reactions
Hydrochlorothiazide (Esidrix, Ezide, Hydrochlor, Hydro-DIURIL, Hydro-Par, Microzide, Oretic)	• Edema • Hypertension	• Pancreatitis • Renal failure • Aplastic anemia, agranulocytosis, leukopenia, thrombocytopenia • Hypersensitivity reactions, anaphylaxis
Metolazone (Diulo, Mykrox, Zaroxolyn)	• Edema (heart failure or renal failure) • Hypertension	• Dizziness, headache, fatigue, vertigo, paresthesia, weakness, restlessness, drowsiness, anxiety, depression, nervousness, blurred vision • Aplastic anemia, agranulocytosis, leukopenia • Hepatitis
Loop diuretics *Bumetanide (Bumex)*	• Edema (heart failure, hepatic and renal disease), postoperative edema; premenstrual syndrome, disseminated cancer • Pediatric heart failure • Hypertension	• Renal failure • Thrombocytopenia
Ethacrynate sodium, ethacrynic acid (Edecrin)	• Acute pulmonary edema • Edema • Hypertension	• Pancreatitis • Agranulocytosis, neutropenia, thrombocytopenia
Furosemide (Lasix)	• Acute pulmonary edema • Edema • Hypertension • Hypercalcemia	• Pancreatitis • Renal failure • Agranulocytosis, leukopenia, thrombocytopenia, azotemia, anemia, aplastic anemia

*Common or life-threatening only

Special considerations

- Therapeutic response may be delayed several weeks in patients with hypertension.
- Drug may interfere with tests for parathyroid function; discontinue drug before such tests.
- Tell the patient to avoid sudden posture changes and to rise slowly to avoid orthostatic hypotension.

- Contraindicated in patients with anuria or hepatic coma.
- Drug isn't effective if creatinine clearance is less than 50 ml/minute.
- Watch for signs of hypokalemia, such as muscle weakness and cramps.
- Monitor blood uric acid levels, especially in patients with history of gout.

- Contraindicated in patients with anuria or hepatic coma or precoma.
- Metolazone is used as an adjunct in furosemide-resistant edema.
- The rapid-acting form (Mykrox) isn't interchangeable with other forms of metolazone. Dosage and uses vary.

- Contraindicated in patients with anuria or hepatic coma, and those in states of severe electrolyte depletion.
- Give I.V. bumetanide slowly, over 1 to 2 minutes, for I.V. infusion.
- With increased doses, monitor the patient for ototoxicity.
- Weigh patient daily to monitor fluid status.

- Contraindicated in patients with anuria, hypotension, dehydration with hyponatremia, and metabolic alkalosis with hypokalemia. Also contraindicated if azotemia, oliguria, electrolyte imbalance, or severe watery diarrhea occurs during therapy.
- Give drug slowly over 20 to 30 minutes, by I.V. infusion or by direct I.V. injection over several minutes; rapid injection may cause hypotension.
- Don't give drug with whole blood or blood products; hemolysis may occur.

- Contraindicated in patients with anuria, hepatic coma, or severe electrolyte depletion. Contraindicated if increased azotemia, oliguria, or progressive renal disease occur during therapy.
- Give I.V. furosemide slowly, over 1 to 2 minutes. For I.V. infusion, dilute furosemide in D_5W, normal saline solution, or lactated Ringer's solution, and use within 24 hours. If high-dose furosemide therapy is needed, administer as a controlled infusion not exceeding 4 mg/minute.

(continued)

Diuretics *(continued)*

Drug	Indications	Adverse effects*
Potassium-sparing diuretics **Amiloride hydrochloride (Midamor)**	• Hypertension; edema related to heart failure, usually in patients who are also taking thiazide or other potassium-wasting diuretics	• Encephalopathy • Anorexia, diarrhea, vomiting • Aplastic anemia, neutropenia
Spironolactone (Aldactone)	• Edema • Hypertension • Diuretic-induced hypokalemia • Heart failure in patients receiving an ACE inhibitor and a loop diuretic with or without a cardiac glycoside	• Agranulocytosis • Hyperkalemia
Triamterene (Dyrenium)	• Edema	• Agranulocytosis, thrombocytopenia • Hyperkalemia • Anaphylaxis
Osmotic diuretic **Mannitol (Osmitrol, Resectisol)**	• Testing for marked oliguria or suspected inadequate renal function • Treatment of oliguria • Prevention of oliguria or acute renal failure • Treatment of edema and ascites • Reduction of intraocular pressure or intracranial pressure • Promotion of diuresis in drug intoxication	• Seizures • Heart failure

*Common or life-threatening only

Special considerations

- Contraindicated in patients with elevated serum potassium level (over 5.5 mEq/L).
- Contraindicated in patients with anuria, acute or chronic renal insufficiency, or diabetic nephropathy.
- Monitor the patient for signs of hyperkalemia, including paresthesia, muscular weakness, and ECG abnormalities.

- Contraindicated in patients with anuria, acute or progressive renal insufficiency, or hyperkalemia and in those receiving amiloride or triamterene.
- Drug's diuretic effect may be delayed 2 to 3 days if drug is used alone; maximum antihypertensive effect may be delayed 2 to 3 weeks.

- Contraindicated in patients receiving other potassium-sparing drugs and in patients with anuria, severe or progressive renal disease or dysfunction, severe hepatic disease, or hyperkalemia.
- To minimize excessive rebound potassium excretion, expect to discontinue drug gradually.
- Monitor blood pressure, CBC, blood uric acid, blood glucose, BUN, and serum electrolyte levels; watch for blood dyscrasia.
- The patient's urine may turn blue.

- Contraindicated in patients with anuria, severe pulmonary congestion, frank pulmonary edema, severe heart failure, severe dehydration, metabolic edema, progressive renal disease or dysfunction, or active intracranial bleeding except during craniotomy.
- Monitor vital signs (including CVP) hourly. Monitor intake and output, weight, renal function, fluid balance, and serum and urine sodium and potassium levels daily.
- Give drug I.V. via an in-line filter with great care to avoid extravasation.
- Don't give with whole blood; agglutination will occur.
- Don't use solutions with undissolved crystals.
- Don't give more than 1 L of fluids in excess of urine output daily.

Dosage calculation formulas and common conversions

Common calculations

$$\text{Body surface area in m}^2 = \sqrt{\frac{\text{height in cm} \times \text{weight in kg}}{3,600}}$$

$$\text{mcg/ml} = \text{mg/ml} \times 1,000$$

$$\text{ml/minute} = \frac{\text{ml/hour}}{60}$$

$$\text{gtt/minute} = \frac{\text{volume in ml to be infused}}{\text{time in minutes}} \times \text{drip factor in gtt/ml}$$

$$\text{mg/minute} = \frac{\text{mg in bag}}{\text{ml in bag}} \times \text{flow rate} \div 60$$

$$\text{mcg/minute} = \frac{\text{mg in bag}}{\text{ml in bag}} \div 0.06 \times \text{flow rate}$$

$$\text{mcg/kg/minute} = \frac{\text{mcg/ml} \times \text{ml/minute}}{\text{weight in kilograms}}$$

Common conversions

1 kg = 1,000 g

1 g = 1,000 mg

1 mg = 1,000 mcg

1 L = 1,000 ml

1 ml = 1,000 microliters (µl)

1 tsp = 5 ml

1 tbs = 15 ml

2 tbs = 30 ml

8 oz = 240 ml

1 oz = 30 g

1 lb = 454 g

2.2 lb = 1 kg

1″ = 2.54 cm

Drugs and the QT interval

Many drugs can prolong the QT interval, especially when combined with substances that affect the metabolism of the drug. This QT interval prolongation can lead to torsades de pointes, a life-threatening polymorphic ventricular tachycardia. The list here shows some drugs that may affect the QT interval.

Anesthetic
- Halothane

Antiarrhythmics
- Disopyramide
- Procainamide
- Quinidine
- Amiodarone
- Sotalol

Antibiotics
- Azithromycin
- Clarithromycin
- Erythromycin
- Metronidazole
(with alcohol)
- Moxifloxacin

Antidepressants
- Amitriptyline
- Clomipramine
- Imipramine
- Dothiepin
- Doxepin

Antifungals
- Fluconazole
(in cirrhosis)
- Ketoconazole

Antimalarials
- Chloroquine
- Mefloquine

Antipsychotics
- Risperidone
- Fluphenazine
- Haloperidol
- Clozapine
- Thioridazine
- Ziprasidone
- Pimozide
- Droperidol

Antivirals
- Nelfinavir

Other drugs
- Probucol

QT$_c$ interval normals

Heart rate (per minute)	QT$_c$ interval normal range (seconds)
40	0.41 - 0.51
50	0.38 - 0.46
60	0.35 - 0.43
70	0.33 - 0.41
80	0.32 - 0.39
90	0.30 - 0.36
100	0.28 - 0.34
120	0.26 - 0.32
150	0.23 - 0.28
180	0.21 - 0.25
200	0.20 - 0.24

Electrolyte components of I.V. solutions

Solution	Sodium (mEq/L)	Potassium (mEq/L)	Osmolarity (mOsm/L)	Tonicity
Aminosyn 3.5% M	47	13	477	hypertonic
Aminosyn 7% with electrolytes	70	66	1,013	hypertonic
Aminosyn 8.5% with electrolytes	70	66	1,160	hypertonic
Dextrose 2.5% in half-strength lactated Ringer's injection	65	2	265	isotonic
Dextrose 5% in electrolyte no. 48	25	20	348	isotonic
Dextrose 5% in electrolyte no. 75	40	35	402	hypertonic
Dextrose 5% in sodium chloride 0.11%	19	—	290	isotonic
Dextrose 5% in sodium chloride 0.2%	34 or 38.5	—	320 - 330	isotonic
Dextrose 5% in sodium chloride 0.33%	51 or 56	—	355 - 365	isotonic
Dextrose 50% with electrolyte pattern A	84	40	2,800	hypertonic
Dextrose 50% with electrolyte pattern N	90	80	2,875	hypertonic
Dextrose 50% with electrolyte no. 1	110	80	2,917	hypertonic
5% Travert and electrolyte no. 2	56	25	449	hypertonic
FreAmine III 3% with electrolytes	35	24.5	405	hypertonic
Ionosol B in dextrose 5% in water	57	25	426	hypertonic
Ionosol MB in dextrose 5% in water	25	20	352	hypertonic
Ionosol T in dextrose 5% in water	40	35	432	hypertonic
Isolyte E	140	10	310	isotonic
Isolyte G with dextrose 5%	65	17	555	hypertonic
Lactated Ringer's injection	130	4	275	isotonic
Normosol-M in dextrose 5%	40	13	363	hypertonic

Calcium (mEq/L)	Magnesium (mEq/L)	Chloride (mEq/L)	Acetate (mEq/L)	Phosphate (millimoles)	Other (mEq/L)
—	3	40	58	3.5	amino acids 3.5%
—	10	96	124	30	amino acids 7%
—	10	98	142	30	amino acids 8.5%
1.4 - 1.5	—	54 - 55	—	—	lactate 14
—	3	24	—	3	lactate 23
—	—	48	—	15	lactate 20
—	—	19	—	—	—
—	—	34 or 38.5	—	—	—
—	—	51 or 56	—	—	—
10	16	115	—	—	gluconate 13 sulfate 16
—	16	150	—	28	sulfate 16
—	16	140	36	24	—
—	6	56	—	12.5	lactate 25
—	5	41	44	3.5	amino acids 3%
—	5	49	—	7	lactate 25
—	3	22	—	3	lactate 23
—	—	40	—	15	lactate 20
5	3	103	49	—	citrate 8
—	—	149	—	—	ammonium 70
2.7 - 3	—	109 or 110	—	—	lactate 28
—	3	40	16	—	—

(continued)

Electrolyte components of I.V. solutions *(continued)*

Solution	Sodium (mEq/L)	Potassium (mEq/L)	Osmolarity (mOsm/L)	Tonicity
Plasma-Lyte A	140	5	294	isotonic
Plasma-Lyte R	140	10	312	isotonic
ProcalAmine	35	24	735	hypertonic
Ringer's injection	147 or 147.5	4	310	isotonic
Sodium bicarbonate	598	—	1,190 - 1,203	hypertonic
Sodium chloride 0.45%	77	—	154	hypertonic
Sodium chloride 0.9%	154	—	308	isotonic
Sodium chloride 3%	513	—	1,030	hypertonic
Sodium chloride 5%	855	—	1,710	hypertonic
Sodium lactate 1/6 M	167	—	330	isotonic
Travasol 3.5% with electrolytes	25	15	450	hypertonic
Travasol 5.5% with electrolytes	70	60	850	hypertonic
Travasol 8.5% with electrolytes	70	60	1,160	hypertonic
Fat emulsion 10%, 20%, 30%	—	—	258 - 3310	isotonic

Calcium (mEq/L)	Magnesium (mEq/L)	Chloride (mEq/L)	Acetate (mEq/L)	Phosphate (millimoles)	Other (mEq/L)
—	3	98	27	—	gluconate 23
5	3	103	47	—	lactate 8
3	5	41	47	3.5	amino acids 3% glycerin 3%
4 or 4.5	—	155 or 156	—	—	—
—	—	—	—	—	—
—	—	77	—	—	—
—	—	154	—	—	—
—	—	513	—	—	—
—	—	855	—	—	—
—	—	—	—	—	lactate 167
—	5	25	52	7.5	—
—	10	70	102	30	—
—	10	70	141	30	—
—	—	—	—	—	—

Factors that affect preload and afterload

Preload

Preload refers to the passive stretching force exerted on the ventricular muscle at the end of diastole by the amount of blood in the chamber. According to Starling's law, the more cardiac muscles are stretched, the more forcefully they contract in systole.

Factors that increase preload

● Increased blood volume returning to the heart
● Control of the fluid loss with replacement therapy such as I.V. or transfusion therapy; fluid overload
● Decreased ventricular compliance
● Mitral stenosis or insufficiency
● Venous congestion, such as with cardiac tamponade and heart failure
● Poor contractility of the right ventricle, such as from infarction or pericarditis
● Conditions associated with high pulmonary vascular resistance, such as pulmonary edema or chronic obstructive pulmonary disease

Factors that decrease preload

● Fluid losses, such as with hemorrhage, excessive diaphoresis, vomiting, or diarrhea
● Third-space shifting
● Diuresis
● Fluid and sodium restriction
● Extreme vasodilation
● Medications, such as loop diuretics, nitrates, and cardiac glycosides

Afterload

Afterload refers to the pressure the ventricular muscles must generate to overcome the higher pressure in the aorta. Normally, end-diastolic pressure in the left ventricle is 5 to 10 mm Hg; in the aorta, however, it's 70 to 80 mm Hg. This difference means that the ventricle must develop enough pressure to force open the aortic valve.

Factors that increase afterload

● Peripheral vasoconstriction
● Decreased stroke volume
● Hypovolemia
● Hypothermia
● Hypertension
● Cardiogenic shock
● Cardiac tamponade
● Massive pulmonary embolism
● Vasopressor agents, such as epinephrine, norepinephrine, and dopamine

Factors that decrease afterload

● Peripheral vasodilation
● Increased stroke volume
● Medications, such as angiotensin-converting enzyme inhibitors (captopril [Capoten] and enalapril [Vasotec]), hydralazine (Apresoline), and sodium nitroprusside (Nitropress)
● Early septic shock

Glasgow Coma Scale

The Glasgow Coma Scale provides an easy way to describe a patient's baseline mental status and to help detect and interpret changes from baseline findings. To use the Glasgow Coma Scale, test the patient's ability to respond to verbal, motor, and sensory stimulation, and grade your findings according to the scale. A score of 15 indicates that the patient is alert, can follow simple commands, and is oriented to time, place, and person. A decreased score in one or more categories may signal an impending neurologic crisis. A score of 7 or less indicates severe neurologic damage.

Test	Score	Patient response
Eye opening response		
Spontaneously	4	Opens eyes spontaneously
To speech	3	Opens eyes when told to
To pain	2	Opens eyes only to painful stimulus
None	1	Doesn't open eyes in response to stimuli
Motor response		
Obeys	6	Shows two fingers when asked
Localizes	5	Reaches toward painful stimulus and tries to remove it
Withdraws	4	Moves away from painful stimulus
Abnormal flexion	3	Assumes a decorticate posture (shown here)
Abnormal extension	2	Assumes a decerebrate posture (shown here)
None	1	No response; just lies flaccid (an ominous sign)
Verbal response to question, *"What year is this?"*		
Oriented	5	Tells correct date
Confused	4	Tells incorrect year
Inappropriate words	3	Replies randomly with incorrect words
Incomprehensible	2	Moans or screams
No response	1	No response
Total score		

Heart sound abnormalities

Auscultation sites

When auscultating for heart sounds, place the stethoscope over four different sites. Follow the same auscultation sequence during every cardiovascular assessment:
- Place the stethoscope in the aortic area, the second intercostal space along the right sternal border, as shown. In the aortic area, blood moves from the left ventricle during systole, crossing the aortic valve and flowing through the aortic arch.
- Move to the pulmonary area, located in the second intercostal space at the left sternal border. In the pulmonary area, blood ejected from the right ventricle during systole crosses the pulmonic valve and flows through the main pulmonary artery.

- In the third auscultation site, assess the tricuspid area, which lies in the fifth intercostal space along the left sternal border. In the tricuspid area, sounds reflect blood movement from the right atrium across the tricuspid valve, filling the right ventricle during diastole.
- Finally, listen in the mitral area, located in the fifth intercostal space near the midclavicular line. (If the patient's heart is enlarged, the mitral area may be closer to the anterior axillary line.) In the mitral (apical) area, sounds represent blood flow across the mitral valve and left ventricular filling during diastole.

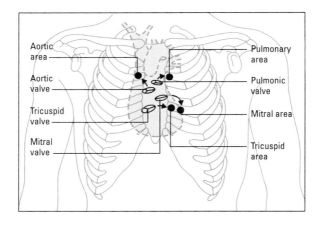

Implications of abnormal heart sounds

Upon detecting an abnormal heart sound, you must accurately identify the sound as well as its location and timing in the cardiac cycle. This information will help you identify the possible cause of the sound. The chart below lists abnormal heart sounds with their possible causes.

Abnormal heart sound	Timing	Possible causes
Accentuated S_1	Beginning of systole	Mitral stenosis; fever
Diminished S_1	Beginning of systole	Mitral insufficiency; severe mitral regurgitation with calcified immobile valve; heart block
Accentuated S_2	End of systole	Pulmonary or systemic hypertension
Diminished or inaudible S_2	End of systole	Aortic or pulmonic stenosis
Persistent S_2 split	End of systole	Delayed closure of the pulmonic valve, usually from overfilling of the right ventricle, causing prolonged systolic ejection time
Reversed or paradoxical S_2 split that appears on expiration and disappears on inspiration	End of systole	Delayed ventricular stimulation; left bundle-branch block or prolonged left ventricular ejection time
S_3 (ventricular gallop)	Early diastole	Normal in children and young adults; overdistention of ventricles in rapid-filling segment of diastole; mitral insufficiency or ventricular failure
S_4 (atrial gallop or presystolic extra sound)	Late diastole	Forceful atrial contraction from resistance to ventricular filling late in diastole; left ventricular hypertrophy; pulmonic stenosis; hypertension; coronary artery disease; and aortic stenosis
Pericardial friction rub (grating or leathery sound at left sternal border; usually muffled, high pitched, and transient)	Throughout systole and diastole	Pericardial inflammation
Click	Early systole or midsystole	Aortic stenosis; aortic dilation; hypertension; chordae tendineae damage of the mitral valve
Opening snap	Early diastole	Mitral or tricuspid valve abnormalities
Summation gallop	Diastole	Tachycardia

Hemodynamic variables

Parameter	Normal value	Formula
Mean arterial pressure (MAP)	70 to 105 mm Hg	$\dfrac{\text{Systolic blood pressure (BP)} + 2\,(\text{Diastolic BP})}{3}$
Central venous pressure (CVP; right atrial pressure [RAP])	2 to 6 cm H_2O; 2 to 8 mm Hg	N/A
Right ventricular pressures	20 to 30 mm Hg (systolic); 0 to 8 mm Hg (diastolic)	N/A
Pulmonary artery pressures (PAP)	20 to 30 mm Hg (systolic; PAS) 8 to 15 mm Hg (diastolic; PAD) 10 to 20 mm Hg (mean; PAM)	N/A
Pulmonary artery wedge pressure (PAWP)	6 to 12 mm Hg	N/A
Cardiac output (CO)	4 to 6 L/minute	Heart rate (HR) $\times$ stroke volume (SV)

Potential causes of elevated values	Potential causes of low values
• Vasoconstriction • Use of inotropic agents • Polycythemia • Cardiogenic or hypovolemic shock • Atherosclerosis	• Vasodilation • Moderate hypoxemia • Anemia • Nitrate drug therapy • Calcium channel blocker therapy • Septic shock • Neurogenic shock • Anaphylactic shock
• Fluid overload • Pericardial tamponade • Pulmonary hypertension • Heart failure • Left ventricular myocardial infarction (MI) (could be high normal to elevated range) • Right ventricular MI • Pulmonary embolism • Cardiogenic shock	• Dehydration • Hypovolemia • Diuretic therapy • Hemorrhage • Arrhythmias • Third-space fluid shifting
• Fluid overload • Pulmonary hypertension	• Dehydration • Diuretic therapy • Hemorrhage • Arrhythmias • Third-space fluid shifting
• Hypertension • Vasoconstriction • Pulmonary edema • Pulmonary hypertension	• Dehydration • Diuretic therapy • Calcium channel blocker therapy • Pulmonary embolism
• Hypertension • Fluid overload • Pulmonary hypertension • Mitral valve regurgitation • Left-sided heart failure • MI • Cardiac tamponade	• Dehydration • Hypovolemia • Pulmonary embolism • Right-sided heart failure • MI • Vasodilation • Diuretic therapy • Afterload reduction
• Sepsis	• Irregularities in heart rate • Hypovolemia • Pulmonary hypertension • Pericardial tamponade • MI • Pulmonary embolism • Decreased contractility • Decreased preload or increased afterload

(continued)

Hemodynamic variables *(continued)*

Parameter	Normal value	Formula
Cardiac index (CI)	2.5 to 4 L/minute/m²	$$\frac{CO}{Body\ surface\ area\ (BSA)}$$
Stroke volume (SV)	60 to 100 ml/beat	$$\frac{CO}{HR}$$
Stroke volume index (SVI)	30 to 60 ml/beat/m²	$$\frac{SV}{BSA}$$
Systemic vascular resistance (SVR)	900 to 1,200 dynes/sec/cm⁻⁵	$$\frac{MAP - RAP \times 80}{CO}$$
Systemic vascular resistance index (SVRI)	1,360 to 2,200 dynes/sec/cm⁻⁵/m²	$$\frac{MAP - RAP \times 80}{CI}$$
Pulmonary vascular resistance (PVR)	60 to 100 dynes/sec/cm⁻⁵	$$\frac{PAM - PAWP \times 80}{CO}$$

Potential causes of elevated values	Potential causes of low values
• Sepsis	• Irregularities in heart rate • Hypovolemia • Heart failure • Pulmonary embolism • Pulmonary hypertension • MI • Cardiac tamponade • Decreased contractility • Decreased preload or increased afterload
• Positive inotropic drug therapy • Exercise • Bradycardia	• Cardiac tamponade • Widespread vasodilation • Arrhythmias • Tachycardia
• Bradyarrhythmias • Positive inotropic drug therapy	• Hypovolemic shock • Vasodilation • Cardiogenic shock
• Cardiogenic shock • Hypovolemic shock • Pericardial tamponade • Pulmonary embolism • Vasopressor therapy • Systemic hypertension • MI	• Septic shock • Anaphylaxis • Vasodilator therapy • Cirrhosis • Arteriovenous fistulas • Thyrotoxicosis
• Positive inotropic drug therapy • Polycythemia • Vasoconstriction • Cardiogenic shock • MI • Hypovolemic shock • Pericardial tamponade • Pulmonary embolism • Heart failure	• Anemia • Nitrate therapy • Calcium channel blocker therapy • Septic shock • Neurogenic shock • Anaphylactic shock • Moderate hypoxemia
• Pulmonary hypertension • Pulmonary edema • Pulmonary embolism • Valvular heart disease • Congenital heart disease • Hypoxemia • Acid-base disturbance	• Prostacycline therapy

(continued)

Hemodynamic variables *(continued)*

Parameter	Normal value	Formula
Pulmonary vascular resistance index (PVRI)	< 425 dynes/sec/cm^{-5}/m^2	$\dfrac{MAP - CVP \times 80}{CI}$
Right ventricular stroke work index (RVSWI)	5 to 10 g/m^2/beat	[SVI (MPAP – RAP)] $\times$ 0.136
Left ventricular stroke work index (LVSWI)	40 to 70 g/m^2/beat	[SVI (MAP – PAWP)] $\times$ 0.136
Arterial oxygen content (Cao$_2$)	20 ml/O$_2$/dl	{(Hemoglobin [Hb] $\times$ 1.34) + Oxygen saturation (Sao$_2$)} $\times$ (0.003 $\times$ Pao$_2$)
Venous oxygen content (Cvo$_2$)	15 ml/O$_2$/dl	[(Hb $\times$ 1.34) $\times$ Svo$_2$] + (Pvo$_2$ $\times$ 0.003)
Oxygen delivery (Do$_2$)	800 to 1,000 ml/minute	Cao$_2$ $\times$ CO $\times$ 10
Oxygen delivery index (Do$_2$I)	500 to 600 ml/minute/m^2	Cao$_2$ $\times$ CI $\times$ 10
Arteriovenous oxygen content difference (C[a – v]o$_2$)	4 to 6 ml/volume % or ml/dl	Cao$_2$ – Cvo$_2$

Potential causes of elevated values	Potential causes of low values
• Hypercapnia • Pulmonary edema • Pulmonary embolism • Hypoxia • Chronic obstructive pulmonary disease • Mitral stenosis • Cardiogenic shock	• Nitrate therapy • Septic shock • Neurogenic shock • Anaphylactic shock • Vasodilation
• Aerobic metabolism • Loss of less than 40% of functional myocardial tissue • Increased preload	• MI • Beta blocker therapy • Calcium channel blocker therapy • Hyponatremia • Hyperkalemia • Anaerobic metabolism • Decreased preload • Loss of greater than 40% of functional myocardial tissue
• Aerobic metabolism • Loss of less than 40% of functional myocardial tissue • Increased preload	• MI • Hyponatremia • Hyperkalemia • Beta blocker therapy • Calcium channel blocker therapy • Anaerobic metabolism • Decreased preload • Loss of greater than 40% of functional myocardial tissue
• Polycythemia	• Anemia • Hypovolemia
• Polycythemia	• Anemia • Cardiac failure • Hypoxemia
• Increased CO, secondary to increased oxygen demand	• Cardiac failure • Anemia • Hypoxemia
• Increased CO, secondary to increased oxygen demand	• Cardiac failure • Anemia • Hypovolemic shock
• Cardiac failure • MI • Pericardial tamponade • Pulmonary embolism • Pulmonary hypertension	• Thyrotoxicosis • Shunt • Sepsis

(continued)

Hemodynamic variables *(continued)*

Parameter	Normal value	Formula
Oxygen consumption (Vo₂)	200 to 250 ml/minute	$CO \times 10 \times C[a-v]o_2$
Oxygen consumption index (Vo₂I)	115 to 165 ml/minute/m²	$CI \times 10 \times C[a-v]o_2$
Mixed venous oxygen saturation (S̄vo₂)	60% to 80%	$(CO \times Cao_2 \times 10) - Vo_2$
Cerebral perfusion pressure (CPP)	70 to 80 mm Hg	MAP − Intracranial pressure (ICP)
ICP	0-10 mm Hg	N/A

Potential causes of elevated values	Potential causes of low values
• Sepsis	• Hypovolemic shock • Sepsis • Cardiogenic shock
• Sepsis	• Cardiogenic shock • Sepsis • Hypovolemic shock
• Increased oxygen supply • Decreased oxygen demand • Decreased use of oxygen by tissues • Hypertension	• Decreased oxygen supply • Increased oxygen demand • Hypovolemic shock • MI • Pericardial tamponade • Pulmonary embolism
• Hypertension	• Acute hydrocephalus • Intracranial hematoma • Cerebral edema • Arrhythmias • MI • Dehydration • Osmotic drugs • Diabetes insipidus • Blood pressure medications (antihypertensives)
• Cerebral edema • Acute hydrocephalus • Intracranial hematoma • Ischemia	• Glaucoma

Infusion flow rates

Epinephrine infusion rates
Mix 1 mg in 250 ml (4 mcg/ml).

Dose (mcg/min)	Infusion rate (ml/hr)
1	15
2	30
3	45
4	60
5	75
6	90
7	105
8	120
9	135
10	150
15	225
20	300
25	375
30	450
35	525
40	600

Isoproterenol infusion rates
Mix 1 mg in 250 ml (4 mcg/ml).

Dose (mcg/min)	Infusion rate (ml/hr)
0.5	8
1	15
2	30
3	45
4	60
5	75
6	90
7	105
8	120
9	135
10	150
15	225
20	300
25	375
30	450

Nitroglycerin infusion rates

Determine the infusion rate in ml/hr using the ordered dose and the concentration of the drug solution.

Dose (mcg/min)	25 mg/250 ml (100 mcg/ml)	50 mg/250 ml (200 mcg/ml)	100 mg/250 ml (400 mcg/ml)
5	3	2	1
10	6	3	2
20	12	6	3
30	18	9	5
40	24	12	6
50	30	15	8
60	36	18	9
70	42	21	10
80	48	24	12
90	54	27	14
100	60	30	15
150	90	45	23
200	120	60	30

(continued)

Infusion flow rates *(continued)*

Dobutamine infusion rates
Mix 250 mg in 250 ml of D_5W (1,000 mcg/ml). Determine the infusion rate in ml/hr using the ordered dose and the patient's weight in pounds or kilograms.

Dose (mcg/kg/min)	lb 88	99	110	121	132	143	154	165	176	187	198	209	220	231	242
	kg 40	45	50	55	60	65	70	75	80	85	90	95	100	105	110
2.5	6	7	8	8	9	10	11	11	12	13	14	14	15	16	17
5	12	14	15	17	18	20	21	23	24	26	27	29	30	32	33
7.5	18	20	23	25	27	29	32	34	36	38	41	43	45	47	50
10	24	27	30	33	36	39	42	45	48	51	54	57	60	63	66
12.5	30	34	38	41	45	49	53	56	60	64	68	71	75	79	83
15	36	41	45	50	54	59	63	68	72	77	81	86	90	95	99
20	48	54	60	66	72	78	84	90	96	102	108	114	120	126	132
25	60	68	75	83	90	98	105	113	120	128	135	143	150	158	165
30	72	81	90	99	108	117	126	135	144	153	162	171	180	189	198
35	84	95	105	116	126	137	147	158	168	179	189	200	210	221	231
40	96	108	120	132	144	156	168	180	192	204	216	228	240	252	264

Dopamine infusion rates
Mix 400 mg in 250 ml of D_5W (1,600 mcg/ml). Determine the infusion rate in ml/hr using the ordered dose and the patient's weight in pounds or kilograms.

Dose (mcg/kg/min)	lb 88	99	110	121	132	143	154	165	176	187	198	209	220	231
	kg 40	45	50	55	60	65	70	75	80	85	90	95	100	105
2.5	4	4	5	5	6	6	7	7	8	8	8	9	9	10
5	8	8	9	10	11	12	13	14	15	16	17	18	19	20
7.5	11	13	14	15	17	18	20	21	23	24	25	27	28	30
10	15	17	19	21	23	24	26	28	30	32	34	36	38	39
12.5	19	21	23	26	28	30	33	35	38	40	42	45	47	49
15	23	25	28	31	34	37	39	42	45	48	51	53	56	59
20	30	34	38	41	45	49	53	56	60	64	68	71	75	79
25	38	42	47	52	56	61	66	70	75	80	84	89	94	98
30	45	51	56	62	67	73	79	84	90	96	101	107	113	118
35	53	59	66	72	79	85	92	98	105	112	118	125	131	138
40	60	68	75	83	90	98	105	113	120	128	135	143	150	158
45	68	76	84	93	101	110	118	127	135	143	152	160	169	177
50	75	84	94	103	113	122	131	141	150	159	169	178	188	197

Nitroprusside infusion rates

Mix 50 mg in 250 ml of D_5W (200 mcg/ml). Determine the infusion rate in ml/hr using the ordered dose and the patient's weight in pounds or kilograms.

Dose (mcg/kg/ min)	lb 88	99	110	121	132	143	154	165	176	187	198	209	220	231	242
	kg 40	45	50	55	60	65	70	75	80	85	90	95	100	105	110
0.3	4	4	5	5	5	6	6	7	7	8	8	9	9	9	10
0.5	6	7	8	8	9	10	11	11	12	13	14	14	15	16	17
1	12	14	15	17	18	20	21	23	24	26	27	29	30	32	33
1.5	18	20	23	25	27	29	32	34	36	38	41	43	45	47	50
2	24	27	30	33	36	39	42	45	48	51	54	57	60	63	66
3	36	41	45	50	54	59	63	68	72	77	81	86	90	95	99
4	48	54	60	66	72	78	84	90	96	102	108	114	120	126	132
5	60	68	75	83	90	98	105	113	120	128	135	143	150	158	165
6	72	81	90	99	108	117	126	135	144	153	162	171	180	189	198
7	84	95	105	116	126	137	147	158	168	179	189	200	210	221	231
8	96	108	120	132	144	156	168	180	192	204	216	228	240	252	264
9	108	122	135	149	162	176	189	203	216	230	243	257	270	284	297
10	120	135	150	165	180	195	210	225	240	255	270	285	300	315	330

Inotropic and vasopressor agents

Drug	Indications	Adverse effects*
Dobutamine hydrochloride (Dobutrex)	• Increase in cardiac output in short-term treatment of cardiac decompensation caused by depressed contractility	• Increased heart rate, hypertension, PVCs • Asthmatic episodes • Anaphylaxis
Dopamine hydrochloride (Intropin)	• Adjunct in shock to increase cardiac output, blood pressure, and urine flow • Short-term treatment of severe, refractory, chronic heart failure	• Hypotension, bradycardia • Anaphylactic reactions
Epinephrine (Bronkaid Mist, EpiPen, EpiPen Jr., Sus-Phrine); epinephrine hydrochloride (Adrenalin Chloride, AsthmaNefrin, Epifrin, Glaucon, microNefrin, Vaponefrin)	• Bronchospasm, hypersensitivity reactions, anaphylaxis • Restoration of cardiac rhythm in cardiac arrest	• Nervousness, tremor, headache, drowsiness, cerebral hemorrhage, stroke • Palpitations, hypertension, ventricular fibrillation, shock, arrhythmias • Nausea, vomiting
Inamrinone lactate (Inocor)	• Short-term management of heart failure • Cardiac life support in patients in whom other preferred drugs can't be used for pump failure and acute pulmonary edema	• Arrhythmias • Thrombocytopenia • Hypersensitivity reactions (pericarditis, ascites, myositis vasculitis, pleuritis)

*Common or life-threatening only

Special considerations

- Contraindicated in patients with idiopathic hypertrophic subaortic stenosis.
- Dobutamine is incompatible with alkaline solution (sodium bicarbonate).
- Don't mix with or give through same I.V. line as heparin, hydrocortisone, cefazolin, or penicillin.
- The concentration of infusion solution shouldn't exceed 5,000 mcg/ml; use the solution within 24 hours. Rate and duration of infusion depend on patient response.
- Monitor serum electrolytes, especially potassium.
- Most patients experience an increase of 10 to 20 mm Hg in systolic blood pressure; some show an increase of 50 mm Hg or more. Most also experience an increase in heart rate of 5 to 15 beats/minute; some show increases of 30 or more beats/minute.

- Contraindicated in patients with uncorrected tachyarrhythmias, pheochromocytoma, or ventricular fibrillation.
- Use cautiously in patients with occlusive vascular disease, cold injuries, diabetic endarteritis, and arterial embolism; in those taking MAO inhibitors; and in pregnant women.
- Reduce dosage gradually because severe hypotension may result with abrupt withdrawal of infusion. Administer I.V. fluids, as ordered, to expand blood volume
- Don't mix other drugs in dopamine solutions. Discard solutions after 24 hours.
- Give drug in a large vein to prevent the possibility of extravasation.
- If extravasation occurs, stop infusion and infiltrate site promptly with 10 to 15 ml saline injection containing 5 to 10 mg phentolamine. Use syringe with a fine needle, and infiltrate area liberally with phentolamine solution.

- Contraindicated in patients with angle-closure glaucoma, shock (other than anaphylaxis), organic brain damage, cardiac dilation, arrhythmias, coronary insufficiency, or cerebral arteriosclerosis.
- Contraindicated in patients with sulfite allergies (some commercial products contain sulfites) except when epinephrine is being used for treatment of serious allergic reactions or other emergencies.
- Use with extreme caution in patients with long-standing bronchial asthma and emphysema in whom degenerative heart disease has developed. Also use cautiously in elderly patients and in those with hyperthyroidism, cardiovascular disease, hypertension, psychoneurosis, and diabetes.
- Administer breathing treatment with first symptoms of bronchospasm. Patient should use the fewest number of inhalations that provide relief. To prevent excessive dosage, at least 1 or 2 minutes should elapse before taking additional inhalations of epinephrine. Dosage requirements vary.

- Contraindicated in patients with severe aortic or pulmonic valvular disease (in place of surgical intervention) and patients in the acute phase of an MI.
- Keep in mind that inamrinone is prescribed primarily for patients who haven't responded to therapy with cardiac glycosides, diuretics, and vasodilators.
- Administer drug as supplied, or dilute in normal or half-normal saline solution to concentration of 1 to 3 mg/ml. Don't dilute drug with solutions containing dextrose because a slow chemical reaction occurs over 24 hours. However, inamrinone can be injected into running dextrose infusions through Y-connector or directly into tubing. Use diluted solution within 24 hours.
- Don't administer furosemide in I.V. lines containing inamrinone because a chemical reaction occurs immediately.
- Monitor platelet counts. A count below 150,000/µl necessitates dosage reduction.

(continued)

Inotropic and vasopressor agents *(continued)*

Drug	Indications	Adverse effects*
Milrinone lactate (Primacor)	• Short-term I.V. therapy for heart failure	• Nonsustained ventricular tachycardia, sustained ventricular tachycardia, ventricular fibrillation • Thrombocytopenia
Norepinephrine bitartrate* (Levophed) ―――――― *formerly levarterenol bitartrate	• Maintenance of blood pressure in acute hypotensive states • GI bleeding	• Bradycardia, severe hypertension, arrhythmias • Asthmatic episodes • Anaphylaxis
Phenylephrine hydrochloride, (Neo-Synephrine)	• Hypotensive emergencies during spinal anesthesia • Mild to moderate hypotension • Paroxysmal supraventricular tachycardia • Adjunct in the treatment of severe hypotension or shock	• Headache • Bradycardia, arrhythmias, PVCs, palpitations, tachycardia • Asthmatic episodes • Anaphylaxis, decreased organ perfusion (with prolonged use)

*Common or life-threatening only

Special considerations

- Contraindicated in patients with severe aortic or pulmonic valvular disease (in place of surgical correction), and patients in the acute phase of an MI.
- Use cautiously in patients with atrial fibrillation or flutter.
- Be sure to dilute milrinone further before I.V. administration. Acceptable diluents include half-normal saline solution, normal saline solution, and D_5W.
- Don't administer furosemide in an I.V. line that contains milrinone.

- Contraindicated in patients with mesenteric or peripheral vascular thrombosis, profound hypoxia, hypercapnia, or hypotension resulting from blood volume deficit and during cyclopropane and halothane anesthesia.
- To treat extravasation, infiltrate site promptly with 10 to 15 ml saline solution containing 5 to 10 mg phentolamine, using a fine needle.
- Observe the patient constantly during norepinephrine administration. Obtain baseline blood pressure and pulse before therapy, and repeat every 2 minutes until stabilization. Repeat every 5 minutes during administration.

- Injectable form is contraindicated in those with severe hypertension or ventricular tachycardia.
- Use injectable form cautiously in patients with severe atherosclerosis, bradycardia, partial heart block, myocardial disease, or allergy to sulfites.
- Give I.V. through large veins, and monitor flow rate. To treat extravasation ischemia, infiltrate site promptly and liberally with 10 to 15 ml saline solution containing 5 to 10 mg phentolamine through fine needle. Topical nitroglycerin has also been used.
- During I.V. administration, monitor pulse, blood pressure, and CVP every 2 to 5 minutes.

I.V. drip rates

When calculating the flow rate of I.V. solutions, remember that the number of drops required to deliver 1 ml varies with the type of administration set you're using. To calculate the drip rate, you must know the calibration of the drip rate for each manufacturer's product. As a quick guide, refer to the chart below. Use this formula to calculate specific drip rates:

$$\frac{\text{volume of infusion (in ml)}}{\text{time of infusion (in min)}} \times \text{ drip factor (in drops/ml)} = \text{drops/min}$$

		Ordered volume		
		500 ml/24 hr or 21 ml/hr	*1,000 ml/24 hr or 42 ml/hr*	*1,000 ml/20 hr or 50 ml/hr*
Administration set	**Drops/ml**	**Drops/min to infuse**		
Macrodrip				
Abbott	15	5	10	12
Baxter Healthcare	10	3	7	8
Cutler	20	7	14	17
IVAC	20	7	14	17
McGaw	15	5	10	12
Microdrip				
Various manufacturers	60	21	42	50

1,000 ml/10 hr or 100 ml/hr	1,000 ml/8 hr or 125 ml/hr	1,000 ml/6 hr or 166 ml/hr
25	31	42
17	21	28
34	42	56
34	42	56
25	31	42
100	125	166

I.V. fluids

I.V. solution	Components	Considerations
Dextrose 5% and water (D₅W)	• 50 g glucose • (isotonic — 260 mOsm/L)	• Rehydration or replace plasma volume • Common vehicle for other I.V. medication administration such as potassium • Aids in renal excretion of solutes • Doesn't replace electrolyte deficits • Contraindicated in head injuries—may increase intracranial pressure
Normal saline (0.9% NaCl; 0.9% NS)	• 154 mEq sodium • 154 mEq chloride • (isotonic — 308 mOsm/L)	• Restoration of extracellular fluid volume • Replacement of sodium and chloride deficits • Doesn't supply calories • Given primarily for blood transfusions and to replace large fluid losses such as in GI fluid loss • Contraindicated in heart failure, pulmonary edema, renal impairment, and sodium retention
Lactated Ringer's (LR)	• 130 mEq sodium • 4 mEq potassium • 3 mEq calcium • 109 mEq chloride • 28 mEq lactate • (isotonic — 275 mOsm/L)	• Fluid of choice for acute blood loss replacement • Rehydration (similar to electrolyte composition of blood serum or plasma) • Hypovolemia • Burns • Mild metabolic acidosis • Sodium depletion • Doesn't supply calories • Contraindicated in heart failure, renal impairment, head injury, liver disease, alkalosis
0.45 sodium chloride (0.45 NaCl; ½ NS)	• 77 mEq sodium • 77 mEq chloride • (hypotonic — 154 mOsm/L)	• Establishment of renal function • Doesn't supply calories • Not for replacement therapy
Dextrose 5% in 0.45% normal saline (D₅ ½ NS; D₅ 0.45 NaCl	• 77 mEq sodium • 77 mEq chloride • 170 calories • (hypertonic — 406 mOsm/L)	• Hypovolemia • Maintenance fluid of choice if no electrolyte abnormalities • Maintenance of fluid intake
Dextrose 5% in normal saline (D₅NS; D₅0.9% NaCl)	• 170 calories • 154 mEq sodium • 154 mEq chloride • (hypertonic — 560 mOsm/L)	• Fluid replacement • Sodium, chloride, and calorie replacement • Temporary treatment of hypovolemia if plasma expander not available

I.V. fluids *(continued)*

I.V. solution	Components	Considerations
Dextrose 5% in Lactated Ringer's (D_5LR)	• 130 mEq sodium • 4 mEq potassium • 3 mEq calcium • 109 mEq chloride • 28 mEq lactate • 170 calories • (hypertonic — 575 mOsm/L)	• Rehydration (similar to electrolyte composition of blood serum or plasma) • Hypovolemia • Burns • Mild metabolic acidosis • Doesn't supply calories • Sodium depletion
3% normal saline (3% NS; 3% NaCl)	• 513 mEq sodium • 513 mEq chloride • (hypertonic— 810 mOsm/L)	• Hyponatremia • Elimination of intracellular fluid excess
Dextran 40 in normal saline or dextrose 5% in water	• 170 calories • (isotonic— 252 mOsm/L when combined with dextrose 5%; 308 mOsm/L when combined with normal saline)	• Expansion of plasma volume in early shock when blood products unavailable • Improvement of microcirculation • Doesn't have electrolyte components

Los Angeles prehospital stroke screen

The Los Angeles prehospital stroke screen (LAPSS) is used to evaluate acute, noncomatose, nontraumatic, neurologic complaints. If items 1 through 6 are all checked "yes" (or "unknown"), notify the facility that a potential stroke patient is about to arrive. If any item is checked "no," return to the appropriate treatment protocol.

To interpret the criteria, note that 93% of patients with stroke will have a positive LAPSS score (sensitivity = 93%), and 97% of those with a positive LAPSS score will have a stroke (sensitivity = 97%). Note that the patient may still be experiencing a stroke even if the LAPSS criteria aren't met.

Criteria	Yes	Unknown	No
Age 45 years	☐	☐	☐
History of seizures or epilepsy absent	☐	☐	☐
Symptom duration < 24 hours	☐	☐	☐
At baseline, patient isn't wheelchair bound or bedridden	☐	☐	☐
Blood glucose level is between 60 and 400 mg/dL	☐	☐	☐

Obvious asymmetry (right versus left) in any of the following 3 categories (must be unilateral)	Equal	R weak	L weak
Facial smile/grimace	☐	☐ Droop	☐ Droop
Grip	☐	☐ Weak grip	☐ Weak grip
	☐	☐ No grip	☐ No grip
Arm strength	☐	☐ Drifts down	☐ Drifts down
	☐	☐ Falls rapidly	☐ Falls rapidly

Source: *AHA Provider Manual,* from Kidwell, C.S., et al. "Design and retrospective analysis of the Los Angeles prehospital stroke screen," *Prehospital Emergency Care,* 1998, 2:267-73.

Murmurs

Identify a heart murmur by first listening closely to determine its timing in the cardiac cycle. Then determine its other characteristics one at a time, including its quality, pitch, location, and radiation. Use the chart below to identify the underlying condition.

Timing	Quality	Pitch	Location	Radiation	Condition
Midsystolic (systolic ejection)	Harsh, rough	Medium to high	Pulmonary	Toward left shoulder and neck, possibly along left sternal border	Pulmonic stenosis
	Harsh, rough	Medium to high	Aortic and suprasternal notch	Toward carotid arteries or apex	Aortic stenosis
Holosystolic (pansystolic)	Harsh	High	Tricuspid	Precordium	Ventricular septal defect
	Blowing	High	Mitral, lower left sternal border	Toward left axilla	Mitral insufficiency
	Blowing	High	Tricuspid	Toward apex	Tricuspid insufficiency
Early diastolic	Blowing	High	Mid-left sternal edge (not aortic area)	Toward sternum	Aortic insufficiency
	Blowing	High	Pulmonary	Toward sternum	Pulmonic insufficiency
Middiastolic to late diastolic	Rumbling	Low	Apex	Usually none	Mitral stenosis
	Rumbling	Low	Tricuspid, lower right sternal border	Usually none	Tricuspid stenosis

Neuromuscular blocking agents

Drug	Indications	Adverse effects*
Depolarizing		
Succinylcholine (Anectine)	• Adjunct to general anesthesia to aid endotracheal (ET) intubation • Induction of skeletal muscle paralysis during surgery or mechanical ventilation	• Bradycardia, arrhythmias, cardiac arrest • Postoperative muscle pain • Respiratory depression, apnea, bronchoconstriction • Malignant hyperthermia, increased intraocular pressure, flushing
Nondepolarizing		
Atracurium besylate (Tracrium)	• Adjunct to general anesthesia, to facilitate ET intubation, and to provide skeletal muscle relaxation during surgery or mechanical ventilation	• Flushing, bradycardia • Prolonged dose-related apnea, bronchospasm, laryngospasm • Anaphylaxis
Cisatracurium besylate (Nimbex)	• Adjunct to general anesthesia, to facilitate ET intubation, and to provide skeletal muscle relaxation during surgery or mechanical ventilation in the CCU • Maintenance of neuromuscular blockade in the CCU	
Pancuronium bromide (Pavulon)	• Adjunct to anesthesia to induce skeletal muscle relaxation, facilitate intubation and ventilation, and weaken muscle contractions in induced seizures	• Residual muscle weakness • Prolonged, dose-related respiratory insufficiency or apnea • Allergic or idiosyncratic hypersensitivity reactions

*Common or life-threatening only

Special considerations

- Contraindicated in patients with history of malignant hyperthermia, myopathies associated with creatinine phosphokinase, acute angle-closure glaucoma, and penetrating eye injuries.
- Monitor the patient for histamine release and resulting hypotension and flushing.

- Drug doesn't affect consciousness or relieve pain. Be sure to keep the patient sedated. Have emergency respiratory support readily available.
- Drug has little or no effect on heart rate and doesn't counteract or reverse the bradycardia caused by anesthetics or vagal stimulation. Thus, bradycardia is seen more frequently with atracurium than with other neuromuscular blocking agents. Pretreatment with anticholinergics (atropine or glycopyrrolate) is advised.
- Use drug only if ET intubation, administration of oxygen under positive pressure, artificial respiration, and assisted or controlled ventilation are immediately available.
- Use a peripheral nerve stimulator to monitor responses during ICU administration; it may be used to detect residual paralysis during recovery and to avoid atracurium overdose.

- Drug isn't compatible with propofol injection or ketorolac injection for Y-site administration. Drug is acidic and also may not be compatible with an alkaline solution having a pH greater than 8.5, such as barbiturate solutions for Y-site administration. Don't dilute in lactated Ringer's injection because of chemical instability.
- Drug isn't recommended for rapid sequence ET intubation because of its intermediate onset of action.
- In patients with neuromuscular disease (myasthenia gravis and myasthenic syndrome), watch for possible prolonged neuromuscular block. The use of a peripheral nerve stimulator and a dose not exceeding 0.02 mg/kg is recommended to assess the level of neuromuscular block and to monitor dosage requirements.
- Burn patients may develop resistance to nondepolarizing neuromuscular blockers; they may need dosage increases and may exhibit shortened duration of action.
- Monitor the patient's acid-base balance and electrolyte levels. Acid-base or serum electrolyte abnormalities may potentiate or antagonize the action of cisatracurium.

- If using succinylcholine, allow its effects to subside before giving pancuronium.
- Don't mix in same syringe or give through same needle with barbiturates or other alkaline solutions.
- Reduce dosage when ether or other inhalation anesthetics that enhance neuromuscular blockade are used.
- Large doses may increase frequency and severity of tachycardia.

(continued)

Neuromuscular blocking agents *(continued)*

Drug	Indications	Adverse effects*
Tubocurarine chloride	● Adjunct to general anesthesia to induce skeletal muscle relaxation, facilitate intubation, and reduce fractures and dislocations ● Assistance with mechanical ventilation ● Weakening of muscle contractions in pharmacologically or electrically induced seizures	● Arrhythmias, cardiac arrest, bradycardia ● Respiratory depression or apnea, bronchospasm ● Hypersensitivity reactions
Vecuronium bromide (Norcuron)	● Adjunct to anesthesia, to facilitate intubation, and to provide skeletal muscle relaxation during surgery or mechanical ventilation	● Prolonged, dose-related respiratory insufficiency or apnea

*Common or life-threatening only

Special considerations

- The margin of safety between a therapeutic dose and a dose causing respiratory paralysis is small.
- Give drug I.V. slowly over 60 to 90 seconds or I.M. by deep injection in deltoid muscle.
- Assess baseline tests of renal function and serum electrolyte levels before drug administration. Electrolyte imbalance, particularly of potassium and magnesium, can potentiate effects of drug.

- Administer by rapid I.V. injection or I.V. infusion. Don't give I.M.
- Diluent supplied by manufacturer contains benzyl alcohol, which isn't intended for use in newborns.
- Recovery time may double in patients with cirrhosis or cholestasis.
- Assess baseline serum electrolyte levels, acid-base balance, and renal and hepatic function before administration.

Oxygen therapy

Various types of devices may be used to deliver oxygen therapy. Regardless of the type, always be sure to assess the patient closely and check the results of pulse oximetry or arterial blood gas analysis 20 to 30 minutes after adjusting the flow rate.

Delivery device	Oxygen concentration administered
Nasal cannula	Low flow, 1 to 6 L/minute (24% to 40% fraction of inspired oxygen [FIO_2])
Simple mask	Oxygen at 5 to 8 L/minute (40% to 60% FIO_2)
Partial rebreather mask	Oxygen at 6 to 10 L/minute (40% to 60% FIO_2)
Nonrebreather mask	Oxygen at 6 to 8 L/minute (60% to 80% FIO_2)

Administration guidelines

- Ensure patency of nostrils with flashlight.
- Hook the cannula tubing behind the patient's ears and under his chin, sliding the adjuster upward under the chin to secure.
- Alternatively, position elastic strap over the patient's ears and around the back of his head; avoid applying too tightly, which can cause pressure on the facial structures and occlude the cannula.
- With this device, oral breathers achieve the same oxygen delivery as nasal breathers.
- Headache may occur if flow rate is greater than 6 L/minute.

- Ensure proper fitting mask for the patient.
- Place mask over the patient's nose, mouth, and chin, molding the flexible metal edge to the bridge of his nose.
- Adjust elastic band around the patient's head to hold the mask firmly but comfortably in place.
- If necessary, tape gauze pads to the mask over the patient's cheek area to make an airtight seal.
- If the mask doesn't fit snugly, room air will dilute the oxygen, interfering with the delivery of the prescribed concentration.
- A minimum of 5 L/minute is required in all masks to flush carbon dioxide from it so that the patient doesn't rebreathe it.

- Follow the measures as for a simple mask with these additions:
- Monitor the reservoir bag collapse; if it collapses more than slightly during inspiration, raise the flow rate until only a slight deflation is seen.
- Marked or complete deflation indicates insufficient oxygen flow, which could possibly lead to carbon dioxide accumulation in the mask.
- Keep the reservoir bag from twisting or kinking.
- Ensure free expansion of the bag by keeping it outside of the patient's gown and bedcovers.

- This type of mask delivers the highest percentage of oxygen without intubation and mechanical ventilation.
- Follow the measures as for a simple mask with these additions:
- Make sure the mask fits snugly and the one-way valves are secure and functioning.
- Watch for possible signs of carbon dioxide buildup due to a malfunctioning valve.
- Monitor the deflation of the reservoir bag; if it collapses more than slightly during inspiration, raise the flow rate until only a slight deflation is seen.
- Marked or complete deflation indicates insufficient oxygen flow, which could possibly lead to carbon dioxide accumulation in the mask.
- Keep the reservoir bag from twisting or kinking.
- Ensure free expansion of the bag by keeping it outside of the patient's gown and bedcovers.

(continued)

Oxygen therapy *(continued)*

Delivery device	Oxygen concentration administered
Venturi mask	Oxygen at 4 to 10 L/minute (24% to 55% FIO_2)
Continuous positive airway pressure (CPAP) mask	Variable
Transtracheal oxygen	Variable
Aerosols	Variable; high-humidity oxygen that can be heated or cooled delivered by a jet nebulizer

Administration guidelines

- Follow the measures as for a simple mask with these additions:.
- – Ensure that the proper device is used and that the oxygen flow rate is set at the amount specified on each mask.
- – Make sure that the Venturi valve is set for the desired FIO_2.
- – Ensure a snug but comfortably fitting mask; a loose fit or twisting, kinking, or blocked oxygen ports may alter the oxygen concentration being given.
- – Keep the patient's skin dry; condensation may collect on the tubing and drip on the patient when humidification is used.

- This system allows the spontaneously breathing patient to receive CPAP with or without an artificial airway.
- This type of mask is contraindicated in patients with chronic obstructive pulmonary disease, bullous lung disease, low cardiac output, or tension pneumothorax.
- Place one strap behind the patient's head and the other strap over it to ensure a snug fit.
- Assess the patient's respiratory, cardiac, circulatory, and GI function hourly.

- This catheter device supplies oxygen throughout the respiratory cycle.
- After insertion, obtain a chest X-ray as ordered to confirm placement of the catheter.
- Assess the patient for bleeding, respiratory distress, pneumothorax, pain, coughing, or hoarseness.
- Don't use the catheter for approximately 1 week after insertion to reduce the risk of subcutaneous emphysema.

- Be alert for condensation buildup in the tubing; empty the tubing at frequent intervals.
- Ensure that condensate doesn't enter the trachea.
- Monitor the tracheostomy tube site (if the patient has one) for signs of irritation and pressure.
- When using a high-output nebulizer, watch for signs of overhydration, pulmonary edema, crackles, and electrolyte imbalances.

Pain management agents

Drug	Indications	Adverse effects*
Acetaminophen (Acephen, Anacin Aspirin Free, Tylenol)	• Mild pain • Fever	• Neutropenia, leukopenia, pancytopenia, thrombocytopenia • Severe liver damage • Hypoglycemia
Aspirin (ASA, Ascriptin, Bufferin)	• Mild pain • Fever • Transient ischemic attacks and thromboembolic disorders • Treatment or reduction of the risk of MI in patients with previous MI or unstable angina • Pericarditis following acute MI • Prevention of reocclusion in coronary revascularization procedures • Stent implantation	• Tinnitus, hearing loss • Nausea, GI distress, occult bleeding, dyspepsia, GI bleeding • Acute renal insufficiency • Leukopenia, thrombocytopenia, prolonged bleeding time • Liver dysfunction, hepatitis • Rash • Hypersensitivity reactions (anaphylaxis, asthma), Reye's syndrome, angioedema
Codeine phosphate; codeine sulfate	• Mild to moderate pain • Nonproductive cough	• Sedation, clouded sensorium, euphoria, dizziness, light-headedness • Hypotension, bradycardia • Nausea, vomiting, constipation, dry mouth, ileus • Urine retention • Respiratory depression • Diaphoresis
Fentanyl citrate (Sublimaze); Fentanyl Transdermal System (Duragesic-25, Duragesic-50, Duragesic-75, Duragesic-100)	• Preoperative analgesic • Adjunct to general anesthetic; low-dose regimen for minor procedures; moderate-dose regimen for major procedures; high-dose regimen for complicated procedures • Postoperative analgesic • Management of chronic pain in patients who can't be managed by lesser means • Management of breakthrough cancer pain	• Sedation, somnolence, clouded sensorium, confusion, asthenia • Arrhythmias • Nausea, vomiting, constipation, dry mouth • Urine retention • Respiratory depression, apnea

*Common or life-threatening only

Special considerations

- Use cautiously in patients with history of chronic alcohol abuse because hepatotoxicity has occurred after therapeutic doses. Also use cautiously in patients with hepatic or cardiovascular disease, renal function impairment, or viral infection.
- Know patient's total daily intake of acetaminophen, especially if he's also taking other prescribed drugs containing this component, such as Percocet. Toxicity can occur.
- Monitor the PT and INR values in patients receiving oral anticoagulants and sustained acetaminophen therapy.

- Contraindicated in patients with G6PD deficiency or bleeding disorders such as hemophilia, von Willebrand's disease, or telangiectasia. Also contraindicated in patients with NSAID-induced sensitivity reactions.
- Use cautiously in patients with GI lesions, impaired renal function, hypoprothrombinemia, vitamin K deficiency, thrombotic thrombocytopenic purpura, or hepatic impairment.
- Use cautiously in patients with history of GI disease (especially peptic ulcer disease), increased risk of GI bleeding, or decreased renal function.
- Give 8 oz (240 ml) of water or milk with salicylates to ensure passage into stomach. Have patient to sit up for 15 to 30 minutes after taking salicylates to prevent lodging of salicylate in esophagus.
- Monitor vital signs frequently, especially temperature.
- Salicylates may mask the signs and symptoms of acute infection (fever, myalgia, erythema); carefully evaluate patients at risk for infections, such as those with diabetes.
- Monitor CBC, platelets, PT, BUN, serum creatinine, and liver function studies periodically during salicylate therapy to detect abnormalities.
- Assess the patient for signs and symptoms of hemorrhage, such as petechiae, bruising, coffee-ground vomitus, and black, tarry stools.

- Use cautiously in elderly or debilitated patients and in those with impaired renal or hepatic function, head injuries, increased intracranial pressure, increased CSF pressure, hypothyroidism, Addison's disease, acute alcoholism, CNS depression, bronchial asthma, COPD, respiratory depression, or shock.
- Don't mix with other solutions because codeine phosphate is incompatible with many drugs.
- Patients who become physically dependent on drug may experience acute withdrawal syndrome if given a narcotic antagonist.
- The drug may delay gastric emptying, increase biliary tract pressure resulting from contraction of the sphincter of Oddi, and interfere with hepatobiliary imaging studies.

- Use cautiously in elderly or debilitated patients and in those with head injuries, increased CSF pressure, COPD, decreased respiratory reserve, compromised respirations, arrhythmias, or hepatic, renal, or cardiac disease.
- Give an anticholinergic, such as atropine or glycopyrrolate, to minimize possible bradycardic effect of fentanyl.
- Gradually adjust dosage in patients using the transdermal system. Reaching steady state levels of a new dose may take up to 6 days; delay dose adjustment until after at least two applications.
- When reducing opiate therapy or switching to a different analgesic, expect to withdraw the transdermal system gradually. Because the serum level of fentanyl decreases very gradually after removal, give half of the equianalgesic dose of the new analgesic 12 to 18 hours after removal.

(continued)

Pain management agents *(continued)*

Drug	Indications	Adverse effects*
Hydromorphone hydrochloride (Dilaudid)	• Moderate to severe pain • Cough	• Sedation, somnolence, clouded sensorium, dizziness, euphoria • Hypotension, bradycardia • Nausea, vomiting, constipation • Urine retention • Respiratory depression, bronchospasm
Ibuprofen (Advil, Motrin, Motrin IB, Nuprin)	• Arthritis, gout • Mild to moderate pain, headache, backache, minor aches associated with the common cold • Fever reduction	• Acute renal failure • Neutropenia, pancytopenia, thrombocytopenia, aplastic anemia, leukopenia, agranulocytosis • Bronchospasm • Stevens-Johnson syndrome
Ketorolac tromethamine (Toradol)	• Short-term management of severe, acute pain • Short-term management of moderately severe, acute pain when switching from parenteral to oral administration	• Drowsiness, sedation, dizziness, headache • Arrhythmias • Nausea, dyspepsia, GI pain • Renal failure • Thrombocytopenia
Morphine sulfate (Astramorph PF, Avinza, Duramorph, Infumorph, Kadian, MS Contin, MSIR, MS/L, MS/S, OMS Concentrate, Oramorph SR, RMS Uniserts, Roxanol)	• Severe pain • Severe, chronic pain related to cancer • Preoperative sedation and adjunct to anesthesia • Postoperative analgesia • Control of pain caused by acute MI • Control of angina pain • Adjunctive treatment of acute pulmonary edema	• Seizures (with large doses), dizziness, nightmares (with long-acting oral forms), light-headedness • Hypotension, bradycardia, shock, cardiac arrest • Nausea, vomiting, constipation, ileus, dry mouth, biliary tract spasms, anorexia • Urine retention • Thrombocytopenia • Respiratory depression, apnea, respiratory arrest • Diaphoresis, edema • Physical dependence, decreased libido

*Common or life-threatening only

Special considerations

- Contraindicated in patients with intracranial lesions caused by increased intracranial pressure, and whenever ventilator function is depressed, such as in status asthmaticus, COPD, cor pulmonale, emphysema, and kyphoscoliosis.
- Use cautiously in elderly or debilitated patients and in those with hepatic or renal disease, Addison's disease, hypothyroidism, prostatic hyperplasia, or urethral strictures.
- For a better analgesic effect, give drug before the patient has intense pain.
- Give by direct injection over no less than 2 minutes, and monitor the patient constantly. Keep resuscitation equipment available. Respiratory depression and hypotension can occur with I.V. administration.
- Drug may worsen or mask gallbladder pain. Increased biliary tract pressure resulting from contraction of the sphincter of Oddi may interfere with hepatobiliary imaging studies.

- Contraindicated in patients who have the syndrome of nasal polyps, angioedema, and bronchospastic reaction to aspirin or other NSAIDs. Contraindicated during the last trimester of pregnancy because it may cause problems with the fetus or complications during delivery.
- Use cautiously in patients with impaired renal or hepatic function, GI disorders, peptic ulcer disease, cardiac decompensation, hypertension, or coagulation defects. Because chewable tablets contain aspartame, use cautiously in patients with phenylketonuria.
- Monitor auditory and ophthalmic functions periodically during ibuprofen therapy.
- Observe the patient for possible fluid retention.
- Patients older than age 60 may be more susceptible to the toxic effects of ibuprofen, especially adverse GI reactions. Use lowest possible effective dose. The effect of drug on renal prostaglandins may cause fluid retention and edema, a significant drawback for elderly patients, especially those with heart failure.

- Contraindicated in patients with active peptic ulcer disease, recent GI bleeding or perforation, advanced renal impairment, risk of renal impairment due to volume depletion, suspected or confirmed cerebrovascular bleeding, hemorrhagic diathesis, incomplete hemostasis, or high risk of bleeding.
- Use cautiously in patients with impaired renal or hepatic function.
- The combined duration of ketorolac I.M., I.V., or P.O. shouldn't exceed 5 days. Oral use is only for continuation of I.V. or I.M. therapy.

- Contraindicated in patients with conditions that would preclude administration of opioids by I.V. route (acute bronchial asthma or upper airway obstruction).
- Use cautiously in elderly or debilitated patients and in those with head injury, increased intracranial pressure, seizures, pulmonary disease, prostatic hyperplasia, hepatic or renal disease, acute abdominal conditions, hypothyroidism, Addison's disease, or urethral strictures.
- For I.V. use, morphine 25 mg/ml is diluted to 0.1 to 1 mg/ml in D_5W. A higher concentration may be used for patients with fluid restriction.
- Long-term therapy in patients with advanced renal disease may lead to toxicity as a result of accumulation of the active metabolite.

Sedatives

Drug	Indications	Adverse effects*
Lorazepam (Ativan)	• Anxiety, tension, agitation, irritability, especially in anxiety neuroses or organic (especially GI or cardiovascular) disorders • Status epilepticus	• Drowsiness, sedation, • Acute withdrawal syndrome (after sudden discontinuation in physically dependent patients)
Midazolam hydrochloride (Versed)	• Preoperative sedation (to induce sleepiness or drowsiness and relieve apprehension) • Conscious sedation • Continuous infusion for sedation of intubated and mechanically ventilated patients as a component of anesthesia or during treatment in a critical care setting • Sedation, anxiolysis, and amnesia before diagnostic, therapeutic, or endoscopic procedures or before induction of anesthesia	• Pain • Cardiac arrest • Nausea • Hiccups, decreased respiratory rate, apnea, respiratory arrest
Propofol (Diprivan)	• Induction and maintenance of sedation in mechanically ventilated patients	• Hypotension, bradycardia • Hyperlipidemia • Apnea

*Common or life-threatening only

Special considerations

- Contraindicated in patients with acute angle-closure glaucoma.
- Use cautiously in patients with pulmonary, renal, or hepatic impairment and in elderly, acutely ill, or debilitated patients.
- Parenteral lorazepam appears to possess potent amnesic effects.
- For the oral concentrated solution, add dose to 30 ml or more of water, juice, or soda, or to semisolid foods.
- For I.V. administration, dilute lorazepam with an equal volume of a compatible diluent, such as D_5W, sterile water for injection, or normal saline solution.
- Inject the drug directly into a vein or into the tubing of a compatible I.V. infusion, such as normal saline solution or D_5W solution. The rate of lorazepam I.V. injection shouldn't exceed 2 mg/minute. Have emergency resuscitative equipment available when administering I.V.
- Monitor hepatic function studies to prevent cumulative effects and to ensure adequate drug metabolism.
- Parenteral administration of drug is more likely to cause apnea, hypotension, bradycardia, and cardiac arrest in elderly patients.

- Contraindicated in patients with acute angle-closure glaucoma and in those experiencing shock, coma, or acute alcohol intoxication.
- Use cautiously in patients with uncompensated acute illnesses, in elderly or debilitated patients, and in patients with myasthenia gravis or neuromuscular disorders and pulmonary disease.
- Closely monitor cardiopulmonary function; continuously monitor patients who have received midazolam to detect potentially life-threatening respiratory depression.
- Have emergency respiratory equipment readily available. Laryngospasm and bronchospasm, although rare, may occur.
- Midazolam can be mixed in the same syringe with morphine, meperidine, atropine, and scopolamine. Solution is stable for 30 minutes. Solutions compatible with midazolam include D_5W, normal saline solution, and lactated Ringer's solution

---

- Contraindicated in patients hypersensitive to propofol or components of the emulsion, including soybean oil, egg lecithin, and glycerol. Because drug is administered as an emulsion, administer cautiously to patients with a disorder of lipid metabolism (such as pancreatitis, primary hyperlipoproteinemia, and diabetic hyperlipidemia). Use cautiously if the patient is receiving lipids as part of a total parenteral nutrition infusion; I.V. lipid dose may need to be reduced. Use cautiously in elderly or debilitated patients and in those with circulatory disorders.
- Although the hemodynamic effects of drug can vary, its major effect in patients maintaining spontaneous ventilation is arterial hypotension (arterial pressure can decrease as much as 30%) with little or no change in heart rate and cardiac output. However, significant depression of cardiac output may occur in patients undergoing assisted or controlled positive pressure ventilation.
- Don't mix propofol with other drugs or blood products. If it's to be diluted before infusion, use only D_5W and don't dilute to a concentration of less than 2 mg/ml. After dilution, drug appears to be more stable in glass containers than in plastic.
- If used for sedation of a mechanically ventilated patient, wake him every 24 hours.

Therapeutic drug monitoring guidelines

Drug	Laboratory test monitored	Therapeutic ranges of test
Aminoglycoside antibiotics (amikacin, gentamicin, tobramycin)	Amikacin peak trough Gentamicin/tobramycin peak trough Creatinine	20 to 25 mcg/ml 5 to 10 mcg/ml 4 to 8 mcg/ml 1 to 2 mcg/ml 0.6 to 1.3 mg/dl
Amphotericin B	Creatinine BUN Electrolytes (especially potassium and magnesium) Liver function CBC with differential and platelets	0.6 to 1.3 mg/dl 5 to 20 mg/dl Potassium: 3.5 to 5 mEq/L Magnesium: 1.5 to 2.5 mEq/L Sodium: 135 to 145 mEq/L Chloride: 98 to 106 mEq/L * *****
Digoxin	Digoxin Electrolytes (especially potassium, magnesium, and calcium) Creatinine	0.8 to 2 ng/ml Potassium: 3.5 to 5 mEq/L Magnesium: 1.7 to 2.1 mEq/L Sodium: 135 to 145 mEq/L Chloride: 98 to 106 mEq/L Calcium: 8.6 to 10 mg/dl 0.6 to 1.3 mg/dl
Diuretics	Electrolytes Creatinine BUN Uric acid Fasting glucose	Potassium: 3.5 to 5 mEq/L Magnesium: 1.7 to 2.1 mEq/L Sodium: 135 to 145 mEq/L Chloride: 98 to 106 mEq/L Calcium: 8.6 to 10 mg/dl 0.6 to 1.3 mg/dl 5 to 20 mg/dl 2 to 7 mg/dl 70 to 110 mg/dl
Ethosuximide	Ethosuximide	40 to 100 mcg/ml
Gemfibrozil	Lipids	Total cholesterol: < 200 mg/dl LDL: < 130 mg/dl HDL: Women: 40 to 75 mg/dl Men: 37 to 70 mg/dl Triglycerides: 10 to 160 mg/dl

Note: ***** For those areas marked with asterisks, these values can be used:

Hemoglobin: Women: 12 to 16 g/dl
            Men: 14 to 18 g/dl
Hematocrit: Women: 37% to 48%
            Men: 42% to 52%
RBCs: 4 to 5.5 x 10^6/mm^3
WBCs: 5 to 10 x 10^3/mm^3

Differential: Neutrophils: 45% to 74%
              Bands: 0% to 8%
              Lymphocytes: 16% to 45%
              Monocytes: 4% to 10%
              Eosinophils: 0% to 7%
              Basophils: 0% to 2%

Monitoring guidelines

Wait until the administration of the third dose to check drug levels. Obtain blood for peak level 30 minutes after I.V. infusion or 60 minutes after I.M. administration. For trough levels, draw blood just before next dose. Dosage may need to be adjusted accordingly. Recheck after three doses. Monitor creatinine and BUN levels and urine output for signs of decreasing renal function.

Monitor creatinine, BUN, and electrolyte levels at least weekly during therapy. Also, regularly monitor blood counts and liver function test results during therapy.

Check digoxin levels at least 12 hours, but preferably 24 hours, after the last dose is administered. To monitor maintenance therapy, check drug levels at least 1 to 2 weeks after therapy is initiated or changed. Make any adjustments in therapy based on entire clinical picture, not solely on drug levels. Also, check electrolyte levels and renal function periodically during therapy.

To monitor fluid and electrolyte balance, perform baseline and periodic determinations of electrolyte, calcium, BUN, uric acid, and glucose levels.

Check drug level 8 to 10 days after therapy is initiated or changed.

Therapy is usually withdrawn after 3 months if response is inadequate. Patient must be fasting to measure triglyceride levels.

(continued)

* For those areas marked with one asterisk, these values can be used:

ALT: 7 to 56 U/L

AST: 5 to 40 U/L

Alkaline phosphatase: 17 to 142 U/L

LDH: 60 to 220 U/L

GGT: < 40 U/L

Total bilirubin: 0.2 to 1 mg/dl

Therapeutic drug monitoring guidelines *(continued)*

Drug	Laboratory test monitored	Therapeutic ranges of test
Heparin	Activated partial thromboplastin time (aPTT)	1.5 to 2 times control
HMG-CoA reductase inhibitors (fluvastatin, lovastatin, pravastatin, simvastatin)	Lipids Liver function	Total cholesterol: < 200 mg/dl LDL: < 130 mg/dl HDL: Women: 40 to 75 mg/dl Men: 37 to 70 mg/dl Triglycerides: 10 to 160 mg/dl *
Insulin	Fasting glucose Glycosylated hemoglobin	70 to 110 mg/dl 5.5% to 8.5% of total hemoglobin
Lithium	Lithium Creatinine CBC Electrolytes (especially potassium and sodium) Fasting glucose Thyroid function tests	0.5 to 1.4 mEq/L 0.6 to 1.3 mg/dl ***** Potassium: 3.5 to 5 mEq/L Magnesium: 1.7 to 2.1 mEq/L Sodium: 135 to 145 mEq/L Chloride: 98 to 106 mEq/L 70 to 110 mg/dl TSH: 0.2 to 5.4 microU/ml T3: 80 to 200 ng/dl T4: 5.4 to 11.5 mcg/dl
Methotrexate	Methotrexate CBC with differential Platelet count Liver function Creatinine	Normal elimination: < 10 micromol 24 hours postdose < 1 micromol 48 hours postdose < 0.2 micromol 72 hours postdose ***** 150 to 450 $\times$ 10^3/mm^3 * 0.6 to 1.3 mg/dl
Phenytoin	Phenytoin CBC	10 to 20 mcg/ml *****

Note: ***** For those areas marked with asterisks, these values can be used:

Hemoglobin: Women: 12 to 16 g/dl
        Men: 14 to 18 g/dl
Hematocrit: Women: 37% to 48%
        Men: 42% to 52%
RBCs: 4 to 5.5 x 10^6/mm^3
WBCs: 5 to 10 x 10^3/mm^3

Differential: Neutrophils: 45% to 74%
        Bands: 0% to 8%
        Lymphocytes: 16% to 45%
        Monocytes: 4% to 10%
        Eosinophils: 0% to 7%
        Basophils: 0% to 2%

Monitoring guidelines

When drug is given by continuous I.V. infusion, check aPTT every 4 hours in the early stages of therapy. When drug is given by deep S.C. injection, check aPTT 4 to 6 hours after injection.

Perform liver function tests at baseline, 6 to 12 weeks after therapy is initiated or changed, and periodically thereafter. If adequate response isn't achieved within 6 weeks, consider changing the therapy.

Monitor response to therapy by evaluating glucose and glycosylated hemoglobin levels. Glycosylated hemoglobin level is a good measure of long-term control. A patient's home monitoring of glucose levels helps measure compliance and response.

Checking lithium levels is crucial to the safe use of the drug. Obtain lithium levels immediately before next dose. Monitor levels twice weekly until stable. Once at steady state, levels should be checked weekly; when the patient is on the appropriate maintenance dose, levels should be checked every 2 to 3 months. Monitor creatinine, electrolyte, and fasting glucose levels; CBC; and thyroid function test results before therapy is initiated and periodically during therapy.

Monitor methotrexate levels according to dosing protocol. Monitor CBC with differential, platelet count, and liver and renal function test results more frequently when therapy is initiated or changed and when methotrexate levels may be elevated, such as when the patient is dehydrated.

Monitor phenytoin levels immediately before next dose and 2 to 4 weeks after therapy is initiated or changed. Obtain a CBC at baseline and monthly early in therapy. Watch for toxic effects at therapeutic levels. Adjust the measured level for hypoalbuminemia or renal impairment, which can increase free drug levels.

(continued)

* For those areas marked with one asterisk, these values can be used:

ALT: 7 to 56 U/L
AST: 5 to 40 U/L
Alkaline phosphatase: 17 to 142 U/L

LDH: 60 to 220 U/L
GGT: < 40 U/L
Total bilirubin: 0.2 to 1 mg/dl

Therapeutic drug monitoring guidelines *(continued)*

Drug	Laboratory test monitored	Therapeutic ranges of test
Procainamide	Procainamide N-acetylprocainamide CBC	4 to 8 mcg/ml (procainamide) 5 to 30 mcg/ml (combined pro- cainamide and NAPA) *****
Quinidine	Quinidine CBC Liver function Creatinine Electrolytes (especially potassium)	2 to 6 mcg/ml ***** * 0.6 to 1.3 mg/dl Potassium: 3.5 to 5 mEq/L Magnesium: 1.7 to 2.1 mEq/L Sodium: 135 to 145 mEq/L Chloride: 98 to 106 mEq/L
Sulfonylureas	Fasting glucose Glycosylated hemoglobin	70 to 110 mg/dl 5.5% to 8.5% of total hemoglobin
Theophylline	Theophylline	10 to 20 mcg/ml
Thyroid hormone	Thyroid function tests Vancomycin	TSH: 0.2 to 5.4 microU/ml T3: 80 to 200 ng/dl T4: 5.4 to 11.5 mcg/dl
Vancomycin	Creatinine	20 to 35 mcg/ml (peak) 5 to 10 mcg/ml (trough) 0.6 to 1.3 mg/dl
Warfarin	INR	For an acute MI, atrial fibrillation, treatment of pulmonary embolism, prevention of systemic embolism, tissue heart valves, valvular heart disease, or prophylaxis or treatment of venous thrombosis: 2 to 3 For mechanical prosthetic valves or recurrent systemic embolism: 2.5 to 3.5

Note: ***** For those areas marked with asterisks, these values can be used:

Hemoglobin:	Women: 12 to 16 g/dl	Differential: Neutrophils: 45% to 74%
	Men: 14 to 18 g/dl	Bands: 0% to 8%
Hematocrit:	Women: 37% to 48%	Lymphocytes: 16% to 45%
	Men: 42% to 52%	Monocytes: 4% to 10%
RBCs: 4 to 5.5 x 10^6/mm^3		Eosinophils: 0% to 7%
WBCs: 5 to 10 x 10^3/mm^3		Basophils: 0% to 2%

Monitoring guidelines

Measure procainamide levels 6 to 12 hours after a continuous infusion is started or immediately before the next oral dose. Combined (procainamide and NAPA) levels can be used as an index of toxicity when renal impairment exists. Obtain CBC periodically during longer-term therapy.

Obtain levels immediately before next oral dose and 30 to 35 hours after therapy is initiated or changed. Periodically obtain blood counts, liver and kidney function test results, and electrolyte levels.

Monitor response to therapy by periodically evaluating fasting glucose and glycosylated hemoglobin levels. Patient should monitor glucose levels at home to help measure compliance and response.

Obtain theophylline levels immediately before next dose of sustained-release oral product and at least 2 days after therapy is initiated or changed.

Monitor thyroid function test results every 2 to 3 weeks until appropriate maintenance dose is determined.

Vancomycin levels may be checked with the third dose administered, at the earliest. Draw peak levels ½ hour after the I.V. infusion is completed. Draw trough levels immediately before the next dose is administered. Renal function can be used to adjust dosing and intervals.

Check INR daily, beginning 3 days after therapy is initiated. Continue checking it until therapeutic goal is achieved, and monitor it periodically thereafter. Also, check levels 7 days after any change in warfarin dose or concomitant, potentially interacting therapy.

* For those areas marked with one asterisk, these values can be used:

ALT: 7 to 56 U/L	LDH: 60 to 220 U/L
AST: 5 to 40 U/L	GGT: < 40 U/L
Alkaline phosphatase: 17 to 142 U/L	Total bilirubin: 0.2 to 1 mg/dl

Thrombolytic enzymes

Thrombolytic enzymes dissolve clots by accelerating the formation of plasmin by activated plasminogen. Plasminogen activators, found in most tissues and body fluids, help plasminogen (an inactive enzyme) convert to plasmin (an active enzyme), which dissolves the clot. Doses of the enzymes listed here may vary according to the patient's condition.

Drug	Action
Alteplase	Directly converts plasminogen to plasmin
Reteplase	Enhances the cleavage of plasminogen to generate plasmin
Streptokinase	Indirectly activates plasminogen, which converts to plasmin
Tenecteplase	Directly converts plasminogen to plasmin
Urokinase	Directly converts plasminogen to plasmin

Troubleshooting arterial monitoring catheters

Problem	Possible causes	Interventions
Damped waveform	● Air in the system	● Check system for air, especially at tubing and transducer's diaphragm. ● Aspirate air or force it from the system through a stopcock port. ● Never flush any fluid containing air bubbles into the patient.
	● Loose connection	● Check all connections. ● Tighten as necessary.
	● Clotted catheter tip	● Check your facility's policy and, if permitted, attempt to aspirate the clot; if successful, flush the catheter line. ● Don't flush if the clot can't be aspirated; notify the physician.
	● Catheter tip resting against arterial wall	● Reposition catheter by carefully rotating it or pulling it back slightly. ● Anticipate possible change in catheter placement site, and assist as necessary.
	● Kinked tubing	● Inspect tubing for kinks, and straighten.
	● Inadequately inflated pressure infuser bag	● Check pressure on bag; inflate the bag to 300 mm Hg.
Drifting waveform	● Temperature change in flush solution	● Allow temperature of flush solution to stabilize before using.
	● Kinked or compressed monitor cable	● Check cable for kinks, and relieve kink or compression.
Inability to flush line or withdraw blood	● Incorrectly positioned stopcocks	● Check stopcocks and reposition.
	● Kinked tubing	● Check for kinks, and straighten as necessary.
	● Inadequately inflated pressure infuser bag	● Check pressure on infuser bag, and inflate to 300 mm Hg.
	● Clotted catheter tip	● Check your facility's policy and, if permitted, attempt to aspirate the clot; if successful, flush the catheter line. ● Don't flush if the clot can't be aspirated; notify physician.
	● Catheter tip resting against arterial wall	● Reposition catheter by carefully rotating it or pulling it back slightly. ● Anticipate possible change in catheter placement site, and assist as necessary.

(continued)

Troubleshooting arterial monitoring catheters *(continued)*

Problem	Possible causes	Interventions
Inability to flush line or withdraw blood *(continued)*	● Position of insertion site	● Check position of insertion area, and change as indicated. ● Use an armboard if the area is the brachial or radial site. ● Elevate the head of the bed at a 45-degree angle or less for femoral site to prevent kinking.
Artifact	● Electrical interference	● Check other electrical equipment in the patient's room, and remove or move away as appropriate.
	● Patient movement	● Ask the patient to lie quietly while you're reading the monitor.
	● Catheter whip or fling	● Shorten the tubing, if possible.
False high-pressure alarm	● Improper calibration	● Recalibrate the system.
	● Transducer positioned below phlebostatic axis	● Relevel the transducer.
	● Catheter kinked	● Check catheter for kinks, and straighten.
	● Clotted catheter tip	● Check your facility's policy and, if permitted, attempt to aspirate the clot; if successful, flush the catheter line. ● Don't flush if the clot can't be aspirated; notify the physician.
	● Catheter tip resting against arterial wall	● Flush the catheter, if appropriate, or reposition catheter by carefully rotating it or pulling it back slightly. ● Anticipate possible change in catheter placement site, and assist as necessary.
	● I.V. tubing too long	● Shorten tubing by removing extension tubing if used, or replace with administration set of a shorter length.
	● Small air bubbles in tubing close to patient	● Remove air bubbles.
False low-pressure reading	● Improper calibration	● Recheck to ensure that the reading is accurate. ● Recalibrate the system.

Troubleshooting arterial monitoring catheters *(continued)*

Problem	Possible causes	Interventions
False low-pressure reading *(continued)*	• Transducer positioned above level of phlebostatic axis	• Relevel the transducer.
	• Loose connections	• Check all connections, and tighten as necessary.
	• Catheter kinked	• Check catheter for kinks, and straighten.
	• Catheter tip resting against arterial wall	• Flush the catheter, if appropriate, or reposition catheter by carefully rotating it or pulling it back slightly. • Anticipate possible change in catheter placement site, and assist as necessary.
	• I.V. tubing too long	• Shorten the tubing by removing extension tubing (if used), or replace with administration set of a shorter length.
	• Large air bubble close to transducer	• Reprime the transducer.
No waveform	• No power supply	• Check power supply, and turn on.
	• Stopcocks turned off to patient	• Check positioning of stopcocks, and reposition properly as necessary. • Make sure that the transducer is open to the stopcock.
	• Transducer disconnected from monitor module	• Reconnect transducer to the module.
	• Occluded catheter	• Attempt to aspirate the clot. If successful, flush the line; if unsuccessful, don't flush — notify the physician.
	• Catheter tip resting against arterial wall	• Flush the catheter, if appropriate, or reposition catheter by carefully rotating it or pulling it back slightly. • Anticipate possible change in catheter placement site, and assist as necessary.

Troubleshooting intra-aortic balloon pumps

Problem	Possible causes	Interventions
High gas leak (automatic mode only)	• Balloon leakage or abrasion	• Check for blood in the tubing. • Stop pumping. • Notify the physician to remove the balloon.
	• Condensation in extension tubing, volume limiter disk, or both	• Remove condensate from tubing and volume limiter disk. • Refill, autopurge, and resume pumping.
	• Kink in balloon catheter or tubing	• Check catheter and tubing for kinks and loose connections; straighten and tighten any found. • Refill and resume pumping.
	• Tachycardia	• Change wean control to 1:2 or operate on "manual" mode. • Keep in mind that alarms are off when pump is in manual mode. • Autopurge balloon every 1 to 2 hours, and monitor balloon pressure waveform closely.
	• Malfunctioning or loose volume limiter disk	• Replace or tighten disk. • Refill, autopurge, and resume pumping.
	• System leak	• Perform leak test.
Balloon line block (in automatic mode only)	• Kink in balloon or catheter	• Check catheter and tubing for kinks and loose connections; straighten and tighten any found. • Refill and resume pumping.
	• Balloon catheter not unfurled; sheath or balloon positioned too high	• Notify physician immediately to verify placement. • Anticipate need for repositioning or manual inflation of balloon.
	• Condensation in tubing, volume limiter disk, or both	• Remove condensate from tubing and volume limiter disk. • Refill, autopurge, and resume pumping.
	• Balloon too large for aorta	• Decrease volume control percentage by one notch.
	• Malfunctioning volume limiter disk or incorrect volume limiter disk size	• Replace volume limiter disk. • Refill, autopurge, and resume pumping.
No ECG trigger	• Inadequate signal	• Adjust ECG gain, and change lead or trigger mode.
	• Lead disconnected	• Replace lead.

Troubleshooting intra-aortic balloon pumps *(continued)*

Problem	Possible causes	Interventions
No ECG trigger *(continued)*	• Improper ECG input mode (skin or monitor) selected	• Adjust ECG input to appropriate mode (skin or monitor).
No atrial pressure trigger	• Arterial line damped	• Flush line.
	• Arterial line open to atmosphere	• Check connections on arterial pressure line.
Trigger mode change	• Trigger mode changed while pumping	• Resume pumping.
Irregular heart rhythm	• Patient experiencing arrhythmia, such as atrial fibrillation or ectopic beats	• Change to R or QRS sense (if necessary to accommodate irregular rhythm). • Notify physician of arrhythmia.
Erratic atrioventricular (AV) pacing	• Demand for paced rhythm occurring when in AV sequential trigger mode	• Change to pacer reject trigger or QRS sense.
Noisy ECG signal	• Malfunctioning leads	• Replace leads. • Check ECG cable.
	• Electrocautery in use	• Switch to atrial pressure trigger.
Internal trigger	• Trigger mode set on internal 80 beats/minute	• Select alternative trigger if patient has a heartbeat or rhythm. • Keep in mind that internal trigger is used only during cardiopulmonary bypass or cardiac arrest.
Purge incomplete	• Off button pressed during autopurge, interrupted purge cycle	• Initiate autopurging again, or initiate pumping.
High fill pressure	• Malfunctioning volume limiter disk	• Replace volume limiter disk. • Refill, autopurge, and resume pumping.
	• Occluded vent line or valve	• Attempt to resume pumping. • If unsuccessful, notify physician and contact manufacturer.
No balloon drive	• No volume limiter disk	• Insert volume limiter disk, and lock securely in place.
	• Tubing disconnected	• Reconnect tubing. • Refill, autopurge, and pump.

(continued)

Troubleshooting intra-aortic balloon pumps *(continued)*

Problem	Possible causes	Interventions
Incorrect timing	• INFLATE and DEFLATE controls set incorrectly	• Place INFLATE and DEFLATE controls at set mid-points. • Reassess timing and readjust.
Low volume percentage	• Volume control percentage not 100%	• Assess cause of decreased volume, and reset, if necessary.

Troubleshooting intracranial pressure monitors

Problem	Possible causes	Interventions
Damped or absent waveform	● Transducer needs recalibration	● Turn stopcock off to the patient. ● Open transducer's stopcock to air and balance transducer. ● Recalibrate transducer and monitor.
	● Air in line	● Turn stopcock off to the patient. ● Flush air out through an open stopcock port with a syringe and sterile normal saline solution. ● Don't use heparin to flush because some of the drug could inadvertently be injected into the patient and cause bleeding. ● Rebalance and recalibrate transducer and monitor.
	● Loose connection	● Check tubing and stopcocks for possible moisture, which may indicate a loose connection. ● Turn stopcock off to the patient, and then tighten all connections. ● Make sure tubing is long enough to allow the patient to turn head without pulling on the tubing.
	● Disconnection in the line	● Turn stopcock off to the patient immediately. ● Keep in mind that with a ventricular catheter, rapid cerebrospinal fluid loss may allow intracranial pressure to drop precipitously, causing brain herniation. ● Replace equipment to reduce the risk of infection.
	● Change in the patient's position	● Reposition transducer's balancing port level with the foramen of Monro. ● Rebalance and recalibrate transducer and monitor. ● Remember to rebalance and recalibrate at least once every 4 hours and whenever the patient is repositioned.
	● Tubing, catheter, or screw occluded with blood or brain tissue	● Notify the physician, because he may want to irrigate the screw or catheter with a small amount of sterile normal saline. ● Never irrigate the screw or catheter by yourself.
False pressure readings, high or low	● Air in line	● Turn stopcock off to the patient. ● Flush air out through an open stopcock port with a syringe and sterile normal saline solution. ● Rebalance and recalibrate transducer and monitor.

(continued)

Troubleshooting intracranial pressure monitors *(continued)*

Problem	Possible causes	Interventions
***False pressure readings, high or low** (continued)*	● Transducer placed too low (causing high pressure reading) or too high (causing low pressure reading)	● Reposition transducer's balancing port level with the foramen of Monro. ● Rebalance and recalibrate transducer and monitor.

Troubleshooting pulmonary artery catheters

Problem	Possible causes	Interventions
No waveform	• Transducer not open to the catheter	• Check the stopcock, and make sure that it's open to the patient. • Reevaluate waveform.
	• Transducer or monitor improperly set up	• Recheck all connections and components of the system to ensure that they're set up properly. • Rebalance the transducer. • Replace the system, if necessary.
	• Clotted catheter tip	• Attempt to aspirate the clot with a syringe, if your facility's policy permits. • If successful, flush the line. • Don't attempt to flush if the clot can't be aspirated; notify the physician.
Overdamped waveform	• Air in the line	• Check the system for air. • Aspirate air, or force it through a stopcock port.
	• Clotted catheter tip	• Attempt to aspirate the clot with a syringe according to your facility's policy. • If successful, flush the line. • Don't attempt to flush if the clot can't be aspirated; notify the physician.
	• Catheter tip lodged against vessel wall	• Reposition the catheter by gently rotating it or pulling it back slightly according to your facility's policy. • Reposition the patient, if necessary. • Ask the patient to cough and breathe deeply to help move the catheter.
Noisy or erratic waveforms	• Incorrectly positioned catheter	• Anticipate need for a chest X-ray to verify catheter position. • Reposition catheter by gently rotating it or pulling it back slightly, according to your facility's policy. • Reposition the patient, if necessary. • Ask the patient to cough and breathe deeply to help move the catheter.
	• Loose connections	• Check all connections, and tighten as necessary.
	• Faulty electrical circuit	• Check to make sure that the power supply is turned on. • Reconnect transducer to the monitor as necessary.

(continued)

Troubleshooting pulmonary artery catheters *(continued)*

Problem	Possible causes	Interventions
Erratic waveform	• Catheter fling	• Reposition the patient according to your facility's policy. • Shorten tubing, if possible.
False pressure readings	• Improper calibration or positioning of the transducer	• Recalibrate the system. • Relevel the transducer.
Arrhythmia	• Catheter irritation of ventricular endocardium or heart valves	• Confirm arrhythmia via ECG. • Notify the physician. • Administer antiarrhythmics as ordered.
Ventricular waveform tracing	• Catheter migration into the right ventricle	• Inflate the balloon with 1.5 cc of air to move the catheter back to the pulmonary artery. • If unsuccessful, notify the physician to reposition the catheter.
Continuous pulmonary artery wedge pressure (PAWP) waveform	• Catheter migration or inflated balloon	• Reposition the patient. • Ask the patient to cough and breathe deeply to help move the catheter. • Keep the balloon inflated for no longer than two respiratory cycles or 15 seconds.
Missing PAWP waveform	• Catheter malposition	• Reposition the patient. • Ask the patient to cough and breathe deeply to help move the catheter.
	• Inadequate air in balloon tip	• Reinflate the balloon, wait for balloon to deflate passively, and then instill the correct amount of air.
	• Ruptured balloon	• Note the balloon competence (resistance during inflation). • Keep in mind that the syringe's plunger should spring back after the balloon inflates. • Check for blood leaking from the balloon. • If ruptured, turn the patient to his left side, tape the balloon inflation port, and notify the physician.

Troubleshooting ventilator alarms

Problem	Possible causes	Interventions
Low pressure	• Tube disconnected from ventilator	• Reconnect tube to the ventilator.
	• Endotracheal (ET) tube displaced above vocal cords or tracheostomy tube extubated	• With displacement or extubation, open the patient's airway. • Manually ventilate the patient. • Notify the physician.
	• Leaking tidal volume from low cuff pressure (from an underinflated ET cuff or a leak in the cuff or one-way valve)	• Listen for a whooshing sound (air leak) around the tube. • Check cuff pressure. • If pressure can't be maintained, anticipate the need for insertion of a new tube.
	• Ventilator malfunction	• Disconnect the patient from ventilator. • Manually ventilate as necessary. • Obtain a new ventilator as soon as possible, and reconnect the patient.
	• Leak in ventilator circuit (from loose connection or hole in tubing, loss of temperature sensing device, or cracked humidification container)	• Check all connections to make sure that they're intact. • Inspect the humidification container and tubing for leaks or cracks, and replace as necessary.
High pressure	• Increased airway pressure or decreased lung compliance due to worsening of disease process	• Auscultate lungs for evidence of increasing lung consolidation, barotrauma, or wheezing. • Notify physician as indicated.
	• Patient biting on ET tube	• Insert a bite block as necessary.
	• Secretions in airway	• Have the patient cough. • Suction airway.
	• Condensate in tubing	• Disconnect tubing and empty condensate.
	• Intubation of right mainstem bronchus	• Check tube position. • If tube has slipped, notify physician to reposition.
	• Patient coughing, gagging, or trying to talk	• If the patient is fighting the ventilator, anticipate the need for additional sedation or neuromuscular blocking agent and administer as ordered.

(continued)

Troubleshooting ventilator alarms *(continued)*

Problem	Possible causes	Interventions
High pressure *(continued)*	• Chest wall resistance	• Reposition the patient if his position interferes with chest-wall expansion. • If unsuccessful, administer analgesia as ordered.
	• Malfunctioning high pressure relief valve	• Replace faulty equipment.
	• Bronchospasm, pneumothorax, or barotrauma	• Assess the patient for cause. • Notify physician and institute measures to treat cause as ordered.
Spirometer or low exhaled tidal volume, or low exhaled minute volume	• Power interruption	• Check all electrical connections. • Reconnect as necessary.
	• Loose connection or leak in delivery system	• Check all connections, and tighten as necessary. • Inspect for leaks, and replace any defective equipment.
	• Leaking chest tube	• Check all chest tube connections to make sure they're secure. • Ascertain that the water seal is intact. • Notify physician of findings.
	• Leaking cuff or inadequate cuff seal	• Listen for leak with stethoscope. • Reinflate cuff according to your facility's policy. • Replace cuff, if needed.
	• Increased airway resistance in a patient on a pressure-cycled ventilator	• Auscultate lungs for signs of airway obstruction, barotrauma, or lung consolidation. • Notify physician of findings.
	• Disconnected spirometer	• Reconnect as necessary.
	• Malfunctioning volume-measuring device	• Notify respiratory therapy for replacement of device.
High respiratory rate	• Anxious patient	• Assess the patient for cause. • Note the patient's fears, and dispel if possible. • Anticipate the need for sedation.
	• Patient in pain	• Reposition the patient comfortably. • Administer analgesics as ordered.

Troubleshooting ventilator alarms *(continued)*

Problem	Possible causes	Interventions
High respiratory rate *(continued)*	● Secretions in airway	● Suction the patient.
Low positive end-expiratory pressure or continuous positive airway pressure	● Leak in system	● Inspect system for leaks. ● Check that all connections are secure. ● Inspect for holes in tubing, and replace as necessary.
	● Mechanical failure	● Discontinue, and notify respiratory therapy for replacement; inform physician.

Vasodilators

Drug	Indications	Adverse effects*
Amlodipine besylate (Norvasc)	• Chronic stable angina, vasospastic angina (Prinzmetal's or variant angina) • Hypertension • Management of Prinzmetal's or variant angina or chronic stable angina pectoris • Hypertension • Atrial fibrillation or flutter, paroxysmal SVT	• Headache • Edema
Diltiazem hydrochloride (Cardizem, Cardizem CD, Cardizem SR, Cartia XT, Dilacor XR, Diltia XT, Tiazac)	• Treatment or prophylaxis of acute anginal attacks; treatment of chronic ischemic heart disease (by preload reduction) • Adjunctive treatment of heart failure • Diffuse esophageal spasm without gastroesophageal reflux	• Headache • Arrhythmias, bradycardia, heart failure • Nausea, constipation
Isosorbide dinitrate (Apo-ISDN, Coronex, Dilatrate-SR, Isordil, Isordil Titradose, Novosorbide, Sorbitrate, Sorbitrate SA)	• Prevention of angina pectoris caused by coronary artery disease (but not to abort acute anginal attacks)	• Headache (sometimes with throbbing) • Flushing, orthostatic hypotension, tachycardia, palpitations, ankle edema • Hypersensitivity reactions
Isosorbide mononitrate (Imdur, ISMO, Isotrate ER, Monoket)	• Hypertension, management of chronic stable angina • Short-term management of hypertension when oral therapy isn't feasible or possible	• Headache (sometimes with throbbing) • Flushing, orthostatic hypotension, tachycardia, palpitations, ankle edema • Hypersensitivity reactions
Nicardipine hydrochloride (Cardene, Cardene I.V., Cardene SR)	• Management of Prinzmetal's (variant) angina or chronic stable angina • Hypertension	• Peripheral edema, palpitations, flushing
Nifedipine (Adalat, Adalat CC, Procardia, Procardia XL)	• Improvement of neurologic deficits after subarachnoid hemorrhage from ruptured congenital aneurysms • Migraine headache	• Dizziness, light-headedness, headache, weakness • Peripheral edema, heart failure, MI, flushing • Nausea

*Common or life-threatening only

Special considerations

- Monitor the patient closely for complaints of chest pain. Some patients, especially those with severe obstructive coronary artery disease, have developed increased frequency, duration, or severity of angina or even acute MI after calcium channel blocker therapy starts or dosage increases.
- Give sublingual nitroglycerin as needed for acute anginal symptoms.

- Contraindicated in patients with sick sinus syndrome or second- or third-degree AV block in the absence of an artificial pacemaker; in patients with SVTs linked to a bypass tract, such as in Wolff-Parkinson-White syndrome or Lown-Ganong-Levine syndrome; and in patients with left-sided heart failure, hypotension, acute MI, or pulmonary congestion (documented by X-ray).
- If systolic blood pressure is less than 90 mm Hg or heart rate is less than 60 beats/minute, withhold the dose until the patient is further evaluated.
- Tell the patient to report feelings of light-headedness or dizziness and to avoid sudden position changes.

- Contraindicated in patients with severe hypotension, shock, or acute MI with low left ventricular filling pressure.
- Maintenance of continuous 24-hour plasma levels may result in refractory tolerance. Dosing regimens should include dose-free intervals.
- Abrupt discontinuation may cause coronary vasospasm.

- Contraindicated in patients with severe hypotension, shock, or acute MI with low left ventricular filling pressure.
- A drug-free interval sufficient to avoid tolerance to drug isn't completely defined.
- Methemoglobinemia has occurred in patients receiving other organic nitrates.
- Don't crush or break extended-release tablets.

- Contraindicated in patients with advanced aortic stenosis.
- When treating hypertension, measure blood pressure at trough level (about 8 hours after dose or just before next dose). Because prominent effects may occur during peak levels, measure blood pressure 1 to 2 hours after conventional dose and 2 to 4 hours after extended-release dose. Base dosage adjustment on blood pressure 2 to 4 hours after oral dose.

- Use cautiously in elderly patients and those with heart failure or hypotension.
- Use cautiously in patients with unstable angina who aren't currently taking a beta blocker because a higher risk of MI has been reported.
- Initial doses and increased dosage may worsen angina briefly.
- Don't break or crush capsules.

(continued)

Vasodilators *(continued)*

Drug	Indications	Adverse effects*
Nimodipine (Nimotop)	• Prophylaxis against chronic anginal attacks • Relief of acute angina pectoris, prophylaxis to prevent or minimize anginal attacks when taken immediately before stressful events • Hypertension, heart failure, angina	• Headache • Decreased blood pressure
Nitroglycerin (glyceryl trinitrate)	• Acute MI • Hypertensive crisis	• Headache, sometimes with throbbing; dizziness • Orthostatic hypotension, tachycardia, flushing, palpitations, fainting • Hypersensitivity reactions
Nitroprusside sodium (Nipride, Nitropress)	• Hypertensive emergencies • Acute heart failure	• Headache, dizziness, loss of consciousness, apprehension, increased intracranial pressure, restlessness • Bradycardia, hypotension, tachycardia, palpitations, ECG changes, flushing • Nausea, abdominal pain, ileus • Acidosis, methemoglobinemia, hypothyroidism • Muscle twitching • Irritation at infusion site • Thiocyanate toxicity, cyanide toxicity, venous streaking
Verapamil hydrochloride (Calan, Calan SR, Covera-HS, Isoptin, Isoptin SR, Verelan, Verelan PM)	• Management of Prinzmetal's or variant angina or unstable or chronic stable angina pectoris • SVTs • Control of ventricular rate in digitalized patients with chronic atrial flutter or fibrillation • Prophylaxis of repetitive paroxysmal SVT • Hypertension	• Transient hypotension, heart failure, pulmonary edema, bradycardia, AV block, ventricular asystole, ventricular fibrillation, peripheral edema • Constipation

*Common or life-threatening only

Special considerations

- Use cautiously in patients with hepatic failure.
- Unlike other calcium channel blockers, nimodipine isn't used for angina pectoris or hypertension.
- Use lower doses in patients with hepatic cirrhosis.
- Closely monitor blood pressure and heart rate.
- If the patient can't swallow capsules, puncture ends of liquid-filled capsule with an 18G needle and draw the contents into syringe. Instill dose into patient's nasogastric tube, and rinse tube with 30 ml of normal saline solution.
- Advise the patient to rise from supine position slowly to avoid dizziness and hypotension, especially at start of therapy.
- Advise the patient to take drug 1 hour before or 2 hours after meals; food decreases absorption.

- Contraindicated in patients with early MI (sublingual form), severe anemia, increased intracranial pressure, angle-closure glaucoma, orthostatic hypotension, and allergy to adhesives (transdermal form). I.V. form is contraindicated in patients hypersensitive to I.V. form, cardiac tamponade, restrictive cardiomyopathy, or constrictive pericarditis. Extended-release preparations shouldn't be used in patients with organic or functional GI hypermotility or malabsorption syndrome.
- Remove transdermal patch before defibrillation. Aluminum backing may cause patch to explode when exposed to electric current.
- When administering I.V. infusion, use special nonabsorbent tubing supplied by manufacturer; regular plastic tubing may absorb up to 80% of drug. Prepare infusion in a glass bottle or container.

- Contraindicated in patients with compensatory hypertension (as in arteriovenous shunt or coarctation of the aorta), inadequate cerebral circulation, congenital optic atrophy, or tobacco-induced amblyopia.
- Hypertensive patients are more sensitive to nitroprusside than normotensive patients. Also, patients taking other antihypertensives are extremely sensitive to nitroprusside.
- Prepare solution using D_5W solution. Because of light sensitivity, foil-wrap I.V. solution (but not tubing). Fresh solutions have faint brownish tint.
- After reconstitution, further dilute the concentrated solution in 250, 500, or 1,000 ml 5% dextrose injection to produce 200, 100, or 50 mcg/ml, respectively.
- Monitor blood pressure at least every 5 minutes at start of infusion and every 15 minutes thereafter during infusion.
- Check serum thiocyanate levels every 72 hours; nitroprusside can cause cyanide toxicity. Levels above 100 µg/ml are linked to cyanide toxicity.

- Contraindicated in patients with severe left ventricular dysfunction, cardiogenic shock, second- or third-degree AV block or sick sinus syndrome except in presence of functioning pacemaker, atrial flutter or fibrillation and accessory bypass tract syndrome, severe heart failure (unless secondary to verapamil therapy), and severe hypotension. In addition, I.V. verapamil is contraindicated in patients receiving I.V. beta blockers and in those with ventricular tachycardia.
- If verapamil is started in the patient receiving carbamazepine, a 40% to 50% reduction in carbamazepine dosage may be needed. Monitor the patient closely for signs of toxicity.
- If verapamil is added to therapy of the patient receiving digoxin, anticipate reduction in digoxin dosage by half and monitor subsequent serum drug levels.
- Monitor ECG and blood pressure continuously in patients receiving I.V. verapamil.
- Give I.V. doses over at least 3 minutes to minimize risk of adverse effects.

Index

A

Abdominal aortic aneurysm, 16-17, 18, 19i. *See also* Aortic aneurysm.

Abrasion, 575, 576. *See also* Traumatic wound care.

Accelerated idioventricular rhythm, 44

Acebutolol, 602-603t

Acephen, 674-675t

Acetaminophen, 674-675t
  antidote for, 615t
  assessment findings in overdose of, 537t
  toxic effects of, 535

Acquired immunodeficiency syndrome, 545-546, 547-549. *See also* Human immunodeficiency virus infection.
  conditions associated with, 548
  opportunistic infections in, 550t

Acute adrenal crisis, 460-466
  progression of, 463i

Acute coronary syndromes, 2-15

Acute idiopathic polyneuritis. *See* Guillain-Barré syndrome.

Acute renal failure, 418-430
  causes of, 419
  classifying, 419-420
  drugs and, 423
  imbalances associated with, 426-429t

Acute respiratory failure, 166-171

Adalat, 700-701t

Adalat CC, 700-701t

Addisonian crisis. *See* Acute adrenal crisis.

Addison's disease, 460, 461, 463-464. *See also* Acute adrenal crisis.

Adenocard, 592-593t

Adenosine, 592-593t

Adrenalin chloride, 656-657t

Adrenal insufficiency. *See* Addison's disease.

Adult respiratory distress syndrome, 172-178
  phases of, 174i
  stages of, 173, 175

Advil, 676-677t

Afterload, factors that affect, 640

AIDS. *See* Acquired immunodeficiency syndrome.

Airway maintenance, forms of, 193-199, 200-201i

Alcohols, toxic effects of, 535

Aldactone, 630-631t

Allogeneic transplant donation, 512

Alteplase, 686t

Amicar, 582-583t

Amikacin, 584t
  monitoring guidelines for, 680-681t

Amiloride hydrochloride, 630-631t

Aminocaproic acid, 582-583t

Aminoglycosides, 584t
  monitoring guidelines for, 680-681t

Amiodarone hydrochloride, 590-591t

Amlodipine besylate, 700-701t

Amoxicillin, 585t

Amoxicillin/clavulanic acid, 585t

Amphetamine overdose, assessment findings in, 537t

i refers to an illustration; t refers to a table.

i refers to an illustration; t refers to a table.

Great vessel rupture, chest trauma as
cause of, 188-189t
Groshong catheter, 610-611t
Grunting, assessing, 601t
Guillain-Barré syndrome, 298-303
sensorimotor nerve degeneration
and, 299

H

Hardwire monitoring, 79, 80, 81i, 82.
See also Continuous cardiac
monitoring.
Harris tube, 382i
Hashimoto's thyroiditis, 483
Head injury, 303-312
types of, 306-309t
Heart failure, 101-107
causes of, 102t
Heart murmurs, characteristics of, 665t
Heart sounds
abnormal, implications of, 643t
auscultation sites for, 642i
Heart transplantation. *See* Cardiac
transplantation.
Heat cramps, 552t, 553. *See also*
Hyperthermia.
Heat exhaustion, 552t, 553. *See also*
Hyperthermia.
Heatstroke, 551, 552t, 553. *See also*
Hyperthermia.
Heat syndrome. *See* Hyperthermia.
Hemodialysis, 435-445. *See also*
Peritoneal dialysis.
access sites for, 436i
with atrioventricular shunt, 441-442
with double-lumen catheter, 440-441
mechanics of, 435, 438-439i
type of dialyzers for, 438-439i
Hemophilus influenza, 219t
Hemorrhagic stroke, 337, 338-339,
338t. *See also* Stroke.
Hemostatic devices, 50
Hemothorax, chest trauma as cause of,
186-187i

Heparin
antidote for, 615t
monitoring guidelines for, 682-683t
Hepatic encephalopathy, 393-394. *See
also* Hepatic failure.
Hepatic failure, 392-399
Hepatitis A, 394t
Hepatitis B, 394t
Hepatitis C, 394t
Hepatitis D, 395t
Hepatitis E, 395t
Hepatitis G, 395t
Hepatorenal syndrome, 393. *See also*
Hepatic failure.
HHNS. *See* Hyperglycemic hyperosmolar
nonketotic syndrome.
Hickman-Broviac catheter, 610-611t
Hickman catheter, 610-611t
HIV. *See* Human immunodeficiency virus
infection.
HMG-CoA reductase inhibitors, moni-
toring guidelines for, 682-683t
Hospital-acquired pneumonia, 218,
220-221t. *See also* Pneumonia.
Household equivalents, 619t
Human immunodeficiency virus
infection, 545-551
forms of, 547
Hydrocephalus as cerebral aneurysm
rupture complication, 288t
Hydrochlor, 628-629t
Hydrochlorothiazide, 628-629t
HydroDIURIL, 628-629t
Hydromorphone hydrochloride,
676-677t
Hydro-Par, 628-629t
Hygroton, 628-629t
Hyperglycemic hyperosmolar nonketotic
syndrome, 477-482
differentiating, from DKA, 479i
Hyperkalemia, acute renal failure and,
426-427t
Hypermagnesemia, acute renal failure
and, 428-429t

i refers to an illustration; t refers to a table.

i refers to an illustration; t refers to a table.

i refers to an illustration; t refers to a table.

i refers to an illustration; t refers to a table.

i refers to an illustration; t refers to a table.

i refers to an illustration; t refers to a table.